THE NATION'S HEALTH

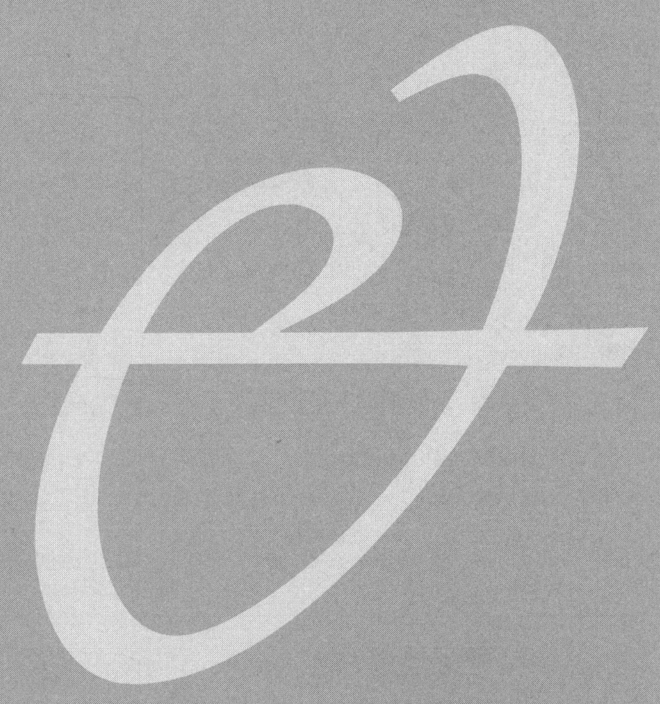

SEVENTH EDITION

THE NATION'S HEALTH

Edited by

PHILIP R. LEE

Institute for Health Policy Studies
School of Medicine
University of California, San Francisco
and
Program in Human Biology
Stanford University

CARROLL L. ESTES

Institute for Health and Aging
School of Nursing
University of California, San Francisco

FÁTIMA M. RODRÍGUEZ

Assistant Editor

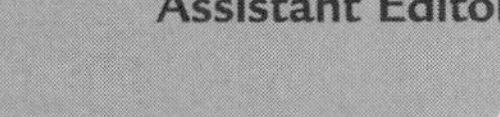

JONES AND BARTLETT PUBLISHERS

Sudbury, Massachusetts

BOSTON   TORONTO   LONDON   SINGAPORE

World Headquarters
Jones and Bartlett Publishers
40 Tall Pine Drive
Sudbury, MA 01776
978-443-5000
info@jbpub.com
www.jbpub.com

Jones and Bartlett Publishers
Canada
6339 Ormindale Way
Mississauga, ON L5V 1J2
CANADA

Jones and Bartlett Publishers
International
Barb House, Barb Mews
London W6 7PA
UK

Jones and Bartlett's books and products are available through most bookstores and online booksellers. To contact Jones and Bartlett Publishers directly, call 800-832-0034, fax 978-443-8000, or visit our website at www.jbpub.com.

Substantial discounts on bulk quantities of Jones and Bartlett's publications are available to corporations, professional associations, and other qualified organizations. For details and specific discount information, contact the special sales department at Jones and Bartlett via the above contact information or send an email to specialsales@jbpub.com.

ISBN-13: 978-0-7637-0759-0
ISBN-10: 0-7637-0759-7

Production Credits
Acquisitions Editor: Kristin L. Ellis
Production Editor: Julie C. Bolduc
Editorial Assistant: Nicole Quinn
Associate Marketing Manager: Ed McKenna
Manufacturing Buyer: Therese Bräuer
Composition: International Typesetting and Composition
Cover Design: Kristin E. Ohlin
Cover Photographs: (l) © Digital Vision, (c) and (r) © PictureQuest
Printing and Binding: Malloy Lithographing, Inc.
Cover Printing: Malloy Lithographing, Inc.

Library of Congress Cataloging-in-Publication Data
The nation's health / [edited by] Philip R. Lee, Carroll L. Estes, Fátima M. Rodríguez.—7th ed.
p. ; cm.
Includes bibliographical references and index.
ISBN 0-7637-0759-7 (alk. paper)
1. Public health—United States. 2. Medical policy—United States. 3. Health care reform—United States.
[DNLM: 1. Public Health—trends—United States. 2. Delivery of Health Care—United States. 3. Health Policy—United States. 4. Long-Term Care—United States. 5. Terrorism—prevention & control—United States. 6. Women's Health Services—United States. WA 100 N284 2003] I. Lee, Philip R. (Philip Randolph), 1924– II. Estes, Carroll L. III. Rodríguez, Fátima M.
RA445 .N36 2003
362.1′0973—dc21 2002154017
6048

Printed in the United States of America

10 09 08 07 10 9 8 7 6 5

Contents

PREFACE

The nation's health is a continuing concern, yet a source of great pride because of the improvement in the health of the American people during the twentieth century. This volume—edited by two of the nation's leading health and aging policy experts, with three younger colleagues—looks at the complex web of issues, policies, controversies, and proposed solutions that surrounds health policy, public health, community health, and health care in the United States. This seventh edition includes a practical, in-depth guide to the factors affecting the health of Americans and the role of public health, medical care, and the community in ensuring the nation's health. It also includes a new section on the threat of bioterrorism.

Health care reform was the top domestic priority when the fourth edition was published a decade ago. A polarized political debate that resulted in little action at the federal level was followed by incremental gains in insuring children and reforming Medicare. In the three years since the publication of the sixth edition, federal policy has focused on bioterrorism, the public health infrastructure, progress in earlier incremental reforms, such as the State Child Health Insurance Program (SCHIP), and the debate on prescription drug coverage and Medicare. Limited progress was made in some areas affecting health: tobacco, immunization, HIV/AIDS, environmental health (e.g., water, pesticides), physical activity, and food safety. There is a continuing set of questions related to the epidemic of obesity, the increase in diabetes, and such wild cards as the West Nile virus. After a brief respite in the 1990s, concerns about health care costs and the quality of health care returned. New issues have arisen related to women's health, including the role of mammograms in the detection of breast cancer and the use of estrogens to control menopausal symptoms and postmenopausal osteoporosis. In addition, Medicare has again risen to the top of the health policy agenda because of rising costs and the lack of outpatient coverage for prescription drugs.

The policy environment changed rapidly after September 11, 2001. Bioterrorism moved to the top of the health policy agenda following the terrorist attacks and the anthrax mailings in the autumn of 2001. It has become apparent that an effective defense against bioterrorism must be based on improved medical care and public health systems. First responders to bioterrorist attacks are likely to be emergency room physicians or other health professionals rather than fire, police, or military personnel. The seventh edition of *The Nation's Health* devotes particular attention to bioterrorism, public health, and community health.

Other important questions addressed in this volume include the following: What is the relationship of socioeconomic status and health? Why do Americans spend over twice as much per capita for health care than people in most other industrialized countries and yet rank far behind in infant mortality, life expectancy, and other measures of health status? How do we eliminate medical care that is wasteful, inefficient, and unnecessary and improve the quality of health care?

The seventh edition of *The Nation's Health* represents part of a multidisciplinary program for advanced training and education in health policy and health services research that is conducted by the Institute for Health Policy Studies, School of Medicine, and the Institute for Health and Aging, School of Nursing, University of California, San Francisco (UCSF), and the undergraduate Program in Human Biology, Stanford University.

During 2002, when this book was being prepared, Philip R. Lee served as an active Emeritus Professor of Social Medicine on the UCSF faculty and as Consulting Professor in the Human Biology Program at Stanford University, where he teaches undergraduate students about health care, health policy, federal health programs, and international health care systems and policies, including an undergraduate course on the nation's health. While serving as Assistant Secretary for Health in the Clinton administration from 1993 to 1997, he played a key role in the national effort to restate the nation's health care agenda in response to many of the problems and issues described in this book and in keeping with many of its themes.

Professor Carroll L. Estes served as Professor of Sociology and Director of the Institute for Health and Aging (Emeritus), UCSF. She continues her active role in teaching graduate and postdoctoral students at UCSF and her research on aging and long-term care.

Special appreciation goes to Fátima M. Rodríguez, MPH, for her work as Assistant Editor and her critical role throughout the entire process, from review and selection of articles to writing and final publication. We also express our appreciation to Cindy Lin, the Research Assistant for Professor Lee, particularly for her contribution to Chapters 6 and 9; to Tracy Weitz, MPA, Projects Director, UCSF Center for Reproductive Health Research and Policy, for her contribution to Chapter 10; and to Mauro Hernandez, PhD candidate, who assisted Professor Estes, particularly on Chapter 11.

Although *The Nation's Health* is a project of the Institute for Health Policy Studies and the Institute for Health and Aging, UCSF, and the Program in Human Biology at Stanford University, the views expressed are those of the authors only and do not necessarily reflect those of the University of California or Stanford University.

INTRODUCTION

The seventh edition of *The Nation's Health* continues the emphasis of earlier editions on the health of the population, the determinants of health, women's health, long-term care, and the precarious set of circumstances faced by the nation's public health and health care systems at the beginning of the 21st century. We intend this book to represent a range of views about determinants of health; the current state of public health, health care, community health, and long-term care; and prospects for the future, with particular emphasis on the current issues, such as bioterrorism, and on proposals for change.

To make some sense of the massive literature on health, population health, community health, public health, and health care, we have organized the book into seven parts, with one to two chapters per part. The seven parts are as follows:

I. The Health of the Nation and Determinants of Health
II. Health Policy and the Politics of Health
III. Identifying, Understanding, and Addressing Population Health Problems
IV. Preparing for Terrorism: A Public Health Response
V. Health Care, Health Care Organization, Health Care Financing, and Quality of Care
VI. Women's Health and the Health Care System
VII. Aging and Long-Term Care

In addition to the material contained in the chapters (40 articles, including excerpts from book chapters, chartbooks, and issue briefs), we have included a list of recommended readings for each chapter and information about the authors.

DEFINITIONS OF HEALTH, POPULATION HEALTH, AND PUBLIC HEALTH

In general, there is broad agreement about the importance of health; however, there tends to be much less agreement about the definition of health. While the World Health Organization's (WHO) definition of health as a "state of complete physical, mental and social well being and not merely the absence of disease or infirmity" (WHO, 1958) has been in use for more than 50 years, it has often proved difficult to measure and apply to a population. At the time the WHO definition was first introduced, the germ theory was the dominant paradigm and most of the emphasis was on measures to control infectious diseases. Vicente Navarro has noted that the WHO definition of health "was an enormous break with the traditional understanding of health and medicine, putting both in their proper context" (Navarro, 1998). While broadening the conceptual basis for defining health, the WHO definition still presents a challenge in its practical application. How can a society go about ensuring the health, so defined, of all of its members?

Over 20 years ago, Lee and Franks (1980) reviewed the many definitions and concepts of health. They noted that the English word *health* is derived from the root word *Kailo*, meaning whole or intact. The Greek *hygienos* means sound or wholesome. In Latin, the word *sanitas*, health, came from sound. Similar ideas have been expressed in Hebrew, Hindi, and Chinese. The Hippocratic concept of health and disease also stresses the concept of balance. The review by Lee and Franks included more than twenty modern definitions or concepts of health. These ranged from an "absence of disease" to health as a "continuity, perfect adjustment of the organism to its environment."

Health is often equated with access to medical care, which primarily meets the needs of individuals. While the public supports many public health measures (e.g., immunizations, food safety), there is little understanding among the general populace of the terms *public health* and *population health*.

In recent years, the term *population health* has been used frequently as a substitute for the health of the population. In Canada, the work of Evans and Stoddart (1990) and Evans, Barer, and Marmor (1994) of the Canadian Institute for Advanced Research's Program in Population Health defined the term as a conceptual framework for thinking about the multiple determinants of health. However, in the United States, the term *population health* has not been widely used.

On the other hand, *public health* is widely used, but it is a poorly understood term. Public health usually refers to the wide array of programs and services provided by the federal, state, or local governments that are designed to protect, promote, and restore the health of the population. The Institute of Medicine (IOM), in its 1988 report *The Future of Public Health*, defined the mission of public health broadly as

> fulfilling society's interest in assuring the conditions in which people can be healthy. Its aim is to generate organized community effort to address the public interest in health by applying scientific and technological knowledge to prevent disease and promote health.

> The mission of public health is addressed by private organizations and individuals as well as public agencies. But the government public health agency has a unique function: to see to it that vital elements are in place and the mission is adequately addressed (IOM, 1988, p. 7).

The committee also stated that the core functions of public health agencies at all levels of government are assessment, policy development, and assurance.

A NEW FRAMEWORK FOR HEALTH POLICY

The evolution of health policies during the past 50 years from an emphasis on medical care and biomedical research to the health of the population has been slow. The absence of a clear framework within which to develop policies that focused on the nation's health has resulted in an overemphasis on the role of medical care and a serious fragmentation of public health programs.

Corrective measures, particularly the effort to develop a health policy framework based on the determinants of health, began prior to the first edition of *The Nation's Health* in 1981. Canada had preceded the United States with the 1974 Lalonde report, *A New Perspective on the Health of Canadians*, published by the Canadian Department of National Health and Welfare. The Lalonde report marked an important step in shaping the current thinking about health policy. It made very clear that health does not equal medical care. The central focus of the Lalonde report was on the "health field concept," which divided the health field into four broad determinants: human biology, environment, lifestyle, and health care organization. While the report proposed a number of intervention strategies, the subsequent emphasis was on health promotion, which stressed health education and greater individual responsibility for healthy behaviors. Although the report had little immediate impact on health policies in Canada, it did begin to change the way people thought about the issues.

In the United States, the *Surgeon General's Report on Health Promotion and Disease Prevention* (U.S. Department of Health and Human Services [DHHS], 1977) set goals to reduce mortality among infants, children, adolescents, and adults and increase independence among older adults. A process was thereby set in motion to establish a more balanced health policy. *Promoting Health/Preventing Disease: Objectives for the Nation in the U.S. Public Health Service* (DHHS, 1980) was published in 1980, setting goals for 1990. *Healthy People 2000: National Health Promotion and Disease Prevention Objectives* (DHHS, 1990) followed in 1990. Most recently, *Healthy People 2010: Objectives, Goals*, released in January 2000 (DHHS, 2000a), proposed two primary goals: (1) to increase quality and years of healthy life, and (2) to eliminate health disparities. This is now a broad-based process involving the federal, state, and local governments and hundreds of private-sector organizations.

A second concept that is gaining wider acceptance and is contributing to the development of a new framework for health policy is the idea of population health. In his book *Population Health Concepts and Methods* (1998), T. K. Young used the term *population health* as a less cumbersome substitute for "the health of populations." About the term *population health*, he noted:

> In 1990 the phrase has taken on a new connotation, especially in Canada and the United Kingdom. It refers to a conceptual framework for thinking about why some people are healthier than others as well as the policy development, research agenda, and the resource allocations that flow from it. The difference between "population health" and terms such as community health and public health, which have been around a long time, is subtle (p. 4).

We agree with others that the term *population health* is broader than traditional public health and includes greater attention to the determinants of health and the social inequities (e.g., income, occupation, education) that are important contributors to the health status of populations. In his book *Purchasing Population Health* (1997), David A. Kindig draws on many different disciplines to propose a different approach to purchasing health care services. Kindig drew primarily on the work of the Canadian Institute for Advanced Research's multidisciplinary group in population health. The product of their efforts, *Why Are Some People Healthy and Others Not? The Determinants of Health of Populations* (Evans, Barer, and Marmor, 1994), summarized a great deal of what is known and stimulated a great deal of thinking about population health.

THE HEALTH OF THE NATION AND THE DETERMINANTS OF HEALTH

In this volume, as in the sixth edition, we give significant attention to population health, the determinants of health, and the evolving role of public health. This edition begins with a review of improvements in the health of the nation during the past 100 years and the factors that have contributed to this improvement. Special attention is given to socioeconomic status (SES) and health, disparities in health status, and the goals of Healthy People 2010. As *Healthy People 2010: Understanding and Improving Health* (DHHS, 2000b) demonstrates, disparities in health status related to socioeconomic status and race/ethnicity require particular attention. For instance, infant mortality related to lack of access to appropriate health services is considerably higher for the poor than for the rich. It is also higher among blacks than among whites, largely because of the continuing prevalence of low-birth-weight infants among blacks. Infant mortality is higher in the United States than in 21 other industrialized countries. Furthermore, sophisticated treatments such as coronary artery bypass graft surgery, coronary angioplasty, and total hip replacement are less available to many poor people and racial/ethnic minorities, even when insured. Other services are also often less available or inaccessible to these populations, including clinical preventive services and programs for the management of chronic conditions. These services are often critical to good health and to the functional capacity and well-being of individuals.

At the same time that the health care delivery crisis is playing out, a number of health and social problems are affecting the lives of many and straining the capacity of the public health and health care systems. At issue are the problems of terrorism, environmental quality, violence, substance abuse, HIV/AIDS, homelessness, chronic mental illness, and unintended pregnancy, as well as the growing problem of asthma, particularly among African American children, and the increasing burden of type 2 diabetes. Each of these problems carries a high price tag in terms of human health and well-being. To deal with these problems effectively, as noted in *Healthy People 2010: Understanding and Improving Health* (DHHS, 2000b), the collaborative efforts of the community as well as public health and medicine are required. Some health issues that have begun to be dealt with in a more promising systematic manner include tobacco use, immunization, HIV/AIDS, food safety, newly emerging infections, unintended pregnancy (especially among adolescents), and certain chronic illnesses such as asthma and diabetes mellitus. Yet concurrent with these advances, the number of chronically ill elderly continues to increase, highlighting the lack of provision in our health care system for adequately meeting their special needs.

HEALTH POLICY AND THE POLITICS OF HEALTH

After opening with a consideration of the health of the nation and the determinants of health, we move to the section on health policy and the politics of health. Chapter 3 contains overview pieces by Beaufort Longest (1998) and Paul Sabatier (1993) on current concepts of health policy, with an emphasis on Sabatier's thesis about advocacy coalitions and policy-oriented learning.

We then move on to a consideration of health policy and the politics of health in Chapter 4 with articles by Mark Peterson (2001); Barr, Lee, and Benjamin (1999); and Estes, Weiner, Goldberg, and Goldenson (1999). Peterson describes the dramatic change in the politics of health after the enactment of Medicare and Medicaid in 1965. Not only did the dominant role of the American Medical Association decline rapidly, but the politics became more complicated because of the rise of multiple interest groups and the increasing number of organizations involved in the politics of health. The result has been formidable barriers standing in the way of even incremental reforms. Many of these obstacles are based on strongly held values, including antigovernment ideologies that have been recurrent themes in American politics over many years (see also Article 3 by Sabatier in Chapter 3 and Article 2 by Barr, Lee, and Benjamin in Chapter 4). Interest groups, often reflecting these antigovernment sentiments, also exert a strong influence on health policy.

Article 3 by Carroll L. Estes, Joshua M. Weiner, Sheryl C. Goldberg, and Susan M. Goldenson delves into the politics of long-term care and provides important lessons learned from the attempt to reform long-term care during the Clinton administration. It also deals with policy issues that have been stressed in the early years of the George W. Bush administration, as they were in the Reagan administration more than 20 years ago.

IDENTIFYING, UNDERSTANDING, AND ADDRESSING POPULATION HEALTH PROBLEMS

Next, we devote considerable attention to public health and community health. Part III begins with a report from the Centers for Disease Control and Prevention (CDC), which provide a brief review of the developments in the public health system during the 20th century (see Chapter 5). In spite of significant advances in the past 20 years, serious problems remain in public health. Among these, of prominent concern are the serious underinvestment in the nation's public health infrastructure (e.g., information systems, laboratories, training public health workers) and a continued emphasis on categorical disease control programs. These situations need to be rectified if we expect to achieve the goals set in Healthy People 2010 and if the nation is to respond to the threat of terrorism, particularly bioterrorism.

We have added Article 2, "Broadening Participation in Community Problem Solving: A Multidisciplinary Model to Support Collaborative Practice and Research," by Roz Lasker and Elisa S. Weiss (2003). This critically important article replaces the excerpt in the sixth edition from Lasker's monograph *Medicine and Public Health: The Power of Collaboration* (1997), which is listed in the Recommended Reading. Lasker's 1997 monograph stressed the increasing importance of collaboration between medicine and public health in achieving the nation's health goals for the future. Article 2 by Lasker and Weiss moves beyond that to describe a new conceptual model for effective collaboration to improve health at the community level.

PREPARING FOR TERRORISM: A PUBLIC HEALTH RESPONSE

Part IV, Preparing for Terrorism: A Public Health Reponse, is new and was added because of the issues that have risen to the forefront of health policy since the September 11, 2001, terrorist attacks on the World Trade Center and the Pentagon and the anthrax attacks that followed. We focus our readings on the issues related to public health, the medical response to a terrorist attack, and ethical issues raised by limitations that may be placed on civil liberties in the name of a public health response to terrorism.

HEALTH CARE, HEALTH CARE ORGANIZATION, HEALTH CARE FINANCING, AND QUALITY OF CARE

In this edition, we do not deal explicitly with the position that health care is a social or public good (which is based on the concept that all members of society benefit when health care is provided for all individuals) rather than a market good. The view that health care is a social good is widely accepted in other Western industrialized democracies and is indeed prevalent among the nations of the Organization of Economic Cooperation and Development (OECD). Every other country in the OECD, except the United States, bases the provision and financing of health care for their populations on this premise. In the United States, health care is perceived by many policymakers as a market good.

Many contributors to this volume argue that the nation is confronted by an outmoded personal health care system that is the result of failed policies and continued technological expansion at the expense of the provision of sound basic care for all and effective nationwide programs of disease prevention, health protection, and health promotion. Those who are well insured are the lucky benefactors of a comprehensive delivery system. Meanwhile, those who suffer most from a lack of adequate public health protection and access to personal health care are poor children, some of whom are unable to obtain even basic care, such as immunizations. Also left behind are the disabled and those suffering from debilitating chronic illnesses. Finally, across all age groups and geographic areas, the working poor are consistently disadvantaged by our current system.

In Part V, we provide two broad overviews of the health care system by Fogel and Lee and by Oberlander. As it was more than a decade ago, the health care system remains a "paradox of excess and deprivation" (Enthoven and Kronick, 1991). While Fogel and Lee suggest some incremental reforms, Oberlander is "doubtful that incremental health reform will significantly ameliorate these problems" (2002, p. 163). In addition, we have included a review of managed care by Dudley and Luft and materials from the Henry J. Kaiser Family Foundation.

Part V contains 11 articles related to health care, health care financing, health care systems, managed care, and quality of health care. We provide an updated review from the *New England Journal of Medicine* and the Henry J. Kaiser Family Foundation on Medicare and Medicaid in Chapter 8. In 1997, with the Balanced Budget Act, Congress authorized the State Child Health Insurance Program (SCHIP). After five years of slow progress in expanding enrollment, "the states are at a critical funding impasse created by the downturn in the economy and the financing structure of the SCHIP statute, and unnecessary disenrollment from the program has emerged as a key barrier to maintaining SCHIP's effectiveness in providing health coverage for uninsured children and families" (Ryan, 2002, Article 4, Chapter 8).

Issues related to quality of care are continuing to receive attention. We devote Chapter 9 to these issues. Measuring the effects of medical interventions is a complex and imprecise science. Increasingly, clinicians are asked to interpret medical findings, and they tend to be ill equipped to make such evaluations. As a result, this leads to variations in treatments prescribed by clinicians. Issues related to inappropriate care are being investigated today. We include three articles by leaders in the field of quality of care, including an important article by Davies, Washington, and Bindman (2002) that raises important questions about the widespread use of report cards.

WOMEN'S HEALTH, AGING, AND LONG-TERM CARE

Part VI contains five articles on women's health issues. The chapter includes articles on particularly important women's health issues: aging and gender (Article 2), racial/ethnic variations in women's health (Article 3), estrogen therapy (Article 4), and mammography (Article 5).

Finally, Part VII deals with aging and long-term care. Similar to the health status of women, the health status of older individuals is a mixed story. Improvements in health status, described in Chapter 1, have extended life, but the advances have been experienced unevenly. Because of the importance of aging in our society, we have included a substantial section on aging, with an emphasis on long-term care. Four articles are included in Chapter 11. There has been anxiety among federal policymakers about the impact of the aging population on federal entitlement programs, but the issues are more complex. In addition, aging is not gender neutral: Women have a disproportionate need for long-term care and are more likely to enter nursing homes. Equally important, from a policy perspective, women constitute a larger percentage of Medicare beneficiaries than men; consequently, they rely on Medicare for more years. They also bear a greater burden of chronic illness and are more likely to have lower incomes and to be living alone in their later years. Through cumulative disadvantages associated with the intersection of age, race, gender, and class, "multiple jeopardy" intensifies the need for long-term care for women while increasing access barriers to needed services.

Structural characteristics of the U.S. long-term care system contribute to the persistence of problems associated with the provision of poor-quality services, uneven regulatory oversight, and inadequate reimbursement for publicly funded long-term care services. As highlighted in this chapter, the provision of and payment for long-term care services need to become increasingly more responsive to a movement toward greater direction and control of these services by their consumers.

SUMMARY

This book critically examines the nation's health; the determinants of health; the roles of both public health (population-based intervention) and personal health care; and the role of the community in protecting and ensuring the health of the population. Rather than merely emphasizing the care of the sick, the financing of care, and public health, we look at the complex web of issues, policies, controversies, hazards, problems, and proposed solutions to protect and promote the nation's health. Despite improvements in health, America must confront critical issues if it is to maintain its leadership role in science and become a world leader in public health, health care, and the health of its population. We believe the message of the first edition is as relevant today as it was 22 years ago:

> Despite the complexity of the issues, one clear message rings through: Americans over the decades have abdicated a large portion of responsibility for their health to physicians, drugs, hospitals and modern technology. Individuals and health professionals in our society have pursued an imbalanced vision to well being that is rapidly heading toward a dead end. We have distorted the relationship between medicine and health. Health is not just a matter for science and medicine: it also involves social, economic, philosophical, and ethical issues—issues that cut to the core of American values and institutions (Lee, 1981, pp. xix–xx).

A major change is needed in the way we think about the health of the population and policies to protect and improve the health of the population. We hope that the seventh edition of *The Nation's Health* can help to stimulate that change.

REFERENCES

Enthoven, A. C., and Kronick, R. (1991). Universal health insurance through incentive reform. *Journal of the American Medical Association, 265* (19), 2532–2536.

Evans, R. G., Barer, M. L., and Marmor, T. R. (Eds.). (1994). *Why are some people healthy and others not? The determinants of health of populations*. New York: Aldine de Gruyter.

Evans, R. G., and Stoddart, G. (1990). Producing health, consuming health care. *Social Science and Medicine, 31* (12), 1347–1363.

Institute of Medicine. (1988). *The future of public health: Summary and recommendations*. Washington, DC: National Academy Press.

Kindig, D. A. (1997). *Purchasing population health: Paying for results*. Ann Arbor: University of Michigan Press.

Lalonde, M. (1974). *A new perspective on the health of Canadians*. Ottawa: Government of Canada.

Lasker, R. D., and the Committee on Medicine and Public Health. (1997). *Medicine and public health: The power of collaboration*. Chicago: Health Administration Press.

Lee, P. R. (1981). Prologue. In P. R. Lee, N. Brown, and I. U. S. W. Red (Eds.), *The nation's health* (p. xix). San Francisco: Boyd and Fraser.

Lee, P. R., and Franks, P. E. (1980). Health and disease in the community. In J. Froj (Ed.), *Primary care* (pp. 3–34). London: William Heinemann.

Navarro, V. (1998). A historical review (1965–1997) of studies of class health, quality of life: A personal account. *International Journal of Health Services, 3*, 389–406.

Oberlander, J. (2002). The U.S. health care system: On a road to nowhere? *Canadian Medical Association Journal, 167* (2), 163–168.

Ryan, J. M. (2002, August 15). *SCHIP turns 5: Taking stock, moving ahead* (Issue Brief 781, pp. 2–13). Washington, DC: National Health Policy Forum Issue.

U.S. Department of Health and Human Services. (1977). *Surgeon general's report on health promotion and disease prevention.* Washington, DC: Public Health Service.

U.S. Department of Health and Human Services. (1980). *Surgeon general's report on promoting health/preventing disease: Objectives for the nation in the U.S. Public Health Service.* Washington, DC: Public Health Service.

U.S. Department of Health and Human Services. (1990). *Healthy People 2000: National health promotion and disease prevention objectives.* Washington, DC: Public Health Service.

U.S. Department of Health and Human Services. (2000a). *Healthy People 2010: Objectives, goals* (2nd ed.). Washington, DC: U.S. Government Printing Office.

U.S. Department of Health and Human Services. (2000b). *Healthy People 2010: Understanding and improving health* (2nd ed.). Washington, DC: U.S. Government Printing Office.

World Health Organization. (1958). Constitution of the World Health Organization. In *The first ten years of the World Health Organization.* Geneva: World Health Organization.

Young, T. K. (1998). *Population health concepts and methods.* New York: Oxford University Press.

ACKNOWLEDGMENTS

CHAPTER 1

William G. Rothstein. (1995). Trends in mortality in the twentieth century. In W.G. Rothstein (Ed.), *Readings in American Health Care* (pp. 71–86). Madison, Wisconsin: The University of Wisconsin Press. Reprinted by permission of The University of Wisconsin Press.

Centers for Disease Control and Prevention. (1999). Achievements in public health, 1900–1999: Control of infectious disease. *MMWR, 48* (29), 621–629. Reprinted by permission of the publisher.

Centers for Disease Control and Prevention. (1999). Achievements in public health, 1900–1999: Healthier mothers and babies. *MMWR, 48* (38), 849–857. Reprinted by permission of the publisher.

Centers for Disease Control and Prevention. (1999). Achievements in public health, 1900–1999: Decline in deaths from heart disease and stroke—United States, 1900–1999. *MMWR, 48* (29), 649–656. Reprinted by permission of the publisher.

U.S. Department of Health and Human Services. (2000). *Healthy People 2010: Understanding and Improving Health*, (pp. 1–4, 7, 8, 10–16).Washington, DC: U.S. Department of Health and Human Services, Government Printing Office, 2000. Reprinted and abridged by permission of the publisher.

CHAPTER 2

Bruce G. Link and Jo C. Phelan. (2002). McKeown and the idea that social conditions are fundamental causes of disease. *American Journal of Public Health, 92* (5), 730–732. Reprinted by permission of the American Public Health Association (APHA).

Michael Marmot. (2002). The influence of income on health: Views of an epidemiologist. *Health Affairs, 21* (2), 31–45. Reprinted by permission of the publisher.

Gary W. Evans and Elyse Kantrowitz. (2002). Socioeconomic status and health: The potential role of environmental risk exposure. *Annual Review of Public Health, 23*, 303–331. Reprinted with permission from the *Annual Review of Public Health,* Volume 23. Copyright 2002 by Annual Reviews, www.annualreviews.org. Permission to abridge from the authors.

CHAPTER 3

Beaufort B. Longest, Jr. (1998). The process of public policymaking: A conceptual model. In *Health Policymaking in the United States* (2nd ed.). Chicago: Health Administration Press, pp. 55–61. Reprinted by permission of the author.

Hank C. Jenkins-Smith and Paul A. Sabatier. (1993). The Study of public policy processes. In Paul A. Sabatier and Hank C. Jenkins-Smith (Eds.), *Policy Change and Learning: An advocacy coalition approach.* Boulder, CO: Westview Press, pp. 1–6. Copyright 1993 by Westview Press. Reprinted by permission of Westview Press, a member of Perseus Books, L.L.C.

Paul A. Sabatier. (1993). Policy change over a decade or more. In Paul A. Sabatier and Hank C. Jenkins-Smith (Eds.), *Policy Change and Learning: An advocacy coalition approach.* Boulder, CO: Westview Press, pp.13–39. Copyright 1993 by Westview Press. Reprinted by permission of Westview Press, a member of Perseus Books, L.L.C.

CHAPTER 4

Mark A. Peterson. (2001). From trust to political power: Interest groups, public choice, and health care. *Journal of Health Politics, Policy and Law, 26* (5), 1145–1163. Copyright 2001 by Duke University Press. All rights reserved. Used by permission of the publisher.

Donald A. Barr, Philip R. Lee, and A.E. Benjamin. (1999). Health care and health care policy in a changing world. In: Helen Wallace et al. (Eds.), *Health and welfare for families in the 21st century* (pp. 13–29). Sudbury, MA: Jones and Bartlett, www.jbpub.com. Reprinted by permission of the publisher.

Carroll L. Estes, Joshua M. Wiener, Sheryl C. Goldberg, and Susan Goldenson. (1999). *The politics of long-term care reform under the Clinton health plan: Lessons for the future* (pp.1–18). Washington, DC/San Francisco: Health Policy Center/Institute, The Urban Institute, Institute for Health and Aging, University of California, San Francisco. Reprinted by permission of the authors.

CHAPTER 5

Centers for Disease Control and Prevention. (1999). Achievements in public health, 1900–1999: Changes in the public health system. *MMWR, 48* (50), 1141–1147. Reprinted by permission of the publisher.

Roz D. Lasker and Elisa S. Weiss. (2003). Broadening participation in community problem solving: A multidisciplinary model to support collaborative practice and research. *Journal of Urban Health,* March 2003, *80* (1). Published with permission from Oxford University Press.

CHAPTER 6

Kenneth C. Hyams, Frances M. Murphy, and Simon Wessely. (2002). Responding to chemical, biological, or nuclear terrorism: The indirect and long-term health effects may present the greatest challenge. *Journal of Health Politics, Policy and Law, 27* (2), 274–291. Copyright 2002 by Duke University Press. All rights reserved. Used by permission of the publisher.

Julie Louise Gerberding, James M. Hughes, and Jeffrey P. Koplan. (2002). Bioterrorism preparedness and response: Clinicians and public health agencies as essential partners. *Journal of the American Medical Association, 287* (7), 898–900. Copyright 2002 by the American Medical Association. All rights reserved. Reprinted by permission of the publisher.

James G. Hodge, Jr. (2002, Summer). Bioterrorism law and policy: Critical choices in public health. *Journal of Law, Medicine & Ethics, 30* (2), 254–261. Copyright 2002. Reprinted with the permission of the American Society of Law, Medicine & Ethics. All rights reserved.

George J. Annas. (2002). Bioterrorism, public health, and civil liberties. *New England Journal of Medicine, 346* (17), 1337–1342. Copyright 2002 Massachusetts Medical Society. All rights reserved. Reprinted by permission of the publisher.

CHAPTER 7

Robert W. Fogel and Chulhee Lee. (2002, Winter). Who gets health care? *Daedalus*, 107–117. Reprinted by permission of the authors.

Jonathan Oberlander. (2002). The US health care system: On a road to nowhere? *Canadian Medical Association Journal, 167* (2), 163–168. Copyright 2002 Canadian Medical Association. Reprinted and abridged by permission of the publisher.

Robert J. Mills. (2001). Health insurance coverage: 2000. *Current Population Reports* (pp. 1–12). Washington, DC: U.S. Census Bureau. Reprinted and abridged by permission of the publisher.

R. Adams Dudley and Harold S. Luft. (2002). Managed care in transition. *New England Journal of Medicine, 344* (14), 1087–1092. Copyright 2002 Massachusetts Medical Society. All rights reserved. Reprinted by permission of the publisher.

CHAPTER 8

Marilyn Moon. (2001). Medicare. *New England Journal of Medicine, 344* (12), 928–931. Copyright 2001 Massachusetts Medical Society. All rights reserved. Reprinted by permission of the publisher.

Becky Briesacher, Bruce Stuart, and Dennis Shea. (2002). *Drug coverage for Medicare Beneficiaries: Why protection may be in jeopardy (Issue Brief 505).* New York: The Commonwealth Fund. Reprinted and abridged by permission of the publisher.

Sara Rosenbaum. (2002). Medicaid. *New England Journal of Medicine, 346* (8), 635–640. Copyright 2002 Massachusetts Medical Society. All rights reserved. Reprinted by permission of the publisher.

Jennifer M. Ryan. (2002). SCHIP Turns 5: Taking stock, moving ahead (Issue Brief 781, pp. 1–12). Washington, DC: National Health Policy Forum. Reprinted by permission of the publisher.

CHAPTER 9

Thomas Bodenheimer. (1999). The American health care system: The movement for improved quality in health care. *New England Journal of Medicine, 340*, 488–492. Copyright 1999 Massachusetts Medical Society. All rights reserved. Reprinted by permission of the publisher.

Elizabeth A. McGlynn and Robert H. Brook. (2002). Keeping quality on the policy agenda. *Health Affairs, 20* (30), 82–90. Reprinted by permission of the publisher.

Huw T.O. Davies, A. Eugene Washington, and Andrew B. Bindman. (2002). Health care report cards: Implications for vulnerable patient groups and the organizations providing them care. *Journal of Health Politics, Policy and Law, 27* (3), 379–399. Copyright 2002 by Duke University Press. All rights reserved. Used by permission of the publisher.

CHAPTER 10

Alina Salganicoff, J. Zoë Beckerman, Roberta Wyn, and Victoria D. Ojeda. (2002). *Women's Health in the United States: health coverage and access to care* (Executive Summary, pp. vii–xii). Menlo Park, CA: Kaiser Family Foundation. Reprinted and abridged by permission of the publisher.

Tracy Weitz and Carroll L. Estes. (2001). Adding aging and gender to the women's health agenda. *Journal of Women and Aging, 13* (2), 3–20. Reprinted by permission of The Haworth Press, Inc. Copyright 2001, Birmingham, New York. Article copies available from the Haworth Document Delivery Service: 1-800-HAWORTH. E-mail address: docdelivery@haworthpressinc.com.

David R. Williams. (2002). Racial/ethnic variations in women's health: The social embeddedness of health. *American Journal of Public Health, 92* (4), 588–597. Reprinted and abridged by permission of the American Public Health Association (APHA).

Suzanne W. Fletcher and Graham A. Colditz. (2002). Failure of estrogen plus progestin therapy for prevention. *Journal of the American Medical Association, 288* (3), 366–368. Copyright 2002 American Medical Association. All rights reserved. Reprinted by permission of the publisher.

Virginia L. Ernster. (2002, February 14). Mammograms and personal choice. *New York Times,* p. A35. Reprinted by permission of *The New York Times* Agency. Originally published in *The New York Times*, February 14, 2002.

CHAPTER 11

Steven P. Wallace, Emily K. Abel, Pamela Stefanowicz, and Nadereh Pourat. (2001). Long-term care and the elderly population. In R.M. Andersen, T.H. Rice, and G.F. Kominski (Eds.), *Changing the U.S. health care system: Key issues in health services, policy, and management* (2nd ed., pp. 205–222). San Francisco: Jossey-Bass. Copyright 2001 Wiley Publishers. This material is used by permission of John Wiley & Sons, Inc. Permission to abridge from the authors. See original article for the full list of references.

Judith Feder. (2001). Long-term care: A public responsibility. *Health Affairs (Millwood), 20* (6), 112–113. Reprinted by permission of the publisher.

Charlene Harrington. (2001). Regulating nursing homes: Residential nursing facilities in the United States. *British Medical Journal, 323* (7311), 507–510. Reprinted by permission of *BMJ* Publishing Group.

Marty Lynch, Carroll L. Estes, and Mauro Hernandez. (2002). *Consumer empowerment issues in chronic and long-term care.* Institute for Health and Aging, University of California San Francisco, originally prepared for the National Academy of Social Insurance Study Panel on Medicare and Chronic Care in the 21st Century. Reprinted by permission of the authors.

ABOUT THE AUTHORS

CHAPTER 1

William G. Rothstein is Professor of Sociology at the University of Maryland, Baltimore County. He is the author of *American Physicians in the Nineteenth Century: From Sects to Science* (Johns Hopkins University Press, 1992) and *American Medical Schools and the Practice of Medicine* (Oxford University Press, 1987). He is also the Editor of *Readings in American Health Care*.

The Centers for Disease Control and Prevention (CDC) in Atlanta, Georgia is the principal public health agency in the U.S. Department of Health and Human Services.

Healthy People 2010 is an initiative headed by the Office of Disease Prevention and Health Promotion, Public Health and Science, Office of the Assistant Secretary for Health, U.S. Department of Health and Human Services, Washington, DC.

CHAPTER 2

Bruce G. Link, PhD, is Professor of Public Health at the Mailman School of Public Health, Columbia University. He is also with the New York State Psychiatric Institute in New York, New York.

Jo C. Phelan, PhD, is Assistant Professor of Public Health in the Mailman School of Public Health at Columbia University in New York, New York.

Sir Michael Marmot, PhD, is Professor and Head of the Department of Epidemiology and Public Health, and Director of the International Centre for Health and Society at University College, London.

Gary W. Evans, PhD, is Professor of Design and Environmental Analysis in the College of Ecology at Cornell University.

Elyse Kantrowitz, MS, is currently Research Assistant in Marketing Communications at Hillier, the fourth-largest architecture firm in the United States.

CHAPTER 3

Beaufort B. Longest, Jr., PhD, FACHE, is the M. Allen Pond Professor of Health Policy and Management in the Graduate School of Public Health and the Founding Director of the Health Policy Institute, University of Pittsburgh in Pittsburgh, Pennsylvania.

Hank C. Jenkins-Smith, PhD, is Professor of Public Policy at the George Bush School of Government and Public Service at Texas A&M University in College Station, Texas. He holds the Joe R. and Teresa Lozano Long Chair of Business and Government at the Bush School.

Paul A. Sabatier, PhD, MA, is Professor in the Department of Environmental Science and Policy at the University of California, Davis. He is the author or coauthor of numerous publications on the public policy process. One of his special areas of interest is environmental health policy.

CHAPTER 4

Mark A. Peterson, PhD, is Professor of Policy Studies and Political Science in the School of Public Policy and Social Research at the University of California, Los Angeles. Dr. Peterson is also Editor of the *Journal of Health Politics, Policy and Law*.

Donald A. Barr, MD, PhD, is Associate Professor (Teaching) of Sociology and Human Biology at Stanford University, Stanford, California. He is Founder and Director of Stanford's undergraduate health policy curriculum and author of *Introduction to U.S. Healthy Policy: The Organization, Financing, and Delivery of Health Care in America* (Pearson Education, Inc., 2002).

Philip R. Lee, MD, is Professor of Social Medicine (Emeritus), Department of Medicine, and Founding Director (Emeritus), Institute for Health Policy Studies, School of Medicine, University of California, San Francisco, and Consulting Professor, Human Biology Program, Stanford University. He is author or coauthor of eight books and over 120 articles. From 1993 to 1997, he served as Assistant Secretary for Health, U.S. Department of Health and Human Services.

A. E. Benjamin, PhD, is Professor, School of Public Policy and Social Research at the University of California, Los Angeles. He has been the author or coauthor of numerous publications on health policy and long-term care policy.

Carroll L. Estes, PhD, is Professor of Sociology in the Institute for Health and Aging, where she was first and Founding Director, and in the Department of

Social and Behavioral Sciences, School of Nursing, at the University of California, San Francisco. Author of *Social Policy & Aging* (Sage, 2001), *The Aging Enterprise* (Jossey-Bass, 1979), and seven other books, she is past president of the Gerontological Society of America, the American Society of Aging, and the Association for Gerontology in Higher Education.

Joshua M. Wiener, PhD, is Principal Research Associate of the Health Policy Center, Urban Institute, Washington, DC.

Sheryl C. Goldberg, PhD, MSW, is Visiting Assistant Research Sociologist at the Institute for Health and Aging, University of California, San Francisco.

Susan Goldenson, MPP, is Health Care Specialist at Mercer Human Resource Consulting, where her research focuses on group health care and employee benefits issues, including health plan design, cost trends, and insurance coverage. Prior to joining Mercer, she was a research associate at the Urban Institute's Health Policy Center, where she worked on long-term care studies and state Medicaid managed care evaluations.

CHAPTER 5

The Centers for Disease Control and Prevention (CDC) in Atlanta, Georgia is the principal public health agency in the U.S. Department of Health and Human Services.

Roz D. Lasker, MD, is Director of the Public Health Division and the Center for the Advancement of Collaborative Strategies in Health, Division of Public Health at The New York Academy of Medicine in New York, New York. She is also the principal author of *Medicine and Public Health: The Power of Collaboration* (Health Administration Press, 1997).

Elisa S. Weiss, PhD, is Associate Director of the Center for the Advancement of Collaborative Strategies in Health, Division of Public Health, at the New York Academy of Medicine in New York, New York.

CHAPTER 6

Kenneth C. Hyams, MD, is the Chief Consultant for Occupational and Environmental Health for the U.S. Department of Veterans Affairs.

Frances M. Murphy, MD, MPH, is Deputy Under Secretary for Health in the Department of Veterans Affairs, Washington, DC. As such, she serves as the second-highest official in the Veterans Health Administration, and is responsible for oversight and operation of the nation's largest integrated health care system.

Simon Wessely, MD, is Professor of Epidemiological and Liaison Psychiatry at Guy's, King's, and St. Thomas' School of Medicine and Institute of Psychiatry in London, England.

Julie Louise Gerberding, MD, MPH, is the newly appointed Director for the Centers for Disease Control and Prevention, U.S. Department of Health and

Human Services. She is also an Associate Clinical Professor of Medicine (Infectious Diseases) at Emory University.

James M. Hughes, MD, is Director of the National Centers for Infectious Diseases of the Centers for Disease Control and Prevention, U.S. Department of Health and Human Services.

Jeffrey P. Koplan, MD, MPH, is the Vice President for Academic Health Affairs at Emory University's Woodruff Health Sciences Center. He served as the Director for the Centers for Disease Control and Prevention, U.S. Department of Health and Human Services from October 1998 to April 2002.

James G. Hodge, Jr., JD, LLM, is Adjunct Professor of Law at Georgetown University Law Center. He is also Scientist and Project Director for the Center for the Law and the Public's Health at Johns Hopkins Bloomberg School of Public Health.

George J. Annas, JD, MPH, is Edward R. Utley Professor of Health Law and Chair of the Health Law Department, School of Public Health, Boston University in Boston, Massachusetts, and author of twelve books.

CHAPTER 7

Robert W. Fogel, PhD, is the Charles R. Walgreen Distinguished Service Professor of American Institutions and Director of the Center for Population Economics at the University of Chicago Graduate School of Business. He is also a member of the Department of Economics and of the Committee on Social Thought at the University of Chicago.

Chulhee Lee, PhD, MA, is Associate Professor of Economics in the School of Economics at Seoul National University in Seoul, Korea.

Jonathan Oberlander, PhD, is Assistant Professor in the Departments of Social Medicine and Political Science at the University of North Carolina at Chapel Hill, North Carolina.

Robert Mills, PhD, is Statistician for the U.S. Census Bureau, U.S. Department of Commerce.

R. Adams Dudley, MD, MBA, is Assistant Professor of Medicine and Health Policy at the University of California, San Francisco. Dr. Dudley is active in the Institute for Health Policy Studies and has served as a consultant on health policy issues to the Institute of Medicine, the American Thoracic Society, and other medical societies.

Harold S. Luft, PhD, is Professor of Health Economics and Director of the Institute for Health Policy Studies, School of Medicine, University of California, San Francisco. He has authored or coauthored numerous publications, including *Health Maintenance Organizations: Dimensions of Performance* (Transaction Books, 1987) and "The Volume Outcome Relationship: Practice Makes Perfect or Selective Referral Patterns?" (1987).

CHAPTER 8

Marilyn Moon, PhD, is Senior Fellow of the Urban Institute in Washington, DC. Dr. Moon is also Program Director for the Commonwealth Fund's Program on Medicare's Future.

Becky Briesacher, PhD, is Director of Research of the Peter Lamy Center on Drug Therapy and Aging at the University of Maryland. Her research focuses on prescription drug coverage, prescribing problems, and barriers to care.

Bruce Stuart, PhD, is Professor and Executive Director of the Peter Lamy Center on Drug Therapy and Aging at the University of Maryland. Dr. Stuart is an economist and health services researcher, with expertise in research design, analysis of large datasets, outcomes research, surveys, econometric analysis, cost-effectiveness analysis, program evaluation, and policy analysis.

Dennis Shea, PhD, is Professor of Health Policy and Administration in the College of Health and Human Development and Senior Research Associate, Center for Health Policy Research, Institute for Policy Research and Evaluation, at the Pennsylvania State University.

Sara Rosenbaum, JD, is Professor of Health Services Management and Policy Director for the Center For Health Policy Research at The George Washington University Medical Center in Washington, DC.

Jennifer M. Ryan is Senior Research Associate of the National Health Policy Forum at The George Washington University in Washington, DC.

CHAPTER 9

Thomas Bodenheimer, MD, MPH, is Associate Clinical Professor in the Department of Family and Community Medicine, School of Medicine, at the University of California, San Francisco.

Elizabeth A. McGlynn, PhD, is Director of the Center for Research on the Quality of Health Care at RAND Health in Santa Monica, California.

Robert H. Brook, MD, ScD, is a Vice President and Corporate Fellow at RAND, and the Director of RAND Health. He also directs the Robert Wood Johnson Clinical Scholars Program at the University of California, Los Angeles (UCLA), and is Professor of Medicine and Health Services at the Center for Health Sciences, UCLA.

Huw T.O. Davies, MA, MSc, PhD, is Professor of Health Care Policy & Management; Director, Centre for Public Policy and Management; Director, Research Unit for Research Utilisation; and Associate Director, PharmacoEconomics Research Centre at the University of St. Andrews in Scotland.

A. Eugene Washington, MD, MSc, is Professor and Chair of the Department of Obstetrics, Gynecology and Reproductive Sciences; Professor of Epidemiology and Health Policy; and Director of the Medical Effectiveness

Research Center for Diverse Populations at the University of California, San Francisco. He is also Director of the UCSF-Stanford Evidence-based Practice Center.

Andrew B. Bindman, MD, is Associate Professor of Medicine, Epidemiology, and Biostatistics at the University of California, San Francisco. Dr. Bindman is also Chief of the Division of General Internal Medicine at San Francisco General Hospital and the Director of the Primary Care Research Center in UCSF's Department of Medicine.

CHAPTER 10

Alina Salganicoff, PhD, is Director and Vice President for Women's Health Policy at the Henry J. Kaiser Family Foundation in Menlo Park, California.

J. Zoë Beckerman, MPH, is Senior Policy Analyst for Women's Health Policy at the Henry J. Kaiser Family Foundation in Washington, DC.

Roberta Wyn, PhD, is Associate Director at the University of California, Los Angeles, Center for Health Policy Research. Her areas of expertise include access to health insurance coverage and health care for women, ethnic populations, and lower-income populations.

Victoria D. Ojeda, MPH, is Project Manager and Research Assistant at the University of California, Los Angeles, Center for Health Policy Research.

Tracy Weitz, MPA, is Projects Director at the Center for Reproductive Health Research and Policy, University of California, San Francisco, and a Tish Sommers Scholar.

Carroll L. Estes, PhD, is Professor of Sociology in the Institute for Health and Aging, where she was first and Founding Director, and in the Department of Social and Behavioral Sciences, School of Nursing, at the University of California, San Francisco.

David R. Williams, PhD, MPH, is Professor of Sociology; Senior Research Scientist, Survey Research Center, Institute for Social Research; and Faculty Associate of the African American Mental Health Research Center and the Center for Afro-American and African Studies at the University of Michigan.

Suzanne W. Fletcher, MD, MSc, is Professor in the Department of Ambulatory Care and Prevention at Harvard Medical School and the Department of Epidemiology, Harvard School of Public Health. She is also appointed in Medicine at the Brigham and Women's Hospital in Boston, Massachusetts.

Graham A. Colditz, DrPH, MD, is Professor in the Department of Epidemiology, Harvard School of Public Health, and Professor of Medicine at Harvard Medical School.

Virginia L. Ernster, PhD, is Professor of Epidemiology and Biostatistics at the University of California, San Francisco (UCSF), and Associate Director for Epidemiology, Prevention and Control, UCSF Cancer Center.

CHAPTER 11

Steven P. Wallace, PhD, is Professor in the Department of Community Health Sciences at the School of Public Health, University of California, Los Angeles (UCLA), and Associate Director of the UCLA Center for Health Policy Research.

Emily K. Abel, PhD, is Professor in the Department of Health Services, UCLA School of Public Health and Women's Studies. She has published several books, including *Hearts of Wisdom: American Women Caring for Kin, 1850–1940* (2000) and *Who Cares for the Elderly? Public Policy and the Experiences of Adult Daughters* (1991).

Pamela Stefanowicz, MPH, is a former doctoral student in the Department of Health Services at the UCLA School of Public Health, where she studied home care workers.

Nadereh Pourat, PhD, is Adjunct Assistant Professor of Health Services at the UCLA School of Public Health and Senior Researcher at the UCLA Center for Health Policy Research.

Judith Feder, PhD, is a political scientist, Professor, and Dean of Policy Studies at the Georgetown Public Policy Institute, Georgetown University. During the Clinton administration, she played a leadership role in health care reform efforts. Dr. Feder is a widely published health policy researcher.

Charlene Harrington, PhD, RN, FAAN, is Professor of Social and Behavioral Science for the Department of Social and Behavioral Sciences, School of Nursing, University of California, San Francisco.

Marty Lynch, PhD, is currently the Chief Executive Officer of LifeLong Medical Care, a Berkeley-based, nonprofit community health center. Dr. Lynch also teaches in the School of Social Welfare at the University of California, Berkeley.

Carroll L. Estes, PhD, is Professor of Sociology in the Institute for Health and Aging, where she was first and Founding Director, and in the Department of Social and Behavioral Sciences, School of Nursing, at the University of California, San Francisco.

Mauro Hernandez is a doctoral student in the Department of Social and Behavioral Sciences, School of Nursing, University of California, San Francisco, and is the Medicaid Waiver Analyst for the San Francisco Department of Aging and Adult Services.

PART I

THE HEALTH OF THE NATION AND DETERMINANTS OF HEALTH

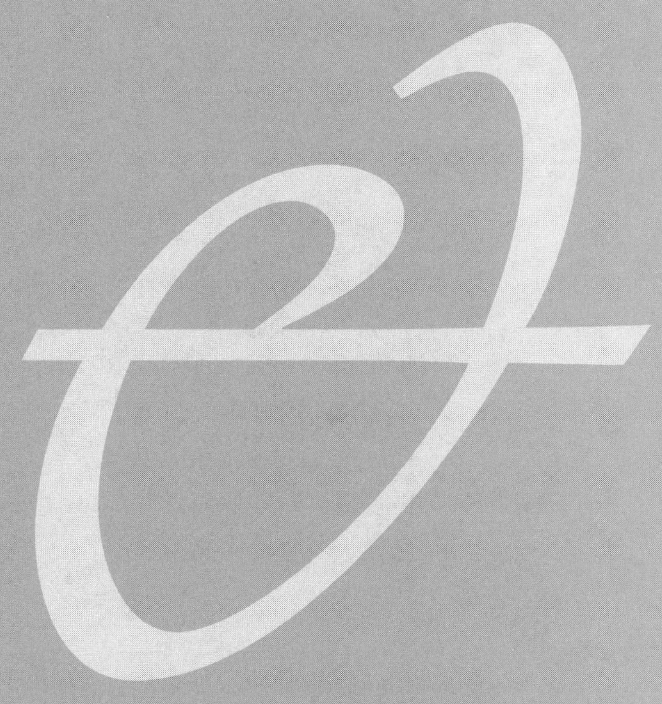

CHAPTER 1

THE HEALTH OF THE NATION

This chapter describes the changing health status of the population in the United States over the past 100 years, as well as the ways in which the health status of the population is measured and the challenges we face at the dawn of the 21st century.

EPIDEMIOLOGICAL TRENDS AND CONCEPTS: MORTALITY AND MORBIDITY

Chapter 1 begins with Rothstein's review of the dramatic improvements in the health status of the U.S. population during the 20th century (Article 1). In the last 100 years, there has been a sharp decline in deaths due to infectious disease, particularly among infants and children, and a rapid increase in life expectancy at birth. The initial dramatic decline in mortality, particularly from infectious diseases, can be attributed primarily to improved socioeconomic conditions (e.g., nutrition, housing) and public health measures (safe water supplies, waste disposal, pasteurization of milk). Later, immunizations began to have an effect. The introduction of sulfonamides in the mid-1930s, penicillin in the early 1940s, and a host of other antibiotics contributed to the sharp drop in mortality from the mid-1930s to the late 1950s. Thereafter, the rate of decline slowed. In addition to penicillin and the sulfonamides, the most important antimicrobial drug developed in the late 1940s was streptomycin, which proved to be the first drug to effectively treat tuberculosis.

Except for the 500,000 deaths in the United States caused by the influenza pandemic of 1918 to 1919, the mortality rate for most infectious diseases declined throughout the 20th century. However, in the late 1980s, the mortality rate increased and life expectancy decreased, largely because of the HIV/AIDS epidemic. This trend has now been reversed with antiviral drugs, the widespread application of prevention programs, and improved treatment of opportunistic infection in persons with AIDS.

The dramatic decline in mortality from infectious diseases is summarized in the excerpt from the Centers for Disease Control and Prevention (CDC) report (Article 2).

As noted by Rothstein and described in more detail in the CDC report "Healthier Mothers and Babies" (Article 3), the greatest decline in age-specific mortality in the 20th century was for infants. In 1900, 1 of 6 infants died in the first year of life. Currently, fewer than 1 in 110 infants dies before the age of one. Although not emphasized by Rothstein, the decline in maternal mortality has been significant since the 1920s, when improvements in obstetrical practice became widely applied. Article 3 provides a brief historical overview of changes in obstetric education, delivery practices, and medical advances and their role in reducing maternal mortality.

Although death from infectious disease has become much less significant, there has been a concomitant increase in what are known as the "diseases of Western civilization," such as cancer, coronary heart disease, stroke, diabetes mellitus, and emphysema. To explain this phenomenon, two related processes have been proposed. The first is often referred to as the "demographic transition," which describes the shift from a society with high fertility and high mortality to one with low mortality and low fertility. During a demographic transition, the mortality rate falls, often dramatically, followed by a fall in the fertility rate. What Young (1998) calls a "companion theory" is the theory of "health or epidemiologic transitions." It describes and explains the long-term temporal changes in the patterns of health and disease in populations. The health transition has three stages: (1) the age of pestilence and famines, (2) the age of receding pandemics, and (3) the age of degenerative and manmade diseases (Young, 1998, p. 42). This transition is observed when a nation's life expectancy increases as mortality from infectious disease declines, and mortality from chronic and degenerative diseases predominates. Because chronic diseases are more prevalent (*prevalence* refers to the proportion of people who have a certain disease either at a point in time or within a specific time period) with increasing age, this is an area of increasing importance, particularly with the aging of the U.S. population.

Article 4, "Decline in Deaths from Heart Disease and Stroke," describes the decline in mortality from heart disease, including coronary artery disease, during the past 40 years and the decline in stroke mortality throughout the 20th century. Although the causes for the dramatic decline in coronary artery disease death rates are not well understood, it is generally attributed to behavior change (e.g., reduced dietary fat), public health efforts (e.g., tobacco control regulations), and improvements in medical care (e.g., treatment of hypertension). It is important to note that the mortality rate from stroke has been declining since the turn of the 20th century and that declines could not be attributed to medical interventions until after mid-century. Although the widespread use of penicillin to treat streptococcal infection had a dramatic impact on the incidence of rheumatic fever and rheumatic heart disease, again, this did not occur until after mid-century. *Incidence* is defined as the number of new cases of a disease that occur during a specified period of time in a population at risk for developing the disease (Gordis, 2000) and should not be confused with prevalence.

MEASURING HEALTH STATUS: MORTALITY, MORBIDITY, AND OUTCOME MEASURES

During much of the 20th century, the health status of the population was measured in terms of deaths: the total number and distributions by age, disease, gender, and geographic area. Life expectancy at birth and at particular ages (e.g., age 65 years) was also measured. Mortality rates were the most commonly used measure of health status, as Rothstein noted, "because all deaths and their causes have been reported to local or state government agencies for many years" (Article 1).

Rothstein deals with some important measures of health status, such as crude death rates, age-specific death rates, infant mortality rates, age-adjusted death rates, and life expectancy. A much wider range of measures is used by the National Center for Health Statistics of the CDC, as illustrated in Table 1.

Morbidity, which concerns illness, is another term that has been used historically to measure health status. Morbidity is defined in the *Oxford American Dictionary* as "caused by or indicating disease" (Ehrlich et al., 1980, p. 578). The most useful data on morbidity relate to infectious diseases because they have also been reported to local and state governments for many years.

TABLE 1

Measures of Health Status

Infant mortality rates	Motor vehicle–related injury and deaths	Five-year relative survival rates for selected cancer cases
Neonatal mortality rates	Suicide	Firearm-related injuries and deaths
Postnatal mortality rates	Homicide	Measures of health behavior (e.g., smoking, substance abuse, alcohol consumption)
Age-adjusted death rates	Occupational disease rates	Physiologic measures (e.g., blood pressure, blood cholesterol, body weight)
Life expectancy	Selected notable disease rates	Environmental measures (ambient air quality)
Years of potential life lost	Acquired immunodeficiency syndrome (AIDS) cases	
Leading cause of death	Age-adjusted cancer incidence rates	

Source: National Center for Health Statistics (2001).

HEALTHY PEOPLE 2010

Chapter 1 concludes with an excerpt from *Healthy People 2010: Understanding and Improving Health* (U.S. Department of Health and Human Services [DHHS], 2000b), which provides an overview of the health status of the population and the two overarching goals for the next decade: to increase quality of life and years of healthy life, and to eliminate health disparities by 2010. The selection replaces *Healthy People 2010: Objectives, Goals* (U.S. DHHS, 2000a), which was included in the sixth edition. The process of setting national health goals began in 1977 under the leadership of Dr. Julius Richmond, Surgeon General and Assistant Secretary for Health (U.S. DHHS, 1977). The process for establishing health objectives for 1990 included not only the federal government but also state and local governments and a wide range of private-sector organizations. Goals and objectives were initially set for 1990 and, more recently, for 2000 and 2010. The Healthy People publications and process now engage literally thousands of people in setting goals, implementing programs, and evaluating progress.

HEALTH DISPARITIES AND HEALTHY PEOPLE 2010

A major change occurred between the goals of Healthy People 2000 (U.S. DHHS, 1990) and the goals of Healthy People 2010, namely, the addition of the goal to "eliminate health disparities." This will not be an easy task. In recent years, increasing attention has been paid to health disparities within the population. The impact of socioeconomic status (SES) on health and health disparities is considered in more detail in Chapter 2 and in the data summarized in *Socioeconomic Status and Health Chartbook: Health, United States* (Pamuck et al., 1998; see the Recommended Reading list at the end of this book). Infant mortality and life expectancy are related to SES and education. The CDC report "Healthier Mothers and Babies" (Article 3) notes:

> Although overall rates have plummeted, black infants are more than twice as likely to die as white infants; this ratio has increased in recent decades. The higher risk for infant mortality among blacks compared to whites is attributed to higher LBW [low birth weight] incidence and preterm births and to higher risk of death among normal birthweight infants.... American Indian/Alaska Native infants have higher death rates than whites because of higher SIDS [sudden infant death syndrome] rates. Hispanics of Puerto Rican origin have higher death rates than white infants because of higher LBW rates (p. 854).

This problem continues to pose a major challenge to communities, the public health system, and medical care systems. The evidence for health disparities includes not only health status but also exposure to environmental hazards (see Chapter 2) and access to appropriate health care (see Chapters 7 and 8). The SES of the population, education, and occupations all play important roles and are inversely related to death rates for chronic diseases, communicable diseases, and injuries among persons aged 25 to 64. Less-educated men and women also have higher suicide rates. Cigarette smoking is more prevalent among those of lower socioeconomic status, and death rates for lung cancer and heart disease are higher. Unintended pregnancy is another significant risk factor for women and their infants. According to the CDC report "Healthier Mothers and Babies":

> Approximately half of all pregnancies in the United States are unintended, including approximately three quarters among women aged less than 20 years. Unintended pregnancy is associated with increased morbidity and mortality for the mother and infant. Lifestyle factors (e.g., smoking, drinking alcohol, unsafe sex practices, and poor nutrition) and inadequate intake of foods containing folic acid pose serious health hazards to the mother and fetus and are more common among women with unintended pregnancies (p. 854).

The Recommended Reading list includes excerpts from the Commonwealth Fund's *U.S. Minority Health: A Chartbook* (Collins, Hall, and Neuhaus, 1999). By almost every measure (e.g., infant mortality, life expectancy, self-reported health status), the health of minorities is worse than that of the non-Hispanic, white population. Within minority groups, such as Hispanics, there are differences, with Cubans usually in better health and living longer than Puerto Ricans or Mexican Americans. Certain problems, such as low birth weight, particularly afflict African Americans. Although a number of the differences between the health status of minorities and the majority of the population (whites) are related to socioeconomic status, not all of the differences are due to socioeconomic factors.

The "Highlights" in the *Socioeconomic Status and Health Chartbook: Health, United States* and the Commonwealth Fund's *U.S. Minority Health: A Chartbook* review some of the evidence related to SES and health status and give a clue as to why it will be a challenge to eliminate health disparities by 2010.

FEDERAL AGENCIES INVOLVED IN HEALTH DATA COLLECTION, ANALYSIS, AND REPORTING

The health of the nation is measured and reported by a wide range of federal agencies. The National Center for Health Statistics (NCHS) of the Centers for Disease Control and Prevention, U.S. Department of Health and Human Services, is the nation's primary health statistics agency. The NCHS collects and publishes data on a wide variety of health care topics. The NCHS manages the National Linked File of Live Births and Deaths and the Compressed Mortality File. The National Vital Statistics System within the NCHS also collects and publishes data on births, deaths, marriages, and divorces in the United States. In addition, the NCHS conducts periodic, large-scale surveys, including the National Survey of Family Growth, the National Health Interview Survey (NHIS), the National Health and Nutrition Examination Survey (NHANES), the National Health Provider Inventory, the National Nursing Home Survey, the National Home and Hospice Care Survey, the National Hospital Discharge Survey, the National Survey of Ambulatory Surgery, the National Ambulatory Medical Care Survey, and the National Hospital Ambulatory Medical Care Survey (NCHS, 2001).

The DHHS oversees more than 100 other health information and data systems, including program-specific information systems and information systems related to disease surveillance, health behavior, medical care expenditures, drug use, health professions, health facilities, mental health, and Medicare and Medicaid. However, there is a lack of coordination and integration among many of these information and data systems.

Other departments and agencies collect health-related information, including the Department of Commerce (Bureau of the Census), the Department of Labor (Bureau of Labor Statistics), the Department of Veteran Affairs, and the Environmental Protection Agency (EPA). The Office of Management and Budget (OMB) is the oversight agency responsible for the coordination of these efforts. The OMB reviews multiple surveys and approves budget proposals for all of the statistical agencies.

In summary, the past century resulted in dramatic improvements in the health status of the population. Particularly important were the declines in infant mortality and infectious disease. Despite the improvement in health status, there remain significant disparities in health status within the population related to socioeconomic status, race/ethnicity, education, and occupation.

REFERENCES

Centers for Disease Control and Prevention. (1999). Achievements in public health, 1900–1999: Control of infectious disease. *MMWR, 48* (29), 621–622.

Centers for Disease Control and Prevention. (1999). Achievements in public health, 1900–1999: Decline in deaths from heart disease and stroke — United States, 1900–1999. *MMWR, 48* (29), 649–650.

Centers for Disease Control and Prevention. (1999). Achievements in public health, 1900–1999. Healthier mothers and babies. *MMWR, 48* (38), 849–855.

Collins, K. S., Hall, A., and Neuhaus, C. (1999). *U.S. minority health: A chartbook.* New York: The Commonwealth Fund.

Ehrlich, E., Flexner, S. B., Carruth, G., and Hawkins, J. M. (Eds.). (1980). *Oxford American Dictionary*. New York: Avon Books.

Gordis, L. (2000). *Epidemiology* (2nd ed.). Philadelphia: W.B. Saunders.

National Center for Health Statistics, Centers for Disease Control and Prevention. (2001). *Health, United States, 2001* (DHHS Publication No. PHS 01-1232). Washington, DC: Department of Health and Human Services.

Pamuk, E., Makuc, D., Heck, K., Reuben, C., and Lochnen, K. (1998). *Socioeconomic status and health chartbook: Health, United States,* 1998. Hyattsville, MD: National Center for Health Statistics.

Rothstein, W. G. (1995). Trends in mortality in the twentieth century. In W. G. Rothstein, *Readings in American health care: Current issues in socio-historical perspective* (pp. 71–86). Madison: University of Wisconsin Press.

U.S. Department of Health and Human Services. (1977). *Surgeon general's report on health promotion and disease prevention*. Washington, DC: Public Health Service, U.S. Department of Health and Human Services.

U.S. Department of Health and Human Services. (1990). *Healthy People 2000: National health promotion and disease prevention objectives*. Washington, DC: Public Health Service, U.S. Department of Health and Human Services.

U.S. Department of Health and Human Services. (2000a). *Healthy People 2010: Objectives, goals* (2nd ed.). Washington, DC: U.S. Government Printing Office.

U.S. Department of Health and Human Services. (2000b). *Healthy People 2010: Understanding and improving health* (2nd ed.). Washington, DC: U.S. Government Printing Office.

Young, T. K. (1998). *Population health: Concepts and methods*. New York: Oxford University Press.

ARTICLE 1

Trends in Mortality in the Twentieth Century

William G. Rothstein

This article examines one of the most remarkable transformations in the history of mankind. The twentieth century has witnessed the greatest and most rapid changes in both death rates and causes of death in recorded history. At the beginning of the century, infectious diseases were the paramount cause of death in all societies, killing millions of infants, children, and young adults. After 1900 death rates from these diseases declined rapidly in advanced countries, enabling many more people to live to old age. The increasing number of the elderly died from chronic and degenerative diseases, especially heart disease, cancer, and stroke. In recent decades, death rates from heart disease and stroke have declined, while those from cancer have not. The reasons for these trends have been the subject of continuing conjecture and debate.

DISEASES IN HUMAN HISTORY

Infectious diseases first became common thousands of years ago when human beings settled in villages to farm the land, tend domestic animals, and trade with residents of other villages. When those events occurred, enough people had contact with each other to enable the microorganisms that cause diseases to find a continuing reservoir of uninfected individuals and thereby survive indefinitely. In earlier hunting and gathering societies, the populations were so small that any pathogenic microorganisms soon ran out of uninfected individuals and died out. From the onset of village societies until early in the twentieth century, human beings fell victim to a growing number of infectious diseases, which became the major cause of death in all societies. Most of the victims of these diseases were children and young adults.[1]

The situation worsened when international and intercontinental travel dispersed diseases around the world, beginning in the late fifteenth century. The early European explorers spread tuberculosis, smallpox, measles, scarlet fever, and other infectious diseases to the Americas, the Pacific Islands, and other parts of the world that had never known them. They returned to Europe bringing yellow fever, cholera, and other infectious diseases from Africa and Asia. International travel also spread previously regional epidemics around the world as infected travelers unknowingly brought the diseases to different countries and continents.

Urbanization and industrialization in the eighteenth and nineteenth centuries forced the laboring classes of western nations to live in unsanitary housing, drink polluted water and milk, suffer diseases caused by unhygienic methods of sewage disposal, and eat a less nutritious diet than was available in many rural areas. Children suffered most from this unhealthy environment. In some American and European cities in the nineteenth century, one out of every four infants died before their first birthday.

Three fundamental changes were necessary to improve the health of the population. One was a higher standard of living to strengthen resistance to disease. This required better food, housing, and clothing, healthier home and work environments, lower birth rates, and a level of education that would enable people to understand and adopt the growing scientific knowledge about health care. The second change was improved public health measures by government to prevent diseases from infecting people. The third was effective clinical medicine, for the treatment of individual patients.

Perhaps the best available historical evidence concerning a society's standard of living is the height of its children and adults. A slow rate of growth during childhood and a short ultimate height that continues for decades in a society is clear evidence of a low standard of living. A study of the heights of British boys, adolescents, and military recruits found a slow but steady increase in the heights of those born from about 1750 to about 1840, a decline in their heights to the 1870s, a gradual return to early nineteenth-century heights by the end of the century, and a rapid increase in heights in the twentieth century. The study also found much taller heights among the children of the wealthy than other children before the twentieth century, indicating that heights throughout the period were strongly affected by the standard of living. Less comprehensive data showed that American men were one to two inches taller than the British (and other European) mean throughout this period, but experienced the same growth trends as British men.[2]

These trends suggest that industrialization and urbanization had a deleterious effect on human health during the middle of the nineteenth century. Industrialization and world trade also lowered the standard of living of many rural people, whose cottage industry and small-scale farming could not compete with goods produced on a large scale elsewhere. A lower birth rate at the end of the nineteenth century and greater national wealth in the twentieth century increased the overall standard of living.[3]

Public health and clinical medicine advanced in the late nineteenth century due to better microscopes and related technologies that enabled scientists to explore the world invisible to the naked eye. During and after the 1870s, the disease-causing roles of many bacteria and other parasites were discovered. Government officials soon developed public health programs to keep bacteria from infecting human beings. Sewerage systems prevented sewage from contaminating water supplies and coming into contact with human beings, water supplies were chemically purified to destroy bacteria, milk and foods were made to conform to standards of bacteriological cleanliness, vectors of infectious diseases like mosquitoes and rodents were controlled, and housing standards were gradually raised.

The first effective clinical treatments for many diseases were developed about the same time. Surgery was revolutionized in the 1880s after it was discovered that antiseptic procedures and sterilization prevented the wounds from becoming infected. Diphtheria antitoxin, discovered in 1894, was the first effective treatment for a major infectious disease. In the ensuing decades, treatments were developed for diabetes, pellagra, and pernicious anemia. The most revolutionary improvements occurred in the late 1930s with the discovery of the sulfa drugs, the first general antibiotics. Penicillin, streptomycin, and other antibiotics followed in the 1940s.

Vaccines to immunize individuals against infectious diseases were also developed. Smallpox vaccination was developed in the late 1790s, but it remained unique until well into the twentieth century, when vaccines were developed for infectious diseases like diphtheria, tetanus, polio, rubella, and measles.

As fewer individuals died in childhood and early adulthood from infectious diseases, they lived to older ages and contracted diseases related to the aging process, such as heart disease, cancer, diseases of the blood vessels, and diseases of individual organs like diabetes, emphysema, or kidney disease. These chronic and degenerative diseases have become the major causes of death in advanced societies. The change in causes of death from infectious diseases to chronic and degenerative diseases, often called an "epidemiological revolution," has had a momentous effect on our society. The remainder of this article will examine the nature of these changes.

BASIC CONCEPTS

Two kinds of statistics are used to describe the state of health of a population. One concerns deaths or *mortality*. The other concerns illnesses or *morbidity*. Historical data on mortality are the most frequently used measures of trends in the health of the population because all deaths and their causes have been reported to local or state government agencies for many years. Reliable historical data on morbidity exist for only a small number of diseases, mostly communicable diseases, that must be reported to the government. Morbidity data also pose problems because illnesses vary in the degree and permanence of the disability they produce. The health impact of a common cold, a heart attack, and diabetes vary so greatly that it makes little sense to group them together in a single category.

In examining mortality trends in a population, we use death *rates* rather than numbers of deaths. The number of deaths are unsatisfactory because they increase or decrease with changes in the size of the population regardless of any change in its health status. Death rates enable us to compare populations of different sizes.

A mortality rate is a fraction in which the numerator consists of the number of persons who have had the experience in question (in this case, death) and the denominator includes all those who could have had that experience (the population). The formula for the *crude death rate* is the number of deaths in a population during a time period divided by the average population during the time period. The population in question may be the population of a nation, the population of a particular state or city, or the number of persons in a particular group, such as women aged 35–44. The time period is usually a specific year, but it can be a month or any other time period of interest.

Death rates always equal 1 or are less than 1, because the numerator (the number of people who died) can never be larger than the denominator (the population). This entangles us in decimal places. To eliminate this nuisance, we usually list death rates per 1,000 persons. For example, if 60 people in a community of 2,000 persons died in a given year, the crude death rate would be 60 divided by 2,000, which equals 0.03. This means that 3 of every 100 people in the community died in that year. We can change the statistic to the death rate per 1,000 population by multiplying 0.03 by 1,000, which equals 30. This says that 30 out of every 1,000 people in the community died in that year. The first number (0.03) gives us the death rate per person; the second (30) gives us the death rate per 1,000 persons.

Death rates per 1,000 persons are useful for examining total deaths, but most individual diseases produce so few deaths that we use death rates per 100,000 persons to eliminate the decimal point. For example, if 800 persons in a population of 20,000,000 died of a particular disease in a given year, the crude death rate equals 800 divided by 20,000,000, or .00004. If we multiply .00004 by 100,000, we get a death rate of 4 per 100,000.

Death rates can be very deceptive because of these arithmetic manipulations. It is easy to forget that the 4 in the above example represents 4 deaths from that disease per 100,000 persons in a given year. In a city of one million persons, only 40 would die from that disease in a year. Such statistics become even more misleading when people speak of changes like a doubling of the death rate. If the death rate just cited doubled in a year, which sounds quite alarming, the number of deaths from that disease would rise from 4 per 100,000 persons to 8 per 100,000 persons, or from 40 deaths per year in the city of one million to 80 deaths per year. Very few people would notice such a change.

One way to assess changes in the health status of the population is to compare death rates at different times. Because crude death rates disregard changes in the age distribution of the population, they can be misleading when used in this way. An increase in the crude death rate over time may indicate only that there were more old people and fewer young people in the population at the end of the period, not that the population was less healthy.

In order to deal with changes in the age distribution of a population, epidemiologists use age-specific and age-adjusted death rates. *Age-specific* death rates are death rates for specific age groups in the population, such as persons 1–4 years of age or 65–74 years of age. By examining death rates for specific age groups, we need not be concerned about changes in the age distribution. *Age-adjusted* death rates adjust the death rate in a population so that the age distribution in every year studied corresponds to the age distribution that existed in a base year chosen for convenience (1940 in most U.S. government statistics). The population for every year except the base year is mathematically adjusted so that the percentage of the population in each age group is the same as in the base year. Although the resulting data do not describe the actual death rates in the population in any year except the base year, they permit comparisons between death rates in different years while holding constant the age distribution of the population.

In addition to total death rates, we are also interested in death rates from specific causes, such as cancer, AIDS, or accidents. Death rates from specific causes are subject to several problems that do not occur with overall death rates.

Information about causes of deaths are obtained from death certificates filled out at the time of death by the patient's physician, or in some cases a medical examiner or a coroner. The death certificate requires the physician to list both the "immediate" and "underlying" causes of death, which might be pneumonia and a stroke, respectively. The physician selects the specific causes of death from the current revision of the *International Classification of Diseases.*

Several factors reduce the utility of time trends for causes of death for specific diseases. Many diseases, like heart attacks, cancer, stroke, and tuberculosis, are diagnosed differently now than they were early in the century, which makes it difficult to compare death rates at different periods. Physicians also tend to be more sensitive to diseases that are prevalent in the community. Early in the century, when heart disease was less prevalent than it is today, physicians often overlooked or misdiagnosed it. At the same time, they sometimes attributed deaths from other causes to tuberculosis, which was extremely common. Another problem, that has become more important in recent years, is that elderly people often have two or more serious diseases at the time of death, which makes it difficult to know the exact cause of death.

Nation-wide statistics on death rates were first gathered in the U.S. in 1900, but included only 10 states, the District of Columbia, and a number of cities in other states. This "Death Registration Area" was steadily expanded as more states gathered the necessary statistics until it covered the entire continental U.S. in 1933. Birth registration statistics (which are used to calculate infant mortality rates) were first listed in 1915 and did not include the entire continental U.S. until 1933 also. The original Death Registration Area consisted of the urbanized and older states, which had lower death rates than the nonreporting states, so that U.S. death rates before 1933 are very slightly lower than would have been the case had all states reported.[4]

THE DECLINE IN MORTALITY RATES

A remarkable decline in the crude death rate has occurred in the twentieth century. In 1900, there were 17.2 deaths for every 1,000 persons in the nation (for those states and cities in the Death Registration Area). In 1930, the rate dropped to 11.3 deaths per 1,000 persons, in 1960 to 9.5, and in 1991 to 8.6 deaths for every 1,000 persons. We may illustrate the significance of the decline in this way: In 1991, 2,169,000 persons died in the U.S.[5]; had the death rate of 1900 remained unchanged, 4,338,000 persons would have died in 1991. Thus, over 2 million lives were saved in 1991 compared to 1900 due to the decline in the death rate.

The decline was most rapid early in the century and has slowed in recent decades. Between 1900 and 1930 the death rate dropped by 5.9 deaths per 1000 persons, while between 1960 and 1991 the decline was only 0.9 deaths per 1000 persons.

Deaths throughout the century have been most likely to occur at the extremes of the life cycle — among the very young and the very old. This has been true from time immemorial. Death rates are high in the first year of life, but they drop very rapidly, so that the death rate over the entire life cycle reaches its nadir between the ages of 5 and 14. It rises slowly during early adulthood, and then ascends quite rapidly among the oldest age groups.

The greatest change in age-specific mortality rates in the twentieth century has been the decline in death rates among the young. In 1900, 162.4 of every 1,000 infants born alive died in the first year of life. This amounted to 1 out of every 6 infants, an appalling toll. The rate has declined steadily to 9.2 per 1,000 in 1991, or 1 out of every 109 infants. The significance of this change may be indicated thus: in 1991 there were 36,766 deaths in the first year of life.[6] Had the 1900 infant mortality rate remained unchanged, there would have been 649,000 deaths in the first year of life in 1991.

The death rate among children 1–4 years of age also plummeted from 19.8 per 1,000 in 1900 to only 0.5 per thousand in 1989. This age group, which had a higher than average death rate in 1900, now has the second lowest death rate among all age groups.

In 1900 only one age group had a death rate of less than 5.9 deaths per 1000: 5–14 years of age. In 1989, every age group from 1–4 years of age to 45–54 years of age bettered that statistic. Death has now become a rarity among children and young and middle-aged adults.

There have also been impressive declines in death rates among the elderly from 1900 to 1991, but they are less striking than the declines among the young. Among those age 65–74, the drop has been from 56.4 to 26.2 deaths per 1000 persons. Among those 75–84, the drop has been from 123.3 to 58.9 deaths per 1000 persons, and among those 85 and over, the drop has been from 260.9 to 151.1 deaths per 1000 persons.

Another important factor affecting mortality rates is sex. Throughout the century females have had lower death rates than males in all age groups. Among the very youngest, the sex difference has narrowed since 1900, so that female infants and young children now have only a slightly lower death rate than males. At the oldest ages, on the other hand, the sex difference has steadily widened, so that older women now have significantly lower death rates than older men.

Some may conclude that if fewer people are dying today, the American population should be growing at a faster rate than it did in 1900. Population growth depends on three factors: the number of deaths, the number of births, and the migration of people to and from America. Since 1900 both the birth and net migration rates have declined substantially, so that overall population growth has slowed substantially.[7]

INCREASES IN LIFE EXPECTANCY

Life expectancy tables show the average number of *remaining* years of life of a person of a given age. Life expectancy is not based on the actual experience of the people described, because that information will not be available until all of those persons have lived out their lives. Instead, it assumes that persons born now, for example, will have the same probability of being alive when they reach a given age that persons born that many years ago have of being alive now. Even though this is a poor assumption, it is the same throughout the table, so that the comparisons are useful even though the predictions will not be.

Average life expectancy at birth has increased by about 25 years for men and 30 years for women from 1900 to 1989. Life expectancy at birth has increased so greatly because death rates drop sharply after the first year of life. If an infant survives the first year of life, the chances are very good that he or she will live for another 60 years or more. Consequently every infant death that is prevented has a dramatic impact on total life expectancy.

The sex difference in life expectancy at birth has also grown. In 1900 the average female could expect to live 2 years more over her lifespan than the average male; by 1989 this difference had expanded to almost 7 years. Both social and biological factors contribute to this difference. With regard to social factors, men engage in many life-shortening behaviors to a greater extent than women: for example, they are more likely to smoke cigarettes (although the sex difference is narrowing), use beverage alcohol and drugs, commit suicide, and die of violence or injuries sustained at work or in other accidents. Biological factors are believed to have some involvement in women's lower rates of heart disease, stroke, and some other diseases.[8]

When we examine changes between 1900 and 1989 in the average number of years of life remaining at age 65, the increases are considerably smaller, especially for men. In 1900, a 65-year-old man could expect to live an average of 11.5 more years, to age 76.5, while a woman of the same age could expect to live an average of 12.2 more years, to age 77.2. In 1989, men 65 years of age lived an additional 3.7 years on the average (to age 80.2), while women 65 years of age lived an additional 6.6 years on the average (to age 83.8).

These data indicate clearly that a revolutionary decline has occurred in death rates, that this revolution has had its greatest impact on the young and least impact on the elderly, and that females have benefited more than males, especially among the elderly. We will now examine explanations for these remarkable changes.

THE DECLINE IN INFECTIOUS DISEASE DEATH RATES

In order to understand the reasons for the declining death rates of the U.S. population, and particularly the great reduction in death rates among the very young, we must examine the causes of death for the whole population and for individual age groups. These show clearly that a decrease in death rates from infectious diseases among the young has been responsible for most of the decline in mortality.

In 1900, nine categories accounted for 63 percent of all deaths. Five of them, mostly infectious diseases, had their greatest impact on the young. Influenza and pneumonia were major causes of death among infants and very young children, as were gastritis and enteritis, which were caused by bacteria-laden milk, water, and food. The communicable diseases of childhood included diphtheria, measles, scarlet fever, and whooping cough. Tuberculosis was primarily a killer of adolescents and young adults, but it prevented millions from living to old age. Accidents, too, were major killers of the young.

Deaths from these diseases declined markedly from 1900 to 1950. Mortality rates from the infectious diseases in the group — influenza, pneumonia, tuberculosis, diphtheria, measles, scarlet fever, and whooping cough — dropped from 472 deaths per 100,000 persons in 1900 to 55 deaths per 100,000 persons in 1950. Gastritis and enteritis also declined greatly. By 1991 tuberculosis had practically disappeared (although it reappeared in the 1990s in AIDS patients), pneumonia and influenza have become diseases of the elderly rather than diseases of the young, and the other diseases that affect the young have become insignificant as causes of death.

These declines were due more to improvements in the standard of living and public health measures than to better medical treatment of the sick. Gastritis and enteritis were eliminated by measures such as pasteurization of milk and purification of water supplies. Death rates from tuberculosis, pneumonia, and communicable diseases of childhood experienced most of their decline long before effective treatments existed for them. Although public health measures like better housing and quarantine of the infected played a role, most of the decrease appears to have been due to a higher standard of living that strengthened the resistance of people to the diseases and enabled them to survive the diseases if they became ill.[9]

Public education was also important in this revolution. Until well into the twentieth century, millions of Americans drank from metal drinking cups kept next to fountains for all to use, did not sterilize bottles or take other measures necessary for hygienic feeding of infants, let their children sleep in the same bed and play with siblings with contagious diseases like diphtheria and scarlet fever, purchased unrefrigerated and bacteria-laden milk and meat, used polluted wells and water supplies without boiling the water, and took baths in bathtubs after others had used the same water. These and many other similar behaviors have disappeared because the public has been educated about personal hygiene.

One type of medical care that has been related to the decline in infectious diseases is vaccination. It is widely agreed that smallpox vaccination played a role in the decline of that disease and some studies have found that diphtheria vaccine played a much greater role than diphtheria antitoxin in the decline of that disease. Vaccines for measles and polio are believed to have contributed to the decline in those diseases. Support for this view was shown by the rise in the measles case rate when federal support for measles immunization was reduced in the 1980s.

The decline in infectious diseases had important indirect health benefits as well. Nephritis and other kidney diseases are more likely to occur in adults who contracted scarlet fever or other streptococcal infections as children. As the incidence of streptococcal diseases has declined, so has the incidence of kidney diseases, which have dropped from a major cause of death in 1900 to a relatively minor one today.[10]

CHRONIC AND DEGENERATIVE DISEASES AS MAJOR CAUSES OF DEATH

As fewer young persons died from infectious and bacterial diseases, they survived to old age and succumbed to chronic and degenerative diseases like heart disease, cancer, and cerebrovascular disease (stroke). Crude death rates from these three diseases combined increased from 308 per 100,000 in 1900 to 546 per 100,000 in 1991.

In describing recent trends in mortality we can avoid the problems created by changes in the age distribution of the population by using age-specific or age-adjusted death rates. For this reason we will limit the analyses to the years since 1950.

The nine leading causes of death categories in 1991 together accounted for 80 percent of all deaths in 1991. Each category listed (except AIDS) includes a number of specific diseases. For example, within the heart disease category, the most common condition is ischemic (meaning deficient in blood) heart disease (often called coronary heart disease or heart attack), in which the blood supply to the heart muscle is interrupted, killing some heart muscle cells (called a myocardial infarction). Cancer encompasses hundreds of specific diseases involving different organs and types of cell abnormalities. The most common cerebrovascular (meaning the blood vessels of the brain) disease is stroke, which is an interruption of the blood supply to the brain. Chronic obstructive pulmonary (pertaining to the lungs) diseases include emphysema, bronchitis, and asthma, all disorders affecting the supply of air to the lungs. Diabetes encompasses a number of conditions involving excessive urination, the most important of which is diabetes mellitus, a malfunctioning of the cells that produce insulin. The trends shown are for all diseases in each category; trends for specific diseases within a category can vary.

Age-adjusted death rate trends from 1950 to 1991 differ substantially by category. The death rate for heart disease has declined substantially, although it remains the major cause of death. A drop has also occurred in the mortality rate for cerebrovascular diseases and, to a lesser extent, from diabetes. Pneumonia and influenza have continued to decline as causes of death. The death rate from cancer, the second largest cause of death, has increased slightly, and that from chronic pulmonary diseases has shown an ominous rise.

From 1900 to about 1950, overall heart disease death rates rose steadily for each age group (the rates for ischemic heart disease continued to rise until the late 1960s). The growing proportion of older persons could not be responsible for the increase in heart disease death rates, because a larger proportion of people *within* each age group died of heart disease in 1950 than in 1900. It is now recognized that an epidemic of heart disease occurred in the first two-thirds of this century, and that it occurred in all advanced societies, not only the United States.[11] Then, beginning about 1950 for non-ischemic heart disease and in the late 1960s for the more prevalent ischemic heart disease, mortality rates declined steadily for all age groups. Currently heart disease death rates for the 45–54-, 55–64-, and 65–74-year age groups are lower than they were in 1900, and those for the older age groups have declined significantly from their 1950 levels but remain higher than their 1900 levels. A similar trend has occurred in many other advanced nations, although the declines began a few years later in some of them.

Ischemic heart disease mortality rates for both sexes increased from 1950 to 1970 (they actually peaked in the late 1960s) and have declined subsequently. Men have much higher death rates from ischemic heart disease in each age group than do women. The decline in ischemic heart disease mortality rates has benefited women as much as men, even though it is much less prevalent among women.

Understanding these trends has been made more difficult by changes in the diagnosis of heart disease by physicians.[12] Heart disease has no ubiquitous signs or symptoms. Many people have heart attacks without realizing it. Physicians often have difficulty diagnosing heart disease, because routine and even sophisticated diagnostic tests can fail to reveal abnormalities. If physicians do not look carefully for heart disease, they can easily overlook it.

At the beginning of the century, when heart disease was uncommon, physicians overlooked it quite often. As it became more prevalent, physicians became sensitized to it and were more likely to recognize it as a cause of death. The development of the electrocardiograph also made more accurate diagnoses possible. Even after midcentury, however, physicians continued to misdiagnose heart disease. A study in one hospital found that deaths diagnosed as due to heart disease were understated (as measured by autopsy findings) in the 1960s and 1970s compared to the 1980s. These findings suggest that the increase in heart disease death rates between 1900 and midcentury was smaller than the official statistics indicate and that the current decline may be greater.[13]

Regardless of diagnostic improvements, the overall trends are indisputable — heart disease mortality rates rose substantially early in the century and have declined in recent years. The trends occurred in many advanced nations with different systems of training physicians and different ways of recording vital statistics. Careful and thorough studies of trends in heart disease death rates in specific regions and cities in the U.S. and other nations covering a decade or more have shown conclusively that heart disease rates have declined in recent years.[14]

What factors caused the great increase in heart disease death rates from 1900 to midcentury and their subsequent decline? Several possible explanations can be easily dismissed. Both the upward and downward trends occurred so rapidly that they must have been caused by social and environmental changes, not changes in human biology. Both the rise and fall occurred in many advanced nations about the same time, so that they cannot be due to changes unique to American society. The trends occurred for both men and women, so that factors that would benefit one sex more than the other cannot be responsible.

The most frequently advanced reasons for the increase in heart disease death rates early in the century are based on the greater wealth of industrialized societies. Research has shown that "a diet excessive in calories, fat, and salt, sedentary habits, unrestrained weight gain, and cigarette smoking predispose to coronary heart disease."[15] It is claimed that early in the twentieth century higher standards of living enabled people to eat more meat and other fatty foods that occluded their arteries and made them overweight. Changing work and home activities and the use of automobiles and mass transportation resulted in less physical exertion and exercise. Cigarette smoking became popular. These and other changes also increased heart disease death rates indirectly by producing higher rates of hypertension, diabetes, and other conditions that made people more susceptible to heart disease.

The major issue in explaining the recent decline in heart disease death rates is whether it was caused by (1) preventive measures that reduced the incidence of fatal heart disease, or (2) better treatment of heart disease.[16] Are fewer people getting fatal heart disease or are people with heart disease receiving better treatment and so are less likely to die? The prevention theory attributes the decline to the same factors that are considered to have caused the rise in heart disease death rates: changes in diet, more exercise, cessation of smoking, reduced blood cholesterol levels, and, possibly, treatment of high blood pressure. The treatment theory points to pre-hospital life support systems and better hospital and continuing care of cardiac patients as enabling more heart disease patients to survive.

Studies of heart disease deaths in several American cities connect much of the decline in the heart disease mortality rate in recent years to a decline in out-of-hospital deaths.[17] This may indicate that fewer people were having heart attacks or that they were having milder heart attacks, supporting the prevention theory. A less likely but possible interpretation is that heart disease patients were receiving better care and so were less likely to have a fatal recurrence after leaving the hospital, supporting the treatment theory.

None of the explanations for the rise in heart disease mortality rates is entirely persuasive. Changes in diet and lifestyles that are supposed to have caused the increase in heart disease early in the century often did not occur until decades later. Cigarette smoking did not become popular until the 1920s and would not have had a measurable impact on heart disease death rates until the late 1930s. No evidence exists that physical activity decreased at the beginning of the century. The automobile was not widely used as a mode of transportation until the 1920s. Perhaps most puzzling is the fact that the increase occurred in many nations about the same time, but it has not been shown that they all experienced appropriate changes in diet and lifestyles at the same time.

Explanations for the decline in heart disease mortality rates are equally problematic. The decline began before public health programs designed to discourage cigarette smoking and change lifestyles could have had an impact, and it also occurred in nations without such programs. The decline has taken place in nations that have taken little interest in pre-hospital resuscitation, intensive coronary care units, or other methods of care in widespread use in the United States. Even programs to lower mild or moderate hypertension, which reduce the risk of stroke, have not been clearly linked to a reduced risk of coronary heart disease. One review has concluded that "no one has yet established a convincing fit of trends for any risk factor with cardiovascular mortality trends."[18]

The trends for cerebrovascular disease are very similar to those for heart disease, as are the issues involving causes. For those reasons, they will not be discussed here.[19]

When we turn to cancer, we find a disheartening picture. Overall cancer death rates for men aged 45 and over rose steadily from 1940 to 1970, while they declined for women over those years. From 1970 to 1988, cancer death rates declined for both men and women aged 35–44 and 45–54 (attributed to a decline in lung cancer death rates), but they have risen for all older groups of both sexes. Similar patterns have been found in other advanced nations, indicating that these patterns are also international in scope.[20]

Trends in overall cancer mortality rates are difficult to interpret because they can change if the mix of types of cancers changes, even if the mortality rate of each type of cancer does not change. For example, if cancers with higher mortality rates become more prevalent relative to cancers with lower mortality rates, overall cancer mortality rates will increase, even though mortality rates from each individual type of cancer have not changed.

National data on the incidence of cancer (the number of new cases) are available for selected areas in the United States since 1973. They show a steady increase in the age-adjusted rates of new cases of cancer per 100,000 population from 319.8 in 1973 to 376.6 in 1989.[21] The increases have occurred for both men and women.

Significant sex differences exist in cancer mortality rates. In 1988, the overall cancer mortality rate per 100,000 was 215.5 for men and 180.0 per women. With the exception of breast cancer, men had higher mortality rates from every major cancer site. The most important of these sex differences was for lung cancer death rates.[22]

In terms of specific cancer sites, mortality rates from two major kinds of cancer have changed dramatically in most western countries in the last half-century. One is the increase in death rates from lung cancer. The age-adjusted mortality rate from cancer of the respiratory system per 100,000 population increased from 12.8 in 1950 to 28.4 in 1970 and 59.1 in 1991.[23] This is attributed to cigarette smoking, based on three kinds of evidence. One consists of studies showing a strong relationship between smoking and lung cancer in individuals: individuals who smoke more cigarettes or have smoked cigarettes for a longer period of time are more likely to contract lung cancer. The second is that lung cancer, which was a very rare form of cancer in the nineteenth century, became more prevalent about two decades after cigarette smoking became popular, which is about the time it takes for smoking to produce cancer.

The third type of evidence is based on the decline in the proportion of persons 18 years of age and over who smoke cigarettes, from 42 to 25 percent between 1965 and 1990. The reduction has occurred for both sexes and all age groups. Lung cancer mortality rates have declined recently among younger age groups, who would be the first to benefit because they have smoked for fewer years. The mortality rates per 100,000 population for cancers of the respiratory system for those 45 to 54 years of age increased from 22.9 in 1950 to 56.5 in 1980 and then declined to 46.9 in 1991. The comparable rates for those aged 65 to 74 increased from 69.3 in 1950 to 243.1 in 1980 and 300.0 in 1991.[24]

The other dramatic change in cancer mortality rates has been the striking decline in death rates from stomach cancer.[25] Before 1940 stomach cancer was a major cause of cancer mortality for both sexes and all age groups; today it is relatively uncommon.

The decline has occurred in most western nations and Japan, although it has been greater and occurred earlier in the United States than most other nations. The most frequently proposed causal factors involve changes in diet, particularly the decline in the consumption of salted, smoked, and fried foods. Before the canning and freezing of vegetables and refrigeration of foods, human diet in western countries included substantial amounts of salted vegetables, such as pickles and sauerkraut, and meats preserved with salts and nitrates, including sausages, ham, salami, and bologna. Canning, refrigeration, and freezing have reduced the need for these methods of preservation. However, no clear-cut evidence exists to support the diet theory, especially in terms of showing appropriate and timely changes in diet in all the nations that have experienced decline in stomach cancer rates.

As with heart disease, changing methods of diagnosis have affected cancer mortality rates. A British authority on lung cancer concluded that lung cancer death rates were understated early in the century because of the difficulty of diagnosing what was then a rare disease. He believes that lung cancer mortality rates for non-smokers today are probably the same as the overall population rates before smoking became widespread. Consequently he estimates that the rise in lung cancer death rates during the first quarter of the century in England and Wales was due almost entirely to more accurate diagnoses (primarily by the use of chest X-rays) rather than an actual increase in lung cancer mortality.[26]

Most cancer is considered to be environmental in origin. This is based on regional differences in specific types of cancers and on the evidence that people who move from one region to another contract different types of cancer than those who remain. As an example, Japanese women who emigrated to Hawaii have much lower rates of stomach cancer than their grandmothers but much higher rates of breast cancer.[27] The specific environmental factors involved are seldom well understood, however.

The inability to identify the causes of individual cancers and other chronic diseases is due to the complex nature of the diseases. These diseases take decades to develop, are produced by several factors operating simultaneously, and are retarded by still other factors. Researchers must therefore obtain data on many details of an individual's life over many years, which is rarely possible. Furthermore, mortality rates are low enough that it is necessary to study many thousands of people to obtain enough cases for a meaningful study. To avoid these problems, researchers usually study populations rather than individuals, by, for example, comparing the diet of a country or region with a low rate of stomach cancer to the diet of another country or region with a high rate. Because people within each country or region have different diets, the results are much less useful than if only individuals with specified diets were studied. This kind of research produces suggestive rather than definitive findings. Most knowledge about the environmental causes of cancer and heart disease is based on suggestive findings from a number of studies.

Because most cancers cannot be cured, research has focused on trends on the number of years that cancer patients live after diagnosis. The standard measure of cancer survival is the five-year survival rate, which is defined as the number of persons who are alive five years after they have been diagnosed as having cancer, divided by the number of persons diagnosed with the disease at the beginning of the period. Five-year survival rates for individual cancer sites vary widely, from about 10 percent for lung cancer and even less for a few other sites, to over 70 percent for bladder, breast, skin, and prostate cancers.[28]

A major concern is whether five-year survival rates have increased in recent years. A federal government study comparing five-year survival rates in 1950 with those in 1982 found real improvements in a few cancers, mostly rare ones, but only marginal improvement in the most frequent cancer sites. Five-year survival rates have a major methodological limitation. As physicians have become more aware of cancer and have better diagnostic devices, they look for it and diagnose it earlier than they did in the past. Thus patients are more likely to survive for five years because the disease was diagnosed in an earlier stage. For example, if a physician who is not alert to the possibility of cancer diagnoses a case of cancer in 1994, the patient will have survived for five years in 1999. If the physician had been more alert to the disease or had better diagnostic tools and diagnosed the same case a year earlier, in 1993, the patient would have reached the five-year mark a year earlier, in 1998, when the disease was less advanced. Earlier diagnoses will improve five-year survival rates regardless of changes in treatment. Earlier diagnosis is widely believed to be responsible for most of the modest improvements in five-year cancer survival rates.[29]

AIDS is the only major disease cause of death to claim most of its victims among the young. The first cases of human immunodeficiency virus infection were observed in the early 1980s, but no U.S. death rates existed until 1987, when an age-adjusted mortality rate of 5.5 per 100,000 population was recorded. In 1991, the age-adjusted mortality rate reached 11.3 per 100,000 population. AIDS deaths in 1991 were concentrated in the 25–44 year age group, with a mortality rate of 47.3 per 100,000 among men aged 25–44 and 6.4 per 100,000 among women aged 25–44. Deaths from AIDS constituted 18.6 percent of all deaths among men and 6.2 percent of all deaths among women in that age group.[30] The sex difference is expected to diminish in the future.

SOCIAL CLASS AND MORTALITY

For many centuries the rich have been known to have lower mortality rates than the poor. During most of recorded history, the differences have been attributed to the higher standard of living of the rich, their physical separation from the poor that protected them from contagious diseases, and their access to better public health measures, including sewage disposal and uncontaminated water. They received their medical care from better trained physicians, but until the twentieth century this was of little benefit because physicians could do little to prevent death or cure illness.

During the last years of the nineteenth century and the first decades of the twentieth century, improvements in medicine aroused the expectation that equalizing access to medical care would eliminate the differences in mortality rates between the rich and the poor. National governments improved access to health care for the poor, at first in Germany and later in other European nations. National health care programs did not develop in the United States because health care for the poor was a local and state government responsibility (as well as private charity). Local and state governments operated public hospitals and/or reimbursed physicians and voluntary hospitals for the care of charity patients. A few cities (most notably New York City) and states accepted their responsibilities conscientiously, but most were parsimonious in providing medical care to the poor. In 1965, with the enactment of Medicare and Medicaid, the federal government assumed substantial responsibility for the medical care of the poor. These programs improved the quality of health care provided to the poor but did not make it equal to the care given others.

As the poor obtained access to better health care in all countries, it was expected that mortality rates would become more equal among socio-economic status (SES) groups. One possibility was a general narrowing of the differences in mortality rates for all SES groups. Another was a threshold effect, in which the rates for those above a certain SES level would become more similar, but the rates for the lowest SES groups would remain higher.

Data from the United States and England have shown that neither trend has occurred. The mortality rates of all SES groups have declined substantially, but the differences among them have increased. One British study placed men under age 65 in five occupational groups from high to low social status and found that the differences in mortality rates among the groups increased significantly between 1931 and 1981. A study of Americans 25 to 64 years of age found a greater difference in mortality rates between the lowest and highest educational groups and the lowest and highest income groups in 1986 than in 1960. These patterns held for white men, white women, black men, and black women. The same trends have also been found for the major diseases considered individually. For example, studies in several countries have found that the greatest decline in heart disease mortality rates has occurred in the higher educational and occupational groups.[31]

Several aspects of this phenomenon should be emphasized: (1) overall mortality rates for all SES groups have declined steadily over time so that members of all SES groups are living longer today; (2) the differences in mortality rates among SES groups in the U.S. exist for both men and women and for whites and blacks; (3) the differences in mortality rates among SES groups exist for all age groups and are not limited to the elderly or to infants; (4) the differences in mortality rates among SES groups exist for many individual diseases, including heart disease, cancer, and stroke; and (5) many SES factors operate together to cause the differences in mortality, including education, income, occupation, parent's SES (used as a measure of SES during a person's childhood), as well as other unknown factors.

The fundamental issue in mortality differences among SES groups is not the higher mortality rates of the lowest SES groups, for which many plausible explanations have been offered. The issue is the inability to explain the growing differences among the highest SES groups. Surely the second highest SES group, for example, has more than an adequate standard of living, benefits from public health measures, has ready access to high quality medical care, and possesses sufficient education and income to live healthy lifestyles. The differences between their death rates and those of the highest SES group should, therefore, be narrowing, but for unknown reasons they are widening.

SES differences in mortality provide an appropriate context to discuss racial differences in mortality rates. In 1991 white males had an age-adjusted mortality rate of 6.3 deaths per 1000 population, while black males had a rate of 10.5 per 1000 population. The corresponding figures for white and black females were 3.7 per 1000 population and 5.8 per 1000 population. Lower mortality rates for whites existed for all major disease categories except suicides. Socio-economic factors must be responsible for these differences, because no known biological factors can explain them. One study found that these so-called "racial" differences in mortality rates were due to differences in age, sex, marital status, family size, and family income between the white and black populations (married persons have lower mortality rates than unmarried ones and members of smaller families have lower mortality rates than members of large families).[32] Black-white differentials in mortality rates are manifestations of the broader SES and demographic differences that exist in our society.

CONCLUSION

In reflecting on trends in mortality rates during the twentieth century, no conclusion is more remarkable than the astonishing number of unanticipated and unexplained changes that have occurred. Death rates from infectious diseases, the major cause of death in the nineteenth century, declined much more spectacularly than any physician in 1900 would have dared to predict, but no explanations for the decline have received universal acceptance. Death rates from stroke and heart disease rose to epidemic proportions in the first half of the twentieth century. This led observers in the 1950s and 1960s to pontificate that increasing death rates from heart disease and stroke were the inevitable fate of mankind in a post-infectious disease era. Despite these claims, mortality rates from both diseases declined dramatically in recent decades. None of the proposed explanations for these rises and declines are supported by convincing evidence.

Other mortality trends have been less gratifying. Overall cancer death rates have remained stable in recent decades. Two favorable developments stand out: the recent decline in lung cancer rates among younger age groups, almost surely due to a decline in smoking, and the continuing decline in stomach cancer death rates, which has no accepted explanation. The lack of decline in death rates from other types of cancer is especially disappointing when we consider the billions of dollars that have been spent on cancer research. Other discouraging and unexplained trends include the widening differences in mortality rates among SES groups and the growing death rates from chronic obstructive pulmonary diseases, which occur after years of painful disability.

The trends in mortality rates are made more baffling by their multinational nature. Most advanced nations have experienced similar trends in death rates, but they differ in many factors that have been offered as explanations, including their social structures, cultures, diets, housing, industries, sources of energy, modes of transportation, occupations, pollutants, and geographic and physical environments.

When physicians are confronted with such inexplicable trends, they tend to explain them according to their cultural predispositions.[33] American physicians like to attribute the positive trends to medical interventions — new drugs, new types of surgery, new medical and surgical specialties, new health care procedures like intensive care units and helicopter evacuation teams, and new public health initiatives. They like to believe that the problem areas, like cancer, await the expenditure of more money on specialists, more money on research, more money on equipment, more money on treatment. British physicians, on the other hand, note that nations that have spent only a fraction of the money that Americans spend on health care have experienced the same positive and negative trends. They believe that more general social changes — in broad public health measures, in the standard of living, in lifestyles — are responsible.

Useful explanations of mortality trends can never be achieved by studying individual diseases as disconnected entities. The human being is an organism, which means that changes in one part of the organism affect the whole organism. To understand changes in the incidence of any particular disease, we must understand factors that affected the organism in the past or are affecting it currently. These include biological factors, like other diseases that the person had contracted, and social factors, including the society and culture in which the person lives, as well as the interrelationships between the two.

REFERENCES

1. A. Cockburn, *The Evolution and Eradication of Infectious Diseases* (Baltimore: Johns Hopkins Press, 1963).

2. R. Floud, K. Wachter, and A. Gregory, *Height, Health and History: Nutritional Status in the United Kingdom, 1750–1980* (Cambridge, Eng.: Cambridge University Press, 1990); and R. W. Fogel, "The Conquest of High Mortality and Hunger in Europe and America: Timing and Mechanisms," in *Favorites of Fortune: Technology, Growth, and Economic Development since the Industrial Revolution*, ed. P. Hoginnet, D. S. Landes, and H. Rosovsky (Cambridge: Harvard University Press, 1991), 52–54.

3. J. R. Gillis, L. A. Tilly, and D. Levine, eds., *The European Experience of Declining Fertility, 1850–1970: The Quiet Revolution* (Cambridge: Blackwell, 1992).

4. F. E. Linder and R. D. Grove, *Vital Statistics Rates in the United States, 1900–1940* (Washington, DC: GPO, 1943), 95–96 and passim.
5. "Advance Report of Final Mortality Statistics 1991," *Monthly Vital Statistics Report* 42 (31 August 1993), suppl. 2, p. 16.
6. Ibid., 16.
7. See R. Daniels, *Coming to America: A History of Immigration and Ethnicity in American Life* (New York: HarperCollins, 1990).
8. I. Waldron, "Recent Trends in Sex Mortality Ratios for Adults in Developed Countries," *Social Science and Medicine* 36 (1993): 451–62; and L. M. Verbrugge, "The Twain Meet: Empirical Explanations for Sex Differences in Health and Mortality," *Journal of Health and Social Behavior* 30 (1989): 282–304.
9. For a discussion of the causes of the decline, see S. J. Kunitz, "Explanations and Ideologies of Mortality Patterns," *Population and Development Review* 13 (1897): 379–408, and articles in *Milbank Memorial Fund Quarterly* 55 (summer 1977).
10. H. Hansen and M. Susser, "Historic Trends in Deaths from Chronic Kidney Disease in the United States and Britain," *American Journal of Epidemiology* 93 (1971): 413–24.
11. R. Doll, "Major Epidemics of the 20th Century: From Coronary Thrombosis to AIDS," *Journal of the Royal Statistical Society* A 150 (1987): 373–95; T. J. Thom, "International Mortality from Heart Disease: Rates and Trends," *International Journal of Epidemiology* 18 (1989), suppl. 1, pp. S20–S28.
12. L. H. Kuller, "Issues in Measuring Coronary Heart Disease Mortality and Morbidity," and R. B. Wallace, "How Do We Measure the Influence of Medical Care on the Decline of Coronary Heart Disease?" both in *Trends in Coronary Heart Disease Mortality: The Influence of Medical Care*, ed. M. W. Higgins and R. V. Luepker (New York: Oxford University Press, 1988), 44–53, 88–93.
13. W. E. Stehbens, "An Appraisal of the Epidemic Rise of Coronary Heart Disease and its Decline," *Lancet* 1 (1987): 606–11; and B. Burnand and A. R. Feinstein, "The Role of Diagnostic Inconsistency in Changing Rates of Occurrence for Coronary Heart Disease," *Journal of Clinical Epidemiology* 45 (1992): 929–40.
14. See R. Beaglehole, "International Trends in Coronary Heart Disease Mortality, Morbidity, and Risk Factors," *Epidemiologic Reviews* 12 (1990): 1–15.
15. W. B. Kannel and T. J. Thom, "Declining Cardiovascular Mortality," *Circulation* 70 (1984): 332.
16. See T. J. Thom and W. B. Kannel, "Downward Trend in Cardiovascular Mortality," *Annual Review of Medicine* 32 (1981): 427–34; R. I. Levy, "The Decline in Cardiovascular Disease Mortality," *Annual Review of Public Health* 2 (1981): 49–70; L. Goldman and E. F. Cook, "The Decline in Ischemic Heart Disease Mortality Rates," *Annals of Internal Medicine* 101 (1984): 825–36; and Beaglehole, "International Trends."
17. L. H. Kuller et al., "Sudden Death and the Decline in Coronary Heart Disease Mortality," *Journal of Chronic Diseases* 39 (1986): 1001–19; and Beaglehole, "International Trends," 5.
18. Kannel and Thom, "Declining Cardiovascular Mortality," 335.

19. See B. Modan and D. K. Wagener, "Some Epidemiological Aspects of Stroke: Mortality/Morbidity Trends, Age, Sex, Race, Socioeconomic Status," *Stroke* 23 (1992): 1230–36; and J. P. Whisnant, "The Decline of Stroke," *Stroke* 15 (1984): 160–68.

20. R. Doll, "Are We Winning the Fight Against Cancer? An Epidemiological Assessment," *European Journal of Cancer* 26 (1990): 500–508; D. L. Davis et al., "International Trends in Cancer Mortality in France, West Germany, Italy, Japan, England and Wales, and the United States," *Annals of the New York Academy of Sciences* 609 (1990): 5–48.

21. Barry Miller, et al., eds., *Cancer Statistics Review, 1973–1989* (Washington, DC: National Cancer Institute, 1992), part 2, p. 4.

22. U.S. Bureau of the Census, *Statistical Abstract of the United States: 1991* (Washington, DC: GPO, 1991), 84.

23. National Center for Health Statistics, *Health United States, 1991* (Hyattsville, MD: Public Health Service, 1992), 169; and "Advance Report of Final Mortality Statistics 1991," 18.

24. National Center for Health Statistics, *Health United States, 1991*, 203, 169; and "Advance Report of Final Mortality Statistics," 18.

25. See J. Higginson, C. S. Muir, and N. Munoz, *Human Cancer: Epidemiology and Environmental Causes* (Cambridge, Eng.: Cambridge University Press, 1992), 273–82; and C. P. Howson, T. Hiyama, and E. L. Wynder, "The Decline in Gastric Cancer: Epidemiology of an Unplanned Triumph," *Epidemiologic Reviews* 8 (1986): 1–27.

26. Doll, "Major Epidemics," 376–77.

27. Davis et al., "International Trends," 6.

28. National Center for Health Statistics, *Health United States, 1991,* 199.

29. U.S. General Accounting Office, *Cancer Patient Survival: What Progress Has Been Made?* (Washington, DC: GPO, 1987).

30. National Center for Health Statistics, *Health United States, 1991,* 156; and "Update: Mortality Attributable to HIV Infection/AIDS Among Persons Aged 25–44 Years — United States, 1990 and 1991," *Morbidity and Mortality Weekly Report* 42 (2 July 1993): 482.

31. R. G. Wilkinson, "Socio-economic Differences in Mortality," in *Class and Health: Research and Longitudinal Data*, ed. Wilkinson (London, Eng.: Tavistock, 1986), 2; G. Pappas et al., "The Increasing Disparity in Mortality Between Socio-economic Groups in the United States, 1960 and 1986," *New England Journal of Medicine* 329 (1993): 103–9; C. C. Seltzer and S. Jablon, "Army Rank and Subsequent Mortality by Cause: 23-Year Follow-up," *American Journal of Epidemiology* 105 (1977): 559–66; Beaglehole, "International Trends," 4; and J. P. Bunker, D. S. Gomby, and B. H. Kehrer, eds., *Pathways to Health: The Role of Social Factors* (Menlo Park, CA: Henry J. Kaiser Family Foundation, 1989).

32. "Advance Report of Final Mortality Statistics 1991," 15; and R. G. Rogers, "Living and Dying in the U.S.A.: Sociodemographic Determinants of Death among Blacks and Whites," *Demography* 29 (1992): 287–303.
33. Cf. Kunitz, "Explanations and Ideologies."

NB: Tables that were excluded from this article appear in W. G. Rothstein, *Readings in American Health Care: Current Issues in Socio-Historical Perspective* (The University of Wisconsin Press, 1995; 71–86).

ARTICLE 2

ACHIEVEMENTS IN PUBLIC HEALTH, 1900–1999

CONTROL OF INFECTIOUS DISEASES

The Centers for Disease Control and Prevention

Deaths from infectious diseases have declined markedly in the United States during the 20th century (Figure 1). This decline contributed to a sharp drop in infant and child mortality (1,2) and to the 29.2-year increase in life expectancy (2). In 1900, 30.4% of all deaths occurred among children aged less than 5 years; in 1997, that percentage was only 1.4%. In 1900, the three leading causes of death were pneumonia, tuberculosis (TB), and diarrhea and enteritis, which (together with diphtheria) caused one third of all deaths. Of these deaths, 40% were among children aged less than 5 years (1). In 1997, heart disease and cancers accounted for 54.7% of all deaths, with 4.5% attributable to pneumonia, influenza, and human immunodeficiency virus (HIV) infection (2). Despite this overall progress, one of the most devastating epidemics in human history occurred during the 20th century: the 1918 influenza pandemic that resulted in 20 million deaths, including 500,000 in the United States, in less than 1 year — more than have died in as short a time during any war or famine in the world (3). HIV infection, first recognized in 1981, has caused a pandemic that is still in progress, affecting 33 million people and causing an estimated 13.9 million deaths (4). These episodes illustrate the volatility of infectious disease death rates and the unpredictability of disease emergence.

Public health action to control infectious diseases in the 20th century is based on the 19th century discovery of microorganisms as the cause of many serious diseases (e.g., cholera and TB). Disease control resulted from improvements in sanitation and hygiene, the discovery of antibiotics, and the implementation of universal childhood vaccination programs. Scientific and technologic advances played a major role in each of these areas and are the foundation for today's disease surveillance and control systems. Scientific findings also have contributed to a new understanding of the evolving relation between humans and microbes (5).

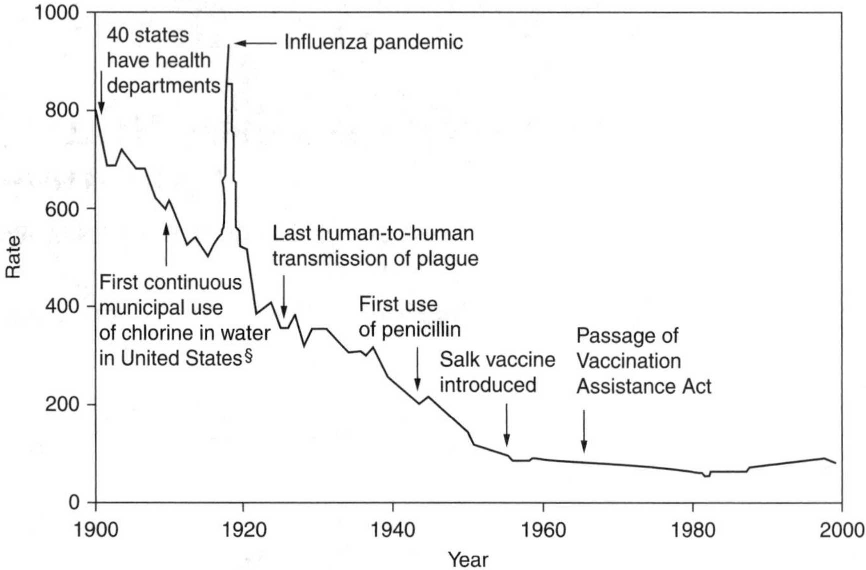

*Per 100,000 population per year.

†Adapted from Armstrong GL, Conn LA, Pinner RW. Trends in infectious disease mortality in the United States during the 20th century. JAMA 1999:281:61–6.

§American Water Works Association. Water chlorination principles and practices: AWWA manual M20. Denver, Colorado: American Water Works Association, 1973.

Figure 1 Crude death rate* for infectious diseases — United States, 1900–1996.†

CONTROL OF INFECTIOUS DISEASES

Sanitation and Hygiene

The 19th century shift in population from country to city that accompanied industrialization and immigration led to overcrowding in poor housing served by inadequate or nonexistent public water supplies and waste-disposal systems. These conditions resulted in repeated outbreaks of cholera, dysentery, TB, typhoid fever, influenza, yellow fever, and malaria.

By 1990, however, the incidence of many of these diseases had begun to decline because of public health improvements, implementation of which continued into the 20th century. Local, state, and federal efforts to improve sanitation and hygiene reinforced the concept of collective "public health" action (e.g., to prevent infection by providing clean drinking water). By 1900, 40 of the 45 states had established health departments. The first county health departments were established in 1908 (6). From the 1930s through the 1950s, state and local health departments made substantial progress in disease prevention activities, including sewage disposal, water treatment, food safety, organized solid waste disposal, and public education about hygienic practices (e.g., foodhandling and handwashing). Chlorination and other treatments of drinking water began in the early 1900s and became widespread public health practices, further decreasing the incidence of waterborne diseases. The incidence of TB also declined as improvements in housing reduced crowding and TB-control programs were initiated. In 1900, 194 of every 100,000 U.S. residents died from TB; most were residents of urban areas. In 1940 (before the introduction of antibiotic therapy), TB remained a leading cause of death, but the crude death rate had decreased to 46 per 100,000 persons (7).

Animal and pest control also contributed to disease reduction. Nationally sponsored, state-coordinated vaccination and animal-control programs eliminated dog-to-dog transmission of rabies. Malaria, once endemic throughout the southeastern United States, was reduced to negligible levels by the late 1940s; regional mosquito-control programs played an important role in these efforts. Plague also diminished; the U.S. Marine Hospital Service (which later became the Public Health Service) led quarantine and ship inspection activities and rodent and vector-control operations. The last major rat-associated outbreak of plague in the United States occurred during 1924–1925 in Los Angeles. This outbreak included the last identified instance of human-to-human transmission of plague (through inhalation of infectious respiratory droplets from coughing patients) in this country.

Vaccination

Strategic vaccination campaigns have virtually eliminated diseases that previously were common in the United States, including diphtheria, tetanus, poliomyelitis, smallpox, measles, mumps, rubella, and *Haemophilus influenzae* type b meningitis (8). With the licensure of the combined diphtheria and tetanus toxoids and pertussis vaccine in 1949, state and local health departments instituted vaccination programs, aimed primarily at poor children. In 1955, the introduction of the Salk poliovirus vaccine led to federal funding of state and local childhood vaccination programs. In 1962, a federally coordinated vaccination program was established through the passage of the Vaccination Assistance Act — landmark legislation that has been renewed continuously and now supports the purchase and administration of a full range of childhood vaccines.

The success of vaccination programs in the United States and Europe inspired the 20th-century concept of "disease eradication" — the idea that a selected disease could be eradicated from all human populations through global cooperation. In 1977, after a decade-long campaign involving 33 nations, smallpox was eradicated worldwide — approximately a decade after it had been eliminated from the United States and the rest of the Western Hemisphere. Polio and dracunculiasis may be eradicated by 2000.*

Antibiotics and Other Antimicrobial Medicines

Penicillin was developed into a widely available medical product that provided quick and complete treatment of previously incurable bacterial illnesses, with a wider range of targets and fewer side effects than sulfa drugs. Discovered fortuitously in 1928, penicillin was not developed for medical use until the 1940s, when it was produced in substantial quantities and used by the U.S. military to treat sick and wounded soldiers.

Antibiotics have been in civilian use for 57 years and have saved the lives of persons with streptococcal and staphylococcal infections, gonorrhea, syphilis, and other infections. Drugs also have been developed to treat viral diseases (e.g., herpes and HIV infection); fungal diseases (e.g., candidiasis and histoplasmosis); and parasitic diseases (e.g., malaria). The microbiologist Selman Waksman led much of the early research in discovering antibiotics. However, the emergence of drug resistance in many organisms is reversing some of the therapeutic miracles of the last 50 years and underscores the importance of disease prevention.

TECHNOLOGIC ADVANCES IN DETECTING AND MONITORING INFECTIOUS DISEASES

Technologic changes that increased capacity for detecting, diagnosing, and monitoring infectious diseases included development early in the century of serologic testing and more recently the development of molecular assays based on nucleic acid and antibody probes. The use of computers and electronic forms communication enhanced the ability to gather, analyze, and disseminate disease surveillance data.

Serologic Testing

Serologic testing came into use in the 1910s and has become a basic tool to diagnose and control many infectious diseases. Syphilis and gonorrhea, for example, were widespread early in the century and were difficult to diagnose, especially during the latent stages. The advent of serologic testing for syphilis helped provide a more accurate description of this public health problem and facilitated diagnosis of infection. For example, in New York City, serologic testing in 1901 indicated that 5%–19% of all men had syphilitic infections (9).

Viral Isolation and Tissue Culture

The first virus isolation techniques came into use at the turn of the century. They involved straining infected material through successively smaller sieves and inoculating test animals or plants to show the purified substance retained disease-causing activity. The first "filtered" viruses were tobacco mosaic virus (1882) and foot-and-mouth disease virus of cattle (1898). The U.S. Army Command under Walter Reed filtered yellow fever virus in 1900. The subsequent development of cell culture in the 1930s paved the way for large-scale production of live or heat-killed viral vaccines. Negative staining techniques for visualizing viruses under the electron microscope were available by the early 1960s.

Molecular Techniques

During the last quarter of the 20th century, molecular biology has provided powerful new tools to detect and characterize infectious pathogens. The use of nucleic acid hybridization and sequencing techniques has made it possible to characterize the causative agents of previously unknown diseases (e.g., hepatitis C, human ehrlichiosis, hantavirus pulmonary syndrome, acquired immunodeficiency syndrome [AIDS], and Nipah virus disease).

Molecular tools have enhanced capacity to track the transmission of new threats and find new ways to prevent and treat them. Had AIDS emerged 100 years ago, when laboratory-based diagnostic methods were in their infancy, the disease might have remained a mysterious syndrome for many decades. Moreover, the drugs used to treat HIV-infected persons and prevent perinatal transmission (e.g., replication analogs and protease inhibitors) were developed based on a modern understanding of retroviral replication at the molecular level.

CHALLENGES FOR THE 21ST CENTURY

Success in reducing morbidity and mortality from infectious diseases during the first three quarters of the 20th century led to complacency about the need for continued research into treatment and control of infectious microbes (10). However, the appearance of AIDS, the re-emergence of TB (including multidrug-resistant strains), and an overall increase in infectious disease mortality during the 1980s and early 1990s (Figure 1) provide additional evidence that as long as microbes can evolve, new diseases will appear. The emergence of new diseases underscores the importance of disease prevention through continual monitoring of underlying factors that may encourage the emergence or re-emergence of diseases.

Molecular genetics has provided a new appreciation of the remarkable ability of microbes to evolve, adapt, and develop drug resistance in an unpredictable and dynamic fashion. Resistance genes are transmitted from one bacterium to another on plasmids, and viruses evolve through replication errors and reassortment of gene segments and by jumping species barriers. Recent examples of microbial evolution include the emergence of a virulent strain of avian influenza in Hong Kong (1997–98); the multidrug-resistant W strain of *M. tuberculosis* in the United States in 1991 (11); and *Staphylococcus aureus* with reduced susceptibility to vancomycin in Japan in 1996 (12) and the United States in 1997 (13,14).

For continued success in controlling infectious diseases, the U.S. public health system must prepare to address diverse challenges, including the emergence of new infectious diseases, the re-emergence of old diseases (sometimes in drug-resistant forms), large foodborne outbreaks, and acts of bioterrorism. Ongoing research on the possible role of infectious agents in causing or intensifying certain chronic diseases (including diabetes mellitus type 1, some cancers [15–17], and heart conditions [18,19]) also is imperative. Continued protection of health requires improved capacity for disease surveillance and outbreak response at the local, state, federal, and global levels; the development and dissemination of new laboratory and epidemiologic methods; continued antimicrobial and vaccine development; and ongoing research into environmental factors that facilitate disease emergence (20).

REFERENCES

1. Department of Commerce and Labor, Bureau of the Census. Mortality Statistics, 1900 to 1904. Washington, DC: US Department of Commerce and Labor, 1906.
2. Hoyert DL, Kochanek KD, Murphy SL. Deaths: final data for 1997. Hyattsville, Maryland: US Department of Health and Human Services, Public Health Service, CDC, National Center for Health Statistics, 1999. (National vital statistics reports, vol 47, no. 19).
3. Crosby AW Jr. Epidemic and peace, 1918. Westport, Connecticut: Greenwood Press, 1976:311.
4. United Nations Program on HIV/AIDS and World Health Organization. AIDS epidemic update: December 1998. Geneva, Switzerland: World Health Organization, 1999. Available at http://www.unaids.org/highband/document/epidemio/wadr98e.pdf.
5. Lederberg J, Shope RE, Oaks SC Jr, eds. Microbial threats to health in the United States. Washington, DC: National Academy Press, 1992.
6. Hinman A. 1889 to 1989: a century of health and disease. *Public Health Rep* 1990;105:374–80.
7. National Office of Vital Statistics. Vital statistics — special reports, death rates by age, race, and sex, United States, 1900–1953; tuberculosis, all forms; vol 43, no. 2. Washington, DC: US Department of Health, Education, and Welfare, 1956.
8. CDC. Status report on the Childhood Immunization Initiative: reported cases of selected vaccine-preventable diseases — United States, 1996. *MMWR* 1997;46:665–71.
9. Morrow PA. Report of the committee of seven of the Medical Society of the County of New York on the prophylaxis of venereal disease in New York City. *N York M J* 1901;74:1146.
10. Institute of Medicine. Emerging infections: microbial threats to health in the United States. Washington, DC: National Academy Press, 1994:vi.
11. Plikaytis BB, Marden JL, Crawford JT, Woodley CL, Butler WR, Shinnick TM. Multiplex PCR assay specific for the multidrug-resistant strain W of *Mycobacterium tuberculosis*. *J Clin Microbiol* 1994;32:1542–6.
12. CDC. Reduced susceptibility of *Staphylococcus aureus* to vancomycin — Japan. 1996. *MMWR* 1997;46:624–6.
13. CDC. *Staphylococcus aureus* with reduced susceptibility to vancomycin — United States, 1997. *MMWR* 1997;46:765–6.
14. CDC. Update: *Staphylococcus aureus* with reduced susceptibility to vancomycin — United States, 1997. *MMWR* 1997;46:813–5.

15. Montesano R, Hainaut P, Wild CP. Hepatocellular carcinoma: from gene to public health. *J Natl Cancer Inst* 1997;89:1844–51.
16. Di Bisceglie AM. Hepatitis C and hepatocellular carcinoma. *Hepatology* 1997;26(3 suppl 1):34S–38S.
17. Muñoz N, Bosch FX. The causal link between HPV and cervical cancer and its implications for prevention of cervical cancer. *Bull Pan Am Health Organ* 1996;30:362–77.
18. Danesh J, Collins R, Peto R. Chronic infections and coronary heart disease: is there a link? *Lancet* 1997;350:430–6.
19. Mattila KJ, Valtonen VV, Nieminen MS, Asikainen S. Role of infection as a risk factor for atherosclerosis, myocardial infarction, and stroke. *Clin Infect Dis* 1998;26:719–34.
20. CDC. Preventing emerging infectious diseases: a strategy for the 21st century. Atlanta, Georgia: US Department of Health and Human Services, Public Health Service, 1998.

---

* Significant progress has been made to eradicate polio worldwide since the Global Polio Eradication Initiative was launched in 1988 by the Forty-first World Health Assembly, consisting then of delegates from 166 Member States. "In 1994, the World Health Organization (WHO) Region of the Americas (36 countries) was certified polio-free, followed by the WHO Western Pacific Region (37 countries and areas including China) in 2000 and the WHO European Region (51 countries) in June 2002" (WHO, 2002). However, polio continues to exist in parts of Africa and south Asia, and the WHO has set 2005 as the new target to certify all WHO regions polio-free.

(Data taken from: Polio Eradication
http://www.polioeradication.org/vaccines/polioeradication/all/news/default.asp)

Dracunculiasis has not yet been eradicated in all parts of the world. In 2000, 75,223 cases were reported, with the majority of cases found in Africa.

ARTICLE 3

ACHIEVEMENTS IN PUBLIC HEALTH, 1900–1999

HEALTHIER MOTHERS AND BABIES

The Centers for Disease Control and Prevention

At the beginning of the 20th century, for every 1000 live births, six to nine women in the United States died of pregnancy-related complications, and approximately 100 infants died before age 1 year (1,2). From 1915 through 1997, the infant mortality rate declined >90% to 7.2 per 1000 live births, and from 1900 through 1997, the maternal mortality rate declined almost 99% to <0.1 reported death per 1000 live births (7.7 deaths per 100,000 live births in 1997) (3) (Figures 1 and 2). Environmental interventions, improvements in nutrition, advances in clinical medicine, improvements in access to health care, improvements in surveillance and monitoring of disease, increases in education levels, and improvements in standards of living contributed to this remarkable decline (1). Despite these improvements in material and infant mortality rates, significant disparities by race and ethnicity persist. This report summarizes trends in reducing infant and maternal mortality in the United States, factors contributing to these trends, challenges in reducing infant and maternal mortality, and provides suggestions for public health action for the 21st century.

INFANT MORTALITY

The decline in infant mortality is unparalleled by other mortality reduction this century. If turn-of-the-century infant death rates had continued, then an estimated 500,000 live-born infants during 1997 would have died before age 1 year; instead, 28,045 infants died (3).

In 1900 in some U.S. cities, up to 30% of infants died before reaching their first birthday (1). Efforts to reduce infant mortality focused on improving environmental and living conditions in urban areas (1). Urban environmental interventions (e.g., sewage and refuse disposal and safe drinking water) played key roles in reducing infant mortality. Rising standards of living, including improvements in economic and

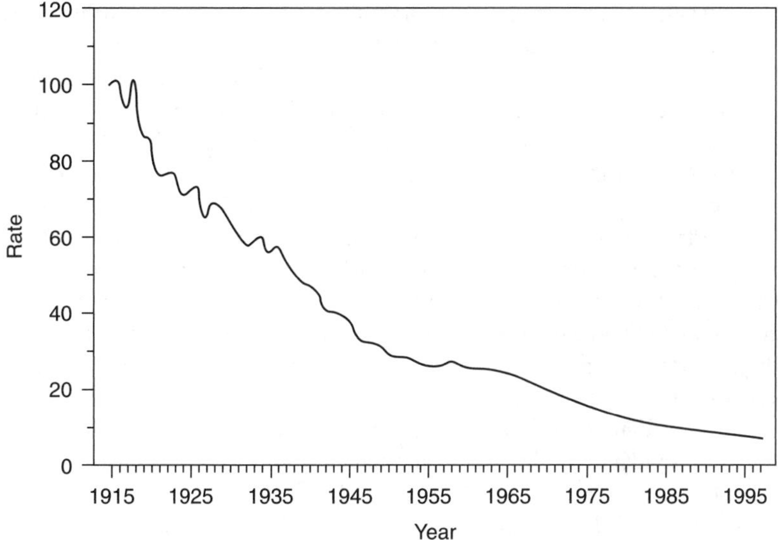

Figure 1 Infant mortality rate,* by year — United States, 1915–1997.

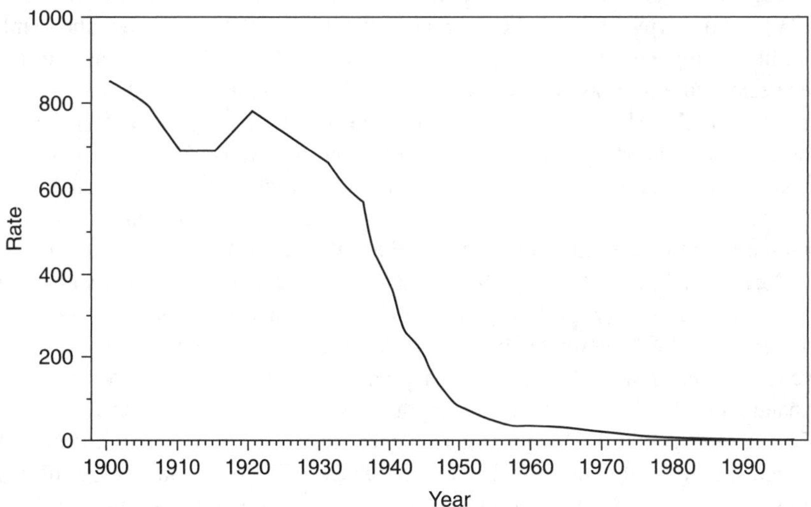

Figure 2 Maternal mortality rate,* by year — United States, 1900–1997.

education levels of families, helped to promote health. Declining fertility rates also contributed to reductions in infant mortality through longer spacing of children, smaller family size, and better nutritional status of mothers and infants (1). Milk pasteurization, first adopted in Chicago in 1908, contributed to the control of milkborne diseases (e.g., gastrointestinal infections) from contaminated milk supplies.

During the first three decades of the century, public health, social welfare, and clinical medicine (pediatrics and obstetrics) collaborated to combat infant mortality (1). This partnership began with milk hygiene but later included other public health issues. In 1912, the Children's Bureau was formed and became the primary government agency to work toward improving maternal and infant welfare until 1946, when its role in maternal and child health diminished; the bureau was eliminated in 1969 (1). The Children's Bureau defined the problem of infant mortality and shaped the debate over programs to ameliorate the problem. The bureau also advocated comprehensive maternal and infant welfare services, including prenatal, natal, and postpartum home visits by health-care providers. By the 1920s, the integration of these services changed the approach to infant mortality from one that addressed infant health problems to an approach that included infant and mother and prenatal-care programs to educate, monitor, and care for pregnant women.

The discovery and widespread use of antimicrobial agents (e.g., sulfonamide in 1937 and penicillin in the 1940s) and the development of fluid and electrolyte replacement therapy and safe blood transfusions accelerated the declines in infant mortality; from 1930 through 1949, mortality rates declined 52% (4). The percentage decline in postneonatal (age 28–364 days) mortality (66%) was greater than the decline in neonatal (age 0–27 days) mortality (40%). From 1950 through 1964, infant mortality declined more slowly (1). An increasing proportion of infant deaths were attributed to perinatal causes and occurred among high-risk neonates, especially low birth weight (LBW) and preterm babies. Although no reliable data exist, the rapid decline in infant mortality during earlier decades probably was not influenced by decreases in LBW rates because the decrease in mortality was primarily in postneonatal deaths that are less influenced by birthweight. Inadequate programs during the 1950s–1960s to reduce deaths among high-risk neonates led to renewed efforts to improve access to prenatal care, especially for the poor, and to a concentrated effort to establish neonatal intensive-care units and to promote research in maternal and infant health, including research into technologies to improve the survival of LBW and preterm babies.

During the late 1960s, after Medicaid and other federal programs were implemented, infant mortality (primarily postneonatal mortality) declined substantially (5). From 1970 to 1979, neonatal mortality plummeted 41% because of technologic advances in neonatal medicine and in the regionalization of perinatal services; postneonatal mortality declined 14%. During the early to mid-1980s, the downward trend in U.S. infant mortality slowed (6). However, during 1989–1991, infant mortality declined slightly faster, probably because of the use of artificial pulmonary surfactant to prevent and treat respiratory distress syndrome in premature infants (7). During 1991–1997, infant mortality continued to decline primarily because of decreases in sudden infant death syndrome (SIDS) and other causes.

Although improvements in medical care were the main force for declines in infant mortality during the second half of the century, public health actions played a role. During the 1990s, a >50% decline in SIDS rates (attributed to the recommendation that infants be placed to sleep on their backs) has helped to reduce the overall infant mortality rate (8). The reduction in vaccine-preventable diseases (e.g., diphtheria, tetanus, measles, poliomyelitis, and *Haemophilus influenzae* type b meningitis) has reduced infant morbidity and has had a modest effect on infant mortality (9). Advances in prenatal diagnosis of severe central nervous system defects, selective termination of affected pregnancies, and improved surgical treatment and management of other structural anomalies have helped reduce infant mortality attributed to these birth defects (10,11). National efforts to encourage reproductive-aged women to consume foods or supplements containing folic acid could reduce the incidence of neural tube defects by half (12).

MATERNAL MORTALITY

Maternal mortality rates were highest in this century during 1900–1930 (2). Poor obstetric education and delivery practices were mainly responsible for the high numbers of maternal deaths, most of which were preventable (2). Obstetrics as a speciality was shunned by many physicians, and obstetric care was provided by poorly trained or untrained medical practitioners. Most births occurred at home with the assistance of midwives or general practitioners. Inappropriate and excessive surgical and obstetric interventions (e.g., induction of labor, use of forceps, episiotomy, and cesarean deliveries) were common and increased during the 1920s. Deliveries, including some surgical interventions, were performed without following the principles of asepsis. As a result, 40% of maternal deaths were caused by sepsis (half following delivery and half associated with illegally induced abortion) with the remaining deaths primarily attributed to hemorrhage and toxemia (2).

The 1933 White House Conference on Child Health Protection, Fetal, Newborn, and Maternal Mortality and Morbidity report (13) demonstrated the link between poor aseptic practice, excessive operative deliveries, and high maternal mortality. This and earlier reports focused attention on the state of maternal health and led to calls for action by state medical associations (13). During the 1930s–1940s, hospital and state maternal mortality review committees were established. During the ensuing years, institutional practice guidelines and guidelines defining physician qualifications needed for hospital delivery privileges were developed. At the same time, a shift from home to hospital deliveries was occurring throughout the country; during 1938–1948, the proportion of infants born in hospitals increased from 55% to 90% (14). However, this shift was slow in rural areas and southern states. Safer deliveries in hospitals under aseptic conditions and improved provision of maternal care for the poor by states or voluntary organizations led to decreases in maternal mortality after 1930. Medical advances (including the use of antibiotics, oxytocin to induce labor, and safe blood transfusion and better management of hypertensive conditions during pregnancy) accelerated declines in maternal mortality. During 1939–1948, maternal mortality decreased by 71% (14). The legalization of induced abortion beginning in the 1960s contributed to an 89% decline in deaths from septic illegal abortions (15) during 1950–1973.

Since 1982, maternal mortality has not declined (16). However, more than half of maternal deaths can be prevented with existing interventions (17). In 1997, 327 maternal deaths were reported based on information on death certificates; however, death certificate data underestimate these deaths, and the actual numbers are two to three times greater. The leading causes of maternal death are hemorrhage, including hemorrhage associated with ectopic pregnancy, pregnancy-induced hypertension (toxemia), and embolism (17).

CHALLENGES FOR THE 21ST CENTURY

Despite the dramatic decline in infant and maternal mortality during the 20th century, challenges remain. Perhaps the greatest is the persistent difference in maternal and infant health among various racial/ethnic groups, particularly between black and white women and infants. Although overall rates have plummeted, black infants are more than twice as likely to die as white infants; this ratio has increased in recent decades. The higher risk for infant mortality among blacks compared with whites is attributed to higher LBW incidence and preterm births and to a higher risk for death among normal birthweight infants (≥5 lbs, 8 oz [≥2500 g]) (18). American Indian/Alaska Native infants have higher death rates than white infants because of higher SIDS rates. Hispanics of Puerto Rican origin have higher death rates than white infants because of higher LBW rates (19). The gap in maternal mortality between black and white women has increased since the early 1900s. During the first decades of the 20th century, black women were twice as likely to die of pregnancy-related complications as white women. Today, black women are more than three times as likely to die as white women.

During the last few decades, the key reason for the decline in neonatal mortality has been the improved rates of survival among LBW babies, not the reduction in the incidence of LBW. The long-term effects of LBW include neurologic disorders, learning disabilities, and delayed development (20). During the 1990s, the increased use of assisted reproductive technology has led to an increase in multiple gestations and a concomitant increase in the preterm delivery and LBW rates (21). Therefore, in the coming decades, public health programs will need to address the two leading causes of infant mortality: deaths related to LBW and preterm births and congenital anomalies. Additional substantial decline in neonatal mortality will require effective strategies to reduce LBW and preterm births. This will be especially important in reducing racial/ethnic disparities in the health of infants.

Approximately half of all pregnancies in the United States are unintended, including approximately three quarters among women aged <20 years. Unintended pregnancy is associated with increased morbidity and mortality for the mother and infant. Lifestyle factors (e.g., smoking, drinking alcohol, unsafe sex practices, and poor nutrition) and inadequate intake of foods containing folic acid pose serious health hazards to the mother and fetus and are more common among women with unintended pregnancies. In addition, one fifth of all pregnant women and approximately half of women with unintended pregnancies do not start prenatal care during the first trimester. Effective strategies to reduce unintended pregnancy, to eliminate exposure to unhealthy lifestyle factors, and to ensure that all women begin prenatal care early are important challenges for the next century.

Compared with the 1970s, the 1980s and 1990s have seen a lack of decline in maternal mortality and a slower rate of decline in infant mortality. Some experts consider that the United States may be approaching an irreducible minimum in these areas. However, three factors indicate that this is unlikely. First, scientists have believed that infant and maternal mortality was as low as possible at other times during the century, when the rates were much higher than they are now. Second, the United States has higher maternal and infant mortality rates than other developed countries; it ranks 25th in infant mortality (22) and 21st in maternal mortality (23). Third, most of the U.S. population has infant and maternal mortality rates substantially lower than some racial/ethnic subgroups, and no definable biologic reason has been found to indicate that a minimum has been reached.

To develop effective strategies for the 21st century, studies of the underlying factors that contribute to morbidity and mortality should be conducted. These studies should include efforts to understand not only the biologic factors but also the social, economic, psychological, and environmental factors that contribute to maternal and infant deaths. Researchers are examining "fetal programming" — the effect of uterine environment (e.g., maternal stress, nutrition, and infection) on fetal development and its effect on health from childhood to adulthood. Because reproductive tract infections (e.g., bacterial vaginosis) are associated with preterm birth, development of effective screening and treatment strategies may reduce preterm births. Case reviews or audits are being used increasingly to investigate fetal, infant, and maternal deaths; they focus on identifying preventable deaths such as those resulting from health-care system failures and gaps in quality of care and in access to care. Another strategy is to study cases of severe morbidity in which the woman or infant did not die. More clinically focused than reviews or audits, such "near miss" studies may explain why one woman or infant with a serious problem died while another survived.

A thorough review of the quality of health care and access to care for all women and infants is needed to avoid preventable mortality and morbidity and to develop public health programs that can eliminate racial/ethnic disparities in health. Preconception health services for all women of childbearing age, including healthy women who intend to become pregnant, and quality care during pregnancy, delivery, and the postpartum period are critical elements needed to improve maternal and infant outcomes (Figure 3).

Prevention measures to reduce maternal and infant mortality and to promote the health of all childbearing-aged women and their newborns should start before conception and continue through the postpartum period. Some of these prevention measures include the following:

Before conception

- Screen women for health risks and pre-existing chronic conditions such as diabetes, hypertension, and sexually transmitted diseases.
- Counsel women about contraception and provide access to effective family planning service (to prevent unintended pregnancies and unnecessary abortions).
- Counsel women about the benefits of good nutrition; encourage women especially to consume adequate amounts of folic acid supplements (to prevent neural tube defects) and iron.
- Advise women to avoid alcohol, tobacco, and illicit drugs.
- Advise women about the value of regular physical exercise.

During pregnancy

- Provide women with early access to high-quality care throughout pregnancy, labor, and delivery. Such care includes risk-appropriate care, treatment for complications, and the use of antenatal corticosteroids when appropriate.
- Monitor and, when appropriate, treat pre-existing chronic conditions.
- Screen for and, when appropriate, treat reproductive tract infections, including bacterial vaginosis, group B streptococcus infections, and human immunodeficiency virus.
- Vaccinate women against influenza, if appropriate.
- Continue counseling against use of tobacco, alcohol, and illicit drugs.
- Continue counseling about nutrition and physical exercise.
- Educate women about the early signs of pregnancy-related problems.

During postpartum period

- Vaccinate newborns at age-appropriate times.
- Provide information about well-baby care and benefits of breastfeeding.
- Warn parents about exposing infants to secondhand smoke.
- Counsel parents about placing infants to sleep on their backs.
- Educate parents about how to protect their infants from exposure to infectious diseases and harmful substances.

Figure 3 Opportunities to reduce maternal and infant mortality.

REFERENCES

1. Meckel RA. Save the babies: American public health reform and the prevention of infant mortality, 1850–1929. Baltimore, Maryland: The Johns Hopkins University Press, 1990.

2. Loudon I. Death in childbirth: an international study of maternal care and maternal mortality, 1800–1950. New York, New York: Oxford University Press, 1992.

3. Hoyert DL, Kochanek KD, Murphy SL. Deaths: final data for 1997. Hyattsville, Maryland: US Department of Health and Human Services, CDC, National Center for Health Statistics, 1999. (*National vital statistics report*; vol 47, no. 20).
4. Public Health Service. Vital statistics of the United States, 1950. Vol I. Washington, DC: US Department of Health and Human Services, Public Health Service, 1954:258–9.
5. Pharoah POD, Morris JN. Postneonatal mortality. *Epidemic Rev* 1979;1:170–83.
6. Kleinman JC. The slowdown in the infant mortality decline. *Pediatr Perinat Epidemiol* 1990;4:373–81.
7. Schoendorf KC, Kiely JL. Birth weight and age-specific analysis of the 1990 US infant mortality drop: was it surfactant? *Arch Pediatr Adolesc Med* 1997;151:129–34.
8. Willinger M, Hoffman H, Wu K, et al. Factors associated with the transition to non-prone sleep positions of infants in the United States: the National Infant Sleep Position Study. *JAMA* 1998;280:329–39.
9. CDC. Status report on the Childhood Immunization Initiative: reported cases of selected vaccine-preventable diseases — United States, 1996. *MMWR* 1997;46: 667–71.
10. CDC. Trends in infant mortality attributable to birth defects — United States, 1980–1995. *MMWR* 1998;47:773–7.
11. Montana E, Khoury MJ, Cragan JD, et al. Trends and outcomes after prenatal diagnosis of congenital cardiac malformations by fetal echocardiography in a well defined birth population, Atlanta, Georgia, 1990–1994. *J Am Coll Cardiol* 1996;27: 1805–9.
12. Johnston RB Jr. Folic acid: new dimensions of an old friendship. In: Advances in pediatrics. Vol 44. St. Louis, Missouri: Mosby-Year Book, 1997.
13. Wertz RW, Wertz DC. Lying-in: a history of childbirth in America. New Haven, Connecticut: Yale University Press, 1989.
14. Children's Bureau. Changes in infant, childhood, and maternal mortality over the decade of 1939–1948: a graphic analysis. Washington, DC: Children's Bureau, Social Security Administration, 1950.
15. National Center for Health Statistics. Vital statistics of the United States, 1973. Vol II, mortality, part A. Rockville, Maryland: US Department of Health, Education, and Welfare, 1977.
16. CDC. Maternal Mortality — United States, 1982–1996. *MMWR* 1999;47:705–7.
17. Berg CJ, Atrash HK, Koonin LM, Tucker M. Pregnancy-related mortality in the United States, 1987–1990. *Obstet Gynecol* 1996;88:161–7.
18. Iyasu S, Becerra JE, Rowley DL, Hogue CJR. Impact of very low birthweight on the black-white infant mortality gap. *Am J Prev Med* 1992;8:271–7.
19. MacDorman MF, Atkinson JO. Infant mortality statistics from the 1997 period linked birth/infant death data set. Hyattsville, Maryland: US Department of Health and Human Services, CDC, National Center for Health Statistics, 1999. (*National vital statistics reports*, vol 47, no. 23).
20. McCormick MC. The contribution of low birth weight to infant mortality and childhood morbidity. *N Engl J Med* 1985;312:80–90.

21. CDC. Impact of multiple births on low birthweight — Massachusetts, 1989–1996. *MMWR* 1999;48:289–92.

22. National Center for Health Statistics. Health, United States, 1998, with socioeconomic status and health chart book. Hyattsville, Maryland: US Department of Health and Human Services, CDC, National Center for Health Statistics, 1998; DHHS publication no. (PHS)98–1232.

23. World Health Organization. WHO revised 1990 estimates of maternal mortality: a new approach by WHO and UNICEF. Geneva, Switzerland: World Health Organization, 1996; report no. WHO/FRH/MSM/96.11.

ARTICLE 4

ACHIEVEMENTS IN PUBLIC HEALTH, 1900–1999

DECLINE IN DEATHS FROM HEART DISEASE AND STROKE — UNITED STATES, 1900–1999

The Centers for Disease Control and Prevention

Heart disease has been the leading cause of death in the United States since 1921, and stroke has been the third leading cause since 1938 (1); together they account for approximately 40% of all deaths. Since 1950, age-adjusted death rates from cardiovascular disease (CVD) have declined 60%, representing one of the most important public health achievements of the 20th century. This report summarizes the temporal trends in CVD, advances in the understanding of risk factors for CVD, development of prevention interventions to reduce these risks, and improvements in therapy for persons who develop CVD.

DECLINE IN CVD DEATH RATES

Age-adjusted death rates per 100,000 persons (standardized to the 1940 U.S. population) for diseases of the heart (i.e., coronary heart disease, hypertensive heart disease, and rheumatic heart disease) have decreased from a peak of 307.4 in 1950 to 134.6 in 1996, an overall decline of 56% (1) (Figure 1). Age-adjusted death rates for coronary heart disease (the major form of CVD contributing to mortality) continued to increase into the 1960s, then declined. In 1996, 621,000 fewer deaths occurred from coronary heart disease than would have been expected had the rate remained at its 1963 peak (1).

Age-adjusted death rates for stroke have declined steadily since the beginning of the century. Since 1950, stroke rates have declined 70%, from 88.8 in 1950 to 26.5 in 1996. Total age-adjusted CVD death rates have declined 60% since 1950 and accounted for approximately 73% of the decline in all causes of deaths during the same period (1).

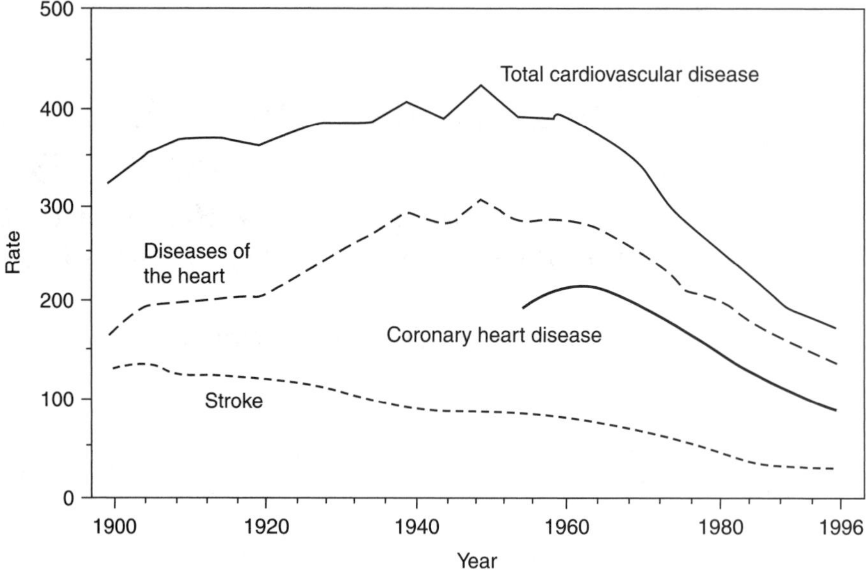

*Per 100,000 population, standardized to the 1940 U.S. population.

†Diseases are classified according to *International Classification of Diseases* (ICD) codes in use when the deaths were reported. ICD classification revisions occurred in 1910, 1921, 1930, 1939, 1949, 1958, 1968, and 1979. Death rates before 1933 do not include all states. Comparability ratios were applied to rates for 1970 and 1975.

Figure 1 Age-adjusted death rates* for total cardiovascular disease, diseases of the heart, coronary heart disease, and stroke,† by year — United States, 1900–1996. (Source: Adapted from reference 1; data provided by the National Heart, Lung and Blood Institute, National Institutes of Health.)

DISEASE EPIDEMIOLOGY

Intensive investigation into the CVD epidemic largely began in the 1940s following World War II, although causal hypotheses about CVD and recognition of geographic differences in disease rates occurred earlier (2–4). Landmark epidemiologic investigations, including the cross-country comparisons of Ancel Keys (5) and the Framingham Heart Study (6), established the major risk factors of high blood cholesterol, high blood pressure, and smoking and dietary factors (particularly dietary cholesterol, fat, and sodium). The risk factor concept — that particular biologic, lifestyle, and social conditions were associated with increased risk for disease — developed out of CVD epidemiology (3,4). In addition to the major risk factors (i.e., high blood pressure, high blood cholesterol, and smoking), other important factors include socioeconomic status, obesity, and physical inactivity (7). Striking regional differences were noted particularly for stroke mortality, with the highest rates observed in the southeastern United States (1). Cross-national and cross-cultural studies highlighted the importance of social, cultural, and environmental factors in the development of CVD.

Coronary heart disease and stroke, the two major causes of CVD-related mortality, are not influenced to the same degree by the recognized risk factors. For example, elevated blood cholesterol is a major risk factor for coronary heart disease, and hypertension is the major risk factor for stroke. Physical activity, smoking cessation, and a healthy diet, which can lower the risk for heart disease, also can help lower the risk for stroke (8).

ADVANCES IN PREVENTION

Early intervention studies in the 1960s sought to establish whether lowering risk factor levels would reduce risk for CVD (2–4). During the 1970s and 1980s, along with numerous clinical trials demonstrating the efficacy of antihypertensive and lipid-lowering drugs, community trials sought to reduce risk at the community level (9). Public health interventions to reduce CVD have benefited from a combination of the "high risk" approach — aimed at persons with increased risk for CVD — and the population-wide approach — aimed at lowering risk for the entire community (10). National programs that combine these complementary approaches and that are aimed at health-care providers, patients, and the general public include the National High Blood Pressure Education Program (11), initiated in 1972, and the National Cholesterol Education Program, initiated in 1985 (12). Although earlier CDC community demonstration projects focused on cardiovascular health (9), CDC established its National Center for Chronic Disease Prevention and Health Promotion in 1989, with a high priority of promoting cardiovascular health.

FACTORS CONTRIBUTING TO THE DECLINE IN CVD DEATHS

Reasons for the declines in heart disease and stroke may vary by period and across region or socioeconomic groups (e.g., age, sex, and racial/ethnic groups). Prevention efforts and improvements in early detection, treatment, and care have resulted in a number of beneficial trends, which may have contributed to declines in heart disease and stroke. These trends include

- a decline in cigarette smoking among adults aged greater than or equal to 18 years from approximately 42% in 1965 to 25% in 1995 (13). Substantial public health efforts to reduce tobacco use began soon after recognition of the association between smoking and CVD and between smoking and cancer and the first Surgeon General's report on smoking and health published in 1964.
- a decrease in mean blood pressure levels in the U.S. population (11,13,14).
- an increase in the percentage of persons with hypertension who have the condition treated and controlled (11,13,14).
- a decrease in mean blood cholesterol levels (12–14).
- changes in the U.S. diet. Data based on surveys of food supply suggest that consumption of saturated fat and cholesterol has decreased since 1909 (15).

Data from the National Health and Nutrition Examination surveys suggest that decreases in the percentage of calories from dietary fat and the levels of dietary cholesterol coincide with decreases in blood cholesterol levels (16).

- improvements in medical care, including advances in diagnosing and treating heart disease and stroke, development of effective medications for treatment of hypertension and hypercholesterolemia, greater numbers of specialists and health-care providers focusing on CVD, an increase in emergency medical services for heart attack and stroke, and an increase in coronary-care units (13,17). These developments have contributed to lower case-fatality rates, lengthened survival times, and shorter hospital stays for persons with CVD (1,17).

CHALLENGES FOR THE 21ST CENTURY

Despite remarkable progress, heart disease and stroke remain leading causes of disability and death. Estimated costs for morbidity and mortality from CVD, including health expenditures and lost productivity, are expected to be $286.5 billion in 1999 (18). In addition, the overall declines in heart disease and stroke mortality mask important differences in rates of decline by race/ethnicity, sex, socioeconomic status, and geographic region. During 1985–1996, for example, heart disease age-adjusted mortality declined 29% among white men, but only 10% among American Indian/Alaska Native women (13). Persons of lower socioeconomic status have higher mortality, morbidity, and risk factor levels for heart disease and stroke than persons of higher socioeconomic status (13,19). In addition, the social class gap in heart disease deaths may be increasing as the rates of heart disease decline faster among higher social classes (19). Geographically, declines in heart disease deaths did not occur at the same time for all communities. Areas with poorer socioeconomic profiles were more likely to experience a later onset of the decline of heart disease (19).

Public health programs at the state level for heart disease and stroke have been limited. In fiscal year 1999, through a new program, CDC funded 11 states with the highest CVD mortality rates to plan, develop, and implement state-based efforts for CVD prevention. In addition to activities such as surveillance, these programs will emphasize policy and environmental interventions, both social and physical, aimed at sustaining positive health behavior change.

Although many trends have been positive, trends for some important indicators have not improved substantially, have leveled off, or are reversing. For example, approximately 70% of persons with hypertension do not have the condition controlled at levels below 140/90 mm Hg, and death rates for stroke have not declined in recent years (1,11,13). Heart failure has emerged as a health concern for older adults (20), and adults who survive a myocardial infarction or other hypertension-related diseases remain at increased risk for heart failure. In addition, the prevalence of obesity has increased among both children and adults in the United States (13).

Major public health challenges for the 21st century include

- reducing risk factor levels and preventing the development of adverse risk factors. Continued research is needed to understand the determinants (social, psychological, environmental, physiologic, and genetic) of CVD risk factors.
- reducing the racial/ethnic disparities in heart disease and stroke mortality.
- increasing the ability to reach underserved groups with appropriate and effective public health messages.
- promoting policy and environmental strategies that enhance healthy behavior.
- determining the relation between genetics and disease. The associations of genetic variants with CVD, and especially the interplay between genetic and environmental factors, may play increasingly important roles in the nation's efforts to prevent CVD.
- identifying new or emerging risk factors and determining their potential for public health intervention. New or emerging risk factors that have been associated with CVD include elevated levels of total homocyst(e)ine, fibrinogen, and C-reactive protein, and infectious agents such as *Helicobacter pylori* and *Chlamydia pneumoniae*.
- focusing on secondary prevention and disability. An aging U.S. population and an increasing number of persons surviving life-threatening cardiovascular conditions require public health programs to focus on issues such as disability and quality of life. Persons with existing cardiovascular conditions are at increased risk for future life-threatening events related to those conditions.
- addressing the needs of the global community. Although CVD death rates are higher in developed nations, most cases occur in developing nations (8). Developing countries may face a double burden of infectious and chronic diseases. International collaboration to improve cardiovascular health (9) will need to continue to reduce the burden of CVD worldwide.

REFERENCES

1. National Heart, Lung and Blood Institute. Morbidity & mortality: 1998 chartbook on cardiovascular, lung, and blood diseases. Rockville, Maryland: US Department of Health and Human Services, National Institutes of Health, 1998.

2. Epstein FH. Contribution of epidemiology to understanding coronary heart disease. In: Marmot M, Elliott P, eds. Coronary heart disease epidemiology: from aetiology to public health. New York: Oxford University Press, 1992:20–32.

3. Epstein FH. Cardiovascular disease epidemiology: a journey from the past into the future. *Circulation* 1996;93:1755–64.

4. Stamler J. Established major coronary risk factors. In: Marmot M, Elliott P, eds. Coronary heart disease epidemiology: from aetiology to public health. New York: Oxford University Press, 1992:35–66.

5. Keys A. Seven countries — a multivariate analysis of death and coronary heart disease. Cambridge, Massachusetts: Harvard University Press, 1980.
6. Dawber TR. The Framingham study: the epidemiology of atherosclerotic disease. Cambridge, Massachusetts: Harvard University Press, 1980.
7. National Heart, Lung and Blood Institute. Report of the task force on research in epidemiology and prevention of cardiovascular diseases. Rockville, Maryland: National Institutes of Health, 1994.
8. Labarthe DR. Epidemiology and prevention of cardiovascular diseases: a global challenge. Gaithersburg, Maryland: Aspen, 1998.
9. CDC/Stanford University School of Medicine. Worldwide efforts to improve heart health: a follow-up of the Catalonia Declaration — selected program descriptions. Atlanta: US Department of Health and Human Services, CDC, 1997.
10. Rose G. The strategy of preventive medicine. New York: Oxford University Press, 1992.
11. National Institutes of Health. The sixth report of the Joint National Committee on Prevention, Detection, Evaluation, and Treatment of High Blood Pressure. Rockville, Maryland: US Department of Health and Human Services, National Institutes of Health, National Heart, Lung, and Blood Institute, November 1997. (NIH publication no. 98–4080).
12. National Cholesterol Education Program. Second report of the expert panel on detection, evaluation and treatment of high blood cholesterol in adults. Rockville, Maryland: US Department of Health and Human Services, National Institutes of Health, 1993. (NIH publication no. 93–3095).
13. National Center for Health Statistics. *Health, United States, 1998 with socioeconomic status and health chartbook.* Hyattsville, Maryland: US Department of Health and Human Services, CDC, 1998.
14. National Center for Health Statistics. Healthy people 2000 review, 1997. Hyattsville, Maryland: US Department of Health and Human Services, CDC, 1997.
15. Gerrior S, Bente L. Nutrient content of the U.S. food supply, 1909–94. Washington, DC: US Department of Agriculture, 1997. (Home economics research report no. 53).
16. Ernst ND, Sempos ST, Briefel RR, Clark MB. Consistency between US dietary fat intake and serum total cholesterol concentrations: the National Health and Nutrition Examination surveys. *Am J Clin Nutr* 1997;66:965S–972S.
17. Higgins M, Thom T. Trends in CHD in the United States. *Int J Epidemiol* 1989;18:S58–S66.
18. American Heart Association. 1999 Heart and stroke statistical update. Dallas, Texas: American Heart Association, 1998.
19. Kaplan GA, Keil JE. Socioeconomic factors and cardiovascular disease: a review of the literature. *Circulation* 1993;88:1973–98.
20. CDC. Changes in mortality from heart failure — United States, 1980–1995. *MMWR* 1998;47:633–7.

ARTICLE 5

HEALTHY PEOPLE 2010

UNDERSTANDING AND IMPROVING HEALTH

U.S. Department of Health and Human Services

INTRODUCTION

Healthy People 2010 outlines a comprehensive, nationwide health promotion and disease prevention agenda. It is designed to serve as a roadmap for improving the health of all people in the United States during the first decade of the 21st century.

Like the preceding Healthy People 2000 initiative — which was driven by an ambitious, yet achievable, 10-year strategy for improving the Nation's health by the end of the 20th century — Healthy People 2010 is committed to a single, overarching purpose: promoting health and preventing illness, disability, and premature death.

The History Behind the Healthy People 2010 Initiative

Healthy People 2010 builds on initiatives pursued over the past two decades. In 1979, *Healthy People: The Surgeon General's Report on Health Promotion and Disease Prevention* provided national goals for reducing premature deaths and preserving independence for older adults. In 1980, another report, *Promoting Health/Preventing Disease: Objectives for the Nation*, outlined 226 targeted health objectives for the Nation to achieve over the next 10 years.

Healthy People 2000: National Health Promotion and Disease Prevention Objectives, released in 1990, identified health improvement goals and objectives to be reached by the year 2000. The Healthy People 2010 initiative continues in this tradition as an instrument to improve health for the first decade of the 21st century.

The Way Healthy People 2010 Goals and Objectives Were Developed

Healthy People 2010 represents the ideas and expertise of a diverse range of individuals and organizations concerned about the Nation's health. The Healthy People Consortium — an alliance of more than 350 national organizations and 250 State public health, mental health, substance abuse, and environmental agencies — conducted 3 national meetings on the development of Healthy People 2010. In addition, many individuals and organizations gave testimony about health priorities at five Healthy People 2010 regional meetings held in late 1998.

On two occasions — in 1997 and in 1998 — the American public was given the opportunity to share its thoughts and ideas. More than 11,000 comments on draft materials were received by mail or via the Internet from individuals in every State, the District of Columbia, and Puerto Rico. All the comments received during the development of Healthy People 2010 can be viewed on the Healthy People Website: http://www.health.gov/healthypeople.

The final Healthy People 2010 objectives were developed by teams of experts from a variety of Federal agencies under the direction of Health and Human Services Secretary Donna Shalala, Assistant Secretary for Health and Surgeon General David Satcher, and former Assistant Secretaries for Health. The process was coordinated by the Office of Disease Prevention and Health Promotion, U.S. Department of Health and Human Services.

The Central Goals of Healthy People 2010

Healthy People 2010 is designed to achieve two overarching goals:

- Increase quality and years of healthy life
- Eliminate health disparities

These two goals are supported by specific objectives in 28 focus areas. Each objective was developed with a target to be achieved by the year 2010. A full explanation of the two goals can be found in the next section of this document: "A Systematic Approach to Health Improvement."

The Relationship between Individual and Community Health

Over the years, it has become clear that individual health is closely linked to community health — the health of the community and environment in which individuals live, work, and play. Likewise, community health is profoundly affected by the collective behaviors, attitudes, and beliefs of everyone who lives in the community.

Indeed, the underlying premise of Healthy People 2010 is that the health of the individual is almost inseparable from the health of the larger community and that the health of every community in every State and territory determines the overall health status of the Nation. That is why the vision for Healthy People 2010 is "Healthy People in Healthy Communities."

How Healthy People 2010 Will Improve the Nation's Health

One of the most compelling and encouraging lessons learned from the Healthy People 2000 initiative is that we, as a Nation, can make dramatic progress in improving the

Nation's health in a relatively short period of time. For example, during the last decade, we achieved significant reductions in infant mortality. Childhood vaccinations are at the highest levels ever recorded in the United States. Fewer teenagers are becoming parents. Overall, alcohol, tobacco, and illicit drug use is leveling off. Death rates for coronary heart disease and stroke have declined. Significant advances have been made in the diagnosis and treatment of cancer and in reducing unintentional injuries.

But we still have a long way to go. Diabetes and other chronic conditions continue to present a serious obstacle to public health. Violence and abusive behavior continue to ravage homes and communities across the country. Mental disorders continue to go undiagnosed and untreated. Obesity in adults has increased 50 percent over the past two decades. Nearly 40 percent of adults engage in no leisure time physical activity. Smoking among adolescents has increased in the past decade. And HIV/AIDS remains a serious health problem, now disproportionately affecting women and communities of color.

Healthy People 2010 will be the guiding instrument for addressing these and other new health issues, reversing unfavorable trends, and expanding past achievements in health.

The Key Role of Community Partnerships

Community partnerships, particularly when they reach out to nontraditional partners, can be among the most effective tools for improving health in communities.

For the past two decades, Healthy People has been used as a strategic management tool for the Federal Government, States, communities, and many other public- and private-sector partners. Virtually all States, the District of Columbia, and Guam have developed their own Healthy People plans modeled after the national plan. Most States have tailored the national objectives to their specific needs.

Businesses; local governments; and civic, professional, and religious organizations have also been inspired by Healthy People to print immunization reminders, set up hotlines, change cafeteria menus, begin community recycling, establish worksite fitness programs, assess school health education curriculums, sponsor health fairs, and engage in myriad other activities.

Everyone Can Help Achieve the Healthy People 2010 Objectives

Addressing the challenge of health improvement is a shared responsibility that requires the active participation and leadership of the Federal Government, States, local governments, policymakers, health care providers, professionals, business executives, educators, community leaders, and the American public itself. Although administrative responsibility for the Healthy People 2010 initiative rests in the U.S. Department of Health and Human Services, representatives of all these diverse groups shared their experience, expertise, and ideas in developing the Healthy People 2010 goals and objectives.

Healthy People 2010, however, is just the beginning. The biggest challenges still stand before us, and we all share a role in building a healthier Nation.

Regardless of your age, gender, education level, income, race, ethnicity, cultural customs, language, religious beliefs, disability, sexual orientation, geographic location, or occupation, Healthy People 2010 is designed to be a valuable resource in determining how you can participate most effectively in improving the Nation's health. Perhaps you will recognize the need to be a more active participant in decisions affecting your own health or the health of your children or loved ones. Perhaps you will assume a leadership role in promoting healthier behaviors in your neighborhood or community. Or perhaps you will use your influence and social stature to advocate for and implement policies and programs that can dramatically improve the health of dozens, hundreds, thousands, or even millions of people.

Whatever your role, this document is designed to help you determine what *you* can do — in your home, community, business, or State — to help improve the Nation's health.

A SYSTEMATIC APPROACH TO HEALTH IMPROVEMENT

Healthy People 2010 is about improving health — the health of each individual, the health of communities, and the health of the Nation. However, the Healthy People 2010 goals and objectives cannot by themselves improve the health status of the Nation. Instead, they should be recognized as part of a larger, systematic approach to health improvement.

This systematic approach to health improvement is composed of four key elements:

- Goals
- Objectives
- Determinants of health
- Health status

Whether this systematic approach is used to improve health on a national level, as in Healthy People 2010, or to organize community action on a particular health issue, such as promoting smoking cessation, the components remain the same. The goals provide a general focus and direction. The goals, in turn, serve as a guide for developing a set of objectives that will actually measure progress within a specified amount of time. The objectives focus on the determinants of health, which encompass the combined effects of individual and community physical and social environments and the policies and interventions used to promote health, prevent disease, and ensure access to quality health care. The ultimate measure of success in any health improvement effort is the health status of the target population.

Healthy People 2010 is built on this systematic approach to health improvement.

HEALTHY PEOPLE 2010 GOALS

Goal 1: Increase Quality and Years of Healthy Life

The first goal of Healthy People 2010 is to help individuals of all ages increase life expectancy *and* improve their quality of life.

Life Expectancy. Life expectancy is the average number of years people born in a given year are expected to live based on a set of age-specific death rates. At the beginning of the 20th century, life expectancy at birth was 47.3 years. Fortunately, life expectancy has dramatically increased over the past 100 years. Today, the average life expectancy at birth is nearly 77 years.

Life expectancy for persons at every age group has also increased during the past century. Based on today's age-specific death rates, individuals aged 65 years can be expected to live an average of 18 more years, for a total of 83 years. Those aged 75 years can be expected to live an average of 11 more years, for a total of 86 years.

Differences in life expectancy between populations, however, suggest a substantial need and opportunity for improvement. At least 18 countries with populations of 1 million or more have life expectancies greater than the United States for both men and women.

There are substantial differences in life expectancy among different population groups within the United States. For example, women outlive men by an average of 6 years. White women currently have the greatest life expectancy in the United States. The life expectancy for African American women has risen to be higher today than that for white men. People from households with an annual income of at least $25,000 live an average of 3 to 7 years longer, depending on gender and race, than people from households with annual incomes of less than $10,000.

Quality of Life. Quality of life reflects a general sense of happiness and satisfaction with our lives and environment. General quality of life encompasses all aspects of life, including health, recreation, culture, rights, values, beliefs, aspirations, and the conditions that support a life containing these elements. *Health-related quality of life* reflects a personal sense of physical and mental health and the ability to react to factors in the physical and social environments. Health-related quality of life is inherently more subjective than life expectancy and therefore can be more difficult to measure. Some tools, however, have been developed to measure health-related quality of life.

Global assessments, in which a person rates his or her health as "poor," "fair," "good," "very good," or "excellent," can be reliable indicators of a person's perceived health. In 1996, 90 percent of people in the United States reported their health as good, very good, or excellent.

Healthy days is another measure of health-related quality of life that estimates the number of days of poor physical and mental health in the past 30 days. In 1998, 82 percent of adults reported having no days in the past month where poor physical or mental health impaired their usual activities. The proportions of days that are reported "unhealthy" are the result more often of mentally unhealthy days for younger adults and physically unhealthy days for older adults.

Years of healthy life is a combined measure developed for the Healthy People initiative. The difference between life expectancy and years of healthy life reflects the average amount of time spent in less than optimal health because of chronic or acute limitations. After decreasing in the early 1990s, years of healthy life increased to a level in 1996 that was only slightly above that at the beginning of the decade (64.0 years in 1990 to 64.2 years in 1996). During the same period, life expectancy increased a full year.

As with life expectancy, various population groups can show dramatic differences in quality of life. For example, people in the lowest income households are five times more likely to report their health as fair or poor than people in the highest income households. A higher percentage of women report their health as fair or poor compared to men. Adults in rural areas are 36 percent more likely to report their health status as fair or poor than are adults in urban areas.

Achieving a Longer and Healthier Life — the Healthy People Perspective. Healthy People 2010 seeks to increase life expectancy and quality of life over the next 10 years by helping individuals gain the knowledge, motivation, and opportunities they need to make informed decisions about their health. At the same time, Healthy People 2010 encourages local and State leaders to develop communitywide and statewide efforts that promote healthy behaviors, create healthy environments, and increase access to high-quality health care. Given the fact that individual and community health are virtually inseparable, it is critical that both the individual and the community do their parts to increase life expectancy and improve quality of life.

Goal 2: Eliminate Health Disparities

The second goal of Healthy People 2010 is to eliminate health disparities among different segments of the population. These include differences that occur by gender, race or ethnicity, education or income, disability, living in rural localities, or sexual orientation. This section highlights ways in which health disparities can occur among various demographic groups in the United States.

Gender. Whereas some differences in health between men and women are the result of biological differences, others are more complicated and require greater attention and scientific exploration. Some health differences are obviously gender specific, such as cervical and prostate cancers.

Overall, men have a life expectancy that is 6 years less than women and have higher death rates for each of the 10 leading causes of death. For example, men are two times more likely than women to die from unintentional injuries and four times more likely than women to die from firearm-related injuries. Although overall death rates for women may currently be lower than for men, women have shown increased death rates over the past decade in areas where men have experienced improvements, such as lung cancer. Women are also at greater risk for Alzheimer's disease than men and twice as likely as men to be affected by major depression.

Race and Ethnicity. Current information about the biologic and genetic characteristics of African Americans, Hispanics, American Indians, Alaska Natives, Asians, Native Hawaiians, and Pacific Islanders does not explain the health disparities experienced by these groups compared with the white, non-Hispanic population in the United States. These disparities are believed to be the result of the complex interaction among genetic variations, environmental factors, and specific health behaviors.

Even though the Nation's infant mortality rate is down, the infant death rate among African Americans is still more than double that of whites. Heart disease death rates are more than 40 percent higher for African Americans than for whites. The death rate for all cancers is 30 percent higher for African Americans than for whites; for prostate cancer, it is more than double that for whites. African American women have a higher death rate from breast cancer despite having a mammography screening rate that is higher than that for white women. The death rate from HIV/AIDS for African Americans is more than seven times that for whites; the rate of homicide is six times that for whites.

Hispanics living in the United States are almost twice as likely to die from diabetes than are non-Hispanic whites. Although constituting only 11 percent of the total population in 1996, Hispanics accounted for 20 percent of the new cases of tuberculosis. Hispanics also have higher rates of high blood pressure and obesity than non-Hispanic whites. There are differences among Hispanic populations as well. For example, whereas the rate of low-birth-weight infants is lower for the total Hispanic population compared with whites, Puerto Ricans have a low-birth-weight rate that is 50 percent higher than that for whites.

American Indians and Alaska Natives have an infant death rate almost double that for whites. The rate of diabetes for this population group is more than twice that for whites. The Pima of Arizona have one of the highest rates of diabetes in the world. American Indians and Alaska Natives also have disproportionately high death rates from unintentional injuries and suicide.

Asians and Pacific Islanders, on average, have indicators of being one of the healthiest population groups in the United States. However, there is great diversity within this population group, and health disparities for some specific groups are quite marked. Women of Vietnamese origin, for example, suffer from cervical cancer at nearly five times the rate for white women. New cases of hepatitis and tuberculosis are also higher in Asians and Pacific Islanders living in the United States than in whites.

Income and Education. Inequalities in income and education underlie many health disparities in the United States. Income and education are intrinsically related and often serve as proxy measures for each other. In general, population groups that suffer the worst health status are also those that have the highest poverty rates and least education. Disparities in income and education levels are associated with differences in the occurrence of illness and death, including heart disease, diabetes, obesity, elevated blood lead level, and low birth weight. Higher incomes permit increased access to medical care, enable one to afford better housing and live in safer neighborhoods, and increase the opportunity to engage in health-promoting behaviors.

Income inequality in the United States has increased over the past three decades. There are distinct demographic differences in poverty by race, ethnicity, and household composition as well as geographical variations in poverty across the United States. Recent health gains for the U.S. population as a whole appear to reflect achievements among the higher socioeconomic groups; lower socioeconomic groups continue to lag behind.

Overall, those with higher incomes tend to fare better than those with lower incomes. For example, among white men aged 65 years, those in the highest income families could expect to live more than 3 years longer than those in the lowest income families. The percentage of people in the lowest income families reporting limitation in activity caused by chronic disease is three times that of people in the highest income families.

The average level of education in the U.S. population has steadily increased over the past several decades — an important achievement given that more years of education usually translate into more years of life. For women, the amount of education achieved is a key determinant of the welfare and survival of their children. Higher levels of education may also increase the likelihood of obtaining or understanding health-related information needed to develop health-promoting behaviors and beliefs in prevention.

But again, educational attainment differs by race and ethnicity. Among people aged 25 to 64 years in the United States, the overall death rate for those with less than 12 years of education is more than twice that for people with 13 or more years of education. The infant mortality rate is almost double for infants of mothers with less than 12 years of education when compared with those with an education of 13 or more years.

Disability. People with disabilities are identified as persons having an activity limitation, who use assistance, or who perceive themselves as having a disability. In 1994, 54 million people in the United States, or roughly 21 percent of the population, had some level of disability. Although rates of disability are relatively stable or falling slightly for people aged 45 years and older, rates are on the rise among the younger population. People with disabilities tend to report more anxiety, pain, sleeplessness, and days of depression and fewer days of vitality than do people without activity limitations. People with disabilities also have other disparities, including lower rates of physical activity and higher rates of obesity. Many people with disabilities lack access to health services and medical care.

Rural Localities. Twenty-five percent of Americans live in rural areas, that is, places with fewer than 2,500 residents. Injury-related death rates are 40 percent higher in rural populations than in urban populations. Heart disease, cancer, and diabetes rates exceed those for urban areas. People living in rural areas are less likely to use preventive screening services, exercise regularly, or wear seat belts. In 1996, 20 percent of the rural population was uninsured compared with 16 percent of the urban population. Timely access to emergency services and the availability of specialty care are other issues for this population group.

Sexual Orientation. America's gay and lesbian population comprises a diverse community with disparate health concerns. Major health issues for gay men are HIV/AIDS and other sexually transmitted diseases, substance abuse, depression, and suicide. Gay male adolescents are two to three times more likely than their peers to attempt suicide. Some evidence suggests lesbians have higher rates of smoking, obesity, alcohol abuse, and stress than heterosexual women. The issues surrounding personal, family, and social acceptance of sexual orientation can place a significant burden on mental health and personal safety.

Achieving Equity — The Healthy People Perspective. Although the diversity of the American population may be one of our Nation's greatest assets, diversity also presents a range of health improvement challenges — challenges that must be addressed by individuals, the community and State in which they live, and the Nation as a whole.

Healthy People 2010 recognizes that communities, States, and national organizations will need to take a multidisciplinary approach to achieving health equity that involves improving health, education, housing, labor, justice, transportation, agriculture, and the environment. However, our greatest opportunities for reducing health disparities are in empowering individuals to make informed health care decisions and in promoting communitywide safety, education, and access to health care.

Healthy People 2010 is firmly dedicated to the principle that — regardless of age, gender, race, ethnicity, income, education, geographic location, disability, and sexual orientation — every person in every community across the Nation deserves equal access to comprehensive, culturally competent, community-based health care systems that are committed to serving the needs of the individual and promoting community health.

CHAPTER 2

The Determinants of Health and Health Disparities

As noted in Chapter 1, there has been a dramatic improvement in the health and life span of Americans during the past 150 years. This largely reflects a general improvement in the socioeconomic status (SES) of the population, improvements in nutrition, changes in reproductive behavior, advances in public health, particularly in environmental sanitation (e.g., chlorination of water supplies, pasteurization of milk), and more recently, improvements in medical care. Until the last 65 years, improvements in medical care had relatively little impact on the decline in mortality, which was mostly a product of the decline in mortality from airborne infectious diseases (e.g., tuberculosis, pneumonia, pertussis, diphtheria, scarlet fever) and waterborne or foodborne diseases (e.g., enteritis, gastritis, cholera). Particularly important were declines in infant mortality.

In his pioneering studies, the late British physician Thomas McKeown analyzed primary data on mortality in England and Wales from the 1700s to the mid-20th century, aiming to understand the impact of improvements in socioeconomic status, particularly nutrition, and changes in reproductive behavior, as well as advances in medical care and public health, on the human life span and quality of life. His papers, published between 1954 and 1978 (McKeown and Brown, 1955; McKeown and Record, 1962; McKeown, 1978), and his two books, *The Modern Rise of Populations* and *The Role of Medicine: Dream, Mirage, or Nemesis*?, published in 1976 and 1979, respectively, stirred great controversy because he concluded that "the rise in the population was due primarily to the decline of mortality, and the most important reason for the decline was an improvement in economic and social conditions" (McKeown and Record, 1962, p. 121).

All analysts, however, do not draw the same conclusions as McKeown from the available data. Some have questioned his conclusions about the important role of nutrition and SES and the minor role assigned to public health in the decline in mortality due to infectious diseases. The controversy stimulated by McKeown has recently been examined by Simon Szreter (2002), James Colgrove (2002), and

Bruce Link and Jo C. Phelan (2002) in the *American Journal of Public Health.* Chapter 2 includes Link and Phelan's article "McKeown and the Idea That Social Conditions Are Fundamental Causes of Disease" (Article 1). Although Link and Phelan basically agree with McKeown in his conclusions regarding the limited role played by medical care in improving the health of the population before the middle of the 20th century, they disagree with his conclusion about the limited role of public health efforts and the importance of a rising standard of living in the declining mortality from infectious diseases.

One of the results of McKeown's work on the determinants of health was the development of the "Health Field" concept, described in the 1974 report *A New Perspective on Health of Canadians* by the Canadian National Department of Health and Welfare in Ottawa, Canada (Lalonde, 1974). The Health Field concept included the factors of lifestyle, environment, human biology, and health care organization. Although produced by the national ministry, the report had little immediate impact on health policy. Slowly, however, there was a greater emphasis on health promotion in the United States.

The Centers for Disease Control and Prevention (CDC) of the U.S. Public Health Service analyzed the relative importance of these four factors on the ten leading causes of premature mortality in the United States (U.S. Department of Health and Human Services, 1980). The first analysis was done in 1977 and repeated in 1990. The contribution of each of the four major determinants of health to premature mortality was examined: Personal behavior/lifestyle accounted for approximately 47 percent, human biology (inherited and genetic factors) 27 percent, environmental factors 16 percent, and inadequacies in health care 10 percent. Although socioeconomic factors influence all other determinants of health, except human biology, the CDC did not include socioeconomic status as a determinant of health.

Taking a different approach that also failed to include an explicit treatment of SES, McGinnis and Foege (1993) found that approximately half of all deaths in 1990 could be attributed to the following nine factors: tobacco (400,000 deaths), diet and sedentary activity patterns (300,000 deaths), alcohol abuse (100,000 deaths), microbial agents (90,000 deaths), toxic agents (60,000 deaths), firearms (35,000 deaths), sexual behavior (30,000 deaths), motor vehicle accidents (20,000 deaths), and illicit drug use (20,000 deaths). Here, again, we see the importance of personal behavior and the environment. Socioeconomic status, although not specifically analyzed by McGinnis and Foege, is clearly a factor related to both behavior and the environment (see also Chapter 1's Recommended Reading, particularly "Highlights" from *The Socioeconomic Status and Health Chartbook: Health, United States, 1998*).

In addition to the research directly related to McKeown's work, well summarized by Colgrove (see Recommended Reading), a wide range of studies were stimulated by McKeown's work and ideas. Very important has been the work of investigators associated with the Population Health Program of the Canadian Institute for Advanced Research (CIAR) (Evans and Stoddart, 1990; Evans, Barer, and Marmor, 1994; Evans, 2002; Power and Hertzman, 1997; Michael Marmot [one of his papers is included as Article 2 in Chapter 2]; Kaplan et al., 1996), as well as Case and Paxson (2002) (see Recommended Reading).

In their seminal article "Producing Health, Consuming Health Care," Evans and Stoddart (1990) present an analytic framework for understanding the determinants of health. Their thinking grew out of the earlier work by McKeown (1976) and the 1974 report *A New Perspective on the Health of Canadians*. They found that it was impossible to include the evidence that had accumulated from many different sources on the determinants of health within the Health Field concept of the Canadian government's 1974 report. A more complex framework that could incorporate findings related to social relationships, socioeconomic status (particularly the gradient in health status across social classes), and stress was required. The framework that they developed reflected this broader understanding. A visual representation can be found in *Purchasing Population Health: Paying for Results* by David A. Kindig (1997; Figure 3 on page 12), reprinted from *Why Are Some People Healthy and Others Not? The Determinants of Health of Populations* (Evans, Barer, and Marmor, 1994).

Evans and colleagues contend that their model is more comprehensive and flexible than the traditional framework, which essentially defines health as the absence of disease or injury and presents the health care system as a feedback mechanism to disease or injury. The authors' broad, complex framework encompasses meaningful categories that are responsive and sensitive to the ways in which a variety of factors interact to determine the health status of individuals and populations. The proposed framework includes a definition of health that reflects the individual's experience as well as the perspective of the health care system. It is therefore of particular relevance to the current policy debate, as it encourages consideration of both behavioral and biological factors and acknowledges the economic trade-offs involved in the allocation of scarce resources.

In his recent monograph, *Interpreting and Addressing Inequalities in Health: From Black to Acheson to Blair to … ?* (2002), Robert Evans brilliantly summarizes and reflects on the evidence that has accumulated since the second major publication of the CIAR's *Why Are Some People Healthy and Others Not? The Determinants of Health* (Evans, Barer, and Marmor, 1994). One of the most important developments is a better understanding of the gradient in health status relating to social class, as demonstrated in the Whitehall Study of British Civil Servants, which began in 1967. A second study, the Whitehall II Study, carried out between 1985 and 1988, confirmed the earlier findings of an inverse association between employment grade and cardiovascular disease and bronchitis.

Marmot and his colleagues have reported these findings in a series of articles. In "Health inequalities among British civil servants," M. G. Marmot and associates (1994) present evidence drawn from the 1985–1988 Whitehall II Study concerning the degree and causes of differences in mortality rates in a cohort of over 10,000 British civil servants. The bearing of social class on health was evident at every level — from the lowest socioeconomic group to the highest of the British civil servants studied in Whitehall II. Those at the top of the social ladder showed lower mortality than the next highest, and so on down the social hierarchy to the lowest social classes, who showed the highest mortality rates. Self-perceived health status and symptoms were also worse in workers in the lower-status jobs.

This concept of a gradient in SES related to health status, as opposed to a threshold below which health is impaired, was a profound advance. Moreover, the inferences that can be drawn from these studies are far-reaching, including factors such as early life environment, leisure-time activity, social networks, housing circumstances, education, and control over the work environment. One of the most important findings relates to the diminished level of healthy behaviors practiced by those in the lower socioeconomic groups, which was reflected in the fact that fewer of those in lower-status jobs believed that they could reduce their risk for a heart attack. This group also demonstrated a higher incidence of smoking, less vigorous exercise, more obesity, less healthy diet patterns, and more stressful life events. Overall, the study has many important policy implications, including the fact that people in lower socioeconomic groups are not benefiting from the vast knowledge available about the close relationship between health status and behavioral factors. Furthermore, it is important to recognize that these socioeconomic factors continue to have a strong influence on this population despite the availability of universal health care through the National Health Service in the United Kingdom.

In the United States, the relationship between socioeconomic status and health was described 30 years ago by Evelyn Kitagawa and Philip Hauser (1973) and two decades later by Gregory Pappas and colleagues (1994). *Healthy People 2010* notes, "Inequalities in income and education underlie many health disparities in the United States" (U.S. Department of Health and Human Services, 2000, p. 12). Adler and Newman (2002) make the point even more strongly: "The most fundamental causes of health disparities are socioeconomic disparities" (p. 61). They examined the most important components of socioeconomic status — education, income, and occupation — and the pathways through which they might influence health. They concluded with consideration of the implications for public policies. Adler and Newman argued that SES-related health effects of the social environment may be even more important than those of the physical environment. Isolation and lack of engagement in social networks are strong predictors of health. The socially isolated have relative risks of mortality ranging from 1.9 to almost 5 times greater than those with better social connections. They also noted how little progress has been made in dealing with the broad range of SES components and the pathways (e.g., behavior, environment) by which they influence health. The emphasis in U.S. policy remains on health care, self-care, health promotion, and biomedical research, with some recent attention to public health. Many of these issues were reviewed in the 1999 Symposium of the New York Academy of Sciences (Adler et al., 1999; see Recommended Reading), as well as in Marmot's recent article (2002; Article 2) and in Evans's recent monograph (2002).

Although a growing number of studies support the view that the relationship between health and SES is best represented as a gradient and not as a threshold phenomenon, the mechanisms underlying this relationship are unclear. Many studies have focused on the behavioral characteristics of individuals of different occupations, educational attainment, income levels, and social class. Where one lives and the environment also matter. In a study of mortality rates in impoverished and nonimpoverished areas, Waitzman and Smith (1996) found in a younger group residing in the poverty area an overall mortality rate 1.5 times those in the nonpoverty area. In their paper "Socioeconomic Status and Health: The Potential Role of Environmental Risk Exposure" (included in Chapter 2 as Article 3), Evans and Kantrowitz (2002) review evidence related to the SES gradient and differential exposure to environmental risk. They documented inverse relationships between income and other indices of SES with a wide range of environmental risk factors — from hazardous wastes to neighborhood conditions. They make the point "that a particularly salient feature of poverty for health consequences is exposure to multiple environmental risk factors" (2002, p. 303).

Income inequality has also been recognized as a factor in life expectancy in industrialized countries. Wilkinson (1992) demonstrated that those industrialized countries with greater equality in income distribution had a proportionately greater increase in life expectancy. In the United States, Kaplan and colleagues (1996) demonstrated a correlation between household income and all causes of mortality, with the less fortunate demonstrating significantly higher mortality rates. Income inequality was associated with higher rates of low birth weights, homicide, violent crimes, work disability, smoking, and sedentary lifestyle. In a special issue of *Health Affairs* (Vol. 21, No. 2, March/April 2002), Marmot reviewed the evidence related to income on health. He noted, "Income is related to health in three ways, through the gross national product of countries, the income of individuals, and the income inequalities among rich nations and among geographic areas" (p. 31). In this paper, he examined two ways in which income could be causally related to health: through a direct effect on material conditions and through an effect on social participation. He concluded with some policy observations. (This paper is reprinted as Article 2 in this chapter.)

A number of studies demonstrate that access to health care alone (e.g., through the National Health Services in the United Kingdom) does not overcome the profound effects of SES on health. Indeed, the gap between the higher and lower socioeconomic groups has grown, particularly in the United States in the past 15 years, with potentially serious implications for the health of the general population.

In addition, Newacheck, Jameson, and Halfon (1994), analyzing data from the National Health Interview Study, found that low-income uninsured children are less likely than nonpoor insured children to receive timely physical and visual examinations and preventive dental care. Poor children with insurance use preventive services at about the same rate as nonpoor children with insurance. The authors conclude:

> These findings suggest expanding the provision of insurance to all low income children could help to close the remaining gaps in the use of preventive services and eventually to eliminate existing disparity in the preventable health problems described earlier (p. 232).

Recent studies by Bunker and his associates (Bunker, Frazier, and Mosteller, 1994; Bunker, 2001) suggest that personal medical care, particularly clinical preventive services, plays a larger role than in the past. They estimated that medical care contributed to 6 of the 30 years of increased life expectancy (20%) since the turn of the century and 3 of the 7 years (43%) since 1950. Medical care not only contributes to reducing premature mortality and increasing life expectancy, but also significantly influences quality of life. Several examples include cataract surgery, total hip replacement and coronary artery bypass graft surgeries, and the treatment of hypertension, stroke, and many chronic illnesses. Together, these studies clearly illustrate the importance of both population-based (public health) and individually directed (personal medical/health care) approaches to the reduction in premature mortality and morbidity.

The issues of race, class, and health status have been examined by Navarro (1990), Pappas and colleagues (1994), Williams and Collins (1995), and Krieger, Williams, and Moss (1997). Although much of the premature mortality in African Americans can be attributed to socioeconomic status, race is of great significance when considering such problems as low birth weight, homicide, diabetes mellitus, and access to medical care. Pappas also notes that the most important factor in the increasing difference in life expectancy between whites and blacks is related to the slower decline in heart disease mortality in blacks in recent decades. Navarro's (1990) analysis suggests that the mortality differentials by social class are greater than mortality differentials due to race. Another poorly understood area is whether and how social differences in health vary by age groups across the life course. Such data are essential to formulating and targeting effective public health policies (Jefferys, 1996).

An important paper by Power and Hertzman (1997) examines the evidence for a pathway linking early life factors and adult disease (see Recommended Reading). Their analysis, which is fairly technical, takes into account "the interrelationships between social and biological risks throughout the life course" (p. 210). They carefully examine the association between birth weight, placenta size, and weight gain in the first year of life with cardiovascular disease in the fifth decade. In addition to this "latency" model, they propose a "pathways" model that relates early life events to subsequent life trajectories. The complex relationships between "latency" and "pathway" effects are illustrated by examination of data from the 1958 birth cohort study in the United Kingdom, in which subjects have been tracked from birth to 33 years as of the most recent follow-up. The data show a clear relationship between social class at birth and health status in early adulthood. The impact of social class differences on health was smallest for males with back pain and greatest for obesity, respiratory symptoms, psychological distress, and poor/fair self-rated health status.

Kuh and Ben-Shlomo (1997) have reviewed the evidence supporting the importance of early life factors for adult chronic disease. They noted that the scientific literature includes a large number of scattered observations that associate a range of early life factors (particularly related to deprivation) with later adult risk factors or disease. Conditions included cardiovascular disease and its risk factors, chronic bronchitis, thyroid function, allergy, stomach cancer, and even suicide. This very interesting book is listed in the Recommended Reading.

In summary, Chapter 2 deals with the growing body of knowledge related to the multiple determinants of the health of populations, particularly the importance of socioeconomic status. Although knowledge of the determinants of health has grown dramatically in the past 30 years and is beginning to influence health policies at the national, state, and local levels, it has had relatively little impact on biomedical research policies or on the allocation of resources to achieve national health goals. Management of the nation's health problems requires different strategies than those that were successful when infectious diseases were the leading killers. We can no longer rely solely on traditional public health and cures of modern medicine but must combine these with measures and policies related to a broad array of socioeconomic factors (e.g., occupation, education, housing). Today, ensuring good health and controlling disease requires a focus on the determinants of health, including the following:

- *Social conditions,* such as socioeconomic status, income disparities, family, and group and community social support.
- *Physical, chemical, and biological hazards in the external environment,* including contaminated food and water, air pollution, radiation, agents used by terrorists (e.g., smallpox, anthrax), and automobiles.
- *Lifestyle* (individual behavior), including diet; physical activity; the use of alcohol, tobacco, and seat belts; and sexual behavior. Unhealthy behaviors such as cigarette smoking and substance abuse are often inversely related to socioeconomic status.
- *Human biology* (e.g., genetics), which governs predisposition to developing clinical illness in relation to environmental exposure.
- *Access to public health and clinical services* for prevention, early detection, and treatment.

The challenge the determinants of health pose to policymakers was well summarized almost a decade ago by Nancy Moss (1995):

> The message of *Why Are Some People Healthy and Others Not?* points to a much broader, deeper, and more difficult policy question: How can we increase equity in occupational hierarchies and occupational positions, reduce disparities of wealth and income, and diminish the contributions of gender and racial/ethnic divisions that cut across and undergird social class to reduce differentials in health and mortality? This challenge, particularly in the current U.S. political environment, makes the recent struggle for health care reform look like a breeze (p. 324).

REFERENCES

Adler, N. E., and Newman, K. (2002). Socioeconomic disparities in health: Pathways and policies. Inequality in education, income, and occupation exacerbates the gaps between the health "haves" and "have-nots." *Health Affairs, 21* (2), 60–76.

Bunker, J. P. (2001). *Medicine matters after all: Measuring the benefits of medical care, a healthy lifestyle, and a just social environment* (J. Nuffield Trust Series No. 15). London: The Stationery Office.

Bunker, J. P., Frazier, H. S., and Mosteller, R. (1994). Improving health: Measuring effects of medical care. *Milbank Quarterly 2,* 225–258.

Colgrove, J. (2002). The McKeown thesis: A historical controversy and its enduring influence. *American Journal of Public Health, 92* (5), 725–729.

Evans, G., and Kantrowitz, E. (2002). Socioeconomic status and health: The potential role of environmental risk exposure. *Annual Review of Public Health, 23,* 303–325.

Evans, R. (2002). *Interpreting and addressing inequalities in health: From black to Acheson to Blair to...*? Whitehall, London: Office of Health Economics.

Evans, R. G., Barer, M. L., and Marmor, T. R. (Eds). (1994). *Why are some people healthy and others not? The determinants of health of populations.* New York: Aldine De Gruyter.

Evans, R. G., and Stoddart, G. (1990). Producing health, consuming health care. *Social Science and Medicine, 31* (12), 1347–1363.

Jefferys, M. (1996). Social inequalities in health: Do they diminish with age? *American Journal of Public Health, 86*, 474–475.

Kaplan, G. A., Pamuk, E. R., Lynch, J. W., Cohen, R. D., and Balfour, J. L. (1996). Inequality in income and mortality in the United States: Analysis of mortality and potential pathways. *British Medical Journal, 312,* 999–1003.

Kindig, D. A. (1997). *Purchasing population health: Paying for results.* Ann Arbor: University of Michigan Press.

Kitagawa, E., and Hauser, P. (1973). *Differential mortality in the United States: A study of socioeconomic epidemiology.* Cambridge, MA: Harvard University Press.

Krieger, N., Williams, D. R., and Moss, N. E. (1997). Measuring social class in U.S. public health research: Concepts, methodologies, and guidelines. *Annual Review of Public Health, 18*, 341–378.

Kuh, D., and Ben-Shlomo, Y. (Eds.). (1997). *A life course approach to chronic disease epidemiology*. Oxford/New York: Oxford University Press.

Lalonde, M. (1974). *A new perspective on the health of Canadians*. Ottawa: National Ministry of Health and Welfare.

Link, B. G., and Phelan, J. C. (2002). McKeown and the idea that social conditions are fundamental causes of disease. *American Journal of Public Health, 92* (5), 730–732.

Marmot, M. (2002). The influence of income on health: Views of an epidemiologist. *Health Affairs, 21* (2), 31–44.

Marmot, M. G., Davey Smith, G., Stansfield, S., Patel, C., North, F., Head, J., White, I., Brunner, E., and Feeney, A. (1994). Health inequalities and social class. In P. R. Lee and C. L. Estes (Eds.), *The nation's health* (4th ed., pp. 34–40). Boston: Jones and Bartlett. Abridged from *Lancet*, 1991;337:1387, under the original title "Health inequalities among British civil servants: The Whitehall II study."

McGinnis, J. M., and Foege, W. H. (1993). Actual causes of death in the United States. *Journal of the American Medical Association, 270,* 2207–2212.

McKeown, T. (1976). *The modern rise of populations.* New York: Academic Press.

McKeown, T. (1978). Determinants of health. *Human Nature,* April 1978.

McKeown, T. (1979). *The role of medicine: Dream, mirage, or nemesis?* Princeton, NJ: Princeton University Press.

McKeown, T., and Brown, R. G. (1955). Medical evidence related to English population changes in the eighteenth century. *Population Studies, 9,* 119–141.

McKeown, T., and Record, R. G. (1962). Reasons for the decline of mortality in England and Wales during the 19th century. *Population Studies, 16,* 94–122.

Moss, N. (1995). Social inequalities in health. *Health Affairs, 14* (2), 321–325.

Navarro, V. (1990). Race or class versus race and class: Mortality differentials in the United States. *Lancet, 336,* 1238–1240.

Newacheck, P., Jameson, W. J., and Halfon, N. (1994). Health status and income: The impact of poverty on child health. *Journal of School Health, 64,* 229–233.

Pappas, G., Queen, S., Hadden, W., Fisher, G. (1994). The increasing disparity in mortality between socioeconomic groups in the United States, 1960 and 1986. *New England Journal of Medicine, 329* (2),103–109.

Power, C., and Hertzman, C. (1997). Social and biological pathways linking early life and adult disease. *British Medical Bulletin, 53* (1), 210–221.

Szreter, S. (2002). Rethinking McKeown: The relationship between public health and social change. *American Journal of Public Health, 92* (5), 722–724.

U.S. Department of Health and Human Services. (1980). *Ten leading causes of death in the United States in 1977.* Atlanta, GA: Centers for Disease Control and Prevention.

U.S. Department of Health and Human Services. (2000). *Healthy People 2010: Understanding and Improving Health.* Washington, DC: U.S. Government Printing Office.

Waitzman, N. J., and Smith, K. R. (1996). *Phantom of the area: poverty, residence and mortality in the U.S.* Paper presented at the Forum on Social and Economic Disparities in Health and Health Care, Salt Lake City, UT.

Wilkinson, R. G. (1992). Income distribution and life expectancy. *British Medical Journal, 304,* 165–168.

Williams, D. R., and Collins, C. (1995). U.S. socioeconomic and racial differences in health: Patterns and explanations. *Annual Review of Sociology, 21,* 349–386.

ARTICLE 1

McKeown and the Idea That Social Conditions Are Fundamental Causes of Disease

Bruce G. Link and Jo C. Phelan

In an accompanying commentary, Colgrove indicates that McKeown's thesis — that dramatic reductions in mortality over the past two centuries were due to improved socioeconomic conditions rather than to medical or public health interventions — has been "overturned" and his theory "discredited."

McKeown sought to explain a very prominent trend in population health and did so with a strong emphasis on the importance of basic social and economic conditions. If Colgrove is right about the McKeown thesis, social epidemiology is left with a gaping hole in its explanatory repertoire and a challenge to a cherished principle about the importance of social factors in health.

We return to the trend McKeown focused upon — post-McKeown and post-Colgrove — to indicate how and why social conditions must continue to be seen as fundamental causes of disease.

The McKeown thesis states that the enormous increase in population and dramatic improvements in health that humans have experienced over the past two centuries owe more to changes in broad economic and social conditions than to specific medical advances or public health initiatives.[1] The thesis gives center stage to social conditions as root causes of the health of populations. On the basis of new data and numerous revisitations, however, Colgrove[2] tells us that the thesis has been "overturned" and the theory "discredited." Whither, then, the idea that social conditions require prominence in any complete understanding of the health of populations? When we turn away from "the thesis," do we accept an "antithesis" asserting that the role of social conditions is insignificant?

WHY SOCIAL CONDITIONS REMAIN IMPORTANT

To answer this question, we turn to a central element of the thesis. McKeown is frequently cited for the relatively small role he assigns to specifically health-directed human agency — to purposive action initiated by medical and public health practitioners. For example, Colgrove characterizes the McKeown thesis as follows: "… the rise in population was due less to human agency in the form of health-enhancing measures than to largely invisible economic forces that changed broad social conditions."[2(p725)] In this construction, if social conditions gain explanatory prominence, human agency loses it. We believe this formulation needs to be turned inside out to assert that as health-directed human agency gains explanatory prominence, so do social conditions.

Our "fundamental social causes" approach argues that, when a population develops the wherewithal to avoid disease and death, individuals' ability to benefit from that wherewithal is shaped by resources of knowledge, money, power, prestige, and beneficial social connections.[3–6] People who command more of these resources are able to gain a health advantage — that is, to benefit from the fruits of "human agency for public health" to a greater extent than people who are less well endowed with respect to these resources. Resources are important in at least two ways. First, resources directly shape individual health behaviors by influencing whether people know about, have access to, can afford, and are supported in their efforts to engage in health enhancing behaviors. Second, resources shape access to broad contexts such as neighborhoods, occupations, and social networks that vary dramatically in associated profiles of risk and protective factors. Housing that poor people can afford is more likely to be located near noise, pollution, and noxious social conditions; blue-collar occupations tend to be more dangerous than white-collar occupations, and social networks with high-status peers are less likely to expose a person to secondhand smoke.

As a consequence of these processes, access to a broad range of circumstances that affect health are shaped by socioeconomic resources. Examples include access to the best doctors; knowing about and asking for beneficial health procedures; having friends and family who support healthy lifestyles; quitting smoking; getting flu shots; wearing seat belts; eating fruits and vegetables; exercising regularly; living in neighborhoods where garbage is picked up frequently, interiors are lead-free, and streets are safe; having children who bring home useful health information from good schools; working in safe occupational circumstances; and taking restful vacations. Critically, the reason social conditions are always prominent and always important is that resources shape access to health-relevant circumstances, whatever the list of such resources happens to contain in a given time or place.

Thus, socioeconomic resources were equally as useful in avoiding the worst sanitation, housing, and industrial conditions of the 19th century as they are in shaping access to the current circumstances just enumerated. In the future, as new discoveries expand our ability to control disease processes, new items will be added to the list of health-enhancing circumstances, and, our theory says, people who command more resources will be advantaged in benefiting from the new knowledge we obtain. For this reason, social conditions have been, are, and will continue to be irreducible determinants of health outcomes and thereby deserve their appellation of "fundamental causes" of disease and death. Social conditions achieve this status not because they are independent from and dominate over human agency but rather because they shape the distribution of the health-enhancing circumstances that health-directed human agency provides. It is effective human agency directed toward enhancing health that ensures the fundamental importance of social conditions in patterns of disease and death.

EXPLAINING GRADIENTS – EXPLAINING LEVELS

But the astute reader will recognize that we have engaged in a shift of focus away from the problem McKeown addressed. McKeown's thesis concerned the importance of social and economic conditions for absolute levels of population health over time. In contrast, the "fundamental cause" perspective seeks to explain the persistence over time of associations between social factors like socioeconomic status (SES) and health outcomes within populations. Figure 1 illustrates this difference — McKeown sought to explain a temporal improvement in life expectancy, among other things, with improving socioeconomic conditions (the upward slope in life expectancy with time), whereas the fundamental cause approach seeks to explain why the gap between high and low SES has been so persistent across time (the gap between the lines). Of course, actual trends have not been as constant or as linear as Figure 1 depicts them — the health gap between high and low SES has been variable and by some accounts increasing in the United States in recent years, and the trend toward improved health has not progressed in lockstep fashion. Still, the figure identifies two major empirical regularities — a prominent SES gap and a general trend toward improved health — to which a thorough social epidemiology must attend. McKeown focused on the second of these empirical regularities while the fundamental cause approach, up until now, has emphasized the first.

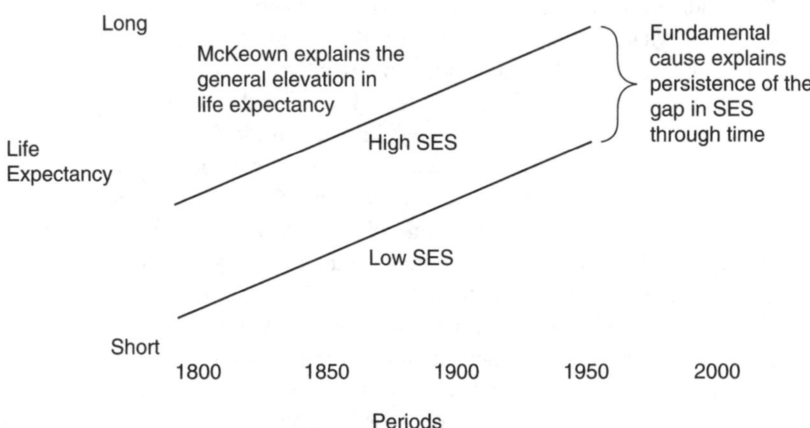

Note: SES = socioeconomic status. The diagram seeks to illustrate the issues and not to precisely describe actual patterns over time.

Figure 1 Illustration of differences between the problem addressed by McKeown and the problem addressed by the fundamental causes approach.

The fundamental cause approach is not alone in its focus on trends that differ from those addressed by McKeown. During the last decade, social epidemiology has been dominated by studies of income inequality in geographic areas and levels of population health in those areas. The idea is that areas with greater income inequality (nations, states, census tracts) experience worse health than areas with less inequality even when the median income of the areas is held constant. Like McKeown, this literature focuses on levels of population health (albeit in geographic areas rather than across time) and therefore might be expected to account for, or at least cohere with, the trends that McKeown addressed. But income inequality turns out to be an unusually poor explanation for trends toward better health over time. If income inequality drives population health, such inequality would need to have been dramatically reduced over time in order to explain the enormous improvements in life expectancy that human beings have experienced. Of course, nothing like such a diminution in inequality has occurred; something else must be driving the powerful trend toward improvements in life expectancy. Thus, if Colgrove is correct and McKeown's thesis has been "overturned," a major trend remains insufficiently examined and insufficiently understood.

POPULATION HEALTH IN A FUNDAMENTAL CAUSE PERSPECTIVE

We return to the question McKeown posed from the vantage point of a fundamental cause perspective and ask whether such a perspective can be usefully applied to this question. We believe the answer is yes if we return with a broadened view of what constitutes public health action or human agency directed toward public health matters. The broadened view asks us to move from a conception of public health action that focuses on what medical and public health operatives do to a conception that focuses more generally on human actions that have important health consequences. Note that, as paraphrased by Colgrove, the McKeown thesis pits the narrower of these two conceptions against largely invisible economic forces. If we apply our broader conception, however, the argument becomes not whether public health action had effects but whose public health action had them. Certainly at some point in the chain of events between improving economic conditions and declining mortality trends, people decided to use newly acquired resources to obtain adequate food, clothing, and shelter for themselves and their families. This did not require a public education effort or some other action by medical or public health operatives. People used resources available to them to garner a health advantage. On the basis of this broader view, we can apply to McKeown's problem two principles from the fundamental cause approach: (1) people with superior resources can use those resources to garner health advantages, and (2) the specific mechanisms that allow advantage to accrue change from place to place and from time to time. Thus, in this formulation, people living in more recent times are akin to people of higher SES — they use their more plentiful resources to gain health outcomes that are superior to those of people living in earlier times. Moreover, the principal reasons for improvement in a population's health change over time. For example, the reasons the US population is doing better now than in 1975 are vastly different from the reasons the US population was better off in 1900 than it was in 1875. What this means is that a thesis like McKeown's that focuses attention on basic needs for nutrition and away from medical and public health actions may have been correct for some — perhaps large — periods of time but is not as helpful at explaining more recent trends in modern industrialized societies. However, at all times, both social conditions and health-directed human agency are key to health improvements — social and economic conditions provide the resources that enable humans to enhance their health. Thus, while we might disagree with some aspects of McKeown's thesis, we are led to agree with his assertion that social conditions are fundamental causes of disease and death.

We end with another lesson the McKeown thesis provides for public health in the modern era. Criticisms of McKeown focus on his minimizing the role of public health and medical interventions, not on the idea that an expansion of economic resources led to improved nutrition and better health. This eminently reasonable aspect of his thesis alerts us that factors not typically conceptualized as relevant to health can have tremendous impacts on health outcome. Thus, we need to be mindful of the potential health impact of the entire array of social, political, and economic policy we humans develop, such as social security, child welfare, education, or the location of potentially polluting industries.[3] When we understand the impact of broad policies like these, we will at least have the possibility of shaping population health through a judicious consideration of the health consequences such policies carry. We believe that it is in this broadening of perspective that public health will find its best response to social conditions that act as fundamental causes of disease.

ACKNOWLEDGMENTS

This work was supported by a Health Policy Investigator Award to both authors from the Robert Wood Johnson Foundation.

We thank Ana Diez-Roux for comments.

REFERENCES

1. McKeown T. *The Role of Medicine: Dream, Mirage or Nemesis?* London, England: Nuffield Provincial Hospitals Trust; 1976.

2. Colgrove J. The McKeown thesis: a historical controversy and its enduring influence. *Am J Public Health.* 2002;92:725–729.

3. Link BG, Phelan JC. Social conditions as fundamental causes of disease. *J Health Soc Behav*. 1995;(extra issue):80–94.

4. Link BG, Phelan JC. Understanding sociodemographic differences in health: the role of fundamental social causes. *Am J Public Health*. 1996;86:471–473.

5. Link BG, Northridge M, Phelan JC, Ganz MC. Social epidemiology and the fundamental cause concept: on the structuring of effective cancer screens by socioeconomic status. *Millbank Q*. 1998;76:375–402.
6. Link BG, Phelan JC. Evaluating the fundamental cause explanation for social disparities in health. In: CE Bird, P Conrad, A Fremont, eds. *Handbook of Medical Sociology*. Upper Saddler River, NJ: Prentice Hall; 2000:33–46.

ARTICLE 2

The Influence of Income on Health

Views of an Epidemiologist

Michael Marmot

DOES MONEY MATTER FOR HEALTH? If so, why? If it does matter, there are at least three ways in which it could be important: not having enough money, maldistribution of money, and spending it on the wrong things. It is also possible that health could matter for money, that the causal direction could be the other way around.

Of course, money could only appear to matter. It may be that poor people have worse health not because they have insufficient money but for some other reason. Similarly, a society characterized by a high degree of income inequality could have poor average health for reasons other than the distribution of income. Or countries that spend more money on surgeons may have better health because they are democratic, not because of the surgery. In each of these cases, money appears to matter because it is a marker for something else.

The distinction between really mattering and appearing to matter is important. For example, if it really matters, a policy devoted to income redistribution could have health benefits. If it only appears to matter, such a policy, whatever other positive or negative features it might have, will not benefit health. This is important for policy, and I return to it after considering the evidence.

In asking if money matters, two types of evidence are relevant: the relation of income to health between and within countries, and the relation of income inequality to health. I also deal with two related debates: the degree to which the apparent relation of income to health should be thought of as a question of poverty or inequality; and the role of material and psychosocial factors in generating inequalities in health. I note that there is evidence that health can affect income, but that it is not the major explanation of the link between income and health. This has been dealt with elsewhere.[1]

I confine my attention largely to the rich countries of the world, not because the problems of health inequalities are absent from poor countries, but because the policy questions are different — lack of sanitation, clean water, and adequate nutrition, for a start — although I suspect that some of the policy questions may not be so different.

ASPECTS OF POVERTY: MATERIAL CONDITIONS AND SOCIAL PARTICIPATION

We cannot discuss income without considering its lack: poverty. There has been a long debate as to the merits of describing poverty in absolute or relative terms.[2] To understand why income may be important for health, it is worth distinguishing two aspects of low income, which for simplicity I label "poor material conditions" and "lack of social participation."

Let me illustrate with a simple thought experiment. Suppose there were a set of material conditions, such as clean water and good sanitation, adequate nutrition, and adequate housing and warmth, that were necessary for good health. Suppose, too, that these material conditions were correlated with income until a threshold was reached. Clean water is necessary for good health. Once water is safe, higher income does not make it safer. Below the threshold, the lower the income, the worse the health because of the link with material conditions. Above the threshold level, differences in material conditions no longer have any plausible connection with differences in pathology. For people above the threshold, there still could be substantial inequalities in health that are related to differing opportunities for social participation, for leading a fulfilling and satisfying life, and for control over one's life. Depending on how society was organized, these opportunities could show a strong direct link with individual income. In this case, income would be causally linked to health, albeit not through material conditions. Alternatively, the link to income of opportunities for participation and control could be more tenuous, in which case, once the threshold was reached, the relation of income to health would be weaker. Other socioeconomic markers, more strongly related to participation and control, would show a stronger relation to health.

One could argue that it mattered little which pathway was important, material conditions or participation. If there were a link between income and health, a policy of equalizing incomes would reduce health inequalities. But what if such a policy were politically unacceptable? Do we not need to understand why incomes might be related to ill health in order to have the possibility to interrupt the chain of causation from economic position to health?

A second reason for making the distinction between material conditions and participation is that the latter constitutes an important part of what people report poverty is about in Britain and other European countries. Poverty includes not having a hobby or leisure activity, not having friends or family around for a snack, not taking children swimming, not having a family holiday. These are related to individual incomes to a greater or lesser extent depending on purchasing power and public provision. They are not "material," in the sense that clean water and good sanitation are.

A third reason for making the distinction is that one can envisage circumstances in which there is a threshold level above which material conditions no longer influence health, but degree of participation and control could show no such threshold. Inequalities in these could account for inequalities in health above a threshold of material provision. Conversely, people who are relatively poor could have good health if their social participation were high.

With these distinctions in mind, it is helpful to develop a little historical perspective on the question of poverty and health.

POVERTY AND HEALTH IN PERSPECTIVE

Infant Mortality

Infant mortality traditionally has been viewed as the measure of health, more strictly ill health, that is most sensitive to poverty. Let us look at one historical example.

Benjamin Seebohm Rowntree was the son of Joseph Rowntree, a chocolate manufacturer, Quaker, and philanthropist in York, England. B.S. Rowntree conducted a study to draw attention to the conditions of what he called the working-class population. He studied three typical areas of the town that housed the working class, grading them according to their degree of poverty.[3]

Infant mortality rates (the number of deaths in the first year of life compared with the number of live births) varied according to area. In the worst-off area the rate was 247 per 1,000 live births; in the middle working-class area, 184 per 1,000; and in the highest, 173. By contrast, among York's "servant-keeping class" it was 94.

Rowntree was ready to attribute the high rate in the poorest area to overcrowding and poor-quality housing. He wondered why the rate in the highest working-class area was double that of the servant-keeping class. In the highest working-class area there was no overcrowding and no back-to-back houses but, rather, wide streets and houses with gardens. To Rowntree, this did not provide a ready explanation. He concluded that the cause must be ignorance — ignorance in the feeding and management of infants "rather than to other causes arising out of the poverty of the people."

Ignorance versus Poor Conditions

This view — that there is no relation between poverty and health and that it is all due to ignorance — was still being propounded in Britain in the 1980s by government ministers. To put it kindly, it was a limited view in the 1980s, as it was eighty years earlier. We now have a different view.

Even were it true that the high infant mortality of the higher working class was due to ignorance, how are we to account for an infant mortality rate of 94 per 1,000 among the wealthiest people of York around 1900? In England and Wales infant mortality in 2000 was 3.7 per 1,000 among infants born to fathers in the top social class and 8.1 among those born into the bottom class.[4] Among single mothers, the rate was 7.6. The richer members of the community at the end of the nineteenth century had infant mortality rates that were much higher than the worst-off members of the community at the end of the twentieth century.

What are the implications of this comparison? The major determinants of high infant mortality are those associated with poverty of material conditions: lack of sanitation; malnutrition; low-quality housing and overcrowding; and lack of medical care including care before, during, and after childbirth. The threefold higher infant mortality rate of the poorest people of York was the result of worse conditions. It is less clear why the best-off people of 1900 should have so much higher rates than the worst-off in the country 100 years later. We can guess that although privileged economically, they were "deprived" of the conditions for low infant mortality: good sanitation, nutrition, and medical care.

Condition of the Community

This is a rather dramatic clue that factors other than individual income play a powerful role in the determinants of health conditions that we associate with poverty. This is a conclusion reached by Sam Preston.[5] Two tentative conclusions from this example run through the discussion that follows. First, we should not view individual incomes in isolation from the community in which people are located. The rich people of York in 1900, in some relevant respects, lived under worse conditions than do poor people in the same city a century later. The community is richer now. Money and technical knowledge have allowed the community to invest in conditions that favor an alleviation of the conditions that lead to high infant mortality. If we are using individual income as a measure of standard of living, then it does only a partial job, because it misses out on the benefits to be derived from living in a richer community.

Black-White Health Differences

The second conclusion relates to the first. In Preston's terms, factors "exogenous" to income have been responsible for much of the health improvement in the twentieth century. Putting the infant mortality of social class V or single mothers for the year 2000, 7.9 per 1,000, beside that of the servant-keeping class of York for 1900 suggests that the problems of ill health due to material deprivation have, to a large extent, been solved in today's industrialized countries. Why then should such countries continue to suffer from large inequalities in health?

One could argue that the "high" infant mortality rate of 15 per 1,000 among U.S. blacks in 2000, although a fraction of the servant-keeper rates of the past, was still due to residual problems of material deprivation: poor sanitation, inadequate nutrition, and poor housing.[6] This is a possibility that must be considered.

But infant mortality is not the main reason for black-white differences in life expectancy in the United States. Arline Geronimus studied sixteen U.S. communities, black and white.[7] In the United States as a whole, the probability of a fifteen-year-old man surviving to age sixty-five was about 77 percent. For a young black man in New York the probability of survival was 37 percent. The three major causes of death contributing to this tragic waste of life were HIV-related factors, homicide, and cardiovascular disease. We do not think that heart disease is related to poor sanitation, malnutrition, and overcrowded conditions in houses without gardens; not, in other words, to material deprivation of 100 years ago. Can material deprivation explain that? If we want to describe coronary heart disease as a disease of poverty, reversing the decades-long practice of describing it as a disease of affluence, we must take a hard look at what we mean by poverty.

POVERTY AND INEQUALITY

Since the 1960s British researchers have been conducting longitudinal studies of British civil servants, the Whitehall studies.[8] A twenty-five-year follow-up from the first Whitehall study found that the higher the position in the occupational hierarchy, the lower the mortality rate from all causes, from coronary heart disease, and from a range of diseases not related to smoking (Figure 1).[9] It should be borne in mind that none of these men was poor in any usual sense of that word. They were all in stable, office-based employment in and around Whitehall, London.

The civil service excludes the richest and poorest of society. Yet among these men there is more than a twofold difference in mortality rates, over the twenty-five years of follow-up, between top and bottom. Also, among these men there is a social gradient in health that runs from top to bottom of the social hierarchy. There is no clear point with good health above and poor health below.

One might assume that something peculiar to the class-based nature of the British civil service accounts for this remarkable social gradient. Not so. For example, a recent publication on British national data classified areas into twentieths according to degree of deprivation.[10] There is no evidence of a threshold, but a clear gradient in mortality for the general population runs from the least to the most deprived.

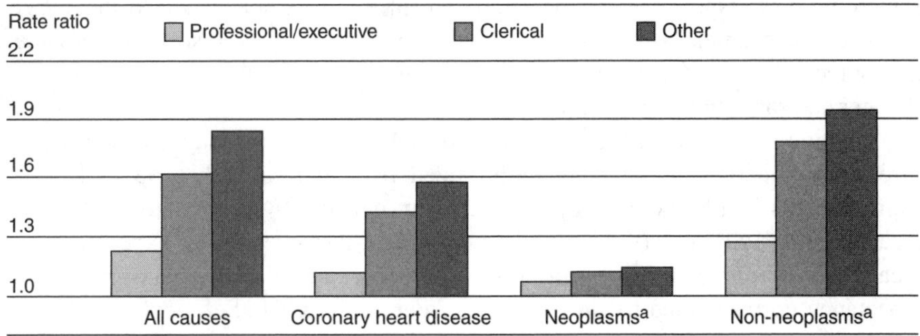

SOURCES: C. van Rossum et al., "Employment Grade Differences in Cause Specific Mortality: Twenty-five Year Follow Up of Civil Servants from the First Whitehall Study," *Journal of Epidemiology and Community Health* (March 2000): 178–184.

NOTE: Ratios are relative to the administrative grade, which equals 1 and is not shown.

[a] Not related to smoking.

Figure 1 Whitehall 25-year mortality (British civil servants), by employment grade.

I have argued, on the basis of the Whitehall findings, that the problem for the rich countries today is inequality in health rather than poverty and health.[11] For me the distinction is important. Doorkeepers and messengers in the British civil service are not poor compared with the working-class poor of late nineteenth-century York. If we are dealing with poverty in Britain and the United States, it is in general a different type of poverty than that of nineteenth-century York or of the poorest countries today. Because health follows a social gradient, if we wish to talk of deprivation, we have to appeal to the concept of relative deprivation.

DIRECT EFFECTS OF INCOME

The question of whether money matters can be approached in two ways: comparison of countries; and studies of the relationship between income and mortality within countries.

Comparisons of Countries

A 1993 World Bank report examined the relationship between life expectancy and gross national product (GNP) per capita in more than 100 countries from about 1900 to 1990.[12] It extended the work of Preston, who showed these relationships for an earlier period.[13] The report makes two key points. First, at low levels of GNP, a small increase in GNP corresponds to a large increase in life expectancy. As GNP increases, the relation levels off. Above about $5,000 per capita in 1991, there is a shallow relationship between a country's average income and life expectancy.

Second, for a given GNP, life expectancy increased during the twentieth century. This suggests that the finding in York was part of a general pattern. In 1900 rich people in York had high infant mortality rates compared with those rates 100 years later. Something was responsible for the improvement that was not related to income. I speculate that even the servant-keepers would have been subject to some of the same environmental insults that we now associate with deprivation. With the improvement of water and sanitation, for example, this was removed.

That improvements in life expectancy in rich countries can happen for reasons unrelated to income was further emphasized by Amartya Sen.[14] He looked at improvements in life expectancy in Britain by decade, from 1901 to 1960. The decades 1911–1921 and 1941–1951 had the fastest increases in life expectancy — decades that embraced the World Wars. These decades of fast expansion in life expectancy corresponded to slow growth of per capita GDP. Sen doubts that it is simply a time lag between economic growth and reduction of mortality rates. He attributes the rapid improvement in life expectancy in the two decades to policies of support: sharing of means of survival, including sharing of health care and the limited food supply (through rationing and subsidized nutrition). The psychology of sharing in beleaguered Britain made radical public arrangements for the distribution of food and health care acceptable and effective. Even the National Health Service (NHS) was born during the war years of World War II.

In the introduction I suggested that the commonalities between rich and poor countries might be greater than they appear. Sen attributes improvements in life expectancy in poor countries despite sluggish economic growth to "support-led" strategies; these include spending on public goods such as education, public health, and basic health care.

Income and Health within Rich Countries

The United States. If average income as measured by GNP is weakly related to overall health among rich countries, what do we find when we make comparisons within these countries? That is, the previous section relates to country averages. Now let us group individuals within one country, such as the United States, according to their income and ask how it relates to health.

Figure 2 shows an example. It comes from the U.S. Panel Study of Income Dynamics, a national sample of people who have been followed since 1972.[15] The high-income group, with average household income greater than $70,000, is the standard to which all others are compared. The low-income group, with household income below $15,000, had 3.9 times the mortality rate of the best-off, but there is a gradient: The higher the income, the lower the mortality. Although the bottom group has particularly high mortality, it accounts for about 7 percent of the population. This means that its members make a relatively modest contribution to all of the deaths that can be attributed to having an income below the highest level. More of the excess death will come from the 30 percent of the population in the $30,001–$50,000 range, who have 59 percent more mortality than is true of the richest group.

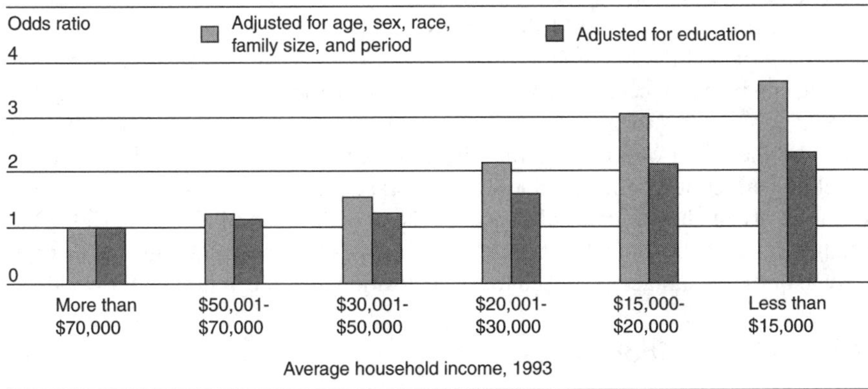

SOURCE: P. McDonough et al., "Income Dynamics and Adult Mortality in the United States, 1972 through 1989," *American Journal of Public Health* (September 1997): 1476–1483.

Figure 2 Risk of death according to household income, shown as odds ratios with and without adjustment for education, persons ages 45–64.

Canada. A similar continuous relation between income and mortality has been shown in Canada.[16] The relative measure means that as you move from the top income to the $30,000–$50,000 range, mortality is multiplied about 1.6 times. As you move down two further categories, to the $15,000–$20,000 range, it is multiplied by about 1.9 again, to give three times higher mortality than is true for the group with the highest income. But this approximately constant relative increase must correspond to an increasing mortality disadvantage if measured on an absolute scale. To illustrate, suppose that the annual mortality rates in the three income categories just described were 1 percent, 1.6 percent, and 3 percent, respectively. The increase in mortality in going from the richest to the $30,000–$50,000 range is 0.6 percent per year. The further increase in going down to the $15,000–$20,000 range is 1.4 percent — more than twice as great.

Impact of Redistribution of Income

Angus Deaton has shown this nonlinear increase in probability of dying with decreasing income.[17] He draws an important implication from this. If at low levels of GNP, a small increase corresponds to a large increase in longevity, then taking some money from rich people will have less effect on their mortality than giving the same money to the poor will affect theirs. Therefore, other things being equal, a population with more egalitarian distribution of income will have better health than another with the same average income but greater income inequality. Whether this would work as a policy depends on losses in the system. I return to this in the next section.

Education Factor

There is another point worth emphasizing about Figure 2. The relative risk of mortality rises in monotonic fashion with falling income throughout the range. This suggests that income is measuring something that is causally related to mortality throughout the range of incomes. Notice that I did not say that income was causally related. One might have gained the impression from the World Bank study that there would be little relation between income and mortality above about $5,000. Yet as Figure 2 shows, the relation is quite strong up to about $50,000. That it may not be income itself is shown by the effect of adjusting for education. Once education is included in the model, the effect of income on mortality is markedly reduced. This may be because education affects health precisely because those with more education have higher incomes. It could, however, be because education is a better indicator than is income of some of the social factors, linked to social position, that are important for health.

Material Deprivation Divide

One way of interpreting the international data is that the level of income of about $5,000 defines material deprivation, as used in this paper. The strong relationship between income and life expectancy below this level results from the relationship of material deprivation to ill health.

This would imply that more or less everyone in the United States is above the level of material deprivation. The relationship between income and mortality up to incomes of $50,000 reflects something other than material deprivation, perhaps participation or the complex of factors that underlies Sen's notion of the "support-led" route to low mortality.

Income as Measure of Social Position

This is consistent with income's defining position in a hierarchy relative to the prevailing standards of society. It may not be income itself that matters, except insofar as it determines ability to participate in the way defined as acceptable by society. To put it more generally, income is an impoverished way of capturing the condition of life that gives rise to health differences. This is illustrated by a comparison of life expectancy among black American men compared with men in Costa Rica. GNP in Costa Rica is around $2,800, and life expectancy for men is seventy-four years.[18] Among U.S. blacks, mean income is around $26,000, and life expectancy is sixty-six years.[19] We can adjust for the fact that a dollar in Costa Rica buys more than a dollar in the United States by using a measure of purchasing power parity, taking the United States as standard. This suggests that we should think of the GNP in Costa Rica as more like $6,600 than $2,800. This comparison suggests that four times the income among U.S. blacks compared with Costa Ricans goes along with eight years fewer in life expectancy.

I am not using this comparison to argue that poverty is not a problem for U.S. black men or that the social conditions under which black people live in the United States are irrelevant to health. I am using it to argue that important as money might be, we need to go beyond absolute measures of income to understand the relation between social position and health — to understand how social factors affect the position in which people find themselves and hence their health.

Occupational Hierarchy. This is even more obviously the case when we return to the social gradient in people who are not below the poverty level. In the Whitehall II study of British civil servants, ten years after the study began we added measures of household income and wealth. Two particular measures of health that we have been studying are a general question of self-perceived health and questions designed to elicit symptoms of depressive illness.[20] It turns out that both of these are related to household income in monotonic fashion: The higher the income, the more likely people are to report themselves in good health and the less likely to report depression. Income is only one measure of social position. In Whitehall II the most powerful predictor has always been position in the occupational hierarchy (that is, grade of employment). A statistician's way of testing out which is more important, grade or income, is to put them both into a predictive equation and see if they still predict. When we do this, income is no longer a predictor of ill health and depression. Grade wins this particular battle.

A tentative conclusion is that in a population above the poverty level, income is important as a predictor of ill health because it is a measure of where a person is in the social hierarchy, rather than because of pounds, dollars, or euros in the pocket.

Consumption. Among other aspects of money that economists consider are wealth and consumption. Attempts have been made in Britain to approach the topic of whether wealth might be related to mortality in addition to other social measures such as an occupation-based measure of social class. At the time of the national census in 1971, about half the population lived in households with access to a car, and about half of adults owned their place of residence. The assumption was made that although some people might have made the conscious choice to own neither car nor house, those who had these things were, on average, wealthier than those who did not. The study in Britain that followed a 1 percent sample of the 1971 national census, known as the Office for National Statistics Longitudinal Study, showed that these wealth measures predicted mortality independent of social class based on occupation.[21]

Household Wealth. In the Whitehall II study, at the same time as asking about household income, we asked participants to estimate household wealth. As with household income this, too, was related positively to reported health (high wealth, better health) and negatively to depression (high wealth, less depression). As with income, this could have been a reflection of the fact that high-status civil servants have more wealth than their low-status colleagues have. It may therefore be a spurious finding, as appeared likely in the case of income. Unlike the findings with income, however, when we tried to make this finding go away by "adjusting" for the correlation between employment grade and wealth, both grade and wealth continued to predict ill health and depression.

Among the several possible interpretations of this finding, it is worth dwelling on three (excluding for the moment the possibility that ill health led to lower household wealth). First, wealth may convey psychosocial benefits. In Whitehall II, for example, wealth was correlated with optimism and a sense of control over future events. In this scenario, wealth may be causal in so far as the psychosocial benefits are directly related to the degree of wealth. Second, wealth may be reflecting accumulation of advantage and disadvantage over the life course. Wealth by itself may or may not be the issue, but it reflects a lifetime of different experiences, good and bad, that may affect health. Third, wealth may be simply acting as a marker for other unmeasured dimensions of socioeconomic position.

INCOME INEQUALITY

Richard Wilkinson drew attention to the apparent contradiction, set out above, that when comparing rich countries, there is little relationship between average income and life expectancy, yet within these countries there is a close relationship between individuals' incomes and their life expectancy and mortality.[22] His resolution of this puzzle was that within a society income was a measure of status, of relative position. This is what was related to mortality. When comparing whole societies, however, relative status has little meaning. Hence, the lack of relationship between mean income and a country's life expectancy was because a country's mean income did not convey the same meaning as the relative income level of people within a country.[23]

Wilkinson then went on to show that the spread of income — income inequality — was related to a country's life expectancy. This finding has generated a great deal of debate.[24] One particular criticism was that the relation was artifactual: For a given level of average income, the higher the income inequality of a society, the higher will be the proportion of people in poverty.[25] If, as discussed above, the relation of absolute mortality rates to income is curvilinear, then although the rich will gain from income inequality and the poor will lose, the health advantage for the rich will be less than the health disadvantage for the poor. In the previous section I quoted Deaton as pointing out that we should not think of this as an artifact. This could be one way that redistribution of income in a more egalitarian way could improve the life expectancy of the whole society.

Impact of Racial Inequality

Wilkinson's thesis is that characteristics of unequal societies lead to worse health in addition to the effect of poverty. One way his finding was tested was within the United States.[26] States with greater income inequality had higher mortality rates than did those with less inequality.[27] Similarly, metropolitan areas with greater income inequality had higher mortality than those with less inequality. Deaton's counter to this is that the state-level correlation between income inequality and mortality could be accounted for by the percentage of the population who were black. He showed that this percentage correlated with mortality rates among whites. When allowance was made for the percentage who were black, income inequality dropped out of the analysis. In Deaton's view, this is a refutation of the thesis that income inequality is causally related to mortality. It does not argue that the social environment is unimportant. As Deaton says, it could be argued that he has replaced income inequality with racial inequality.

Effects of Economic Segregation

Nancy Ross and colleagues, showing a weaker relation between income inequality among Canadian provinces than among U.S. states, conclude that the relation between income inequality and mortality depends on context.[28] There may be a greater degree of economic segregation in the United States than in Canada. This leads to a concentration of people with high social needs in municipalities with low tax bases, which in turn leads to worse provision of public goods and services, such as schools, transportation, health care, and housing. Lack of these public goods leads to worse health in poor areas. The marketplace has a more central role in the allocation of health care and high-quality education in the United States than it has in Canada. Therefore, utilization in the United States tends to be related to ability to pay, whereas these services in Canada are publicly funded and universally available. This Canadian argument appears to have two aspects: Low income and income inequality will both deprive people of access to services more in the United States than they will in Canada.

Social Environment

An important part of the argument that income inequality is a marker of the social environment is that in the United States, areas with high income inequality have not only high mortality but high crime rates, especially of homicide.[29] Ichiro Kawachi and colleagues have interpreted the environment in terms of social capital.[30] They have shown that measures of social capital appear to mediate the relation between income inequality and mortality. Robert Putnam also points to the relation between income inequality and erosion of social capital.[31]

A POLICY FOR INCOME?

My purpose in this paper was to take a noneconomist's view of income and health, not especially to speculate about policy implications. But the causal question and the policy question are interlinked. Crucially, would income redistribution matter to health?

First, for the reasons that Deaton set out, income redistribution would improve overall health by relieving the fate of the poor more than it hurt the rich. Deaton has pointed out to me that the benefits of redistribution would be less than would appear from the simple observation of the link between income and mortality. Economists describe as "deadweight loss" the fact that to redistribute a dollar to a poor person usually takes more than a dollar from a rich person. This happens because people both avoid and evade taxes.

Second, lack of income may not be related to deprivation in the sense of that prevailing in York 100 years ago, but lack of income hinders full participation in society. In a "support-led" society, to use Sen's term, with sharing and public provision of goods and services, income would matter less to social participation and receipt of services. In a society where both participation and receipt of services depend heavily on individual income, its lack is serious.

The data on income inequality by state or country should alert us to the powerful role that the social environment might play in health. We are still feeling our way toward understanding what this means. In Britain, on the basis of the Acheson inquiry, we made a series of recommendations for policy development that were related to improving the quality of the social environment to reduce inequalities in health. One of our three headline recommendations was to use the tax and benefit system to improve the living standards of those who are worst off.[32]

AT THE LOW END OF THE SCALE, individual incomes matter for health because of their link with both material deprivation and restriction on social participation and opportunity to exercise control over one's life. Above a threshold of material deprivation, income may be more important because of its link with these social factors related to social conditions. Pretax income inequalities have increased in many countries. A policy of not redressing this through the tax and benefit system, linked to lack of investment in public goods that brings the benefits of richer communities to all, will damage health.

ACKNOWLEDGMENTS

Sir Michael Marmot is supported by an MRC Research Professorship and by the John D. and Catherine T. MacArthur Foundation Research Network on Socioeconomic Status and Health. The author is grateful to an anonymous reviewer and to Angus Deaton, whose constructive criticisms were invaluable. He also thanks Mandy Feeney for her help with preparation of this paper.

REFERENCES

1. J.P. Smith, "Healthy Bodies and Thick Wallets: The Dual Relationship between Health and Socioeconomic Status," *Journal of Economic Perspectives* (Spring 1999): 145–166.

2. See, for example, papers in D. Gordon and P. Townsend, *Breadline Europe* (Bristol, England: Policy Press, 2000).

3. B.S. Rowntree, "Poverty: A Study of Town Life (1901)," in *Poverty, Inequality, and Health in Britain, 1800–2000: A Reader*, ed. G. Davey Smith, D. Dorling, and M. Shaw (Bristol, England: Policy Press, 2001), 97–106.

4. National Statistics, "Infant and Perinatal Mortality by Social and Biological Factors, 2000," *Health Statistics Quarterly* (Winter 2001): 78–82.

5. S.H. Preston, "The Changing Relation between Mortality and Level of Economic Development," *Population Studies* (March 1974): 19–51.

6. *Healthy People 2010* (Washington: U.S. Department of Health and Human Services, 2000).

7. A.T. Geronimus et al., "Excess Mortality among Blacks and Whites in the United States," *New England Journal of Medicine* (21 November 1996): 1552–1558.

8. M.G. Marmot, M.J. Shipley, and G. Rose, "Inequalities in Death — Specific Explanations of a General Pattern," *Lancet* (5 May 1984): 1003–1006; and M.G. Marmot et al., "Health Inequalities among British Civil Servants: The Whitehall II Study," *Lancet* (8 June 1991): 1387–1393.

9. C. van Rossum et al., "Employment Grade Differences in Cause Specific Mortality: Twenty-five Year Follow Up of Civil Servants from the First Whitehall Study," *Journal of Epidemiology and Community Health* (March 2000): 178–184.

10. C. Griffiths and J. Fitzpatrick, *National Statistics: Geographic Variations in Health* (London: Stationery Office, 2001).

11. M.G. Marmot, "Inequalities in Health," *New England Journal of Medicine* (12 July 2001): 134–136.

12. World Bank, *World Development Report 1993* (New York: Oxford University Press, 1993).

13. Preston, "The Changing Relation between Mortality and Level of Economic Development."

14. A. Sen, *Development as Freedom* (New York: Alfred A. Knopf, 1999).

15. P. McDonough et al., "Income Dynamics and Adult Mortality in the United States, 1972 through 1989," *American Journal of Public Health* (September 1997): 1476–1483.
16. M. Wolfson et al., "Career Earnings and Death: A Longitudinal Analysis of Older Canadian Men," *Journal of Gerontology* (July 1993): 167–179.
17. A. Deaton, "Health Inequality and Economic Development" (Working paper, Princeton University Research Program in Development Studies and Center for Health and Wellbeing, 2001).
18. World Bank, *World Development Report 1999/2000* (New York: Oxford University Press, 2000).
19. D.R. Williams, "Race, Socioeconomic Status, and Health: The Added Effects of Racism and Discrimination," in *Socioeconomic Status and Health in Industrial Nations: Social, Psychological, and Biological Pathways*, ed. N. Adler et al., Annals of the New York Academy of Sciences, Vol. 896 (December 1999), 173–188.
20. P. Martikainen et al., "The Effects of Income and Wealth on GHQ Depression and Poor Self-Rated Health in White-Collar Women and Men in the Whitehall II Study" (Unpublished manuscript, University College London, 2001).
21. P. Goldblatt, *1971–1981 Longitudinal Study: Mortality and Social Organisation* (London: Stationery Office, 1990).
22. R.G. Wilkinson, *Unhealthy Societies: The Afflictions of Inequality* (London: Routledge, 1996).
23. R.G. Wilkinson, *Mind the Gap: Hierarchies, Health, and Human Evolution* (London: Weidenfeld and Nicolson, 2000).
24. For a comprehensive review, see Deaton, *Health Inequality and Economic Development.*
25. H. Gravelle, "How Much of the Relation between Population Mortality and Unequal Distribution of Income Is a Statistical Artefact?" *British Medical Journal* (31 January 1998): 382–385.
26. G.A. Kaplan et al., "Inequality in Income and Mortality in the United States: Analysis of Mortality and Potential Pathways," *British Medical Journal* (20 April 1996): 999–1003.
27. J. Lynch et al., "Income Inequality and Mortality in Metropolitan Areas of the United States," *American Journal of Public Health* (July 1998): 1074–1080.
28. N.A. Ross et al., "Relation between Income Inequality and Mortality in Canada and in the United States: Cross Sectional Assessment Using Census Data and Vital Statistics," *British Medical Journal* (1 April 2000): 898–902.
29. M. Wilson and M. Daly, "Life Expectancy, Economic Inequality, Homicide, and Reproductive Timing in Chicago Neighbourhoods," *British Medical Journal* (26 April 1997): 1271–1274.
30. I. Kawachi et al., "Social Capital, Income Inequalities, and Mortality," *American Journal of Public Health* (September 1997): 1491–1498.
31. R. Putnam, *Bowling Alone: The Collapse and Revival of American Community* (New York: Simon and Schuster, 2000).
32. *Independent Inquiry into Inequalities in Health: Report* (London: Stationery Office, 1998).

ARTICLE 3

SOCIOECONOMIC STATUS AND HEALTH

THE POTENTIAL ROLE OF ENVIRONMENTAL RISK EXPOSURE

Gary W. Evans and Elyse Kantrowitz

Satisfactory explanation for the ubiquitous socioeconomic status-health gradient remains elusive, suggesting, in part, that an adequate model of this relation is probably complex and multifaceted (1, 81). In this paper we provide an overview of data indicating that income is inversely correlated with exposure to suboptimal environmental conditions. By environmental conditions we mean the physical properties of the ambient and immediate surroundings of children, youth, and families, including pollutants, toxins, noise, and crowding as well as exposure to settings such as housing, schools, work environments, and neighborhoods. We also briefly cite evidence that each of these environmental factors, in turn, is linked to health.

The implicit conceptual model under discussion is as follows (Figure 1): As can be seen above, what we discuss is evidence for two necessary prerequisites for this model to be valid — namely that socioeconomic status (SES) is associated with environmental quality and, in turn, that environmental quality affects health. This is not equivalent, however, to the conclusion that SES effects on health are caused by differential exposure to environmental quality. There are few if any data directly testing this proposition. What is necessary to verify the model shown in Figure 1 is that the SES health link is mediated by environmental quality.

In addition to this fundamental shortcoming in the extant database, results on SES and environmental exposure tend to be restricted to income and, in several cases, are not continuous; instead they compare individuals below and above the poverty line. Furthermore, for certain salient environments, especially work and school settings, scant data are available on income-related differential exposures to hazardous, polluted, or inadequate building conditions. The reader should also bear in mind that for several of the income-related environmental exposure results, the data are confounded with ethnicity. Given that there is also evidence that nonwhite individuals, at least in the United States, are more likely to be exposed to health-threatening environmental

SES ⇒ ENVIRONMENTAL ⇒ HEALTH
QUALITY

Figure 1 Basic underlying conceptual model.

conditions than are white individuals, it can be difficult to disentangle associations between income and environmental quality from racism.

There is also a conceptual issue we wish to briefly discuss before overviewing some of the evidence for linkages among SES, environmental quality, and health. Nearly all of the empirical work, and for that matter theoretical discussion about this issue, has examined individual environmental risk factors. Research and discussion tend to be focused on specific pollutants, toxins, or particular ambient conditions such as housing quality and each respective factor's link to income or health. We suspect that the potential of environmental exposure to account for the link between SES and health derives from multiple exposures to a plethora of suboptimal environmental conditions. That is, we would argue that a particularly important and salient aspect of reduced income is exposure to a confluence of multiple, suboptimal environmental conditions. The poor are most likely to be exposed not only to the worst air quality, the most noise, the lowest-quality housing and schools, etc., but of particular consequence, also to lower-quality environments on a wide array of multiple dimensions. We hypothesize that it is the accumulation of exposure to multiple, suboptimal physical conditions rather than any singular environmental exposure that will provide a fruitful explanation for the SES health gradient.

SOCIOECONOMIC STATUS AND ENVIRONMENTAL QUALITY

In this section we overview data on the relations between income or SES and exposure to environmental risks. We examine both individual environmental conditions such as toxic wastes, air pollution, crowding, and noise as well as the physical quality of specific settings such as the home, school, work, and neighborhood.

Hazardous Wastes

The environmental justice movement, launched in the 1980s, called attention to the fact that low-income citizens, and especially low-income, ethnic minority individuals, were much more likely to be exposed to toxic wastes and other forms of health-threatening environmental conditions relative to their more affluent and white fellow citizens (67). An influential book, *Dumping in Dixie* (18), documented the geographic association of toxic waste dumps in the Southeastern region of the United States with low-income, minority neighborhoods. The percentage of families below the federal poverty line in census tracts inclusive of EPA Region IV Hazardous Waste Landfills ranged from 26% (South Carolina) to 42% in Alabama. Twenty-nine percent of families living within one mile of a commercial hazardous waste facility in Detroit are below the poverty line, and 49% of them are nonwhite. More than 1.5 miles away, 10% are poor and 18% are people of color (89). One hundred percent of U.S. Government uranium mining and 4 of the largest 10 coal strip mines are located on Native American reservations (53). Nearly half of Native Americans live below the federal poverty line. More recent analyses of income and race differentials in hazardous waste exposure reveal similar trends (142). Children's body lead burden is strongly associated with both income and race. For example, in a recent EPA Task Force report, "Environmental Equity: Reducing Risk for All Communities" (136), 68% of urban black children in families with incomes below $6000 had blood lead levels that exceeded safe limits in comparison to 15% of the same population with incomes above $15,000. For white children, the comparable data were 36% and 12%. The National Health and Nutrition Survey conducted in 1980 and 1990 documents elevated blood-lead levels in low-income individuals, particularly among inner-city residents (105).

Air Pollution

Ambient pollutant exposure reveals similar race and income-related trends. Figure 2, for example, depicts factory carcinogen emissions in Britain in relation to income (42a). Analogous data have been found for several other common ambient air pollutants (e.g., sulfur oxides, fine particulates) with known pathogenic effects in the United States (42). Exposure to ozone, a principal toxic component of photochemical smog, as well as fine particulate matter in the South Coast Air Basin of California is inversely related to income levels (15). The World Bank has also become interested in environmental justice, publishing sobering statistical summaries about environmental

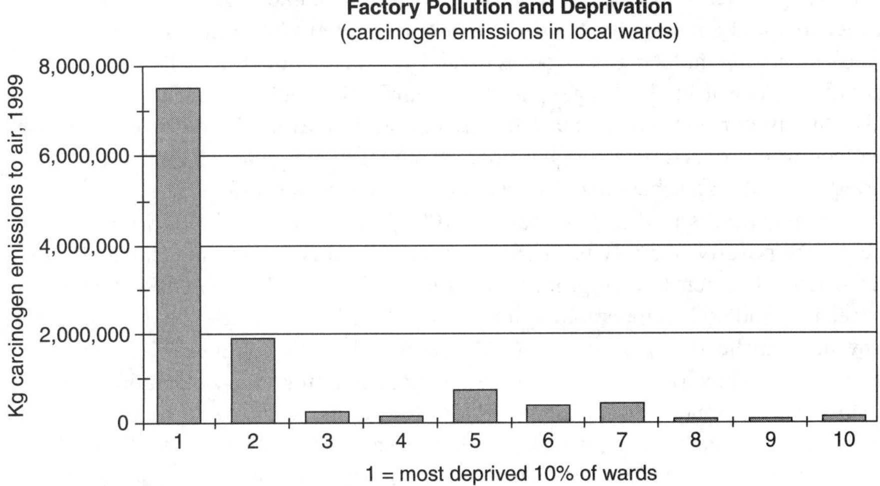

Figure 2 Factory pollution and income in England. (Source: Reprinted by permission from Friends of the Earth, United Kingdom [42a].)

health threats worldwide. For example, in low-income countries from the 1970s to the late 1980s, the average levels of suspended particulate matter in cities increased from approximately 300 μg per cubic meter of air to 325 μg. The total range of measured particulates for all of these cities at both time periods exceeded even marginal, let alone acceptable, limits from a respiratory health standpoint. Cities in middle-income countries over the same time period witnessed improved air quality (from approximately 180 to 150 μg/cubic meter of air) and wealthy countries improved from ~100 to 75 μg per cubic meter of air. Analogous data are provided by the World Bank for water quality (144).

Today increasing interest is focused on exposure to indoor air quality, which may play an even greater role in the respiratory health and well-being of individuals, particularly young children. Levels of several common airborne toxins are higher indoors, and for young children, the duration of exposure is often greater inside relative to the outdoors. Although there are some suggestive data, with the exception of secondary cigarette smoke, little is known about the association between income levels and exposure to indoor air contaminants.

Parental smoking, which is inversely related to income levels, increases children's exposures to a wide variety of indoor toxins. For example, in the United States, 65% of preschool children living in poverty have been exposed to cigarette smoke at home in comparison to 47% of those not in poverty (94). In both the United States and Britain, mothers who are poorer are also less likely to quit and smoke more than their higher-income counterparts (54, 56). Length of tenure on welfare also predicts maternal smoking prevalence and consumption levels (55). Young children's levels of salivary cotinine increase linearly in relation to lower occupational class (27, 69). Cotinine is a metabolite of nicotine and a valid indicator of exposure to environmental tobacco smoke. Moreover, cumulative risk factors associated with poverty increase smoking prevalence in mothers of newborns. Rental occupied housing, lack of higher education, and single-parenthood status are associated with a ninefold increase in smoking among mothers of newborns in the United Kingdom (121). This association is independent of mother's age, parity, and ethnicity. Smoking during pregnancy is also highly correlated with maternal education. For example, 48% of American women who dropped out of high school smoke during pregnancy compared to 12% going beyond high school and 3% who are college graduates (95).

In rental units in the United States, 10% percent of households with incomes below the poverty line rely primarily upon hot air units without ducts, and 4% use unvented gas heaters as their primary heat source. For rental households with incomes exceeding $30,000, comparable figures are 7% and 1% for ductless hot air heat and unvented gas heaters, respectively (123). Toxic indoor air pollutants, NO_2 and CO, related to combustion processes (stoves, heating, smoking), are substantially higher in low-income, inner-city residences relative to U.S. averages (52, 116). Exposure to radon, a known carcinogen, is related to income levels in rural counties in New York state. Chi & Laquatra (22) suggest that income-related differences in radon exposure are probably related to structural deficiencies that provide more permeable vectors for radon to enter into the residence.

Acute respiratory obstructive diseases such as asthma are associated with serum IgE antibodies to dust mite feces, cats, cockroaches, and certain pollens. Exposure to cockroach allergens as well as antibody sensitivity is associated with socioeconomic status with 0%, 26%, and 46% of high-, middle-, and low-SES, respectively, children exposed (114). Positive skin tests data revealed a parallel SES gradient (114). Rosenstreich et al. (109) also found high levels of allergenic reactions to cockroaches in a general population sample of inner-city children, and more than half of low-income asthma patients in several urban, inner-city samples evidenced specific IgE antibodies and positive skin test results to cockroaches (10, 72). Furthermore, dampness in houses, which is inversely associated with household income, is conducive to dust mites as well as molds and fungi, all related to respiratory obstructive disorders (51).

Water Pollution

Although most attention to environmental pollutants and income has been focused on hazardous wastes and air pollution, several case studies suggest higher levels of contaminated water among low-income populations (21). For example, 44% of water supplies for migrant farm workers in North Carolina tested positive for coliform and 26% for fecal coliform. For comparable farm areas in the same region, both levels were at 0% (23). Low-income Chicano populations living along the U.S./Mexico border (Colonias) are plagued by contaminated drinking water. Estimates indicate, for example, that in Texas nearly 50% of the Colonias population lacks safe drinking water, a condition that is largely believed to be the source of the threefold increase in this population's risk for waterborne diseases relative to the overall morbidity rate in Texas (21, pp. 887–88). In 1984, EPA surveyed rural drinking water supplies in the United States and found significantly higher levels of coliform in low-income households (135). Finally, low-SES families are much more likely to swim in polluted beaches (20) as well as consume fish from contaminated waters (141). Statistics on access to safe, clean drinking water do not convey the full picture with respect to public health. For example, in many developing countries people designated as having access to suitable water supplies have to walk long distances to reach them, often averaging 30 minutes or more. Overburdened parents may not have the time or energy to utilize such distant facilities (6).

Ambient Noise

Exposure to ambient noise levels is also associated with income. According to data from the American Housing Survey, low-income residents are nearly twice as likely (9.1%) to report that neighborhood noise is bothersome in comparison to families not in poverty (5.9%) (118). A nationwide survey of major U.S. metropolitan areas found a strong, adverse correlation ($r = -0.61$) between household income and 24-h average sound level exposures (134). Households with incomes below $10,000 had average sound exposure levels more than 10 dBA higher than households above $20,000 annual income. Decibels is a logarithmic scale, with an increase of 10 dBA perceived as approximately twice as loud. A recent analysis of airport noise and children's health and cognitive performance around Heathrow Airport documents linkages between income and actual objective indices of noise exposure. Elementary schools with higher levels of aircraft noise exposure have greater percentages of children eligible for free lunches (58).

Residential Crowding

Residential crowding, which is typically indexed by the ratio of people to number of rooms, is also linked to income. Figure 3 depicts national data from the 1990 census, showing a clear income-related gradient (92). The official U.S. Census definition of a crowded household is greater than one person per room.

Similar trends have been uncovered in economically underdeveloped countries. For example, in 1990 in Monterey, Mexico, 48% of households situated in the lowest income district of the city had one bedroom in comparison to 16% of households in the most affluent district (48). Similar trends have been uncovered in major urban areas in other developing countries (125).

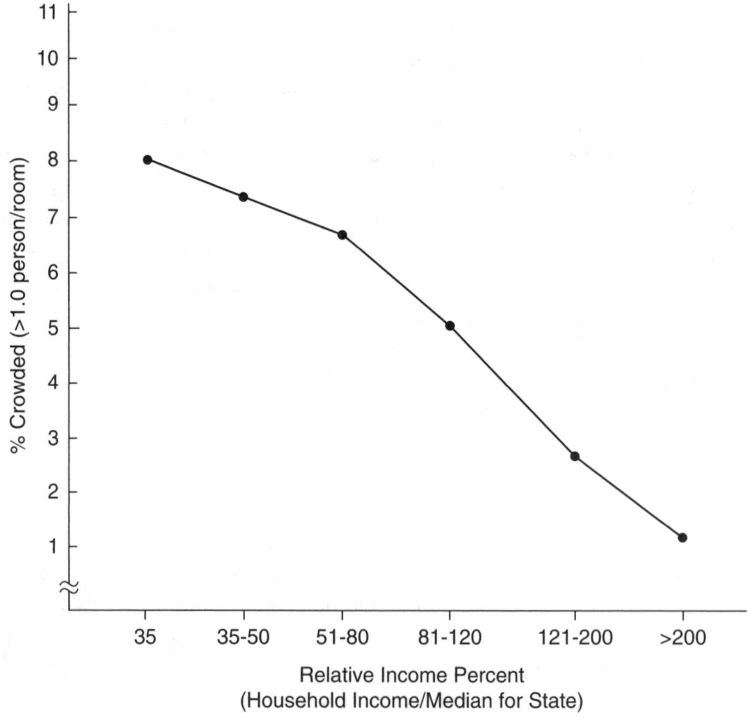

Figure 3 Residential crowding (greater than one person per room) and household income in the United States. (Source: Adapted from Table 1 in Reference 92.)

The quantity and quality of space proximate to residences may also bear upon health and quality of life. Low-income neighborhoods in New York City have 17 square yards of park space per child, whereas all other New York City neighborhoods average 40 square yards of park space per child (118). In the United Kingdom, 86% of professionals and supervisors have access to a private garden at home in comparison to 69% of manual laborers (131). Manual laborers are four times more likely (14%) to have a garden or yard at home too small to sit outside in the sun relative to professionals, managers, or supervisors.

Housing Quality

In addition to examining linkages between constituents of environmental quality and SES, one can also look at bundles of environmental quality as embodied in the overall quality of settings such as housing, schools, work, or neighborhoods. In the United States, housing quality is strongly tied to income levels, which in turn are positively associated with home ownership and negatively correlated with residential mobility (40). For example, approximately three quarters of those above the federal poverty line own their own home compared with 40% of those who are poor. Low-income families are five times more likely to be evicted than their non-poor counterparts. Statistics from the American Housing Survey, conducted by the U.S. Census, indicate that the poor are more than three times as likely to have substandard quality housing than the not poor (22% vs. 7%) (118). Thirty-six percent of all American households with a child under the age of 18 report at least one problem with housing compared to 77% of households at or below 50% of the median income for the surrounding geographic area (133). Income is inversely related to various indicators of housing adequacy.

Analogous trends have been uncovered in a representative national sample of households in the United Kingdom (131). We have also found that housing quality is significantly correlated with the income to needs ratios ($r = -0.39$) of rural families in upstate New York. The income-to-needs ratio is a per capita poverty index formed by taking the ratio of family income to the federally defined poverty index. Thus an income-to-needs ratio of 1 equals the poverty line. The federal formula is adjusted annually to the cost of living index. We used a housing composite scale that relied on raters' assessments of cleanliness/clutter, indoor climate quality, privacy, exposure to safety hazards, and structural quality (38). Social class differentials in childhood injuries from accidents in the home (e.g., falls) are correlated with hazardous characteristics of residential structures (11).

Poor families in America are also much less likely to have basic amenities such as clothes washers (72%), clothes dryers (50%), air conditioning (50%), or telephone (77%) than the not poor (clothes washer, 93%; clothes dryer, 87%; air conditioning, 72%; telephone, 97%) (40, 87). In the Netherlands, the percentage of persons with one or more housing deficiencies (no refrigerator, no washing machine, no clothes dryer, ≥1 person/room) is linearly related to income, ranging from 16% for families in the lowest income sextile to 1% of those in the highest income sextile (126).

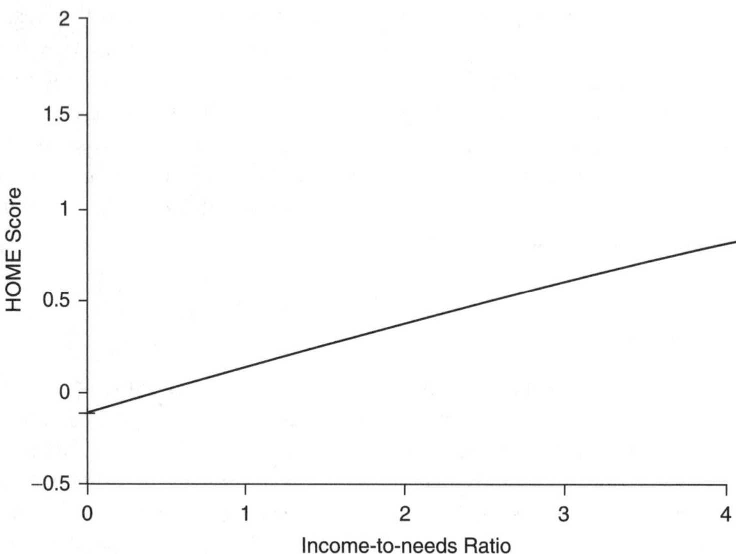

Figure 4 HOME scale values and income. (Source: Adapted from Figure 2, Reference 47, by permission from the University of Chicago.)

Not surprisingly, the situation is even more extreme in the developing world. In Monterey, Mexico, income differences among districts in the city are associated with housing problems such as the absence of a permanent roof, no indoor running water, lack of drainage, and overcrowding (48). Looking at census tracts rather than metropolitan districts, Stephens and colleagues (125) uncovered similar trends in Accra, Ghana, and São Paulo, Brazil. In Accra, 37% of households in the lowest income census tracts have no piped in water, whereas 11% lack this amenity in wealthier areas of the city. In São Paulo, 36% of homes in the lowest income census tracts have no indoor toilets compared to 1% among more affluent tracts in the city.

Developmental psychologists have devised rating instruments to assess dimensions of the home environment of families. These instruments encompass measurements of physical qualities and evaluations of parenting and other aspects of the social environment. Figure 4 depicts a linear relation between the income-to-needs ratio and scores on a common residential environment rating scale, the HOME in the United States (47).

Bradley & Caldwell (13), the principal authors of the HOME scale, reported that the lower the SES, the poorer the HOME scores for infants and two-year-olds in the United States. More recently, Bradley and colleagues (14) examined relations between HOME scores across five biennial waves of a national sample of over 25,000 American children. Parental responsiveness (e.g., answering questions) was lower in poor versus not poor families, and these children had fewer learning resources (e.g., books, tape recorders) in their homes. Low-income homes were also more monotonous, dark, and contained more hazardous conditions. In another analysis using the HOME scale, 6- to 9-year-olds in American families below the poverty line suffered a 34% deficit in overall HOME scores relative to those in families with an income-to-needs ratio above 4 (88). Moreover, the longer the duration of childhood poverty, the stronger the negative association. Dubow & Ippolito (32) found a correlation of –0.54 between HOME scores and the number of years elementary school-aged children lived below the poverty line.

Sherman (118) provides a sobering statistic that may be indicative of the quality of the home environment available to children in the United States. Fifty-nine percent of children ages 3 to 5 who are poor have 10 or more books at home; 81% of children who are not poor have 10 or more books at home. Sadly, only 38% of low-income parents in the United States read on a daily basis to their preschoolers. Although substantially higher, the figure for their more affluent counterparts, 58%, is also dismal (133). Not surprisingly, the higher the socioeconomic status of the family, the more time youth spend reading on a daily basis (75). An interesting companion statistic that may interrelate to reading activity is television watching. Numerous studies have documented an inverse relation between household SES and youth TV viewing (75). For example, the percentage of 13-year-olds in the United States who watch more than five hours of television is 18 and 10, respectively, with household heads who did not graduate from high school or are college graduates (133).

In 1998, 94% of American urban children in predominantly low-income neighborhoods (≥40% below poverty line) versus 57% of urban children living in neighborhoods with little poverty (<10% below poverty line) had no Internet access (73). Eighty-four percent of the former households and 35% of the latter had no access to a computer. Across the entire United States, 52% and 15% of elementary and secondary school children, respectively, who are in the bottom income quintile have computer access at home. This contrasts markedly with the 74% and 79% of elementary and secondary children, respectively, in the highest income quintile who have home computer access (133).

Educational Facilities

An important setting for children are schools and daycare environments. The quality of the school environment is tied to income. Per capita school expenditures vary greatly according to community resources given the reliance of many school districts on local property taxes. In 1999, a federal survey of physical facilities in a representative sample of 903 public elementary and secondary schools (93) found that 20% of schools had a building in less than adequate repair, 43% had at least one infrastructure deficiency (e.g., heating, indoor air quality), and about 10% were seriously overcrowded (greater than 125% capacity). Not surprisingly, predominantly low-income schools suffered a disproportionate burden of inadequate school facilities.

Table 1 provides summary data from the National Center for Education Statistics report on the Condition of America's Public School Facilities: 1999. As is apparent on

TABLE 1

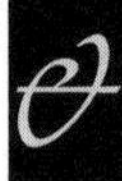

Percentage of Building Components Inadequate in Relation to Percentage of Children in the School Eligible for Free or Subsidized Lunch

	Building Features								
Percentage Eligible Children	*Roof*	*Plumbing*	*Heating*	*Electric Power*	*Lighting*	*Ventilation*	*Indoor Air Quality*	*Acoustics*	*Physical Security*
<20	18	23	28	18	8	24	14	14	17
20–39	21	23	26	20	13	29	20	18	22
40–69	22	23	29	21	10	24	17	15	21
>70	32	32	35	30	19	29	24	25	17

Source: Adapted from Tables 4 and 8 of the National Center for Education Statistics (93).

every dimension, low-income schools fare worst. Moreover, on several indices of facility quality, there appear to be linear gradients in relation to income levels for the school.

Children in schools with a larger proportion of poor children are also more likely to be crowded. Twelve percent of American public schools with more than 70% of their children eligible for subsidized or free lunch programs are above 125% of building capacity in comparison to 6% of schools with less than 20% eligible for lunch programs (93).[1] In terms of health outcomes, low-income children are also more likely to live in seriously overcrowded households, defined as more than one person per room (see Figure 3 p. 98). The adverse impacts of residential crowding are exacerbated among children in more crowded daycare facilities (86).

It is, of course, difficult to disentangle the quality of the physical plant from the social environment of schools. Perhaps the most fundamental resource in a school is the quality of its teachers. Secondary teachers in low-income schools are significantly less likely to have undergraduate majors or minors in the subjects they teach relative to those in more affluent schools. For example, 27% of secondary math teachers in poor school districts majored or minored in mathematics in college compared to 43% in school districts that are not predominantly low income (66). Comparable differences occur in the sciences, whereas the differential in English is smaller.

School safety is associated with income as well. Blue-collar adolescents are twice as likely to report the presence of weapons at school (12%) or fighting in school (32%) as their white-collar counterparts (44).

Recently, several authors have examined the quality of daycare in relation to income levels. The ratio of daycare staff to children as well as expenditure is related to income levels (96, 104). The educational level and pay scales of childcare workers are related to income as well (104). Both of these studies suggest that for the very poor, subsidies appear to offset daycare quality relative to the lower middle and working

[1]The percentage of schools seriously overcrowded in the intermediate ranges of income, 20–39% school lunch eligible and 40–69% school lunch eligible, are 8% and 7%, respectively.

class for institutional daycare center care. For home care, the more typical income-quality gradient is seen, with poorer-quality home daycare associated with reduced family income. Philips and colleagues have also documented that the quality of child-care provider-child interaction (e.g., sensitivity, harshness, detachment) is also correlated with income levels (104).

Work Environments

Outside of home and school, poorer people may be subject to greater health risks on the job. In a large sample of Swedish workers, Lundberg (80) assessed different environmental and behavioral factors believed to account for SES gradients in health. Of particular interest, the strongest predictor of the gradient was poor working conditions, defined as heavy lifting or tasks with repetitive strain plus daily contact with toxins, fumes, dust, explosives, vibration, and the like. Furthermore, in multiple regression models, poor working conditions were the only independent (i.e., entered last after all other factors) predictor of the SES health gradient. Emerging evidence documents pervasive race differentials in occupational exposure to toxins and physically hazardous, risky working conditions (43, 79, 145). For example, steelworkers located in the most hazardous component of the production process (topside of the coke ovens) are nearly three times more likely to be black than white. Among the most notoriously unhealthy labor sectors are seasonal agricultural work and sweatshop garment production — settings predominated by low-income workers. Moses et al. (91) review several studies suggesting a greater body burden of persistent chlorinated hydrocarbons among low-income, Chicano/Latino, and black agricultural workers. Although these substances are now banned in the United States, because they are lipophilic they remain sequestered in fatty tissue for many years. DDE serum levels are related to SES among blacks and whites in Dade County, Florida (30). DDE is a major metabolite of DDT and more indicative of lifelong exposure. Two aspects of these data are noteworthy. First, the data reveal a nearly perfect linear SES gradient, and second, African Americans suffer much higher body-pesticide burdens. DDT concentrations in human breast milk among indigent black women in rural counties in Mississippi and Arkansas averaged 447 ppb. Average levels for middle-class women in Nashville averaged 14 ppb (143). In the National Health and Nutritional Examination Survey II, conducted from 1976–1980, living below the federal poverty line had a significant, independent association with serum DDT (odds ratio = 1.48) and dieldrin (odds ratio = 1.43) levels (124).

Given the robust association of ethnicity and income among American workers, it is reasonable to suspect that differential income-work setting quality relations exist as have been documented with respect to ethnicity. We know with some certainty that work-related injuries are inversely related to wages. Moreover, injury-caused sick days and duration of sick days per injury are both inversely associated with wages (60). Similar trends have been noted in the developing world (106). Occupational status in a large, representative sample of workers in the United Kingdom (131) is inversely related to more difficult working conditions.

Berney and colleagues (9) asked elderly individuals (M = 67.9 years) to retrospectively report the number of years during which they had been exposed to various environmental hazards, including those at work. Exposure to combined occupational hazards (i.e., fumes and dust, physically arduous tasks, lack of job autonomy) was inversely related to class. For example, male manual laborers had more than double the number of years working in hazardous conditions (M = 51.1 years) than nonmanual laborers (M = 20.9 years). Combined occupational hazards are expressed in years, cumulatively across hazards. Thus, for example, an individual exposed to 10 years of dust, 5 years in arduous labor, and 20 years in a job with low autonomy would be assigned a score of 35 hazardous years.

Townsend (131), in his report of occupational class and working conditions in the United Kingdom, developed a composite index of working amenities that included sufficient heat in the winter for those outside, availability of tea/coffee, indoor toilet, facilities for washing/changing clothes, place to buy or eat lunch, secure place to keep coat/spare clothing, lockable personal storage, first-aid kit/facilities, possibility to make at least one call daily, and control over task lighting. He then constructed summary Working Conditions based on the number of amenities available: very poor working conditions, less than four amenities; poor working conditions, between four and six amenities; adequate working conditions, six amenities; and good working conditions, more than six amenities. Table 2 depicts data from this study on men in the United Kingdom working under different levels of overall work quality as a function of occupational status.

Investigation and concern about the plight of child laborers throughout the developing world has largely neglected the environmental conditions these children work in. In addition to long hours and dismal wages, many of these children work in deplorable conditions that are filthy, polluted, hazardous, and unsanitary (115).

Stressful psychosocial conditions of working settings also appear related to occupational status. Marmot and colleagues (83) have shown among British civil servants

TABLE 2

OCCUPATIONAL STATUS AND OVERALL WORK SETTING QUALITY

	Occupational Status			
	Professional	*Manager*	*Supervisory*	*Manual*
Overall work setting quality				
Very poor	0	4	4	13
Poor	2	8	5	17
Adequate	5	22	19	28
Good	93	66	72	42

Source: Adapted from Table A.41 in Reference 131.

that grade level is inversely related to autonomy (decision latitude) on the job, monotonous working conditions, and work pace. The trends are linear in relation to civil service grade (1 to 6) and, in turn, are related to sickness absence and incidence of coronary heart disease.

Neighborhood Quality

In addition to school, work, and home, local surroundings may contribute to health and well-being. Low-income urban neighborhoods suffer poorer basic municipal services [e.g., police, fire, sanitation (138)] and experience greater residential mobility (77) relative to more affluent, urban neighborhoods. Nine- to eleven-year-old children in Sydney, Australia, rated their overall neighborhood quality as higher in relation to an objective composite index of neighborhood risk, based upon census data (64). A primary component of this neighborhood risk index was SES. The higher the neighborhood risk index, the more likely it was that children rated their setting as having too much traffic, being dirty and polluted, too much noise, no safe places to play, and having fewer parks and outdoor play spaces. Even within predominantly low-income areas, family income is positively related to the overall quality of neighborhood housing and other amenities (120).

Macintyre and colleagues (82) found that working-class areas of Glasgow, Scotland, in comparison to upper-middle-class sections, had fewer shops, paid more for food, had dramatically fewer recreational opportunities, were further from mass transit stops in combination with lower rates of car ownership, and had poorer street cleaning and maintenance. As noted earlier, low-income children have less access to parks and suitable nearby nature (e.g., gardens) (118). Furthermore, as shown by the Sydney study, children seem well aware of this (64). Playgrounds in low-income areas are more hazardous (as assessed by independent, trained raters) relative to those in higher-income neighborhoods (127). Moreover, young children of low-income families are much more likely to have no safe play areas nearby their home (131). Income-related rates of child pedestrian injuries appear to be caused by differential exposure to street traffic. For example, children in Montreal from relatively disadvantaged schools cross 50% more streets a day, on average, than their more affluent schoolmates (82a). Basic housing stock is of significantly lower quality (percentage dilapidated housing) in low-income neighborhoods than in middle- or upper-income areas (71). Abandoned lots and boarded up houses also occur more frequently in low-income areas (128, 139).

Rates of exposure to crime are strongly tied to family income levels as well as neighborhood income composition (113). Children from low-SES neighborhoods are more likely to be exposed to aggressive peers than children from higher-income areas (119). Low-income adolescents perceive their neighborhood as more dangerous, violent, and of poorer overall quality (graffiti, cleanliness, housing quality) than their middle-class counterparts (2). Homel & Burns (64), in their Sydney neighborhood study, also found that neighborhood risk was linearly related to young children's judgments about the presence of unfriendly people. Thus, both the immediate residential environment as well as the neighborhood infrastructure of low-income individuals are likely to be of lower overall quality than the home or surroundings of people with more financial resources.

ENVIRONMENTAL QUALITY AND HEALTH

The section above documents pervasive income-related differences in exposure to environmental risks. The present section provides a much briefer summarization of evidence that the disproportionate burden of suboptimal environmental exposure shared by those who are poorer could have health consequences. The amount and quality of research on environmental effects on health and well-being are substantially greater than evidence of income differentials in exposure to poor environmental quality.

Air Quality

A voluminous literature relying on epidemiological studies as well as human and animal experiments demonstrates that ambient air pollutants cause various respiratory problems including bronchitis, emphysema, and asthma. Less well-documented links exist between certain ambient pollutants and lung cancer. Exposure to carbon monoxide may also be a risk factor for coronary heart disease. In addition, ambient air pollution may increase risk for respiratory infection (63, 78, 98). Exposure to ambient pollutants, principally ozone, a toxic component of photochemical smog, has been linked to psychological distress, negative emotional affect, and behaviors including interpersonal attraction and aggression. The latter function appears to be curvilinear, with moderate levels of irritable pollutants causing increased aggression (33, 110). Although a relatively new area of inquiry, there is already an impressive body of literature linking indoor air quality, including environmental tobacco smoke, with various respiratory problems (5, 68, 112).

Environmental Toxins

Environmental toxins, principally heavy metals (e.g., lead), solvents (e.g., cleaning fluids), and pesticides, occur in hazardous waste-disposal facilities and various manufacturing, mining, and agricultural activities. Toxicological effects include cancer, respiratory morbidity, brain damage, and various neurotoxicological difficulties (70, 98, 117). In utero exposure to several toxins also produces teratological effects. Many of these same toxins in much lower doses produce cognitive and behavioral abnormalities, including attentional and memory disorders, lower IQ, and poorer academic achievement. Behavioral problems including impulse control, frustration intolerance, and aggression have also been associated with several toxins (3, 108). The low-dose behavioral toxicological effects appear to be especially dangerous during the critical period of fetal development.

Ambient Noise

Another aspect of environmental quality, ambient noise levels, also appears to threaten health. Links between chronic noise exposure and hearing damage are well documented (74). Both intensity and duration of exposure are important parameters of noise exposure and health. Suggestive data link noise exposure to coronary heart disease and hypertension, but the evidence is not solid (8, 130). Several community studies have shown that children's blood pressure and possibly neuroendocrine stress hormones are elevated when living or attending schools in the flight paths of major airports (34). There are contradictory findings on ambient noise exposure and prematurity and birth defects, as well as a small number of studies suggesting immunosuppression from noise in animal models (34).

Noise clearly interferes with complex task performance (e.g., dual tasks) but has inconsistent effects on simple tasks (e.g., vigilance) (35). Several studies have uncovered evidence that both acute as well as chronic noise exposure can lead to motivational deficits linked to learned helplessness (25, 34). Glass & Singer (50) found, for example, that immediately following exposure to 20 minutes of noxious noise in the laboratory, subjects were less likely to persist at challenging puzzles. Their data also indicate that it is the uncontrollability of noise, in particular, that is problematic for motivation. A large number of studies have shown that chronic noise exposure is linked to reading deficits in young children. The effects on reading are not due to hearing loss. Moreover, some of this effect is due to problems with speech perception in noise-exposed children (36). Noise also has adverse consequences for interpersonal processes including altruism and aggression (26). Conclusions about an association between ambient noise exposure and mental illness are not well substantiated (122).

Residential Crowding

Crowding, like noise, functions as a stressor, elevating blood pressure and neuroendocrine parameters (34). Several studies have indicated that infectious diseases are more likely in relation to crowding among vulnerable subgroups (e.g., prisoners, refugee camps) and that residential crowding (i.e., people per room) is associated with psychological distress in the general population (34). There is no evidence to substantiate the widespread perception of cultural differences in tolerance for crowding (37). Areal indices of density (e.g., people/acre) appear less important than interior density measures such as people per room for understanding health outcomes associated with crowding. Several studies indicate that a principal pathway linking residential crowding to psychological distress is problems with unwanted social interaction (7, 34). Residents of more crowded homes are more socially withdrawn and perceive lower levels of social support in comparison to individuals living in less crowded settings. Parents in crowded homes are also less responsive to their children and tend to employ harsher, more punitive parenting styles (34). Crowding may also interfere with complex task performance and has been linked to learned helplessness (34, 35). Relations between crowding and aggression are unclear but several studies have indicated reduced altruism and more negative interpersonal interactions in more crowded settings (7).

Housing Quality

Concerns about housing quality and physical health are a longstanding interest within the field of public health. Because of the design of research projects investigating housing and health, it is difficult to draw definitive conclusions; nonetheless, the preponderance of evidence suggests that substandard and more hazardous construction is associated with more unintentional injuries, especially among young children and the elderly. Inadequate heating systems and the presence of dampness, molds, and other allergens are also associated with poor respiratory health (19, 65, 85). Epidemic increases in asthma in inner-city settings may be partially attributable to elevated ambient pollutants along with exposure to allergens in the home. The evidence linking housing and health includes several longitudinal analyses of housing improvements and at least one study with random assignment.

Work investigating a possible link between housing quality and mental health is more controversial. The findings are less numerous and consistent than the physical health research. Evidence suggests that high-rise housing may be linked to elevated psychological distress among low-income women with young children as well as with restricted outdoor play activities in young children (39, 49, 59).

There is also a good deal of evidence showing relations between the design of public housing and both fear of crime and actual incidence of crime (128). One of the problems with research on mental health and housing is reliance on housing measurements developed originally to assess physical health. Recent work indicates that scales indexing behaviorally relevant aspects of housing may prove more fruitful in research on housing and psychological well-being (38).

The quality of the home environment has also been linked to children's cognitive development. The provision of adequate learning materials and the absence of chaotic conditions predict better achievement, both cross sectionally and longitudinally (12, 84, 137). The role of structure and predictability in family routines has also been implicated in children's socioemotional development (41).

Educational Facilities

The quality of the research on the physical environment of daycare settings and early school environments and children's development is not sufficiently developed to draw definitive conclusions, but trends indicate that the physical environment may play a role directly affecting children's cognitive and social development and indirectly by way of changes in teachers' behaviors (90, 132). Some of the physical characteristics of schools, in addition to noise and crowding, believed to be important to cognitive development include structure and predictability, arrangement and quality of activity areas, degree of openness, privacy, access to nature, availability and variety of age-appropriate toys and learning aids, and play materials for fine and gross motor development that provide graduated challenge, and natural light (101, 140).

Neighborhood Quality

There has been a recent upsurge of interest in neighborhood effects on well-being, focusing on cardiovascular health, crime and violence, and children's development. Some studies look at neighborhood effects, after statistically controlling for individual variation in SES or income levels. Other studies employ hierarchical linear modeling techniques that account for both individual and areal-level variation in SES or income. Low-SES neighborhood characteristics, independent of household SES, are associated with higher all-cause mortality (29, 57); greater cardiovascular risk in men (29, 61), as well as women (29); cardiovascular disease in men and women (29, 76); and with injury mortality (28). As noted earlier, exposure to urban crime is positively associated with both individual income levels and neighborhood income characteristics (113). Interestingly from a psychological health perspective, a key underlying mechanism to explain the linkage between neighborhood poverty and crime is diminished collective efficacy. Residents of low-income, high-crime neighborhoods perceive less social cohesion and diminished social control in their neighborhoods relative to persons living in lower-crime areas (113). Fear of crime in adults, particularly the elderly population, has reached epidemic proportions in low-income, inner-city neighborhoods (103, 139). Finally, exposure to violence has well-documented, adverse consequences on children's socioemotional development (45, 46, 102, 107).

Children growing up in high-SES neighborhoods have a clear advantage in school readiness and perform better academically, independently of familial income or education (77). Mental health in children and youth, particularly externalizing behaviors (acting out, aggression), is associated with residence in low-income neighborhoods. Studies controlling for individual SES as well as multiple-level analyses converge on these findings. Adolescents in low-income neighborhoods also appear to become sexually active earlier and are more likely to become teenage parents compared to their peers living in more affluent neighborhoods (77).

CONCLUSIONS

We have reviewed data showing that income is associated with exposure to a wide variety of environmental quality indicators in the ambient environment, at home, in school, on the job, and in one's neighborhood. Differential income and racial exposure to environmental health risks constitute an important and emerging field of scholarship and public policy, frequently termed environmental justice. It would be fair to summarize this body of work as showing that the poor and especially the non-white poor bear a disproportionate burden of exposure to suboptimal, unhealthy environmental conditions in the United States. Moreover, the more researchers scrutinize environmental exposure and health data for racial and income inequalities, the stronger the evidence becomes that grave and widespread environmental injustices have occurred throughout the United States. Such findings moved former President Clinton to establish an Office of Environmental Justice in 1992 within EPA (99, 136) and in 1994, to issue an executive order requiring all federal agencies to identify and address disproportionately high and adverse human health or environmental effects of federal programs and policies on minority and low-income populations (24). [See also the Office on Minority Health (100) within the Department of Health and Human Services and the National Institute for Environmental Health Sciences (97) for further information on U.S. Federal environmental justice programs. Friends of the Earth, United Kingdom, has a research and policy program devoted to environmental justice (42b).]

There are several gaping holes in the current database necessary to critically examine whether the SES health gradient could be partly attributed to environmental exposures. First, data on income or SES and environmental exposure are quite thin for several important settings, especially work, schools, and neighborhood settings. In several instances, a dose-response function is not available; rather, measures of environmental risk for low-income individuals are compared to persons above the poverty line. It would be preferable to have data across the continuum of income or SES and environmental risk exposure. In many instances, the poverty/not poverty comparison is entangled with ethnicity. In the cases of exposure to hazardous waste sites and to occupational risk exposure, respectively, the data on ethnic differentials in exposure are better developed than they are for income. Available data are largely confined to North America and Western Europe. The paucity of data on income and environmental risk for residents of developing countries is particularly troublesome given both the greater population size and more adverse environmental risk exposure in many of these countries.

Second, we hypothesize that the likelihood of singular environmental exposure accounting for the SES health gradient is small. We believe that it is the confluence of suboptimal conditions that is most likely to function as a potent mechanism helping to account for SES-related differences in health. Research on cumulative risk exposure among children offers a useful analogue. This work shows that children exposed to one or perhaps two serious risk factors suffer at most modest decrements in psychological or cognitive functioning. However, the accumulation of multiple risk factors dramatically elevates the probability of adverse socioemotional and cognitive developmental outcomes (16, 111). The gap in our analysis of income, environmental risk, and health is such that few data exist showing the relation between income and multiple sources of environmental risk. We do know with some clarity that income is inversely related to exposure to a higher frequency of social stressors and to more adverse social stressors (4, 17) but parallel data for multiple physical stressor exposure do not exist.

Should this multiple exposure, health, and income hypothesis prove correct, then current estimates of the importance of environmental risk to account for some of the SES health gradient are likely conservative. Nearly all of the available data on environmental risk and income emanate from economically developed countries, whereas the greatest convergence of multiple suboptimal environmental conditions with the severest health consequences likely occurs in the less developed world (62, 115).

The third serious deficiency in the current database for claiming that adverse environmental exposure might account for the SES health gradient is the absence of any data testing for the mediational model depicted in Figure 1. To our knowledge, no data indicate that the effects of poverty or income on health are mediated by exposure to multiple environmental risk factors. Therefore what we have shown herein can be summarized as follows:

- Income is often directly related to environmental quality, especially when low-income samples are contrasted with samples that are not poor.
- Environmental quality is inversely related to multiple physical and psychological health outcomes.

Greater progress in addressing the model shown in Figure 1 will require the collection of environmental risk and health data broken down by income or SES levels. Currently, such databases remain the exception. The absence of longitudinal studies also raises the possibility that the relations among income, environmental risk, and health are due to selection factors rather than environmental effects. Such a person-based explanation seems unlikely to account for the wide array of differential, environmental exposure shown herein, but changes in environmental conditions intra-person would provide stronger evidence of an environmentally based mechanism for the SES health gradient than the current preponderance of cross-sectional data. Reliance on cross-sectional data also precludes examination of the temporal course of environmental risk exposure and health in relation to income. Use of hierarchical linear modeling would also enable investigators to tease out nested, ecological niches of environmental exposure (e.g., region, neighborhood, home, work, school) in relation to income, class, or ethnicity (31).

In summary, public health databases need to routinely incorporate information about income and ethnicity. Such databases ideally would be longitudinal, sample across a continuum of income levels, and incorporate whenever possible multiple ecological niches of environmental exposure. Given the income and multiple environmental risk hypothesis, it would also behoove us to construct exposure estimates that include multiple environmental risk factors. This would enable scientists and policy makers to examine whether low-income persons and other disadvantaged individuals are exposed to higher levels of combined environmental risks and, in turn, determine if such multiple risk exposure helps account for their higher levels of morbidity and mortality. Public health professionals should be alert to the reasonable possibility that scrutiny of isolated, distinct physical and/or social risk factors misrepresents the ecology of environmental risk. This misrepresentation might, in turn, lead to underestimation of the contribution of environmental risk exposure to the public's health.

There is clearly consistent evidence that people who are poorer in the United States are more likely to be exposed to multiple environmental risks that portend adverse health consequences. Exposure to multiple, suboptimal environmental risk factors is one viable mechanism among several that could be a partial explanation for the gradient between SES and multiple health outcomes.

ACKNOWLEDGMENTS

We thank Nancy Adler, Urie Bronfenbrenner, and Judith Stewart for their feedback and support of this work. Preparation of this article was partially supported by the John D. and Catherine T. MacArthur Foundation Network on Socioeconomic Status and Health, and the Cornell University Agricultural Experiment Station, Project Nos. NYC 327404 and NYC 327407.

REFERENCES

1. Adler NE, Boyce T, Chesney M, Folkman S, Syme L. 1993. Socioeconomic inequalities in health: no easy solution. *JAMA* 269:3140–45.
2. Aneshensel C, Sucoff C. 1996. The neighborhood context of adolescent mental health. *J. Health Soc. Behav.* 37:293–310.
3. Araki S, ed. 1994. *Neurobehavioral Methods and Effects in Occupational and Environmental Health*. New York: Academic.
4. Attar B, Guerra N, Tolan P. 1994. Neighborhood disadvantage, stressful life events, and adjustment in urban elementary school children. *J. Clin. Child Psychol.* 23:391–400.
5. Bardana E, Montanaro B, eds. 1997. *Indoor Air Pollution and Health*. New York: Marcel Dekker.
6. Bartlett S. 1999. Children's experience of the physical environment in poor urban settlements and the implications for policy, planning, and practice. *Environ. Urban.* 11:63–73.
7. Baum A, Paulus PB. 1987. Crowding. See Ref. 125a, pp. 533–70.
8. Berglund B, Lindvall T. 1995. Community noise. *Arch. Cent. Sens. Res.* 2:1–195.
9. Berney L, Blane D, Davey Smith G, Gunnell D, Holland P, Montgomery S. 2000. Socioeconomic measures in early old age as indicators of previous lifetime exposure to environmental health hazards. *Soc. Health. Ill.* 22:415–30.
10. Bernton H, McMahon T, Brown H. 1972. Cockroach asthma. *Br. J. Dis. Child.* 66:61.
11. Blane D, Barley M, Davey-Smith G. 1997. Disease aetiology and materialist explanations of socioeconomic mortality differentials. *Eur. J. Public Health* 7:385–91.
12. Bradley RH. 1999. The home environment. In *Measuring Environment Across the Lifespan*, ed. SL Friedman, TD Wachs, pp. 31–58. Washington, DC: Am. Psychol. Assoc.
13. Bradley RH, Caldwell B. 1984. The HOME inventory and family demographics. *Dev. Psychol.* 20:315–20.
14. Bradley RH, Corwyn R, McAdoo H, Garcia C. 2001. The home environments of children in the United States Part I: variations by age, ethnicity, and poverty status. *Child Dev.* 72:1844–67.
15. Brajer V, Hall J. 1992. Recent evidence on the distribution of air pollution effects. *Contemp. Policy Issues* 10:63–71.

16. Bronfenbrenner U, Morris P. 1998. The ecology of developmental processes. In *Handbook of Child Psychology*, ed. W Damon, R Lerner, pp. 992–1028. New York: Wiley.
17. Brown L, Cowen E, Hightower A, Lotyczewski B. 1986. Demographic differences among children in judging and experiencing specific stressful life events. *J. Spec. Ed.* 20:339–46.
18. Bullard RD. 1990. *Dumping in Dixie*. Boulder, CO: Westview.
19. Burridge R, Ormandy D, eds. 1993. *Unhealthy Housing*. London: E. F. Spon.
20. Cabelli V, Dufour A. 1983. *Health Effects Criteria for Marine Recreational Waters*. Res. Triangle Park, NC: U.S. EPA, Off. Res. Dev. Res. EPA-600/1-80-031.
21. Calderon R, Johnson C, Craun G, Dufour A, Karlin R, et al. Health risks from contaminated water: Do class and race matter? *Toxicol. Ind. Health* 9:879–900.
22. Chi P, Laquatra J. 1990. Energy efficiency and radon risks in residential housing. *Energy* 15:81–89.
23. Cieselski S, Handzel T, Sobsey M. 1991. The microbiologic quality of drinking water in North Carolina migrant farmer camps. *Am. J. Public Health* 81:762–64.
24. Clinton WJ. 1994. Federal actions to address environmental justice in minority populations and low income populations. *Fed. Regist.* 59:7629–33.
25. Cohen S. 1980. Aftereffects of stress on human performance and social behavior: a review of research and theory. *Psychol. Bull.* 88:82–108.
26. Cohen S, Spacapan S. 1984. The social psychology of noise. In *Noise and Society*, ed. DM Jones, AJ Chapman, pp. 221–45. New York: Wiley.
27. Cook D, Whincup P, Jarvis M, Strachan D, Papacosta O, Bryant A. 1994. Passive exposure to cigarette smoke in children aged 5–7 years: individual, family, and community factors: *Br. Med. J.* 308:384–89.
28. Cubbin C, LeClere F, Davey Smith G. 2000. Socioeconomic status and injury mortality: individual and neighborhood determinants. *J. Epidemiol. Commun. Health* 54:517–24.
29. Davey Smith G, Hart C, Watt G, Hole D, Hawthorne V. 1998. Individual social class, area-based deprivation, cardiovascular disease risk factors, and mortality in Renfrew and Paisley study. *J. Epidemiol. Commun. Health* 52:399–405.
30. Davies J, Edmundson W, Raffonelli A, Cassady J, Morgade C. 1972. The role of social class in human pesticide pollution. *Am. J. Epidemiol.* 96:334–41.
31. Diez-Roux AV. 2000. Multilevel analysis in public health research. *Annu. Rev. Public Health* 21:171–92.
32. Dubow E, Ippolito M. 1994. Effects of poverty and quality of the home environment on changes in the academic and behavioral adjustment of elementary school-age children. *J. Clin. Child Psychol.* 23:401–12.
32a. Duncan GJ, Brooks-Gunn J, eds. 1997. *Consequences of Growing Up Poor*. New York: Russell Sage.
33. Evans GW. 1994. The psychological costs of chronic exposure to ambient air pollution. In *The Vulnerable Brain and Environmental Risks, Vol. 3: Toxins in Air and Water*, ed. RL Isaacson, KF Jensen, pp. 167–82. New York: Plenum.
34. Evans GW. 2001. Environmental stress and health. In *Handbook of Health Psychology*, ed. A Baum, T Revenson, JE Singer, pp. 365–85. Mahwah, NJ: Erlbaum.

35. Evans GW, Cohen S. 1987. Environmental stress. See Ref. 125a, pp. 571–610.
36. Evans GW, Lepore SJ. 1993. Nonauditory effects of noise on children: a critical review. *Child. Environ.* 10:31–51.
37. Evans GW, Lepore SJ, Allen K. 2000. Cross cultural differences in tolerance for crowding: fact or fiction? *J. Pers. Soc. Psychol.* 79:204–10.
38. Evans GW, Wells NM, Chan E, Saltzman H. 2000. Housing and mental health. *J. Consult. Clin. Psychol.* 68:526–30.
39. Evans GW, Wells NM, Moch A. 2002. Housing and mental health: a review of the evidence and a methodological and conceptual critique. *J. Soc. Issues.* In press.
40. Federman M, Garner T, Short K, Cutter W, Levine D, et al. 1996. What does it mean to be poor in America? *Mon. Labor Rev.* May:3–17.
41. Fiese B, Kline C. 1993. Development and validation of the family ritual questionnaire: initial reliability and validation studies. *J. Fam. Psychol.* 6:290–99.
42. Freeman AM. 1972. The distribution of environmental quality. In *Environmental Quality Analysis*, ed. AV Kness, B Bower, pp. 243–80. Baltimore: Johns Hopkins Press.
42a. Friends of the Earth, United Kingdom. 2001. *Pollution and Poverty: Breaking the Link.* London: Friends of the Earth.
42b. Friends of the Earth, United Kingdom. 2001. Environmental justice and inequalities. http://www.foe.co.uk/campaigns/sustainable-development/research-progs/env_just_prog.html.
43. Frumkin H, Walker D. 1998. Minority workers and communities. In *Maxcy Rosenau Last Public Health and Preventative Medicine*, ed. R Wallace, pp. 682–88. Stamford, Conn: Appleton & Lange. 14th ed.
44. Gallup G. 1993. *America's Youth in the 1990's.* Princeton: Gallup Inst.
45. Garbarino J. 1995. *Raising Children in a Socially Toxic Environment.* San Francisco: Jossey-Bass.
46. Garbarino J, Dubrow N, Kostelny K, Pardo C. 1992. *Children in Danger: Coping with the Consequences of Community Violence.* San Francisco: Jossey-Bass.
47. Garrett P, Ng'andu N, Ferron J. 1994. Poverty experiences of young children and the quality of their home environments. *Child Dev.* 65:331–45.
48. Garza G. 1996. Social and economic imbalances in the metropolitan area of Monterey. *Environ. Urban.* 8:31–42.
49. Gifford R. 2002. Satisfaction, health, security and social relations in high rise buildings. In *Social Effects of the Building Environment*, ed. A Seidel, T Heath. London: E. & F. N. Spon. In press.
50. Glass DC, Singer JE. 1972. *Urban Stress.* New York: Academic.
51. Gold D. 1992. Indoor air pollution. *Clin. Chest Med.* 13:215–29.
52. Goldstein I, Andrews L, Hartel D. 1988. Assessment of human exposure to nitrogen dioxide, carbon monoxide and respirable particulates in New York inner city residents. *Atmos. Environ.* 22:2127–39.
53. Goldtooth TBK. 1995. Indigenous nations: summary of sovereignty and its implications for environmental protection. In *Environmental Justice*, ed. B Bryant, pp. 138–48. Washington, DC: Island Press.
54. Graham H. 1995. Cigarette smoking: a light on gender and class inequality in Britain? *Int. J. Soc. Policy* 24:509–27.

55. Graham H, Blackburn C. 1998. The socioeconomic patterning of health and smoking behavior among mothers with young children on income support. *Sociol. Health Ill.* 20:215–40.
56. Groner J, Ahijevych K, Grossman L, Rich L. 1998. Smoking behaviors of women whose children attend an urban pediatric primary care clinic. *Women Health* 8:19–32.
57. Haan M, Kaplan G, Camacho T. 1987. Poverty and health. *Am. J. Epidemiol.* 125:898–908.
58. Haines M, Stansfeld S, Head J, Job RFS. 2002. Multi-level modeling of aircraft noise on national standardized performance tests in primary schools around Heathrow Airport, London. *J. Epidemiol. Commun. Health.* In press.
59. Halpern D. 1995. *More Than Bricks and Mortar*? London: Taylor & Francis.
60. Hamermesh D. 1999. Changing inequality in work injuries and work timing. *Mon. Labor Rev.* Oct.: 22–30.
61. Harburg E, Erfurt J, Hausentstein L, Chape C, Schull W, Schork M. 1973. Socioecological stress, suppressed hostility, skin color, and black-white male blood pressure: Detroit. *Psychosom. Med.* 35:276–96.
62. Hardoy J, Mitlin D, Satterthwaite D. 2001. *Environmental Problems in the Urbanizing World.* London: Earthscan.
63. Holgate S, Samet J, Koren H, Maynard R. 1999. *Air Pollution and Health.* New York: Academic.
64. Homel R, Burns A. 1987. Is this a good place to grow up in? Neighborhood quality and children's evaluations. *Landscape Urban Plan.* 14:101–16.
65. Ineichen B. 1993. *Housing and Health.* London: E & FN Spon.
66. Ingersoll RM. 1999. The problem of under qualified teachers in American secondary schools. *Educ. Res.* 28:26–37.
67. Inst. Med. 1999. *Environmental Justice.* Washington, DC: Natl. Acad. Press.
68. Inst. Med. 2000. *Clearing the Air: Asthma and Indoor Air Exposure.* Washington, DC: Natl. Acad. Press.
69. Jarvis M, Strachan D, Feyerbrand C. 1992. Determinants of passive smoking in children in Edinburgh, Scotland. *Am. J. Public Health* 82:1225–29.
70. Johnson BL. 1999. *Impact of Hazardous Waste on Human Health.* New York: Lewis.
71. Joint Cent. Housing Stud. Harvard Univ. 1999. *The State of the Nation's Housing.* Cambridge, MA: Harvard Univ.
72. Kang B. 1976. Study on cockroach antigen as a probable causative agent in bronchial asthma. *J. Allergy Clin. Immunol.* 58:357–65.
73. Kids Count Data Book 2000. 2000. Seattle: Annie Casey Found.
74. Kryter K. 1994. *The Handbook of Hearing and the Effects of Noise.* New York: Academic.
75. Larson RW, Verma S. 1999. How children and adolescents spend time around the world: work, play and developmental opportunities. *Psychol. Bull.* 125: 701–36.
76. Le Clere FB, Rogers R, Peters K. 1998. Neighborhood context and racial differences in women's heart disease. *J. Health Soc. Behav.* 39:91–107.

77. Leventhal T, Brooks-Gunn J. 2000. The neighborhoods they live in: the effects of neighborhood residence on child and adolescent outcomes. *Psychol. Bull.* 126:309–37.
78. Lippman N. 1992. *Environmental Toxicology.* New York: Van Nostrand.
79. Lucas REB. 1974. The distribution of job characteristics. *Rev. Econ. Stat.* 56:530–40.
80. Lundberg O. 1991. Causal explanations for class inequality in health — an empirical analysis. *Soc. Sci. Med.* 32:385–93.
81. MacArthur Found. 2001. *Network on Socioeconomic Status and Health.* http://www.macses.ucsf.edu.
82. Macintyre S, Maciver S, Sooman A. 1993. Area, class and health: Should we be focusing on places or people? *Int. Soc. Policy* 22:213–34.
82a. Macpheron A, Roberts I, Press IB. 1998. Children's exposure to traffic and pedestrian injuries. *Am. J. Public Health* 88:1840–45.
83. Marmot M, Siegrist J, Theorell T, Feeney A. 1999. Health and the psychosocial environment at work. In *Social Determinants of Health,* ed. M Marmot, RG Wilkinson, pp. 105–31. New York: Oxford Univ. Press.
84. Matheny A, Wachs TD, Ludwig J, Phillips E. 1995. Bringing order out of chaos: psychometric characteristics of the confusion, hubbub, and order scale. *J. Appl. Dev. Psychol.* 16:429–44.
85. Matte T, Jacobs D. 2000. Housing and health: current issues and implications for research and progress. *J. Urban Health Bull. NY Acad. Med.* 77:7–25.
86. Maxwell LM. 1996. Multiple effects of home and day care crowding. *Environ. Behav.* 28:494–511.
87. Mayer SE. 1997. Trends in the economic well-being and life chances of America's children. See Ref. 32a, pp. 49–69.
88. Miller J, Davis D. 1997. Poverty history, marital history, and quality of children's home environments. *J. Marriage Fam.* 59:996–1007.
89. Mohai P, Bryant B. 1992. Environmental racism: reviewing the evidence. In *Race and the Incidence of Environmental Hazards,* ed. B Bryant, P Mohai, pp. 163–76. Boulder, CO: Westview.
90. Moore GT, Lackney J. 1993. School design. *Child. Environ.* 10:99–112.
91. Moses M, Johnson E, Anger W, Burse V, Horstman S, et al. 1993. Environmental equity and pesticide exposure. *Toxicol. Ind. Health* 9:913–59.
92. Myers D, Baer W, Choi S. 1996. The changing problem of overcrowded housing. *J. Am. Plan. Assoc.* 62:66–84.
93. Natl. Cent. Educ. Stat. 2000. *Condition of America's Public School Facilities: 1999.* Washington, DC: U.S. Dep. Educ. NCES 2000–032.
94. Natl. Cent. Health Stat. 1991. Children's exposure to environmental cigarette smoke. *Advance Data from Vital and Health Statistics*: No. 202. Hyattsville, MD.
95. Natl. Cent. Health Stat. 1998. *Socioeconomic Status and Health Chart Book.* Hyattsville, MD: Natl. Cent. Health Stat.

96. Natl. Inst. Child Health Hum. Dev. Early Child Care Res. Network. 1997. Poverty and patterns of child care. See Ref. 32a, pp. 100–31.
97. Natl. Inst. Environ. Health Sci. 2001. *Health disparities research.* http://www.niehs.nih.gov/oc/factsheets/disparity/thome.htm.
98. Natl. Res. Counc. 1991. *Environmental Epidemiology*, Vol. 1. Washington, DC: Natl. Acad. Press.
99. Off. Environ. Justice. Washington, DC: EPA. http://es.epa.gov/oeca/main/ej/publis/html.
100. Off. Minority Health. Washington, DC: Dep. Health Hum. Serv. Closing the gap. http://www.omhrc.gov/ctg/ctg-env.htm.
101. Olds A. 2000. *Child Care Design Guide.* New York: McGraw-Hill.
102. Osofsky J. 1995. The effects of exposure to violence on young children. *Am. Psychol.* 50:782–88.
103. Perkins D, Taylor RB. 1996. Ecological assessments of community disorder: their relationship to fear of crime and theoretical implications. *Am. J. Commun. Psychol.* 24:63–107.
104. Phillips DA, Voran M, Kisker E, Howes C, Whitebook M. 1994. Childcare for children in poverty: opportunity or inequity? *Child Dev.* 65:472–92.
105. Pirkle J, Brody D, Gunter E, Kramer R, Paschal D, et al. 1994. The decline in blood lead levels in the United States. *JAMA* 272:284–91.
106. Pryer J. 1993. The impact of adult ill-health on household income and nutrition in Khulna, Bangladesh. *Environ. Urban.* 5:35–49.
107. Richters JE, Martinez P. 1993. The NIMH community violence project. *Psychiatry* 56:7–21.
108. Riley E, Vorhees C, eds. 1991. *Handbook of Behavioral Teratology.* New York: Plenum.
109. Rosenstreich D, Eggleson P, Kattan M, Baker D, Slavin R, et al. 1997. The role of cockroach allergy and exposure to cockroach allergens in causing morbidity among inner-city children with asthma. *N. Engl. J. Med.* 336:1356–63.
110. Rotton J. 1983. Affective and cognitive consequences of malodorous pollution. *Basic Appl. Soc. Psychol.* 4:171–91.
111. Rutter M. 1981. Protective factors in children's responses to stress and disadvantage. In *Prevention of Psychopathology*, ed. M Kent, J Rold, 1:49–74. Hanover, NH: Univ. Press.
112. Samet J, Spengler J, eds. 1991. *Indoor Air Pollution: A Health Perspective.* Baltimore: Johns Hopkins Press.
113. Sampson R, Raudenbush S, Earls F. 1997. Neighborhoods and violent crime: a multilevel study of collective efficacy. *Science* 277:918–24.
114. Sarpong S, Hamilton R, Eggleston P, Adkinson N. 1996. Socioeconomic status and race as risk factors for cockroach allergen exposure and sensitization in children with asthma. *J. Allergy Clin. Immunol.* 97:1393–401.
115. Satterthwaite D, Hart R, Levy C, Mitlin D, Ross D, et al. 1996. *The Environment for Children.* London: Earthscan.

116. Schwab M. 1990. An examination of intra-SMSA distribution of carbon monoxide exposure. *J. Air Waste Manag. Assoc.* 40:331–36.
117. Scott R. 1990. *Chemical Hazards in the Workplace*. Chelsea, MN: Lewis.
118. Sherman A. 1994. *Wasting America's Future*. Boston: Beacon Press.
119. Sinclair J, Pettit G, Harrist A, Dodge K, Bates J. 1994. Encounters with aggressive peers in early childhood: frequency, age differences, and correlates of risk for behavior problems. *Int. J. Behav. Dev.* 17:675–96.
120. Spencer MB, Mc Dermott P, Burton L, Kochman T. 1997. An alternative approach to assessing neighborhood effects on early adolescent achievement and problem behavior. In *Neighborhood Poverty*, Vol. 2: *Policy Implications in Studying Neighborhoods*, ed. J Brooks-Gunn, GJ Duncan, JL Aber, pp. 145–63. New York: Russell Sage Found.
121. Spencer NJ, Coe C. 2001. *The additive effects of social factors on risk of smoking in households with newborn infants*. Unpubl. Manuscr. Univ. Warwick, UK.
122. Stansfeld S. 1993. Noise, noise sensitivity, and psychiatric disorder: epidemiological and psychophysiological studies. *Psychol. Med. Monogr. Suppl.* 22:1–44.
123. Statistical Universe. 2000. *Income of families and primary individuals by selected characteristics: renter occupied units, 1999*. http://web.lexis-nexis.com/statuniv/.
124. Stehr-Green P. 1989. Demographic and seasonal influences on human serum pesticide residue levels. *J. Toxicol. Environ. Health* 27:405–21.
125. Stephens C, Akerman M, Avle S, Maia P, Campanario P, et al. 1997. Urban equity and urban health: using existing data to understand inequalities in health and environment in Accra, Ghana and Sao Paulo, Brazil. *Environ. Urban.* 9:181–202.
125a. Stokols D, Altman I, eds. 1987. *Handbook of Environmental Psychology*. New York: Wiley.
126. Stronks K, Dike van de Mheen H, Mackenbach J. 1998. A higher prevalence of health problems in low income groups: Does it reflect relative deprivation? *J. Epidemiol. Commun. Health* 52:548–57.
127. Suecoff S, Avner J, Chou K, Drain E. 1999. A comparison of New York City playground hazards in high and low income areas. *Arch. Pediatr. Adolesc. Med.* 153:363–66.
128. Taylor RB, Harrell A. 1999. *Physical Environment and Crime*. Washington, DC: Natl. Inst. Justice.
129. Deleted in proof.
130. Thompson SJ. 1993. Review: extra aural health effects of chronic noise exposure in humans. In *Larm und Krankheit (Noise and disease)*, ed. H Ising, B Kruppa, pp. 107–17. New York: Gustav Fischer Verlag.
131. Townsend P. 1979. *Poverty in the United Kingdom*. Berkeley: Univ. Calif. Press.
132. Trancik A, Evans GW. 1995. Spaces fit for children: competency in the design of daycare center environments. *Child. Environ.* 12:311–19.
133. U.S. Dep. Health Hum. Serv. 2000. *Trends in the Well Being of America's Children and Youth 2000*. Washington, DC: U.S. GPO.

134. U.S. Environ. Prot. Agency. 1977. *The Urban Noise Survey*. Washington, DC: EPA 550/9-77-100.
135. U.S. Environ. Prot. Agency. 1984. *National Statistical Assessment of Rural Water Conditions*. Washington, DC: EPA 570/9-84-004.
136. U.S. Environ. Prot. Agency. 1992. *Environmental Equity: Reducing Risk for All Communities*. Washington, DC: Off. Solid Waste Emerg. Response. EPA 230-R-92-008.
137. Wachs TD, Gruen G. 1982. *Early Experience and Development*. New York: Plenum.
138. Wallace D, Wallace R. 1998. *A Plague on Your Houses*. London: Verso.
139. Wandersman A, Nation M. 1998. Urban neighborhoods and mental health. *Am. Psychol.* 50:647–56.
140. Weinstein C, David T, eds. 1987. *Spaces for Children*. New York: Plenum.
141. West P, Fly J, Marans R, Larkin F. 1989. *Michigan Sports Anglers Fish Consumption Survey*. Ann Arbor, MI: Univ. Mich. Sch. Nat. Resourc., Nat. Resourc. Sociol. Res. Lab. Tech. Rep. 1.
142. White HL. 1998. Race, class, and environmental hazards. In *Environmental Injustices, Political Struggles*, ed. DE Camacho, pp. 61–81. Durham, NC: Duke Univ. Press.
143. Woodard B, Ferguson B, Wilson D. 1976. DDT levels in milk of rural indigent blacks. *Am. J. Dis. Child.* 130:400–3.
144. World Bank. 1992. *World Development Report*. New York: Oxford Univ. Press.
145. Wright BH. 1992. The effects of occupational injury, health, and disease on the health status of black Americans. See Ref. 89, pp. 114.

Part II

Health Policy and the Politics of Health

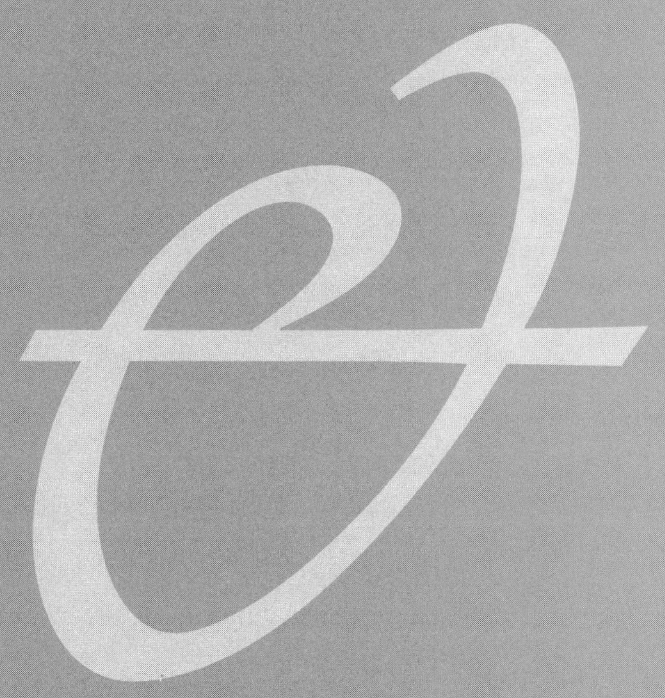

CHAPTER 3

HEALTH POLICY: THEORIES, MODELS, AND CONCEPTS

This edition of *The Nation's Health* places a greater emphasis on health policy and the politics of health. Chapter 3 focuses on the conceptual basis of the health policy process in the United States. Although there is a vast literature on the topic, we have chosen two models to describe the policy process. Article 1 is an excerpt from *Health Policymaking in the United States* by Beaufort B. Longest (1998). Longest presents a stages heuristic model for the complex health policymaking process described by Sabatier (1988) in "An Advocacy Coalition Framework of Policy Change and the Role of Policy-Oriented Learning Therein."

Sabatier's model is reviewed critically by Jenkins-Smith and Sabatier in Article 2. They describe the strengths and limitations of the model and make a distinction between the stages of "problem identification, agenda setting, adoption, implementation, and policy evaluation" (1993, p. 2). Longest uses this model but refers to policy evaluation as policy modification. As described by Longest and analyzed by Jenkins-Smith and Sabatier (1993),

> the stages is a useful heuristic because by dividing the policy process into a set of stages, it provides aid in understanding that process. But it is not a causal theory at all because it contains no clear set of causal factors that drive the process from one stage to the next (p. 9).

HEALTH POLICY CONCEPTS

This chapter introduction uses the term *policy* to describe public policies. Longest describes public policies as "authoritative decisions that are made in the legislative, executive or judicial branches of government. These decisions are intended to direct or influence the actions, behaviors, or decisions of others" (1998, p. 4). The same definition can be applied to long-term care policy, which focuses on such areas as skilled nursing home care, home health care, adult day care, and meals on wheels. Health policy and long-term care decisions are made at the federal, state, and local levels. The various forms of health policy described by Longest include laws, rules and regulations, and judicial decisions.

BASIC PREMISES OF THE ADVOCACY COALITION FRAMEWORK

Sabatier's 1988 paper begins with a description of the elements of policy making in the United States:

> … the importance of problem perception; shifts in elite and public opinion concerning the salience of various problems; periodic struggle over the proper locus of government authority; incomplete attainment of legally-prescribed goals; and an interactive process of policy formulation, problematic implementation, and struggles over reformulation (p. 130).

Next, he outlines the three basic premises of his advocacy coalition framework. The first premise posits that an understanding of the process of policy change requires a time perspective of a decade or more. Sabatier's second premise is that the most useful way to think about policy change over time is to focus on policy subsystems. Douglass Cater and Philip R. Lee described such a subsystem, "the subgovernment of health," more than 30 years ago (Cater and Lee, 1972). The third premise suggests that "public policies (or programs) can be conceptualized in the same manner as belief systems, i.e., as sets of values, priorities, and causal assumptions about how to realize them" (p. 341).

The important point that Sabatier makes about his first premise relates to the role of policy research and analysis, and what Weiss (1977) described as the "enlightenment function" of policy research. Such research can alter the perceptions of policymakers over time. This is evident in the evolving body of knowledge about the determinants of health described in Chapter 2. Prior to McKeown's seminal work from the 1950s to the 1970s and his book *The Role of Medicine: Dream, Mirage, or Nemesis?* (1976), the consensus was that most improvements in health were the result of medical care. Consequently, physicians and organized medicine held a uniquely powerful position with regard to health policy in the United States.

Sabatier's second premise about the role of policy subsystems is based on developments since the enactment of Medicare and Medicaid in 1965 and the proliferation of federal health policies, including those related to environmental health, in the 1960s and 1970s. Sabatier (1993) states:

> We argue that our conception of policy subsystems should be broadened from traditional notions of "iron triangles" limited to administrative agencies, legislative

> committees, and interest groups at a single level of government — to include action at various levels of government active in policy formulation and implementation, as well as journalists, researchers, and policy analysts who play important roles in the generation, dissemination, and evaluation of policy ideas (p. 17).

His third premise is that policy subsystems involve actors from all levels of government. He believes that it is a mistake to exclusively examine the policy process at the national level. The fourth premise is one of his most important:

> Public policies and programs incorporate implicit theories about how to achieve their objectives (Pressman and Wildavsky, 1973; Majone, 1980) and thus can be conceptualized in much the same way as belief systems. They involve value priorities, perceptions of important causal relations, perceptions of world states (including the magnitude of the problem), perceptions of the efficacy of policy instruments, and so on (1993, p. 17).

An important concept within his overall framework is policy-oriented learning, which is "relatively enduring alterations of thought or behavioral interactions that result from experience and are concerned with the attainment (or revision) of policy objectives." Policy-oriented learning may alter secondary aspects of an advocacy coalition's belief system, but not the core aspects of a belief system. The latter, if they are to change, will require changes external to the subsystem, such as macroeconomic conditions.

THE ROLE OF BELIEF SYSTEMS IN THE POLICY PROCESS

Sabatier also deals with the structure of the belief system of the policy elites. He describes the literature in this area as "a mine field of conflicting theories and evidence" (1993, p. 30). His analysis of the structure of belief systems of policy elites is, however, very helpful. He notes that there are three structural categories:

> a deep core of fundamental normative and ontological axioms that defines a person's underlying philosophy, a near (policy) core of basic strategies and policy positions for achieving deep core beliefs in the policy area or subsystem in question, and a set of secondary aspects comprising a multitude of instrumental decisions and information searches necessary to implement a policy core in the specific policy area (1993, p. 30).

The current debate on the coverage of prescription drugs in the Medicare program illustrates differences between the deep (normative) core values of the conservative Republicans and the liberal Democrats and how these have influenced their policy proposals. The Republicans propose a privatized system with individual choice of plans and a major reform of Medicare, changing from a defined benefit guaranteed by the government to a defined contribution by the government with the choice of health insurance plan left to the elderly and disabled beneficiaries. By contrast, the Democrats include prescription drugs as a defined benefit within the traditional Medicare framework.

POLICY THEORY

In discussion of Sabatier's model, Daniel McCool (1995) states that "There is a kind of paradox surrounding subsystems theory; many people like to use it, yet we have made only limited progress in developing it into a coherent, highly specialized and testable theory (see Recommended Reading). Like most policy theory, its potential has yet to be fully developed" (p. 380). McCool adds: "The greatest advantage of subsystem theory is that like the alliance it models, it cuts across innumerable dimensions of policy making" (p. 383). And finally, "subsystem theory tells us something about our governing institutions and how they interact with each other and with non-governing entities such as interest groups, the medical profession, and policy specialists. In this sense, the subsystem theory is potentially the most powerful policy theory of all" (p. 385).

LITIGATION AND THE ROLE OF COURTS IN PUBLIC HEALTH POLICY

Because of limitations of space, we have chosen not to include articles dealing with issues related to litigation and the role of courts in public health policy. Nonetheless, they are important, and there is a growing literature on the topic. The role of litigation in tobacco control policy has been reviewed by Jacobson and Warner (1999, see Recommended Reading). This review describes the dramatic shift in efforts to control tobacco use in the United States, with a shift to litigation by a limited number of states (Florida, Mississippi, Texas, and Minnesota) and the negotiated agreement between the remaining 46 states and the tobacco industry that will result in the payment of $208 billion to the states over the next 25 years by the tobacco companies. Despite this dramatic reversal of the influence of tobacco companies, the authors concluded that "litigation is a second best solution" (p. 769). Litigation is viewed as a "complement to a broader, comprehensive approach to tobacco control policy making rather than as an alternative to the traditional political apparatus of formulating and implementing public health policy" (p. 769).

The second development that has brought increased attention to the courts includes a series of Supreme Court decisions in the past decade that have increasingly restricted the role of the federal government vis-à-vis the states, particularly the role of Congress. These developments have been analyzed by Wendy Parmet (2002) in her article "After September 11: Rethinking Public Health Federalism." Parmet states that although the decisions by the Supreme Court repeatedly limited the role of the federal government, "it has not imposed significant limits on its ability to spend broadly for public health. Nor has the court rejected Congress's ability to attach conditions to State's receipt of federal monies as long as there is a nexus between the conditions imposed and the money received" (p. 206). Restrictions on the federal role are critical in light of the threat of bioterrorism since September 11 and the expanded role that Congress has assigned to the federal government in responding to terrorist attacks. The goal of these actions is to strengthen the partnership between federal, state, and local governments. Some of these issues are dealt with in greater detail in Part IV, "Preparing for Terrorism: A Public Health Response."

CRAFTING WORKABLE POLICY SOLUTIONS

Today, policymakers and citizens continue to debate the relative efficacy of various methods for tackling the fragmentation in financing and provision of public health programs, health care, and long-term care. Because of long-term care's costs, its custodial nature, and the lack of effective treatments for many of the disabling illnesses of old age (e.g., Alzheimer's disease), it has never been a health care priority at the federal or state level.

The formulation of health policy across several levels of government and hundreds of programs is complex. The health policy framework described by Sabatier in this chapter is widely accepted. Barr, Lee, and Benjamin (1999) (see Chapter 4, Article 2) identified four characteristics of the policy process in the United States: (1) the American character, (2) federalism and the role of government in health care, (3) pluralism and the role of special interest groups, and (4) incrementalism as the principal means of health policy. All of these characteristics can fit within the advocacy coalition framework and have contributed to the fragmentation of programs and services at the federal, state, and local levels. Twenty years ago, in her book *The Aging Enterprise* (1979), Estes described the equally fragmented state of politics related to long-term care. The problems remain much the same today. Crafting workable policy solutions is thus a very complex and dynamic endeavor. Although we deal separately with health and long-term care politics, it is important to recognize their interconnection.

In summary, the health policy process is undergoing continuous study and analysis. In our view, the best conceptual model has been developed by Sabatier and has been called an "advocacy coalition approach." We believe it best explains the complex health policy process at the national, state, and local levels.

REFERENCES

Barr, D. A., Lee, P. R., and Benjamin, A. E. (1999). Health care and health care policy in a changing world. In H. Wallace, G. Green, K. J. Jaros, L. L. Paine, and M. Story (Eds.), *Health and welfare for families in the 21st century* (pp. 13–29). Boston: Jones and Bartlett.

Cater, D., and Lee, P. R. (Eds.). (1972) *Politics of health.* Huntington, NY: Robert E. Krieger.

Estes, C. L. (1979). *The aging enterprise: A critical examination of social policies and services for the aged.* San Francisco: Jossey-Bass.

Jenkins-Smith, H. C., and Sabatier, P. A. (1993). The study of policy processes. In P. A. Sabatier and H. C. Jenkins-Smith (Eds.), *Policy change and learning: An advocacy coalition approach* (pp. 1–9). Boulder, CO: Westview Press.

Longest, B. B. (1998). *Health policymaking in the United States* (2nd ed.). Chicago: Health Administration Press.

McCool, D. C. (1995). Discussion [Commentary on "An advocacy coalition framework of policy change and the role of policy-oriented learning therein"]. In D. C. McCool (Ed.), *Public policy theories, models, and concepts. An anthology* (pp. 380–385). Englewood Cliffs, NJ: Prentice Hall.

McKeown, T. (1976). *The role of medicine: Dream, mirage, or nemesis?* London: Provincial Trust.

Parmet, W. E. (2002). After September 11: Rethinking public health federalism. *Journal of Law, Medicine, and Ethics, 30,* 201–211.

Sabatier, P. (1993). Policy change over a decade or more. In P. A. Sabatier and H. C. Jenkins-Smith (Eds.), *Policy change and learning: An advocacy coalition approach* (pp. 13–39). Boulder, CO: Westview Press.

Sabatier, P. (1988). An advocacy coalition framework of policy change and the role of policy-oriented learning therein. *Policy Sciences, 21,* 129–168.

Weiss, C. H. (1977). Research for policy's sake: The enlightenment function of social research. *Policy Analysis, 3,* 531–545.

Article 1

The Process of Public Policymaking

A Conceptual Model

Beaufort B. Longest, Jr.

The most useful way to conceptualize a process as complex and intricate as the one through which public policies are made is through a schematic model of the process. Although such models tend to be oversimplifications of real processes, they nevertheless can accurately reflect the component parts of the process as well as their interrelationships. Figure 1 is a model of the public policymaking process in the United States. A brief overview of this model is presented in this section.

Several general features of the model should be noted. First, as the model clearly illustrates, the policymaking process is distinctly cyclical. The circular flow of the relationships among the various components of the model reflects one of the most important features of public policymaking. The process is a continuous cycle in which almost all decisions are subject to subsequent modification. Public policymaking, including that in the health domain, is a process within which numerous decisions are reached but then revisited as circumstances change. The circumstances that trigger reconsideration of earlier decisions include changes in the way problems are defined as well as in the menu of possible solutions to problems. The new circumstances that trigger modification in previous decisions also routinely include the relative importance attributed to issues by the various participants in the political marketplace where this process plays out over time. For example, a problem with a low priority among powerful participants in the policymaking process may elicit a limited or partial policy solution. Later, if these participants give the problem a higher priority, a policy developed in response to the problem is much more likely. The major changes in Medicare policy made in 1997, for example, reflect a much more widely and deeply shared concern about the implications of this program for the federal budget than was previously the case.

Another important feature of the public policymaking process shown in the model is that the entire process is influenced by factors external to the process itself. This makes the policymaking process an *open system* — one in which the process

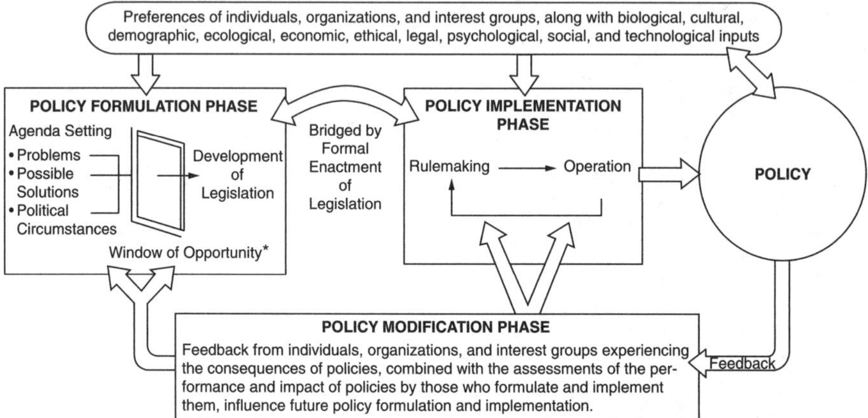

Figure 1 A model of the public policymaking process in the United States.

interacts with and is affected by events and circumstances in its external environment. This important phenomenon is shown in Figure 1 by the impact of the preferences of the individuals, organizations, and interest groups who are affected by policies, along with biological, cultural, demographic, ecological, economic, ethical, legal, psychological, social, and technological inputs, on the policymaking process. Legal inputs include decisions made in the courts that affect health and its pursuit. As was noted earlier, such decisions are themselves policies. In addition, decisions made within the legal system are important influences on the other decisions made within the policymaking process. Legal inputs help shape all other policy decisions, including reversing them on occasion when they are not consistent with the constitution.

A third important feature of the model is that it emphasizes the various distinct component parts of phases of the policymaking process, but also shows that they are highly interactive and interdependent. The conceptualization of the public policymaking process as a set of interrelated phases has been used by a number of authors, although there is considerable variation in what the phases of activities are called in these models as well as in their comprehensiveness. Brewer and de Leon (1983) provide a good generic example; Paul-Shaheen (1990) applies such a model specifically to health policymaking. The public policymaking process includes three interconnected phases:

- policy formulation, which incorporates activities associated with setting the policy agenda and, subsequently, with the development of legislation;
- policy implementation, which incorporates activities associated with rulemaking that help guide the implementation of policies and the actual operationalization of policies; and
- policy modification, which allows for all prior decisions made within the process to be revisited and perhaps changed.

The formulation phase (making the decisions that lead to public laws) and the implementation phase (taking actions and making additional decisions necessary to implement public laws) are bridged by the formal enactment of legislation, which shifts the cycle from its formulation to implementation phase. Once enacted as laws, policies remain to be implemented. Implementation responsibility rests mostly with the executive branch, which includes many departments that have significant health policy implementation responsibilities — for example, the Department of Health and Human Services (DHHS) (http://www.dhhs.gov) and the Department of Justice (DOJ) (http://www.usdoj.gov), and independent federal agencies, such as the Environmental Protection Agency (EPA) (http://www.epa.gov) and the Consumer Product Safety Commission (CPSC) (http://www.cpsc.gov). These and many other departments and agencies in the executive branch of government exist primarily to implement the policies formulated in the legislative branch.

It is important to remember that some of the decisions made within the implementing entities, as they implement policies, become policies themselves. For example, rules and regulations promulgated to implement a law and operational protocols and procedures developed to support a law's implementation are just as much policies as is the law itself. Similarly, judicial decisions regarding the applicability of laws to specific situations or regarding the appropriateness of the actions of implementing organizations are decisions that are themselves public policies. It is important to remember that policies are established within both the policy formulation and the policy implementation phases of the overall process.

The policy modification phase exists because perfection cannot be achieved in the other phases and because policies are established and exist in a dynamic world. Suitable policies made today may become inadequate with future biological, cultural, demographic, ecological, economic, ethical, legal, psychological, social, and technological changes. Pressure to change established policies may come from new priorities or perceived needs by the individuals, organizations, and interest groups that are affected by the policies.

Policy modification, which is shown as a feedback loop in Figure 1, may entail nothing more than minor adjustments made in the implementation phase or modest amendments to existing public laws. In some instances, however, the consequences of implementing certain policies can feed back all the way to the agenda-setting stage of the process. For example, formulating policies to contain the costs of providing health services — a key challenge facing policymakers today — is, to a large extent, an outgrowth of the success of previous policies that expanded access and subsidized an increased supply of human resources and advanced technologies to be used in providing health services.

One feature of the public policymaking process that the model presented in Figure 1 cannot adequately show — but one that is crucial to understanding the policymaking process — is the *political* nature of the process in operation. While there is a belief among many people — and a naive hope among still others — that policymaking is a predominantly rational decision-making process, this is not the case.

The process would no doubt be simpler and better if it were driven exclusively by fully informed consideration of the best ways for policy to support the nation's pursuit of health, by open and comprehensive debate about such policies, and by the rational selection from among policy choices strictly on the basis of ability to contribute to the pursuit of health. Those who are familiar with the policymaking process, however, know that it is not driven exclusively by these considerations. A wide range of other factors and considerations influence the process. The preferences and influence of interest groups, political bargaining and vote trading, and ideological biases are among the most important of these other factors. This is not to say that rationality plays no part in health policymaking. On a good day, it will gain a place among the flurry of political considerations, but "It must be a very good and rare day indeed when policymakers take their cues mainly from scientific knowledge about the state of the world they hope to change or protect" (Brown 1991, 20).

The highly political nature of the policymaking process in the United States accounts for very different and competing theories about how this process plays out. At the opposite ends of a continuum sit what can be characterized as strictly public-interest and strictly self-interest theories of the process. Policies made entirely in the public interest would be those that result when *all* participants act according to what they believe to be the public's interest. Alternatively, policies made entirely through a process driven by the self-interests of the diverse participants in the process would reflect an intricate calculus of the interplay of these various self-interests. Policies resulting from these two hypothetical extremes of the way people might behave in the policymaking process would indeed be very different.

In reality, however, health policies always reflect various mixes of public-interest and self-interest influences. The balance between the public and self-interests being served are quite important to the ultimate shape of health policies. For example, the present coexistence of the extremes of excess (e.g., exorbitant incomes of some physicians and health plan managers, esoteric technologies, and various overcapacities in the healthcare system) alongside true deprivation (e.g., lack of insurance for millions of people and inadequate access to basic health services for millions more) resulting from or permitted by some of the nation's existing health policies suggests that the balance has been tipped too often toward the service of self-interests.

This aside, public policymaking in the health domain in the United States is a remarkably complex and interesting process, although, as in all domains, clearly an imperfect process. The intricacies of the process are explored more thoroughly in the following chapters, where each of its interconnected phases is examined in more detail. One should keep in mind, as the separate components of the public policymaking process are examined individually and in greater detail, that policymaking, in general, is a highly political process; that it is continuous and cyclical in its operation; that it is heavily influenced by factors external to the process; and that the component phases and the activities within the phases of the process are highly interactive and interdependent.

SUMMARY

Health policies, like those in other domains, are made within the context of the political marketplace, where demanders for and suppliers of policies interact. The demanders of policies include all of those who view public policies as a mechanism through which to meet some of their health-related objectives or other objectives, such as economic advantage. Although individuals alone can demand public policies, the far more effective demand emanates from organizations and especially from organized interest groups. The suppliers of health policy include elected and appointed members of all three branches of government as well as the civil servants who staff the government.

The interests of the various and very diverse demanders and suppliers in this market cannot be completely coincident — often they are in open conflict — and the decisions and activities of any participants always affect and are affected by the activities of other participants. Thus, public policymaking in the health domain, as well as in other domains, is very much a human process, a fact with great significance for the outcomes and consequences of the process.

The policymaking process itself is a highly complex, interactive, and cyclical process that incorporates formulation, implementation, and modification phases.

REFERENCES

Alexander, J. A., and L. L. Morlock. 1997. "Power and Politics in Health Services Organizations." In *Essentials of Health Care Management,* edited by S. M. Shortell and A. D. Kaluzny, 256–85. Albany, NY: Delmar Publishers, Inc.

Anderson, G. F. 1992. "The Courts and Health Policy: Strengths and Limitations." *Health Affairs* 11:95–110.

Bauer, R. A., I. de S. Pool, and L. A. Dexter. 1963. *American Business and Public Policy.* New York: Atherton.

Beauchamp, T. L., and J. F. Childress. 1989. *Principles of Biomedical Ethics,* 3rd ed. New York: Oxford University Press.

Bibfeldt, F. 1958. *Paradoxes Observed.* Chicago: Perspective Press.

Brewer, G. D., and P. de Leon. 1983. *The Foundations of Policy Making*. Homewood, IL: Dorsey.

Brown, L. D. 1991. "Knowledge and Power: Health Services Research as a Political Resource." In *Health Services Research: Key to Health Policy,* edited by E. Ginzberg, 20–45. Cambridge, MA: Harvard University Press.

Buchholz, R. A. 1989. *Business Environment and Public Policy: Implications for Management and Strategy Formulation*, 3rd ed. Englewood Cliffs, NJ: Prentice Hall.

Christoffel, T. 1991. "The Role of Law in Health Policy." In *Health Politics and Policy,* 2nd ed., edited by T. J. Litman and L. S. Robins, 135–47. Albany, NY: Delmar Publishers, Inc.

Dye, T. R. 1978. *Understanding Public Policy,* 3rd ed. Englewood Cliffs, NJ: Prentice-Hall.

———. 1990. *Who's Running America? The Bush Era,* 5th ed. Englewood Cliffs, NJ: Prentice-Hall.

Dye, T. R., and H. Zeigler. 1975. *The Irony of Democracy,* 3rd ed. New York: Wadsworth Publishing Company, Inc.

Encyclopedia of Associations. 1993. Detroit, MI: Gale.

Feldstein, P. J. 1996. *The Politics of Health Legislation: An Economic Perspective,* 2nd ed. Chicago: Health Administration Press.

French, J. R. P., and B. H. Raven. 1959. "The Basis of Social Power." In *Studies of Social Power*, edited by D. Cartwright, 150–67. Ann Arbor, MI: Institute for Social Research.

Green, J. 1995. "High-Court Ruling Protects Hospital-bill Surcharges." *AHA News* 31 (18): 1.

Greenberger, D., S. Strasser, R. J. Lewicki, and T. S. Bateman. 1988. "Perception, Motivation, and Negotiation." In *Health Care Management: A Text in Organization Theory and Behavior,* 2nd ed., edited by S. M. Shortell and A. D. Kaluzny, 81–141. New York: John Wiley & Sons.

Keys, B., and T. Case. 1990. "How to Become an Influential Manager." *The Executive* 4 (4): 38–51.

Lineberry, R. L., G. C. Edwards, III, and M. P. Wattenberg. 1995. *Government in America,* 2nd ed. New York: HarperCollins College Publishers.

Lowi, T. J. 1979. *The End of Liberalism,* 2nd ed. New York: Norton.

Marmor, T. R., and J. B. Christianson. 1982. *Health Care Policy: A Political Economy Approach*. Beverly Hills, CA: Sage Publications.

Mintzberg, H. 1983. *Power In and Around Organizations*. Englewood Cliffs, NJ: Prentice-Hall.

Moe, T. 1980. *The Organization of Interests*. Chicago: University of Chicago Press.

Morone, J. A. 1990. *The Democratic Wish: Popular Participation and the Limits of American Government*. New York: Basic Books.

Olson, M. 1965. *The Logic of Collective Action*. Cambridge, MA: Harvard University Press.

Ornstein, N. J., and S. Elder. 1978. *Interest Groups, Lobbying and Policymaking*. Washington, DC: Congressional Quarterly Press.

Paul-Shaheen, P. A. 1990. "Overlooked Connections: Policy Development and Implementation in State-Local Relations." *Journal of Health Policy, Politics and Law* 15 (4): 133–56.

Pear, R. 1993. "Clinton's Health-Care Plan: It's Still Big, But It's Farther Away." *The New York Times.* (June 13): E4.

Peters, B. G. 1986. *American Public Policy: Promise and Performance,* 2nd ed. Chatham, NJ: Chatham House.

Peterson, M. A. 1993. "Political Influence in the 1990s: From Iron Triangles to Policy Networks." *Journal of Health Politics, Policy and Law* 18(2): 395–438.

Potter, M. A., and B. B. Longest, Jr. 1994. "The Divergence of Federal and State Policies on the Charitable Tax Exemption of Nonprofit Hospitals." *Journal of Health Politics, Policy and Law* 19: 393–419.

Rawls, J. 1971. *A Theory of Justice*. Cambridge, MA: The Belknap Press of Harvard University Press.

Starr, P. 1982. *The Social Transformation of American Medicine*. New York: Basic Books, Inc.

Truman, D. 1971. *The Governmental Process,* 2nd ed. New York: Knopf.

Wilsford, D. 1991. *Doctors and the State: The Politics of Health in France and the United States.* Durham, NC: Duke University Press.

Wilson, J. Q. 1973. *Political Organizations*. New York: Basic Books, Inc.

ARTICLE 2

The Study of Public Policy Processes

Hank C. Jenkins-Smith and Paul A. Sabatier

Many who study, teach, or practice policy analysis have experienced a growing dissatisfaction with the widely used concepts and metaphors of the policy process. Those concepts and metaphors — dubbed the "textbook approach" (Nakamura, 1987) — represent a broadly shared way of thinking about public policy. The shared language channels the way scholars frame research projects concerning the policy process and the way practitioners conceive the role of policy analysis. In our view, although the textbook approach has made important contributions and retains some heuristic value, it has outlived its usefulness as a guide to research and teaching.

We will first discuss the historical contributions of the textbook approach to the study of public policy as well as why it has ceased to be a fruitful frame of reference for analyzing the policy process. Next, we shall present the rudiments of an alternative approach — the advocacy coalition framework of policy change — that holds greater promise.

I. THE TEXTBOOK APPROACH AND ITS LIMITS

Policy researchers, practitioners, and teachers have broadly accepted a *stages heuristic* to public policy, derived from the work of Harold Lasswell, David Easton, and others.[1] Briefly put, the familiar stages model breaks the policy process into functionally and temporally distinct subprocesses. Easton (1965) elaborated a "systems model" of politics, which specified the functioning of input, throughput, output, and feedback mechanisms operating within broader "environments" (ecological, biological, social, personality, etc.). Lasswell (1951) developed a more policy-specific set of stages, including intelligence, recommendation, prescription, invocation, application, appraisal, and termination.

The functions and stages set out by Easton and Lasswell have been diffused throughout the literature of public policy, although the specification and content of the stages vary considerably. Among the most authoritative statements of the stages heuristic is Jones's *An Introduction to the Study of Public Policy* (1977) and Anderson's *Public Policy Making* (1979).[2] Both of these works, leaning heavily on Lasswell and Easton, make distinctions among the stages of problem identification, agenda setting, adoption, implementation, and policy evaluation. Both cast these stages within a broader environment characterized by federalism, political institutions, public opinion, political culture, and other constraints. Each of the stages in the process involves distinct periods of time, political institutions, and policy actors.

The widespread acceptance of the stages model results from important contributions made by that heuristic. As it evolved from the works of Easton (1965) and others, the concept of a *process* of policy making, operating across the various institutions of government, has provided an alternative to the institutional approach of traditional political science that emphasized analysis of specific institutions — such as the presidency, Congress, or the courts — or of public opinion. By shifting attention to the "process stream," the stages model has encouraged analysis of phenomena that transcend any given institution. Implementation of federal legislation, for example, typically involves one or more federal agencies, congressional policy and appropriations committees, federal court decisions, a multitude of state and local agencies, and the intervention of interest groups at multiple levels of government.

The reconceptualization accomplished by the stages heuristic has also permitted useful analysis of topics that were less readily perceived from within the institutionalist framework. Perhaps the most important of these has been its focus on policy impacts, that is, the ability of governmental institutions to accomplish policy objectives, such as improving air quality or assuring secure energy supplies, in the real world. Traditional institutional approaches tended to stop at the output of that particular institution — whether it be a law, a court decision, or an administrative agency rule — without specific attention to the ultimate outcome or impact of the policy.

Finally, the stages heuristic has provided a useful conceptual disaggregation of the complex and varied policy process into manageable segments. The result has been an array of very useful "stage focused" research, particularly regarding agenda setting (e.g., Cobb et al., 1972; Kingdon, 1984) and policy implementation (e.g., Pressman and Wildavsky, 1973; Bardach, 1977; Mazmanian and Sabatier, 1989).

In addition to the ready division of scholarly labor, scholars find the stages heuristic congenial because it fits the self-consciously rational method of the policy science disciplines. Bureaucrats find it attractive because it portrays a rational division of labor between the executive and legislative institutions of government, thereby legitimizing the role of the bureaucracy within representative systems. And for policy makers the stages model provides a view of the policy process that is in accord with democratic theory. According to the model, the decision maker draws on the inputs of the broader society to make policy, which is in turn handed over to other government players for implementation.

Despite its conceptual strengths and broad acceptance, we believe the stages heuristic has serious limitations as a basis for research and teaching:

1. First, and most important, the stages model is not really a *causal model* at all. It lacks identifiable forces to drive the policy process from one stage to

another and generate activity within any given stage. Although it has heuristic value in dividing the policy process into manageable units for analysis, it does not specify the linkages, drives, and influences that form the essential core of theoretical models. This lack of a crucial component of causal models is why we prefer to refer to it as the "stages heuristic."

2. Because it lacks causal mechanisms, the stages model *does not provide a clear basis for empirical hypothesis testing*. Absent such a basis, the means for empirically based confirmation, alteration, or elaboration of the model are lacking. For example, even in the most recent edition of his text, Jones (1977) does not provide a coherent set of hypotheses about the conditions under which the policy process will move from one stage to the next.
3. The stages heuristic suffers from *descriptive inaccuracy* in its positing of a sequence of stages starting with agenda setting and passing through policy formulation, implementation, and evaluation. Although proponents often acknowledge deviations from the sequential stages in practice (see, e.g., Jones, 1977:28–29), a great deal of recent empirical study suggests that deviations may be quite frequent: Evaluations of existing programs often affect agenda setting, and policy making occurs as bureaucrats attempt to implement vague legislation (Lowi, 1969; Majone and Wildavsky, 1978; Nakamura and Smallwood, 1980; Barrett and Fudge, 1981; Hjern and Hull, 1982; Kingdon, 1984; but see Sabatier, 1986:31).
4. The stages metaphor suffers from a built-in *legalistic, top-down focus*. It draws attention to a specific cycle of problem identification, major policy decision, and implementation that focuses attention on the intentions of legislators and the fate of a particular policy initiative. Such a top-down view results in a tendency to neglect other important players (e.g., street-level bureaucrats), restricts the view of "policy" to a specific piece of legislation, and may be entirely inapplicable when "policy" stems from a multitude of overlapping directives and actors, none of them dominant (Sabatier, 1986).
5. The stages metaphor inappropriately *emphasizes the policy cycle as the temporal unit of analysis*. Examination of a range of policy areas demonstrates that policy evolution often involves multiple cycles. These are initiated by actors at different levels of government as various formulations of problems and solutions are conceived, partially tested, and reformulated by a range of competing policy elites against a background of change in exogenous events and related policy issue areas (Jones, 1975; Heclo, 1974; Nelson, 1984; Sabatier and Pelkey, 1990). Thus, rather than focus on a single cycle initiated at a given (usually federal) governmental level, a more appropriate model would focus on *multiple, interacting cycles involving multiple levels of government*.
6. The stages metaphor fails to provide a good vehicle for integrating the roles of policy analysis and *policy-oriented learning throughout the public policy process*. The metaphor tends to confine analysis to the evaluation stage and to post-hoc assessments of the impacts of a given policy initiative. This approach is much too simple. Analysis clearly plays a large role in policy adoption (Jenkins-Smith and Weimer, 1985; Jenkins-Smith, 1990), agenda

setting (Kingdon, 1984), and other stages. The practical result, in policy studies, has been to "ghettoize" the perceived role of analysis and learning, as evidenced by the development of two distinct literatures; one that focuses on the interplay of self-interested policy actors pursuing rational strategies in pursuit of predetermined goals (Riker, 1962; Niskanen, 1971, 1975) and another that elaborates the processes by which analysis and learning are integrated into policy making (Weiss, 1977a, 1977b; Caplan et al., 1975).

In general, then, while the stages metaphor served a useful purpose in the 1970s and early 1980s, it has outlived that usefulness and needs to be replaced or substantially revised. We believe that the most promising replacement will be one that attempts to integrate the literature on the politics of the policy process with that on the utilization of policy analysis.

II. TOWARD AN ALTERNATIVE APPROACH TO THE POLICY PROCESS

Over the past two decades, a rather substantial literature has developed dealing with the utilization of policy analysis and other forms of relatively technical information by public-policy makers. Among its major findings have been the following:

1. Substantial cultural differences impede interaction between researchers and governmental officials (Dunn, 1980; Webber, 1983; but see Sabatier, 1984);
2. While policy analyses may seldom influence specific governmental decisions, they often serve an "enlightenment function" by gradually altering the concepts and assumptions of policy makers over time (Caplan et al., 1975; Weiss, 1977a, 1977b);
3. Policy analyses are often used for nonsubstantive reasons, such as to enhance organizational credibility, occupy "turf," and delay undesirable decisions (Rein and White, 1977; Jenkins-Smith and Weimer, 1985);
4. If researchers and policy analysts wish to have a significant impact on policy, they generally must abandon the role of "neutral technician" and instead adopt that of an "advocate" (Meltsner, 1976; Jenkins-Smith, 1982; Nelson, 1987).

While these contributions have been important, one of the most surprising — and distressing — aspects of the literature on knowledge utilization is that its development has been largely independent of the literature in political science on the factors affecting the policy process.[3]

In their efforts to understand public-policy making, political scientists have traditionally stressed such factors as:

1. Individual interests and values (Riker, 1962; Wilson, 1973);
2. Organizational rules and procedures (Kaufman, 1960; Fenno, 1973);
3. The broader socioeconomic environment in which political institutions operate (Easton, 1965; Hofferbert, 1974); and

4. The tendency for legislators, bureaucratic officials, and interest group leaders concerned with a specific policy area to form relatively autonomous policy subsystems (Fritschler, 1983; Hamm, 1983).

When they have dealt with the role of policy analysis — which has not been often — political scientists have generally argued that it is simply another resource used in an advocacy fashion to advance one's interests (Margolis, 1974; Wildavsky and Tenenbaum, 1981).

The advocacy coalition framework (ACF) of the policy process synthesizes many of the major findings of the knowledge utilization literature — particularly those concerning the enlightenment function and the advocacy use of analysis — into the broader literature on public-policy making (Sabatier and Jenkins-Smith, 1988). According to the ACF, policy change over time is a function of three sets of processes. The first concerns the interaction of competing *advocacy coalitions* within a policy subsystem. An advocacy coalition consists of actors from a variety of public and private institutions at all levels of government who share a set of basic beliefs (policy goals plus causal and other perceptions) and who seek to manipulate the rules, budgets, and personnel of governmental institutions in order to achieve these goals over time. The second set of processes concerns *changes external to the subsystem* in socioeconomic conditions, system-wide governing coalitions, and output from other subsystems that provide opportunities and obstacles to the competing coalitions. The third set involves the effects of *stable system parameters* — such as social structure and constitutional rules — on the constraints and resources of the various subsystem actors.

The ACF assumes that, with respect to both belief systems and public policies, one can distinguish "core" from "secondary" elements. Coalitions are organized around common beliefs in core elements; since these common beliefs are hypothesized to be relatively stable over periods of a decade or more, so is coalition composition. Coalitions seek to learn about how the world operates and the effects of various governmental interventions in order to realize their goals over time. Because of resistance to changing core beliefs, however, such "policy-oriented learning" is usually confined to the secondary aspects of belief systems. Changes in core elements of public policies require the replacement of one dominant coalition by another, and this transition is hypothesized to result primarily from changes external to the subsystem.

NOTES

1. *Webster's New Collegiate Dictionary* defines "heuristic" as "providing aid or direction in the solution of a problem but otherwise unjustified." As will be discussed in the following pages, the stages model is a useful heuristic because, by dividing the policy process into a set of stages, it provides aid in understanding that process. But it is not a causal theory at all because it contains no clear set of causal factors that drive the process from one stage to the next.

2. Jones's text was originally published in 1970 and Anderson's in 1975. Among the other public policy texts that rely heavily on the stages metaphor are Brewer and de Leon (1983), Peters (1986), Palumbo (1988), and Rushefsky (1990). Ripley (1985) combines the stages metaphor with Lowi's work on policy arenas.
3. There have been some exceptions, most notably dealing with the use of analysis in specific institutional settings, such as legislatures (Sabatier and Whiteman, 1985; Webber, 1986) and administrative agencies (Sabatier, 1978; Beyer and Trice, 1982).

REFERENCES

Anderson, James (1979). *Public Policy Making,* 2d ed. New York: Holt, Rinehart, and Winston.

Bardach, Eugene (1977). *The Implementation Game: What Happens After a Bill Becomes a Law*? Cambridge, MA: MIT Press.

Barrett, Susan, and Fudge, Colin, eds. (1981). *Policy and Action.* London: Methuen.

Beyer, Janice, and Trice, Harrison (1982). "The Utilization Process: A Conceptual Framework and Synthesis of Empirical Findings," *Administrative Science Quarterly* 27 (December): 591–622.

Brewer, Garry, and de Leon, Peter (1983). *Foundations of Policy Analysis.* Homewood: Dorsey.

Caplan, Nathan, et al. (1975). *The Use of Social Science Knowledge in Policy Decisions at the National Level.* Ann Arbor Institute for Social Research.

Cobb, Roger, et al. (1975). "Agenda Building as a Comparative Process," *American Political Science Review* 70 (March): 126–138.

Dunn, William (1980). "The Two-Communities Metaphor and Models of Knowledge Use," *Knowledge* 1 (June): 515–536.

Easton, David (1965). *A Systems Analysis of Political Life.* New York: John Wiley.

Fenno, Richard (1975). *Congressmen in Committees.* Boston: Little, Brown.

Fritschler, A. Lee (1983). *Smoking and Politics,* 3d ed. Englewood Cliffs: Prentice-Hall.

Hamm, Keith (1983). "Patterns of Influence Among Committees, Agencies and Interest Groups," *Legislative Studies Quarterly* 8 (August): 379–426.

Heclo, Hugh (1974). *Social Policy in Britain and Sweden.* New Haven: Yale Univ. Press.

Hjern, Benny, and Hull, Chris (1982). "Implementation Research as Empirical Constitutionalism," *European Journal of Political Research* 10 (June): 105–116.

Hofferbert, Richard (1974). *The Study of Public Policy.* Indianapolis: Bobbs-Merrill.

Jenkins-Smith, Hank (1982). "Professional Roles for Policy Analysis: A Critical Analysis," *Journal of Policy Analysis and Management* 2 (Fall): 88–100.

Jenkins-Smith, Hank (1990). *Democratic Politics and Policy Analysis.* Pacific Grove, CA: Brooks/Cole.

Jenkins-Smith, Hank, and Welmer, David (1985). "Analysis as Retrograde Action," *Public Administration Review* 45 (July): 485–494.

Jones, Charles (1975). *Clean Air.* Pittsburgh: Univ. of Pittsburgh Press.

Jones, Charles (1977). *An Introduction to the Study of Public Policy,* 3d ed. Belmont, CA: Wadsworth.

Kaufman, Herbert (1960). *The Forest Ranger.* Baltimore: Johns Hopkins Univ. Press.

Kingdon, John (1984). *Agendas, Alternatives, and Public Policies.* Boston: Little, Brown.

Lasswell, Harold (1951). "The Policy Orientation," in D. Lerner and H. Lasswell, eds., *The Policy Sciences.* Stanford: Stanford Univ. Press.

Lowi, Theodore (1969). *The End of Liberalism.* New York: Norton.

Majone, Giandomenico, and Wildavasky, Aaron (1978). "Implementation as Evolution," in Howard Freeman, ed., *Policy Studies Review Annual: 1978.* Beverly Hills: Sage.

Margolis, Howard (1974). *Technical Advice on Policy Issues.* Beverly Hills: Sage.

Mazmanian, Daniel, and Sabatier, Paul (1989). *Implementation and Public Policy.* Lanham, MD: Univ. Press of America.

Meitsner, Arnold (1976). *Policy Analysis in the Bureaucracy.* Berkeley: Univ. of California Press.

Nakamura, Robert (1987). "The Textbook Policy Process and Implementation Research," *Policy Studies Review* (no. 1): 142–154.

Nakamura, Robert, and Smallwood, Frank (1980). *The Politics of Policy Implementation.* New York: St. Martin's.

Nelson, Barbara (1984). *Making an Issue of Child Abuse.* Chicago: Univ. of Chicago Press.

Nelson, Robert (1987). "The Economics Profession and the Making of Public Policy," *Journal of Economic Literature* 25 (March): 42–84. Nevada Gaming Commission, Economic Research Division (1970). *Direct Levies on Gaming in Nevada, FY 2969–70.* Carson City, NV, November.

Niskanen, William (1971). *Bureaucracy and Representative Government.* Chicago: Rand McNally.

———. (1975). "Bureaucrats and Politicians," *Journal of Law and Economics* 18: 617–643.

Palumbo, Dennis (1988). *Public Policy in America.* New York: Harcourt, Brace, Jovanovich.

Peters, Guy (1986). *American Public Policy: Promise and Performance,* 2d ed. Chatham, NJ: Chatham House.

Pressman, Jeffery, and Wildavsky, Aaron (1973). *Implementation.* Berkeley, CA: Univ. of California Press.

Rein, Martin, and White, Sheldon (1977). "Policy Research: Belief and Doubt," *Policy Analysis* 3 (Spring): 239–271.

Riker, William (1962). *The Theory of Political Coalitions.* New Haven: Yale Univ. Press.

Rushefsky, Mark (1990). *Public Policy in the U.S.,* Monterey: Brooks/Cole.

Sabatier, Paul A. (1978). "The Acquisition and Utilization of Technical Information by Administrative Agencies," *Administratives Science Quarterly* 23 (September): 386–411.

Sabatier, Paul A. (1984). "Faculty Interest in Policy-Oriented Advising and Research," *Knowledge* 5 (June): 469–502.

Sabatier, Paul A. (1986). "Top-Down and Bottom-Up Models of Policy Implementation: A Critical Analysis and Suggested Synthesis," *Journal of Public Policy* 6 (January): 21–48.

Sabatier, Paul A., and Jenkins-Smith, Hank (1986). Symposium Volume. "Policy Change and Policy-Oriented Learning," *Policy Sciences* 21 (Summer and Fall): 125–277.

Sabatier, Paul A., and Pelkey, Neil (1990). *Land Development at Lake Tahoe: The Effects of Environmental Controls and Economic Conditions on Housing Construction.* Davis, CA: Institute of Ecology.

Sabatier, Paul A., and Whiteman, David (1985). "Legislative Decision-Making and Substantive Policy Information: Models of Information Flow," *Legislative Studies Quarterly* 10 (August): 395–422.

Webber, David (1983). "Obstacles to the Utilization of Systematic Policy Analysis," *Knowledge* 4 (June): 534–560.

Webber, P. (1985). *Basic Content Analysis.* Beverly Hills: Sage.

Weiss, Carol (1977a). *Using Social Research in Public Policy Making.* Lexington: D.C. Heath.

Weiss, Carol (1977b). "Research for Policy's Sake: The Enlightenment Function of Social Research," *Policy Analysis* 3 (Fall): 531–545.

Wildavsky, Aaron, and Tenenbaum, Ellen (1981). *The Politics of Mistrust.* Beverly Hills: Sage.

Wilson, James O. (1973). *Political Organizations.* New York: Basic Books.

ARTICLE 3

POLICY CHANGE OVER A DECADE OR MORE

Paul A. Sabatier

In the mid-1950s, air pollution was scarcely a subject of public policy debate in the United States. Federal efforts were limited to a tiny program of technical assistance, and only a few states had more than paper programs. Governmental entities with active control programs were largely limited to a few cities — New York, Chicago, Pittsburgh, St. Louis, and Los Angeles — where the problem was perceived as one of dirty air arising primarily from coal combustion.

Ten years later, federal expenditures had risen more than twenty-fold, the number of states with pollution control budgets of more than $100,000 had increased from three to twenty-two, California had instituted the first controls on automobile emissions, and the 1967 Federal Air Quality Amendments had attempted to provide some federal review of state programs (Davies, 1970:105, 129; Krier and Ursin, 1977). But increasing public concern about environmental degradation, criticism of state and federal programs, and partisan competition for the growing environmental constituency led to passage of the 1970 Federal Clean Air Amendments (Jones, 1975; Ingram, 1978). This landmark law transferred principal responsibility for pollution control from local and state governments to Washington and instituted a massive regulatory program designed to dramatically improve air quality by the mid-1970s. Passage of the 1970 Amendments was probably also assisted by the publication of federally sponsored research reports indicating that air quality posed significant health risks to many people in urban areas as well as increasing evidence that industry, utilities, and automobiles — rather than residential space heating — were the major sources of most pollutants (Sabatier, 1975).

The consensus in favor of stringent pollution control soon weakened, however, as new issues (e.g., energy prices) came to the fore and as people became aware of the technical and political difficulties of implementing such ambitious legislation. By the end of the 1970s, while emissions and air quality levels in many areas had improved, the implementation of increasingly stringent automotive emissions standards had been delayed several times. Public-policy makers and scholars increasingly became aware that much of the real authority lay with state and local governments (Ingram, 1977; Mazmanian and Sabatier, 1989:Chap. 4; Downing, 1984:Chaps. 11–13). During the 1980s, air pollution remained a controversial issue: The Reagan administration sought — with very mixed results — to substantially weaken the federal program (Vig and Kraft, 1984; Wood, 1988); economists argued for the replacement of uniform legal standards with more flexible economic incentives (White, 1982; Liroff, 1986); California continued to pioneer in a number of areas, such as alternative-fuel (nongasoline) vehicles; and repeated efforts were made to amend the federal law. These efforts finally bore fruit in the 1990 Clean Air Amendments, which strengthened the program in a number of areas, most notably by the adoption of an economic incentive approach to acid rain and the beginning of federal efforts to stimulate alternative-fuel vehicles (Cohen, 1992).

How is one to understand the incredibly complex process of policy change over a decade or more in air pollution control or any other policy area? On the one hand, the stages heuristic provides some assistance. It draws attention to the iterative process of agenda setting, formulation, implementation, and reformulation — with major changes in federal law in 1967, 1970, 1977, and 1990. On the other hand, the stages heuristic would have difficulty explaining the continuing role of state and local governments — particularly California — in policy innovation. It also neglects the importance *throughout the policy process* of technical information concerning the effects of air pollutants on human health, the principal sources of various pollutants, the causes of acid rain, and the effectiveness of economic incentives as a policy instrument.

The traditional concerns of political scientists also provide some assistance. The dramatic increase in public support for environmental protection in the late 1960s was an important factor in the passage of the 1970 Amendments, and the public's equivocation over the tradeoff between energy security and environmental protection in the 1970s played some role in the 1974 and 1977 congressional approvals of delays in imposing more stringent automobile emissions standards. Likewise, the decentralization of power in Congress from party leaders to subcommittee chairs played a role in the passage of the 1970 Amendments and in the stalemate during the 1980s (Cohen, 1992). And political scientists' focus on "iron triangles" — in this case, the Senate Environment Committee, the House Commerce Committee, the Environmental Protection Agency, and concerned interest groups — certainly constitutes a necessary part of any explanation of federal air pollution policy implemented over the past thirty years. But the traditional preoccupations of political scientists also neglect the critical role of state and local implementing agencies, the continuing importance of California (and several other jurisdictions) as policy innovators, and the importance of technical information in framing the debate over such issues as acid rain, the validity of air quality standards (which substantially drive the entire policy process), and the debate over whether the dominant policy instrument should be uniform emissions regulations or more flexible economic incentives. In short, political scientists' traditional focus on specific governmental institutions (Congress, the presidency, interest groups) or specific types of political behavior (popular voting, legislative roll calls) encounters enormous difficulties when dealing with policy change over several decades. Policy evolution over that span of time usually goes way beyond a few critical institutions or types of political behavior to include hundreds of governmental institutions, dozens of important elections in various jurisdictions, and several dozen "iron triangles" at various levels of government. It also involves entire categories of behavior — particularly technical debates over critical policy issues — neglected by the vast majority of political scientists (Sabatier, 1991a, 1991b).

Both the stages heuristic and the traditional preoccupations of political scientists suffer from at least two major limitations in their ability to explain the evolution of air pollution policy in the United States over the past thirty years. First, they both suffer from severe cases of "Potomac fever," of assuming that almost everything of importance occurs in Washington, D.C. In the process, they dramatically underestimate the considerable discretion exercised by state and local agencies when implementing federal law as well as their ability to generate and implement innovative policies on their own.[1] Second, both neglect the role of ideas — particularly ideas involving the relatively technical aspects of policy debates — in policy evolution.

Fortunately, not everyone has been restricted by the blinders imposed by the stages heuristic or the concerns of most political scientists. A critical contribution to understanding policy change over time was made by Heclo's (1974) analysis of British and Swedish welfare policy during the initial decades of this century. On the one hand, Heclo agreed with political demographers who pointed to the role of changing social and economic conditions — such as population migrations, the emergence of new social movements, critical elections, and macroeconomic changes in inflation and unemployment — in providing the constituency base for major policy changes (Hofferbert, 1974; Hibbs and Fassbender, 1981; Burnham, 1970). Equally important in his view, however, was the interaction of specialists within a specific policy area as they gradually learned more about various aspects of the problem over time and experimented with a variety of means to achieve their policy objectives. In essence, Heclo saw policy change as a product of both (1) large-scale social, economic, and political changes and (2) the interaction of people within a policy community involving both competition for power and efforts to develop more knowledgeable means of addressing various aspects of the policy problem.

In many respects, Chapters 2 and 3 of *Policy Change and Learning: An Advocacy Coalition Approach* (1993) represent an attempt to translate Heclo's basic insight into a reasonably clear conceptual framework of policy change over time. This chapter continues his focus on the interaction of political elites within a policy community or subsystem who attempt to respond to changing socioeconomic and political conditions. The first part presents an overview of the conceptual framework as it applies to policy change over periods of a decade or more. Subsequent sections deal with specific aspects, including external events affecting policy subsystems and the internal structure of subsystems. This chapter touches on the role of policy-oriented learning in policy change, particularly the conditions under which elites from different advocacy coalitions gradually alter their belief systems over time as a result of formal policy analyses and trial-and-error learning.[2]

I. AN OVERVIEW OF THE FRAMEWORK

The advocacy coalition framework (ACF) has at least four basic premises: (1) that understanding the process of policy change — and the role of policy-oriented learning therein — requires a time perspective of a decade or more; (2) that the most useful way to think about policy change over such a time span is through a focus on "policy subsystems," that is, the interaction of actors from different institutions who follow and seek to influence governmental decisions in a policy area; (3) that those subsystems must include an intergovernmental dimension, that is, they must involve all levels of government (at least for domestic policy); and (4) that public policies (or programs) can be conceptualized in the same manner as belief systems, that is, as sets of value priorities and causal assumptions about how to realize them.

The focus on time spans of a decade or more comes directly from findings concerning the importance of the "enlightenment function" of policy research. Weiss (1977a, 1977b) has argued persuasively that a focus on short-term decision making will underestimate the influence of policy analysis because such research is used primarily to alter the perceptions and conceptual apparatus of policy makers over time. A corollary of this view is that it is the *cumulative* effect of findings from different studies and from ordinary knowledge (Lindblom and Cohen, 1979) that has the greatest influence on policy. The literature on policy implementation also points to the need for utilizing time frames of a decade or more, both in order to complete at least one cycle of formulation, implementation, and reformulation and to obtain a reasonably accurate portrait of program success and failure (Mazmanian and Sabatier, 1989). Numerous studies have shown that ambitious programs that appeared after a few years to be abject failures received more favorable evaluations when seen in a longer time frame; conversely, initial successes may evaporate over time (Bernstein, 1955; Kirst and Jung, 1982; Hogwood and Peters, 1983).

The framework's second basic premise is that the most useful aggregate unit of analysis for understanding policy change in modern industrial societies is not any specific governmental institution but rather a policy subsystem, that is, those actors from a variety of public and private organizations who are actively concerned with a policy problem or issue such as air pollution control, mental health, or surface transportation. Following a number of recent authors, we argue that conceptions of policy subsystems should be broadened from traditional notions of "iron triangles" — limited to administrative agencies, legislative committees, and interest groups at a single level of government — to include actors at various levels of government active in policy formulation and implementation as well as journalists, researchers, and policy analysts who play important roles in the generation, dissemination, and evaluation of policy ideas (Heclo, 1978; Dunleavy, 1981; Milward and Wamsley, 1984; Scholz et al., 1991).

The third basic premise is that policy subsystems will normally involve actors from *all* levels of government. To examine policy change only at the national level will, in most instances, be seriously misleading. In the United States and many other countries, policy innovations normally occur first at a subnational level and then may get expanded into nationwide programs; even after national intervention, subnational initiatives normally continue. Air pollution is typical: Cities like Pittsburgh, St. Louis, Chicago, and New York had viable stationary source controls twenty years before any significant federal involvement occurred, and California has consistently been several years ahead of the feds on mobile source controls. Moreover, two decades of implementation research has conclusively demonstrated that state and local implementing officials have substantial discretion in deciding exactly how federal "policy" gets translated into thousands of concrete decisions in very diverse local situations.[3]

The fourth important premise is that public policies and programs incorporate implicit theories about how to achieve their objectives (Pressman and Wildavsky, 1973; Majone, 1980) and thus can be conceptualized in much the same way as belief systems. They involve value priorities, perceptions of important causal relationships, perceptions of world states (including the magnitude of the problem), perceptions of the efficacy of policy instruments, and so on. This ability to map beliefs and policies on the same "canvas" provides a vehicle for assessing the influence of various actors over time, particularly the role of technical information (beliefs) on policy change.

Figure 1 presents a general overview of the framework. On the left side are two sets of exogenous variables — the one fairly stable, the other more dynamic — that

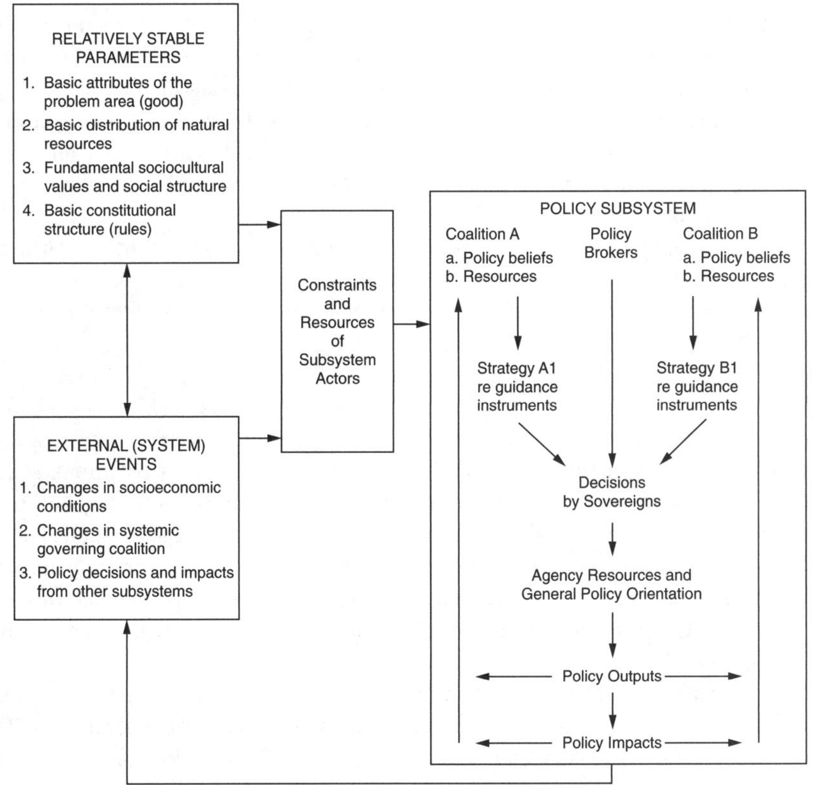

Figure 1 The advocacy coalition framework of policy change.

affect the constraints and opportunities of subsystem actors. Air pollution policy, for example, is strongly affected by the nature of air quality as a collective good, by the geographical contours of air basins, and by political boundaries, which are usually quite stable over time. But there are also more dynamic factors, including changes in socioeconomic conditions (e.g., public opinion and oil prices) and in the systemic governing coalition, which provide some of the principal sources of policy change.

Within the subsystem, it is assumed that actors can be aggregated into a number of advocacy coalitions composed of people from various governmental and private organizations who share a set of normative and causal beliefs and who often act in concert. At any particular point in time, each coalition adopts a strategy envisaging one or more institutional innovations that members feel will further policy objectives. Conflicting strategies from various coalitions are normally mediated by a third group of actors, here termed "policy brokers," whose principal concern is to find some reasonable compromise that will reduce intense conflict. The end result is one or more governmental programs, which in turn produce policy outputs at the operational level (e.g., agency permit decisions). These outputs — mediated by a number of other factors — result in a variety of impacts on targeted problem parameters (e.g., ambient air quality) as well as in various side effects.

On the basis of perceptions of the adequacy of governmental decisions and the resultant impacts as well as new information arising from search processes and external dynamics, each advocacy coalition may revise its beliefs or alter its strategy. The latter may involve the seeking of major institutional revisions at the collective choice level, more minor revisions at the operational level (Kiser and Ostrom, 1982), or even changes in the dominant electoral coalition at the systemic level, an arena outside of the subsystem itself.

Within the general process of policy change, this framework has a particular interest in policy-oriented learning. Following Heclo (1974:306), policy-oriented learning refers to relatively enduring alterations of thought or behavioral intentions that result from experience and are concerned with the attainment (or revision) of policy objectives. Policy-oriented learning involves the internal feedback loops depicted in Figure 1, perceptions concerning external dynamics, and increased knowledge of problem parameters and the factors affecting them. The framework assumes that such learning is instrumental, that is, that members of various coalitions seek to better understand the world in order to further their policy objectives. They will resist information suggesting that their basic beliefs may be invalid or unattainable, and they will use formal policy analyses primarily to buttress and elaborate those beliefs (or attack their opponents' views). Within this assumption of the prevalence of advocacy analysis, Chapter 3 identifies several factors that facilitate learning across advocacy coalitions.

Such learning comprises, however, only one of the forces affecting policy change over time. In addition to this cognitive activity, there is a real world that changes. This world, first of all, involves the realm of system dynamics depicted in Figure 1: Changes in relevant socio-economic conditions and system-wide governing coalitions — such as the 1973 Arab oil embargo or the 1980 election of Ronald Reagan — can dramatically alter the composition and the resources of various coalitions and, in turn, public policy within the subsystem. Turnover in personnel — sometimes resulting from external conditions, sometimes merely from death or retirement — constitutes a second noncognitive source of change that can substantially alter the political resources of various advocacy coalitions and thus the policy decisions at the collective choice and operational levels.

The basic argument of this framework is that, although policy-oriented learning is an important aspect of policy change and can often alter secondary aspects of a coalition's belief system, changes in the core aspects of a policy are usually the results of perturbations in noncognitive factors external to the subsystem, such as macroeconomic conditions or the rise of a new systemic governing coalition. While the framework borrows a great deal from Heclo (1974, 1978), it differs in its emphasis on ideologically based coalitions and its conception of the dynamics of policy-oriented learning. It can also be clearly distinguished from analyses that view formal organizations as the basic actors (e.g., Krasnow et al., 1982) or that focus on individuals seeking to attain their self-interest through the formation of short-term "minimum winning coalitions" (Riker, 1962).

Although in presenting the ACF, we will illustrate relevant concepts and hypotheses with examples from U.S. air pollution policy, the ACF should be applicable to a variety of policy issues in most industrial societies.

II. EXTERNAL FACTORS AFFECTING POLICY CHANGE WITHIN SUBSYSTEMS

Policy making in any political system or policy subsystem is constrained by a variety of social, legal, and resource features of the society of which it is a part (Heclo, 1974; Hofferbert, 1974; Kiser and Ostrom, 1982).

Our concern with the analysis of policy change means that stable external factors must be distinguished from more dynamic ones. In addition, the focus on policy subsystems means that a subsystem's relationship to other subsystems and to the broader political system must be taken into account. Thus, the framework distinguishes between (1) parameters that are relatively stable over several decades and (2) those aspects of the system that are susceptible to significant fluctuations over the course of a few years and thus serve as major stimuli to policy change.

Relatively Stable Parameters

The following set of very stable factors may be either within or external to the policy subsystem. The difficulty of changing these factors discourages actors from making them the object of strategizing behavior. These factors can limit the range of feasible alternatives or otherwise affect the resources and beliefs of subsystem actors.

Basic Attributes of the Problem Area (or "Good"). Public choice theorists have shown how various characteristics of goods, such as excludability, affect institutional (policy) options. For example, ocean fisheries and large underground aquifers give rise to common pool problems that markets cannot deal with efficiently and that make them candidates for governmental regulation (Ostrom, 1990).

Other aspects of the good or problem area (or issue area) affect the degree of policy-oriented learning likely to take place. For example, a problem's susceptibility to quantitative measurement affects the policy maker's ability to ascertain performance gaps. The extent of learning is likewise contingent upon the ease of developing good causal models of the factors affecting a problem. One would thus expect more learning on air pollution than on mental health.

Perceptions of various aspects of a good can change over time, often because of the activities of an advocacy coalition. Thirty years ago, cigarette smoking was widely regarded as a relatively harmless activity and there was virtually no concern with the effects of smoking on nonsmokers. The situation is quite different today, due in large part to a concerted campaign on the part of a public health coalition led by several surgeons general (Fritschler, 1983).

Basic Distribution of Natural Resources. The present (and past) distribution of natural resources strongly affects a society's overall wealth and the viability of different economic sectors, many aspects of its culture, and the feasibility of options in many policy areas. For example, the United States could encourage utilities to switch from oil to coal in the mid-1970s — with its potentially significant effects on sulfur emissions — while the French, lacking abundant coal reserves, turned to nuclear power as an alternative means of generating electricity.

Fundamental Cultural Values and Social Structure. Large-scale nationalization of the means of production is a viable policy option in many European countries, but not in the United States. Although such norms are not immutable, change usually requires decades.

Similarly, political power in most countries tends to be rather highly correlated with income, social class, and large organizations. Significant changes in the influence of various social groups — whether it be blacks and Chicanos or the auto companies — normally take several decades. The political resources (or lack thereof) of many interest groups are slowly changing "facts of life" that actors within a subsystem must take into account in formulating their strategies in the short or medium term.

Basic Legal Structure. In most political systems, basic legal norms are quite resistant to change. The U.S. Constitution has not been significantly altered since the granting of women's suffrage in 1920. The institutions of the French Fifth Republic have remained virtually unchanged for thirty years, those of Great Britain for almost a century. Basic legal traditions — such as the role of the courts and the fundamental norms of administrative law — also tend to be rather stable over periods of several decades.

Constitutional and other fundamental legal norms can also affect the extent of policy-oriented learning. For example, Ashford (1981b:16–17) has argued that the concentration of policy-making authority in the British cabinet and higher civil service — coupled with the secrecy that permeates that system — inhibits outsiders from making intelligent evaluations of present policy. In a similar vein, public choice theorists have long argued that decentralized political systems with relatively autonomous local governments facilitate learning by providing arenas for policy experimentation and realistic points of comparison for evaluating different policy instruments (V. Ostrom, Tiebout, and Warren, 1961; E. Ostrom, 1982).

These relatively stable parameters — the nature of the good, the basic distribution of natural resources, fundamental cultural values and social structure, and basic legal structure — significantly constrain the options available to subsystem actors. Changing them is not impossible, but it is very difficult. Change at this level normally requires a concerted effort by an advocacy coalition for at least a decade — and often several decades. Major changes in public policy within a subsystem are more likely to come from the factors outside the subsystem discussed below.

Dynamic System Events

Changes in the following factors external to a policy subsystem can be substantial over the course of a few years or a decade. Because such changes alter the constraints and opportunities confronting subsystem actors, they constitute the principal dynamic elements affecting policy change. They also present a continuous challenge to subsystem actors, who must learn how to anticipate them and respond to them in a manner consistent with their basic beliefs and interests. The process must be frustrating at times, as actors who have worked for years to gain an advantage over their competitors within a subsystem suddenly find their plans knocked awry by (external) events — such as the Arab oil embargo — over which they have little control.

1. Socioeconomic Conditions and Technology. Changes in these areas can substantially affect a subsystem, either by undermining the causal assumptions of present policies or by significantly altering the political support or various advocacy coalitions. For example, on the one hand, the dramatic rise in public concern with environmental degradation in the late 1960s played an important role in the passage of the 1970 Clean Air Amendments (Ingram, 1978). On the other hand, the Arab oil embargo of 1973–1974 contributed to such a depression in the domestic automobile industry that the United Auto Workers — previously a strong supporter of stringent air pollution programs — began echoing industry calls for a relaxation of costly and allegedly energy-inefficient automotive pollution controls (Mazmanian and Sabatier, 1989:104).

2. Systemic Governing Coalitions. Changes in the dominant coalition at a given level of government, that is, "critical elections" (Burnham, 1970), normally require that the same coalition control the chief executive's office and both houses of the legislature. Such changes in the system-wide governing coalition are quite rare.

More limited changes are more common but also have lesser effects. The 1980 national election, for example, resulted in both the presidency and the Senate changing from relatively liberal Democrats to relatively conservative Republicans. Although air pollution was only a minor issue in the election — a campaign dominated by the issues of stagflation and the Iranian hostage crisis — President Ronald Reagan attempted to fundamentally alter air pollution policy through appointing conservatives to key Environmental Protection Agency (EPA) positions, drastically cutting the EPA's budget, and proposing major amendments to the Clean Air Act (Vig and Kraft, 1984). In the final analysis, however, he failed. Most of his key appointees were forced to resign in scandal after a couple of years, the budget cuts were gradually restored, and his legislative proposals died in Senate committee. The reason is that members of the clean air coalition remained in control in the House, the Senate Environment Committee, and among EPA career officials (Wood, 1988; Cook and Wood, 1989; Waterman, 1989). Because there was no change in the system-wide governing coalition — but only in the presidency and a portion of the Senate — Reagan was unable to bring about a fundamental change within the air pollution subsystem at even the federal level, let alone in the states (Wood, 1991).

3. Policy Decisions and Impacts from Other Subsystems. Subsystems are only partially autonomous. In fact, the decisions and impacts from other policy sectors are principal dynamic elements affecting specific subsystems.

Examples are legion. The search for "energy independence" in the mid-1970s had significant repercussions on U.S. pollution control policy, as the Nixon and Ford administrations sought to require utilities to change from clean-burning natural gas to more abundant coal. Britain's entry into the Common Market (largely on foreign policy and economic grounds) has had repercussions on subsystems from taxation to pollution control because of the need to comply with European Economic Community (EEC) mandates. And there is evidence that drastic reductions in local tax revenues brought about by Proposition 13 have affected California land use policy by encouraging local governments to become more leery of the service costs of dispersed new housing developments (Inan, 1979).

III. POLICY SUBSYSTEMS: INTERNAL STRUCTURE

The complexity of modern society, the expansion of governmental functions, and the technical nature of most policy problems create enormous pressures for specialization. It is exceedingly difficult, except perhaps in small communities, to be knowledgeable about more than one or two policy sectors. When others specialize — as they do in any moderately large political system — generalists find it difficult to compete.

Thus it has long been recognized that political elites concerned with a specific problem or policy area tend to form relatively autonomous subsystems (Griffith, 1961; Fritschler, 1983; Dodd and Schott, 1979; Hamm, 1983). But traditional notions of "whirlpools" and "iron triangles" suffer because they are generally limited to interest groups, administrative agencies, and legislative committees at a single level of government. They need to be expanded to include journalists, analysts, researchers, and others who play important roles in the generation, dissemination, and evaluation of policy ideas as well as actors at other levels of government who play important roles in policy formulation and implementation (Heclo, 1978; Wamsley, 1983; Kingdon, 1984; Sabatier and Pelkey, 1987).

Traditional notions of "iron triangles" also assume that conflict among participants is relatively restrained — which often is not the case. The ACF argues that the level of conflict will vary depending upon whether the relevant actors disagree on "secondary" versus "core" aspects of their belief systems.

Delimiting Subsystem Boundaries

Let us define a policy subsystem as the set of actors who are involved in dealing with a policy problem such as air pollution control, mental health, or energy. Although it is often useful to begin with a networking approach to identify the actors involved at any particular point in time (Hjern and Porter, 1981), one must also be willing to identify potential ("latent") actors who would become active if they had the appropriate information (Balbus, 1971). In fact, activating latent constituencies is often one of the strategies of coalitions.

Latent constituencies are also an important factor in using technical information to affect policy change over time. For example, federal air pollution officials in the late 1960s identified a number of latent supporters of stricter pollution control programs and then developed several information and participation programs to encourage their involvement (Sabatier, 1975). This explicit effort to use information to expand the range of subsystem actors fundamentally altered air pollution politics in Chicago and several other cities.[4]

Origins of Subsystems

The most likely reason for the emergence of new subsystems is that a group of actors become dissatisfied enough with the neglect of a particular problem by existing subsystems to form their own. For example, dissatisfaction with the laissez-faire approach to food safety (e.g., meat inspections) by the agriculture subsystem became so intense in the early 1900s that a new subsystem — centered around what was to become the Food and Drug Administration (FDA) — gradually separated from the agricultural subsystem over a period of several decades (Nadel, 1971:7–17). Whereas this case involved a minority coalition breaking away to form its own subsystem, in other cases a new subsystem is essentially the product of a subset of a dominant coalition becoming large and specialized enough to form its own; an example would be the emergence of a housing subsystem out of the urban policy subsystem during the 1960s (Farkas, 1971).

Subsystem Actors: Advocacy Coalitions and Policy Brokers

Whatever their origins, subsystems normally contain a large and diverse set of actors. For example, the U.S. air pollution control subsystem includes the following:

1. The Environmental Protection Agency;
2. Relevant congressional committees;

3. Portions of peer agencies, such as the Department of Energy, that are frequently involved in pollution control policy;
4. Polluting corporations, their trade associations, unions, and occasionally, consumer associations;
5. The manufacturers of pollution control equipment;
6. Environmental and public health groups at all levels of government;
7. State and local pollution control agencies;
8. Research institutes and consulting firms with a strong interest in air pollution;
9. Important journalists who frequently cover the issue;
10. On some issues, such as acid rain, actors in other countries.

Given the enormous number and range of actors involved, it becomes necessary to find ways of aggregating them into smaller and theoretically useful sets of categories.

After considering several alternatives, I have concluded that the most useful means of aggregating actors in order to understand policy change over fairly long periods of time is by "advocacy coalitions." These are people from a variety of positions (elected and agency officials, interest group leaders, researchers, etc.) who share a particular belief system — that is, a set of basic values, causal assumptions, and problem perceptions — and who show a nontrivial degree of coordinated activity over time.

I find this strategy for aggregating actors superior to the most likely alternative — that of viewing formal institutions as the dominant actors — because in most policy subsystems there are at least fifty to a hundred organizations at various levels of government that are active over time. Developing models involving changes in the positions and interaction patterns of that many units over a period of a decade or more would be an *exceedingly* complex task (Sabatier and Pelkey, 1987). Moreover, institutional models have difficulty accounting for the importance of specific individuals who move about from organization to organization within the same subsystem (Heclo, 1978). Finally, institutional models have difficulty accounting for the huge variation in behavior among individuals within the same institution, such as Congress, the federal district courts, the AFL-CIO, or even the same governmental agency (Mazmanian and Nienaber, 1979; Liroff, 1986). Thus I prefer to utilize advocacy coalitions as a more manageable focus of analysis, while certainly acknowledging that formal institutions have some capacity to constrain their members' behavior. Formal institutions also bring critical resources — such as the authority to make certain types of decisions — to the members of a coalition.

In most subsystems, the number of politically significant advocacy coalitions will be quite small. In quiescent subsystems there may only be a single coalition. In most cases, however, there will be two to four important coalitions — the number being limited by all the factors that push actors to coalesce if they are to form effective coalitions (Jenkins-Smith, personal communication; Kingdon, 1984). If one's opponents pool their resources under a common position, to remain without allies is to invite defeat; but allies create pressures for common positions, which tend to harden over time. This hardening of positions is strengthened by the importance of organizational actors (whose positions are usually slow to change) and by the tendency to perceive one's opponents as being more hostile and powerful than they probably are (Sabatier et al., 1987). This argument suggests, then, that there will be greater fragmentation of beliefs in recently formed subsystems than in more established ones. Since most subsystems have existed for decades, however, one would expect the number of coalitions in each to be relatively small.

For example, the U.S. air pollution subsystem in the 1970s and 1980s was apparently divided into two rather distinct advocacy coalitions. One, which might be termed "the Clean Air Coalition," was dominated by environmental and public health groups, their allies in Congress (e.g., Senator Edmund Muskie, Congressman Henry Waxman), most pollution control officials in the EPA, a few labor unions, many state and local pollution control officials (particularly in large cities with serious problems), and some researchers. It had a belief system that stressed (1) the primacy of human health over economic development and efficiency; (2) a perception that air pollution was a serious health problem in many urban areas; (3) a focus on the inability of markets to deal with "negative externalities" such as air pollution; (4) a causal assumption that state and local governments' preoccupation with competitive advantage in attracting industry made them susceptible to industrial "blackmail" and thus required a strong federal presence; (5) a deep distrust of the motives of corporate officials and a consequent assumption of the necessity of forcing the pace of technological innovation; and (6) a strong preference for a legal command and control approach rather than reliance on economic incentives.

The competing coalition, which I'll call the Economic Feasibility Coalition, was dominated by industrial sources of air pollution, energy companies, their allies in Congress (e.g., Congressmen John Dingell and James Broyhill), several labor unions (particularly after the Arab oil embargo), some state and local pollution control officials, and several economists. Its belief system (1) stressed the need to balance human health against economic development and efficiency; (2) questioned the alleged seriousness of the health problem except in isolated instances; (3) believed that increasing social welfare generally required a deference to market arrangements; (4) generally disapproved of a strong federal role (largely on the assumption that their leverage was greater with local officials); (5) placed great emphasis on legally requiring only what was technologically feasible; and (6) expressed support (at least in principle) for the flexibility and cost-effectiveness of economic incentives rather than general legal commands (Downing, 1984).[5]

Not everyone active in a policy subsystem will "belong to" an advocacy coalition or share one of the major belief systems. Some researchers who are otherwise indifferent to the policy disputes may participate simply because they have certain skills to offer (Meltsner, 1976). The same would hold true for bureaucrats who actually adhere to the tradition of "neutral competence" (Knott and Miller, 1987). In addition, there will almost certainly be a category of actors — here termed "policy brokers" — whose dominant concerns are with keeping the level of political conflict within acceptable limits and reaching some "reasonable" solution to the problem. This is a traditional function of some elected officials (particularly chief executives) and, in some European countries like Britain and France, of high civil servants (Doggan, 1975). The courts, "blue ribbon commissions," and other actors may also play the role of policy broker. The distinction between "advocate" and "broker," however, rests on a continuum. Many brokers will have some policy bent, while advocates may show some serious concern with system maintenance. The framework merely insists that policy brokering is an empirical matter that may or may not correlate with institutional affiliation: While high civil servants may be brokers, they are also often policy advocates — particularly when their agency has a clearly defined mission.

The concept of an advocacy coalition assumes that shared beliefs provide the principal "glue" of politics. Moreover, as shall be discussed shortly, it assumes that people's core beliefs are quite resistant to change. These assumptions lead to one of the critical hypotheses of the entire framework:

> *Hypothesis 1:* On major controversies within a policy subsystem when core beliefs are in dispute, the lineup of allies and opponents tends to be rather stable over periods of a decade or so.[6]

Thus the framework explicitly rejects the view that actors are primarily motivated by their short-term self-interest and thus that "coalitions of convenience" of highly varying composition will dominate policy making over time. This claim is consistent with the evidence from a number of studies, including (1) the history of U.S. energy policy by Wildavsky and Tenenbaum (1981), (2) Marmor's (1970) analysis of the politics of Medicare in the United States, and (3) numerous analyses of the composition of majority coalitions in multiparty European parliaments over the past several decades, which have found that — in contrast to Riker's (1962) "minimum winning coalition" model — coalition formation has been quite constrained by ideology.[7]

Of course, coalition stability could be the result not of stable beliefs but rather of stable economic and organizational interests. This objection raises very thorny methodological issues, in part because belief systems are normally highly correlated with self-interest and the causation is reciprocal.[8] For example, Sierra Club leaders and steel company executives typically have quite different views on air pollution control, but is this (1) because their organizations have quite different (economic) interests or (2) because people join organizations — and put in the effort to rise to prominence in them — out of affinity with the organization's stated goals? This framework uses belief systems, rather than "interests," as its focus because beliefs are more inclusive and more verifiable than interests. Interest models must still identify a set of means and performance indicators necessary for goal attainment; this set of interests and goals, perceived causal relationships, and perceived parameter states constitutes a "belief system." While belief system models can thus incorporate self-interest and organizational interests, they also allow actors to establish goals in quite different ways (e.g., as a result of socialization) and are therefore more inclusive. In addition, I personally have great difficulty in specifying a priori a clear and falsifiable set of interests for most actors in policy conflicts (see also Kingdon, 1988). Instead, it seems preferable to allow actors to indicate their belief systems (via questionnaires and content analyses of documents) and then empirically examine the extent to which these change over time.

Advocacy Coalitions and Public Policy

Coalitions seek to translate their beliefs into public policies or programs (which usually consist of a set of goals and directions, or empowerments, to administrative agencies for implementing those goals). Although pressures for compromise generally result in governmental programs that incorporate elements advocated by different coalitions, the 1970 Federal Clean Air Amendments incorporated to an unusual degree most elements of the belief system of the Clean Air Coalition. The 1977 and 1990 Clean Air Amendments incorporated some compromises sought by the Economic Feasibility Coalition (such as the 1977 delays in imposing more stringent auto emissions standards and the 1990 Amendments' use of economic incentives in the acid rain program), but the overall philosophy of the federal Clean Air Act remains consistent with most beliefs of the Clean Air Coalition.

In any intergovernmental system, however, different coalitions may be in control of various governmental units. For example, the Economic Efficiency Coalition was apparently more powerful in Sun Belt states during most of the 1970s than at the national level. In fact, one of the basic strategies of any coalition is to manipulate the assignment of program responsibilities so that the governmental units that it controls have the most authority (Schattschneider, 1960).

While belief systems will determine the *direction* in which an advocacy coalition (or any other political actor) will seek to move governmental programs, *its ability to do so* will be critically dependent upon its resources. These include such things as money, expertise, number of supporters, and legal authority. With respect to the last, this framework acknowledges one of the central features of institutional models — namely, that rules create authorizations to act in certain ways (Kiser and Ostrom, 1982; Ostrom, 1990). The ACF differs from many institutional theories, however, in viewing these rules as the product of competition among advocacy coalitions and in viewing institutional members as providing resources to different coalitions.

The resources of various coalitions change, of course, over time. Some of this is intentional. In fact, most coalitions seek to augment their budgets, recruit new members (especially those with legal authority, expertise, or money), place their members in positions of authority, and employ the variety of other means long identified by interest group theorists (Truman, 1951; Berry, 1977). Some coalitions have a more difficult time than others in maintaining an effective presence and increasing their resources over time. This is particularly true in consumer and environmental protection, where the groups that originally championed regulation have had more difficulty than the regulated industries in finding sufficient organizational resources to monitor and to intervene in the extended process of policy implementation (Bernstein, 1955; Nadel, 1971; Quirk, 1981). Even more severe difficulties confront economically disadvantaged groups in their efforts to muster the resources necessary to remain active over any extended period of time (Goodwin and Moen, 1981).

Although coalitions will seek to increase their resources, the advocacy coalition framework argues that *major* shifts in the distribution of political resources will usually be the product of events *external* to the subsystem and largely external to activities of subsystem coalitions. For example, members of the Economic Feasibility Coalition attempted to utilize the 1973–1974 oil crisis and the 1980 election of President Reagan to increase their resources, but those changes were not sufficient to enable them to overcome the Clean Air Coalition on issues relating to the policy core incorporated into the 1970 Clean Air Amendments. In contrast, Chapters 4 and 5 of this book explore cases illustrating how subsystem coalitions successfully exploited and amplified opportunities arising from external events.

Policy-Oriented Belief Systems

In its conception of the belief systems of individuals and coalitions, the framework has three basic points of departure. The first is Ajzen and Fishbein's (1980) "theory of reasoned action" — basically an expected utility model in which actors weigh alternative courses of action in terms of their contribution to a set of goals, but in which the preferences of reference groups (such as members of one's coalition) are accorded a more prominent role than in most utilitarian models. Second, rationality is limited rather than perfect. Thus the framework relies heavily upon the work of March and Simon (1958), Nisbett and Ross (1980), Kahneman et al. (1982), and many others in terms of satisficing, placing cognitive limits on rationality, carrying out limited search processes, etc. Third, because subsystems are composed of policy elites rather than members of the general public, there are strong grounds for assuming that most actors will have relatively complex and internally consistent belief systems in the policy area(s) of interest to them (Wilker and Milbrath, 1972; Cobb, 1973; Axelrod, 1976; Putnam, 1976:87–93; Buttel and Flinn, 1978).

These, however, are only starting points, for they tell us very little about what will happen when experience reveals anomalies — such as internal inconsistencies, inaccurate predictions, and invalid assertions — among the beliefs. Assuming some social and psychological pressures for belief consistency and validity, are conflicts resolved in an essentially random process — that is, with all beliefs accorded the same logical status — or are some beliefs more fundamental than others and thus more resistant to change? What, in short, is the *structure* of the belief systems of policy elites?

The literature on political belief systems is a mine field of conflicting theories and evidence.[9] But the most useful approach seems to be a synthesis of Putnam's (1976:81–89) review of the normative and cognitive orientations of political elites, Axelrod's (1976) work on the complexity of their causal assumptions, an adaptation of Lakatos's (1971) distinction between "core" and other elements of scientific belief systems, and Converse's (1964) contention that abstract political beliefs are more resistant to change than specific ones (also Peffley and Hurwitz, 1985; Hurwitz and Peffley, 1987).

Given that the basic strategy of the framework is to use the structure of belief systems to predict changes in beliefs and attempted changes in policy over time, that structure must be stipulated a priori if the argument to come in Hypotheses 2 and 3 is to be falsifiable. The unsettled nature of the field makes this a risky undertaking. Nevertheless, on the assumption that clarity — even if wrong — begets clarity and eventually improved understanding of a phenomenon, the framework proposes the structure of elite belief systems outlined in Table 1.

Table 1 outlines three structural categories: a deep core of fundamental normative and ontological axioms that define a person's underlying personal philosophy, a near (policy) core of basic strategies and policy positions for achieving deep core beliefs in the policy area or subsystem in question, and a set of secondary aspects comprising a multitude of instrumental decisions and information searches necessary to implement the policy core in the specific policy area. The three structural categories are arranged in order of decreasing resistance to change, that is, the deep core is much more resistant than the secondary aspects.

U.S. air pollution policy once again serves as an example, in this case to illustrate the structure of belief systems. The Clean Air Coalition and the Economic Efficiency Coalition have been fundamentally divided over the extent to which the pursuit of individual freedom in a market economy should be constrained in order to protect the health of "susceptible populations" (e.g., those already suffering from respiratory diseases). Members of the Clean Air Coalition argue that the protection accorded susceptible populations should be virtually absolute, while members of the Economic Efficiency Coalition have been more willing to put these populations at some risk in the interests of individual liberty and increased production. This normative difference in the policy core of the two coalitions probably reflected a deep core difference in the relative priority accorded freedom (or efficiency) versus equality, a conflict underlying many policy disputes (Rokeach, 1973: Okun, 1975).

Differences on this issue and others helped members of the two coalitions to adopt quite different positions on such policy core issues as the proper scope of governmental (vs. market) activity, the proper role of the federal government, the advantages of using coercion vs. other policy instruments, the overall seriousness of the air pollution problem in the United States, and so on. These are the sorts of issues that were decided in the 1970 Clean Air Amendments and that, despite numerous attacks, have remained largely unchanged in law since then (Mazmanian and Sabatier, 1989:Chap. 4). While there have been some issues (most notably, nondegradation and acid rain) since 1970 that have involved core disputes, most policy making has focused on secondary aspects, such as determining which air quality standards are adequate to protect susceptible populations, which auto emissions standards would minimize emissions without wrecking the domestic auto industry, the feasibility of using parking surcharges as a tool for reducing vehicle miles traveled, and the technical validity of various techniques for monitoring atmospheric emissions.

It would be absurd to assume that all members of an advocacy coalition have precisely the same belief system. But, based upon the assumption that elite belief systems are hierarchical (i.e., that abstract beliefs are more salient and more resistant to change than more specific ones), the ACF hypothesizes that most members of a coalition will show substantial agreement on the policy core issues outlined in Table 1, which need

TABLE 1

STRUCTURE OF BELIEF SYSTEMS OF POLICY ELITES*

	Deep (Normative) Core	*Near (Policy) Core*	*Secondary Aspects*
Defining characteristics	Fundamental normative and ontological axioms.	Fundamental policy positions concerning the basic strategies for achieving normative axioms of deep core.	Instrumental decisions and information searches necessary to implement policy core.
Scope	Part of basic personal philosophy. Applies to all policy areas.	Applies to policy area of interest (and perhaps a few more).	Specific to policy area/subsystem of interest.
Susceptibility to change	Very difficult: akin to a religious conversion.	Difficult, but can occur if experience reveals serious anomalies.	Moderately easy: this is the topic of most administrative and even legislative policymaking.
Illustrative components	1. The nature of man: i. Inherently evil vs. socially redeemable. ii. Part of nature vs. dominion over nature. iii. Narrow egoists vs. contractarians. 2. Relative priority of various ultimate values: freedom, security, power, knowledge, health, love, beauty, etc. 3. Basic criteria of distributive justice: Whose welfare counts? Relative weights of self, primary groups, all people, future generations, nonhuman beings, etc.	1. Proper scope of governmental vs. market activity. 2. Proper distribution of authority among various units (e.g., levels) of government. 3. Identification of social groups whose welfare is most critical. 4. Orientations on substantive policy conflicts, e.g., environmental protection vs. economic development. 5. Magnitude of perceived threat to those values. 6. Basic choices concerning policy instruments, e.g., coercion vs. inducements vs. persuasion. 7. Desirability of participation by various segments of society: i. Public vs. elite participation. ii. Experts vs. elected officials. 8. Ability of society to solve problems in this policy area: i. Zero-sum competition vs. potential for mutual accommodation. ii. Technological optimism vs. pessimism.	1. Most decisions concerning administrative rules, budgetary allocations, disposition of cases, statutory interpretation, and even statutory revision. 2. Information concerning program performance, the seriousness of the problems, etc.

*The Policy Core and Secondary Aspects also apply to governmental programs.

to be addressed by any belief system. In addition, positions on these issues will be slower to change than those concerning the secondary (implementing) aspects on a belief system. In short:

> *Hypothesis 2:* Actors within an advocacy coalition will show substantial consensus on issues pertaining to the policy core, although less so on secondary aspects.
>
> *Hypothesis 3:* An actor (or coalition) will give up secondary aspects of a belief system before acknowledging weaknesses in the policy core.

While this argument leaves open the precise amount of consensus on the policy core necessary for an advocacy coalition to be said to "exist," its basic thrust should be quite clear. It is also far from self-evident, as it disagrees with those who proclaim the end of ideology (Bell, 1960), perceive the domination of short-term "coalitions of convenience" (Riker, 1962), view specific beliefs as more salient than abstract ones (Wilker and Milbrath, 1972), or see policy change as a muddled process in which policy technocrats play a major role (Heclo, 1978).

Methods for investigating the content of belief systems include elite surveys, panels of knowledgeable observers (Hart, 1976), and content analysis of relevant documents (Axelrod, 1976). Given the rather technical nature of many secondary aspects and the focus on changes in beliefs over a decade or more, content analyses of government documents (e.g., legislative and administrative hearings) and interest-group publications probably offer the best prospects for systematic empirical work on changes in elite beliefs.

The entire notion of a belief system organized around a set of core values and policy strategies, plus implementing activities, assumes some psychological predilection for instrumental rationality and cognitive consistency on the part of policy elites. It does not, however, take issue with the implications of Simon's recent work suggesting that cognitive structures resemble semiautonomous filing cabinets into which one places new information (Newell and Simon, 1972; Simon, 1979). Instead, the framework supposes that policy elites seek to better understand the world within a particular policy area ("filing cabinet") in order to identify means to achieve their fundamental objectives. Such thought produces pressures for evaluative consistency (Tesser, 1978:295).

The framework also presumes some (modest) selection pressures in favor of policy elites with a capacity for reasoned discourse involving the major issues relevant to their policy subsystem (e.g., air pollution control). Insofar as policy discussions among insiders are based on reasoned argument, actors holding blatantly inconsistent or unsubstantiated positions will lose credibility. That loss may not be completely debilitating for their position, but it will force them to expend scarce political resources in its support and will eventually be to their competitive disadvantage (Brewer and de Leon, 1983).

Once something has been accepted as a policy core belief, however, powerful ego-defense, peer-group, and organizational forces create considerable resistance to change, even in the face of countervailing empirical evidence or internal inconsistencies (Festinger, 1957; Argyris and Schon, 1978; Janis, 1983). The literature on cognitive dissonance and selective perception is enormous and far from conclusive (Abelson et al., 1968; Wicklund and Brehm, 1976; Greenwald and Ronis, 1978; Innis, 1978). But, *when* salient beliefs and/or the egos of policy elites are at stake, the evidence of selective perception and partisan analysis is strong enough to warrant a prominent place in any model (Schiff, 1962; Smith, 1968; Steinbruner, 1974; Cameron, 1978; Innis, 1978; Nelkin, 1979; Mazur, 1981; Fiske and Taylor, 1984; Etheredge, 1985).

IV. COALITION LEARNING AND EXTERNAL PERTURBATION

Policy change within a subsystem can be understood as the product of two processes. First, advocacy coalitions within the subsystem attempt to translate the policy cores and the secondary aspects of their belief systems into governmental programs. Although most programs will involve some compromise among coalitions, there will usually be a dominant coalition and one or more minority coalitions (Wamsley, 1983). Each will seek to realize its objectives over time through increasing its political resources and through policy-oriented learning. The second process is one of external perturbation, that is, the effects of *system-wide* events — changes in socioeconomic conditions, outputs from other subsystems, and changes in the system-wide governing coalition — on the resources and constraints of subsystem actors.

The framework argues, however, that the policy core of an advocacy coalition is quite resistant to change over time. This leads to the following hypothesis:

> *Hypothesis 4:* The core (basic attributes) of a governmental program is unlikely to be significantly revised as long as the subsystem advocacy coalition that instituted the program remains in power.

This hypothesis assumes that a coalition seeks power to translate its core beliefs into policy. It will not abandon those core beliefs merely to stay in power, although it may well abandon secondary aspects and even try to incorporate some of the opponents' core as *secondary* aspects of the program.

Likewise, the relative strength of different advocacy coalitions within a subsystem will seldom be sufficiently altered by events *internal* to the subsystem (i.e., by efforts to increase resources or to "outlearn" opponents) to overthrow a dominant coalition. Hence:

> *Hypothesis 5:* The core (basic attributes) of a governmental action program is unlikely to be changed in the absence of significant perturbations external to the subsystem, that is, changes in socioeconomic conditions, system-wide governing coalitions, or policy outputs from other subsystems.

These hypotheses suggest that, while minority coalitions can seek to improve their relative position through augmenting their resources and "outlearning" their adversaries, their basic hope of gaining power within the subsystem resides in waiting for some *external* event to significantly increase their political resources.

If Hypothesis 5 is correct, the type of policy-oriented learning discussed in the next chapter is unlikely by itself to significantly alter the *policy core* attributes of a governmental action program. But it can still lead to substantial changes in the secondary aspects. Learning by a minority coalition may demonstrate such major deficiencies in the core of a program that the majority will acknowledge these deficiencies or, more likely, a system-wide learning process will occur in which system-wide leaders eventually overturn the dominant coalition. A possible example would be the efforts of economists over the past twenty years to demonstrate the inefficiencies of governmental regulation of airline fares and entry — a campaign that eventually led to the abolition of the Civil Aeronautics Board (Derthick and Quirk, 1985; Brown, 1987; Nelson, 1987). The airline deregulation case is analyzed in detail in Chapter 5.[10]

V. CONCLUSION

This chapter has presented the basic features of the advocacy coalition framework (ACF) of policy change over periods of a decade or more.

The ACF starts from three premises that, in my view, are prerequisites for any theory of policy change. First, it deals with periods of sufficient length to incorporate the enlightenment function of policy research and to give some attention to policy-oriented learning. Periods of a decade are also long enough to incorporate at least one policy cycle (consisting of formulation, implementation, and reformulation) at a specific level of government. Second, the ACF focuses on policy subsystems — rather than specific governmental institutions — as the principal unit for understanding policy change. This premise follows a long tradition in the policy literature, although the expansion of the list of subsystem actors beyond traditional iron triangles to include the generators and disseminators of ideas, as well as an intergovernmental dimension, is fairly recent. Third, the ACF emphasizes the intergovernmental nature of policy subsystems. Subsystems will usually include actors from all levels of government, and there is no a priori assumption that national actors are more important than subnational ones.

The ACF then incorporates four additional major building blocks. First, it follows Pressman and Wildavsky (1973) and Majone (1980) in assuming that public policies can be conceptualized in the same manner as political belief systems, that is, as sets of value priorities, perceptions of important causal relationships, perceptions of the seriousness of the problem, and perceptions of the efficacy of various sorts of institutional relationships as means of attaining those value priorities. Second, it builds upon aspects of Majone (1989) and the political belief system literature (Putnam, 1976) in assuming that both policies and belief systems have a structure composed of a very abstract deep core, a policy core relating to that specific subsystem, and a large number of secondary aspects. The abstract levels are hypothesized to be stable, in large part because they are largely normative issues inculturated in childhood and largely impervious to empirical evidence. Third, the ACF chooses advocacy coalitions — that is, sets of actors from both public and private institutions at various levels of government who share critical aspects of a belief system — as the principal vehicle for aggregating individuals into a manageable number of units. It perceives a coalition as seeking to manipulate institutional rules and actors in order to achieve its policy goals. The ACF thus represents a fundamental departure from most political science research, which tends to aggregate by type of institution (such as the Congress, presidency, and interest groups), usually at a single level of government. The choice of advocacy coalitions facilitates a focus on policy-oriented learning, as the actors within a coalition share basic values and search for means to accomplish them. It also facilitates an intergovernmental focus: A coalition doing poorly in Washington is not helpless but instead can focus its efforts at subnational levels where it is more powerful. Fourth, the ACF follows Heclo (1974) in distinguishing the internal dynamics within a subsystem from the perturbations in the broader political system and socioeconomic environment. It goes out on a limb by hypothesizing that the latter are necessary for changes in the core of governmental policy within a subsystem.

The ACF certainly represents a radical departure from the stages metaphor in its focus on belief systems, policy-oriented learning, subsystem vs. external system, and aggregation by advocacy coalitions and in its ability to deal with multiple, interacting sets of cycles, consisting of formulation, implementation, and reformulation, at different levels of government (or in different states or localities at the same level). It also differs from the stages metaphor in that it identifies two specific motors of change: (1) individuals' efforts to achieve their goals over time (with individuals aggregated into coalitions) and (2) the effects of perturbations exogenous to the subsystem (i.e., changes in system-wide governing coalitions, changes in socioeconomic conditions, or policy outputs from other subsystems) on the resources and beliefs of subsystem actors, and eventually on policy change.[11]

The ACF also differs from other major theories of the policy process:

1. ***Lowi's Arenas of Power*** (Lowi, 1964, 1972; Ripley and Franklin, 1982). The ACF ignores the fundamental tenet of this approach, namely, that the policy process differs substantially in distributive, regulatory, and redistributive arenas. Such differences may exist, but they are not deemed important enough to include in the ACF.
2. ***Kingdon's Multiple Streams*** (Kingdon, 1984). Kingdon is one of the few political scientists to deal seriously with the role of ideas and analysis in policy making. But the ACF views the "analytical" stream as much more integrated with the "political" stream than does Kingdon; it deals with the entire policy process, not just agenda setting and policy formulation; and it tries to relate Kingdon's "windows of opportunity" for major policy change to specific types of changes in events exogenous to the policy subsystem (see Sabatier, 1991a).
3. ***Hofferbert's Funnel of Causality*** (Hofferbert, 1974; Mazmainan and Sabatier, 1980). The ACF incorporates Hofferbert's emphasis on the importance of the

socioeconomic environment but differs from him in distinguishing the policy subsystem from the broader political system, emphasizing policy-oriented learning, and stressing intergovernmental relations.

4. ***Statist Theory*** (Skocpol, 1979; Skowronek, 1982). The ACF completely rejects the fundamental tenet of this approach, that there exists a unified, relatively autonomous "state." In fact, this approach strikes me as highly dubious in countries like the United States, given federalism, the diversity of interests and values represented by various governmental institutions, and the permeability of most institutions to external influences. Statist theory is even misleading in supposedly centralized regimes like France (Ashford, 1981a).
5. ***Institutional Rational Choice*** (Kiser and Ostrom, 1982; Ostrom, 1990; Chubb and Moe, 1990). The ACF agrees with these scholars that institutional rules affect individual behavior. But it goes beyond them in viewing such rules as the product of strategies by advocacy coalitions over time. It also expands the range of guidance instruments from institutional rules to include changes in budgets and personnel (Sabatier and Pelkey, 1987). Finally, it gives socioeconomic conditions more importance than do most institutional rational choice scholars.
6. ***Traditional Pluralist Theory*** (Truman, 1951). On the one hand, the ACF accepts Truman's emphasis on the importance of interest-group competition in molding governmental institutions. On the other hand, advocacy coalitions are *not* simply constellations of interest groups; their "members" also include legislators, agency officials, researchers, and journalists. Second, the ACF completely rejects Truman's naive assumption that all latent interests will be effectively represented (Sabatier, 1992). Third, the ACF emphasizes policy-oriented learning and hierarchical belief systems, concepts completely neglected by Truman. Finally, unlike Truman, the ACF does not rely on cross-cutting cleavages to assure system stability; instead, the emphasis is on stable system parameters (e.g., social structure), policy brokers, and stable belief systems.

In short, the ACF differs significantly from not only the stages metaphor but other theories of the policy process as well. While it borrows elements from many of them — particularly Hofferbert, institutional rational choice, and pluralism — the basic insight was taken from Heclo's book on the evolution of welfare policy in Britain and Sweden. Moreover, several of the fundamental elements — including the importance of intergovernmental relations, the role of policy-oriented learning, and the ability to conceptualize public policy as a belief system — are derived primarily from the implementation literature (Pressman and Wildavsky, 1973; Mazmanian and Sabatier, 1981, 1989).

NOTES

1. Fortunately, this situation is changing. A number of recent studies do an excellent job of exploring the intergovernmental dimension in several policy areas (Anton, 1989; Wood, 1991; Scholtz et al., 1991).

2. This chapter borrows heavily from Sabatier (1987, 1988).
3. The debate in the implementation literature between "top-downers" and "bottom-uppers" is *not* over whether "street level bureaucrats" exercise considerable discretion. Everyone agrees on that. Instead, the debate is over whether central decision makers have any real capacity to constrain that discretion or if they should basically accommodate themselves to whatever the street level bureaucrats wish to do (Sabatier, 1986; Palumbo, 1988).
4. On the one hand, the actual activation of latent interests depends upon the perceptions and strategies of actors within the subsystem. On the other hand, an analyst interested in predicting future events within a subsystem would do well to also identify latent constituencies and the circumstances under which they could be mobilized.
5. Beginning in the 1980s, one might consider adding a third, the Economic Efficiency Coalition. Its belief system relies very heavily on principles of welfare economics and includes both (1) critiques of EPA regulations and (2) a preference for substituting economic incentives for command and control regulation. Dominated by research economists such as Bob Hahn, Larry White, and Lester Lave, it would also include many officials in the EPA's Office of Policy Analysis, the Office of Management and Budget (OMB), the Environmental Defense Fund (EDF), and the California Legislative Analyst's Office, as well as a few legislators, notably former Senator Tim Wirth (Liroff, 1986; Cook, 1986; the1988 symposium of the *Columbia Journal of Environmental Law;* Hahn and Hester, 1989). I have chosen not to add it as a third coalition, in part because most economists traditionally have mirrored the views of the Economic Feasibility Coalition (see, for example, White, 1982) and, in part, because it is not clear that the EDF and Wirth share the OMB's passion for critiquing EPA rules on welfare economics principles.
6. A weaker hypothesis would suggest that an advocacy coalition will consist of (1) a set of farily stable members with compatible policy cores and (2) temporary members who float in and out depending upon the particular policy dispute. For example, Ackerman and Hassler (1981) report that the ranks of the Clean Air Coalition were augmented during the mid-1970s by western coal companies, whose supply of low-sulfur coal led them to join environmentalists in seeking stringent emissions controls on utilities (which would give them a competitive advantage against high-sulfur midwestern coal). But this alliance was subsequently disrupted when Congressman Henry Waxman, one of the leaders of the Clean Air Coalition, suggested a uniform nationwide tax on utilities as a means of dealing with the acid rain problem and dealing equitably with the concerns of midwestern coal companies and utilities.
7. The literature on coalition formation in multiparty parliamentary regimes has found both minimum size and ideological constraints to be important factors, with their relative importance varying by country (Browne, 1970; de Swann, 1973; Taylor and Laver, 1973; Dodd, 1976; Warwick, 1979; Hinckley, 1981; Browne and Dreijamis, 1982; Franklin and Mackie, 1984; Zariski, 1984). Unfortunately, the literature on (interest-group) coalitions within subsystems over periods of at least a

decade appears to be remarkably sparse and unsophisticated, with the study by Wildavsky and Tenenbaum (1981) among the more suggestive. The problem probably resides in methodological difficulties in determining what constitutes a coalition when using, for example, legislative and budgetary hearings as a data base.

8. In the case of air pollution control, the willingness of western coal companies to side with environmentalists against midwestern coal companies would be a case of self-interest (competitive market advantage) over laissez-faire ideology (Ackerman and Hassler, 1981). But the reluctance of manufacturers of pollution control equipment to openly ally themselves with environmentalists in most controversies over the past twenty years would suggest that ideology can likewise restrain the pursuit of self-interest.

9. Among the major strands in this literature are (1) the work of Converse (1964) and many others who view the Left-Right continuum as critical; (2) the "operational code" studies examining elite assumptions concerning the nature of political conflict (George, 1969; Putnam, 1973); (3) the work of Axelrod (1976) diagramming the causal assumptions of policy elites; and (4) the work of Conover and Feldman (1984) on "schema theory." For a summary of much of this literature, see Putnam (1976:Chap. 4). The distinction between "secondary aspects" and "core" is rather similar to Steinbruner's (1974) distinction between "cybernetic" and "cognitive" levels of thinking and to Argyris and Schon's (1978) analysis of "single" and "double loop" learning.

10. Brown and Stewart (Chapter 5) conclude that, while the economic critique played a critical role in deregulation, it was not sufficient to bring about a change in the policy core of federal airline policy. In short, their analysis basically supports Hypothesis 5, although they would argue that the distinction between internal and external events is not as clear as I have made it.

11. The basic forces producing change within a policy subsystem are thus similar to biological theories of change within an ecosystem: There are both individuals striving for specific goals and exogenous perturbations. This similarity is quite intentional. The major difference is that the ACF does not identify a single, dominant human goal analogous to biologists' assumption that individual organisms are "seeking" to maximize their reproductive success.

REFERENCES

Abelson, Robert, et al. (1968). *Theories of Cognitive Consistency.* Chicago: Rand McNally.

Ackerman, Bruce, and Hassler, William (1981). *Clean Coal Dirty Air*. New Haven: Yale Univ. Press.

Ajzen, Icek, and Fishbein, Martin (1980). *Understanding Attitudes and Predicting Social Behavior*. Englewood Cliffs: Prentice-Hall.

Anton, Thomas (1989). *American Federalism and Public Policy: How the System Works*. New York: Random House.

Argyris, Chris, and Schon, Donald (1978). *Organizational Learning*. New York: Wiley.

Ashford, Douglas (1981a). *British Dogmatism and French Pragmatism*. London: George Alen & Unwin.

Ashford, Douglas (1981b). *Policy and Politics in Britain*. Philadelphia: Temple Univ. Press.

Axelrod, Robert, ed. (1976). *Structure of Decision*. Princeton: Princeton Univ. Press.

Balbus, Isaac (1971). "The Concept of Interest in Pluralist and Marxian Analysis," *Politics and Society* 1 (February): 151–177.

Bell, Daniel (1960). *The End of Ideology*. New York: Free Press.

Bernstein, Marver (1955). *Regulating Business by Independent Commission*. Princeton: Princeton Univ. Press.

Berry, Jeffrey (1977). *Lobbying for the People*. Princeton: Princeton Univ. Press.

Brewer, Garry, and de Leon, Peter (1983). *Foundations of Policy Analysis*. Homewood: Dorsey.

Brown, Anthony E. (1987). *The Politics of Airline Deregulation*. Knoxville: Univ. of Tennessee Press.

Browne, Eric (1970). *Coalition Theories*. Beverly Hills: Sage.

Browne, Eric, and Dreijams, John, eds. (1982). *Government Coalitions in Western Democracies*. London: Longmans.

Burnham, Walter Dean (1970). *Critical Elections and the Mainsprings of American Politics*. New York: Norton.

Buttel, Frederick, and Flinn, William (1978). "The Politics of Environmental Concern," *Environment and Behavior* 10 (March): 17–36.

Cameron, James (1978). "Ideology and Policy Termination; Restructuring California's Mental Health System," in Judith May and Aaron Wildavsky, eds. *The Policy Cycle*, pp. 301–328. Beverly Hills: Sage.

Crubb, John E., and Moe, Terry M. (1990). *Politics, Markets, and America's Schools.* Washington, DC: Brookings.

Cobb, Roger (1973). "The Belief Systems Perspective," *Journal of Politics* 35 (February): 121–153.

Coher, Richard (1992). *Washington at Work: Back Rooms and Clean Air*. New York: Macmillan.

Conover, Pamela J., and Feldman, Stanley (1984). "How People Organize the Political World: A Schematic Model," *American Journal of Political Science* 28 (February): 95–126.

Converse, Philip (1964). "The Nature of Belief Systems in Mass Publics," in David Apter, ed., *Ideology and Discontent,* pp. 206–261. New York: Free Press.

Cook, Brian (1986). "Characteristics of Administrative Decisions About Regulatory Form," *American Politics Quarterly* 14 (October): 294–316.

Cook, Brian, and Wood, B. Dan (1989). "Principal-Agent Models of Political Controls of Bureaucracy." *American Political Science Review* 83 (September): 965–978.

Davies, J. Clarence (1970). *The Politics of Pollution.* New York: Pegasus.

de Swann, Abram (1973). *Coalition Theories and Cabinet Formations*. Amsterdam: Elsevier.

Derthick, Martha, and Quirk, Paul (1985). *The Politics of Deregulation*. Washington, DC: Brookings.

Dodd, Lawrence (1976). *Coalitions in Parliamentary Governments*. Princeton: Princeton Univ. Press.

Dodd, Lawrence, and Schott, Richard (1979). *Congress and the Administrative State*. New York: John Wiley.

Doggan, Mattei (1975). *The Mandarins of Western Europe*. New York: Wiley.

Downing, Paul (1984). *Environmental Economics and Policy*. Boston: Little, Brown.

Dunleavy, Michael (1981). *The Politics of Mass Housing in Britain, 1945–75*. Oxford: Clarendon Press.

Etheredge, Lloyd (1985). *Can Governments Learn? American Foreign Policy and Central American Relations*. New York: Pergamon Press.

Farkas, Suzanne (1971). *Urban Lobbying*. New York: New York Univ. Press.

Fesneger, Leon (1957). *A Theory of Cognitive Dissonance,* Evansion: Row, Paterson.

Fiske, Susan, and Taylor, Shelley (1984). *Social Cognition*. Reading, MA: Addison-Wesley.

Franklin, Mark, and Mackie, Thomas (1984). "Reassessing the Importance of Size and Ideology for the Formation of Governing Coalitions in Parliamentary Democracies," *American Journal of Political Science* 28 (November): 671–692.

Fritschler, A. Lee (1983). *Smoking and Politics*, 3d ed. Englewood Cliffs: Prentice-Hall.

George, Alexander (1969). "The Operational Code," *International Studies Quarterly* 13 (June): 110–222.

Goodwin, Leonard, and Moen, Phyllis (1981). "The Evolution and Implementation of Federal Welfare Policy," in D. Mazmanian and P. Sabatier, eds., *Effective Policy Implementation*, pp. 147–168. Lexington, MA: D.C. Heath.

Greenwald, Anthony, and Ronis, David (1978). "Twenty-Years of Cognitive Dissonance: Case Study of the Evolution of a Theory," *Psychological Review* 85 (no. 1): 53–57.

Griffith, Ernest (1961). *Congress: Its Contemporary Role*, 3d ed. New York: New York Univ. Press.

Hahn, Robert W., and Hester, Gordon L. (1989). "Where Did All the Markets Go? An Analysis of EPA's Emissions Trading Program," *Yale Journal on Regulation* 6: 109–152.

Hamm, Keith (1983). "Patterns of Influence Among Committees, Agencies and Interest Groups," *Legislative Studies Quarterly* 8 (August): 379–426.

Hart, Jeffrey (1976). Comparative Cognition: Politics of International Control of the Oceans," in R. Axelrod, ed., *Structures of Decision*, Chap. 8. Princeton: Princeton Univ. Press.

Heclo, Hugh (1974). *Social Policy in Britain and Sweden*. New Haven: Yale Univ. Press.

Heclo, Hugh (1978). "Issue Networks and the Executive Establishment," in A. King, ed., *The New American Political System,* Washington, DC: American Enterprise Institute.

Hibbs, Douglas, and Fassbender, H., eds. (1981). *Contemporary Political Economy*. Amsterdam: North Holland.

Hinckley, Barbara (1981). *Coalitions and Politics*. New York: Harcourt, Brace, Jovanovich.

Hjern, Benny, and Porter, David (1981). "Implementation Structures," *Organization Studies* 2: 211–227.

Hofferbert, Richard (1974). *The Study of Public Policy*. Indianapolis: Bobbs-Merrill.

Hogwood, Brian, and Peters, B. Guy (1983). *Policy Dynamics*. New York: St. Martin's.

Hurwitz, Jon, and Peffley, Mark (1987). "How Are Foreign Policy Attitudes Structured? A Hierarchical Model," *American Political Science Review* 81 (December): 1099–1120.

Inan, Michele (1979). "Savior of the Cities — Would You Believe, Howard Jarvis?" *California Journal* 10 (April): 138–139.

Ingram, Helen (1977). "Policy Implementation Through Bargaining: Federal Grants in Aid," *Public Policy* 25 (Fall): 449–526.

Ingram, Helen (1978). "The Political Rationality of Innovation: The Clean Air Act Amendments of 1970," in Ann Friedlaender, ed., *Approaches to Controlling Air Pollution*, pp. 12–67. Cambridge: MIT Press.

Innis, J. M. (1978). "Selective Exposure as a Function of Dogmatism and Incentive," *Journal of Social Psychology* 106: 261–265.

Janis, Irving (1983). *Groupthink*, 2d ed. Boston: Houghton Mifflin.

Jones, Charles (1975). *Clean Air*. Pittsburgh: Univ. of Pittsburgh Press.

Kahneman, Daniel, Slovic, Paul, and Tversky, Amos (1982). *Judgment Under Uncertainty*. Cambridge: Cambridge Univ. Press.

Kingdon, John (1984). Agendas. *Alternatives, and Public Policies*. Boston: Little, Brown.

Kingdon, John (1988). "Ideas, Politics and Public Policies." Paper presented at the 1988 Annual Meeting of the American Political Science Association, Washington, DC.

Kirst, Michael, and Jung, Richard (1982). "The Utility of a Longitudinal Approach in Assessing Implementation: Title I, ESEA," in Walter Williams, ed., *Studying Implementation,* pp. 119–148. Chatham, NJ: Chatham House.

Kiser, Larry, and Ostrom, Elinor (1982). "The Three Worlds of Action," in E. Ostrom, ed., *Strategies of Political Inquiry*, pp. 179–222. Beverly Hills: Sage.

Knott, Jack, and Miller, Gary (1987). *Reforming Bureaucracy. The Politics of Institutional Choice*. Englewood Cliffs: Prentice-Hall.

Krasnow, Erwin G., Longley, Lawrence D., and Terry, Herbert A. (1982). *The Politics of Broadcast Regulation*, 3rd ed. New York: St. Martin's Press.

Krier, James, and Ursin, Edmund (1977). *Pollution and Policy*. Berkeley: Univ. of California Press.

Lakatos, Imre (1971). "History of Science and Its Rational Reconstruction," *Boston Studies in the Philosophy of Science* 5: 42–134.

Lindblom, Charles E., and Cohen, David (1979). *Usable Knowledge*. New Haven: Yale Univ. Press.

Liroff, Richard (1986). *Reforming Air Pollution Regulation: The Toil and Trouble of EPA's Bubble*. Washington, DC: Conservation Foundation.

Lowi, Theodore (1964). "American Business, Public Policy, Case Studies, and Political Theory," *World Politics* 16 (June): 677–715.

Majone, Glandamenico (1980). "Policies as Theories," *Omega* 8: 151–162.

Majone, Glandamenico (1989). *Evidence, Argument, and Persuasion in the Policy Process.* New Haven: Yale Univ. Press.

March, James, and Simon, Herbert (1958). *Organizations*. New York: Wiley.

Marmor, Theodore (1970). *The Politics of Medicare*. Chicago: Aldine.

Mazmanian, Daniel, and Nienaber, Jeanne (1979). *Can Organizations Change?* Washington, DC: Brookings.

Mazmanian, Daniel, and Sabatier, Paul, eds. (1981). *Effective Policy Implementation.* Lexington, MA: D.C. Heath.

Mazmanian, Daniel, and Sabatier, Paul, eds. (1989). *Implementation and Public Policy.* Lanham, MD: Univ. Press of America.

Mazur, Alian (1981). *The Dynamics of Technical Controversy*. Washington, DC: Communications Press.

Meitsner, Arnold (1976). *Policy Analysis in the Bureaucracy*. Berkeley: Univ. of California Press.

Milward, H. Brinton, and Wamsley, Gary (1984). "Policy Subsystems, Networks, and the Tools of Public Management," in Robert Eyestone, ed., *Public Policy Formation and Implementation,* Chap. 1. New York: JAI Press.

Nadel, Mark (1971). *The Politics of Consumer Protection*. Indianapolis: Bobbs-Merrill.

Nelkin, Dorothy (1979). *Controversy: Politics of Technical Decisions*. Beverly Hills: Sage.

Nelson, Robert (1987). "The Economics Profession and the Making of Public Policy," *Journal of Economic Literature* 25 (March): 42–84. Nevada Gaming Commission, Economic Research Division (1970). *Direct Levies on Gaming in Nevada, FY 1969–70*. Carson City, NV, November.

Newell, Allen, and Simon, Herbert (1972). *Human Problem Solving*. Englewood Cliffs: Prentice-Hall.

Nisbit, Richard, and Ross, Lee (1980). *Human Inference: Strategies and Shortcomings of Social Judgment*. Englewood Cliffs: Prentice-Hall.

Okun, Arthur (1975). *Equality and Efficiency. The Big Tradeoff*. Washington, DC: Brookings.

Ostrom, Elinor (1990). *Governing the Commons.* Cambridge, UK: Cambridge Univ. Press.

Ostrom, Vincent, Tiebout, Charles, and Warren, Robert (1961). "The Organization of Government in Metropolitan Areas," *American Political Science Review* 55 (December): 831–842.

Palumbo, Dennis (1988). *Public Policy in America*. New York: Harcourt, Brace, Jovanovich.

Peffley, Mark, and Hurwitz, Jen (1985). "A Hierarchical Model of Attitude Constraint," *American Journal of Political Science* 29 (November): 871–890.

Pressman, Jeffery, and Wildavsky, Aaron (1973). *Implementation*. Berkeley, CA: Univ. of California Press.

Putnam, Robert (1973). *The Beliefs of Politicians.* New Haven: Yale Univ. Press.

Putnam, Robert (1978). *The Comparative Study of Political Elites*. Englewood Cliffs: Prentice-Hall.

Quirk, Paul (1981). *Industry Influence in the Federal Regulatory Agencies*. Princeton, NJ: Princeton Univ. Press.

Riker, William (1962). *The Theory of Political Conditions*. New Haven: Yale Univ. Press.

Ripley, Randall, and Franklin, Grace (1982). *Bureaucracy and Policy Implementation*. Homewood, IL: Dorsey Press.

Rokeach, Milton (1973). *The Nature of Human Values*. New York: Macmillan.

Sabatier, Paul A. (1975). "Social Movements and Regulatory Agencies," *Political Science* 6 (September): 301–342.

———. (1986). "Top-Down and Bottom-Up Models of Policy Implementation: A Critical Analysis and Suggested Synthesis," *Journal of Public Policy* 6 (January): 21–48.

———. (1987). "Knowledge, Policy-Oriented Learning, and Policy Change," *Knowledge: Creation, Diffusion, Utilization* 8 (June): 649–692.

———. (1988). "An Advocacy Coalition Framework of Policy Change and the Role of Policy-Oriented Learning Therein," *Policy Sciences* 21: 129–165.

———. (1991a). "Toward Better Theories of the Policy Process," *PS: Political Science & Politics* 24 (June): 147–156.

———. (1991b). "Political Science and Public Policy," *PS: Political Science & Politics* 24 (June): 144–156.

Sabatier, Paul A., and Pelloey, Neil (1987). "Incorporating Multiple Actors and Guidance Instruments into Models of Regulatory Policy-Making: An Advocacy Coalition Framework," *Administration and Society* 19 (September): 236–263.

Sabatier, Paul A., Hunter, Susan, and McLaughlin, Susan (1987). "The Devil Shift: Perceptions and Misperceptions of Opponents," *Western Political Quarterly* 41 (September): 449–476.

Schattschneider, E. E. (1960). *The Semi-Sovereign People*. New York: Holt, Rinehart and Winston.

Schitt, Ashley (1962). *Fire and Water: Scientific Heresy in the Forest Service*. Cambridge: Harvard Univ. Press.

Scholtz, John T., Twombly, Jim, and Hendrick, Barbara (1991). "Street-level Political Controls over Federal Bureaucracy," *American Political Science Review* 85 (September): 829–850.

Simon, Herbert (1979). *Models of Thought*. New Haven: Yale Univ. Press.

Skocpol, Theda (1979). *States and Social Revolution*. Cambridge, UK: Cambridge Univ. Press.

Skowronek, Stephen (1982). *Building a New American State*. Cambridge, UK: Cambridge Univ. Press.

Smith, Don (1968). "Cognitive Consistency and the Perception of Others' Opinions," *Public Opinion Quarterly* 32: 1–15.

Steinbruner, John D. (1974). *The Cybernetic Theory of Decision*. Princeton: Princeton Univ. Press.

Taylor, Michael, and Laver, Michael (1973). "Government Coalitions in Western Europe," *European Journal of Political Research* 1 (September): 205–248.

Tesser, Abraham (1976). "Self-Generated Attitude Change," *Advances in Experimental Social-Psychology* 11: 289–338.

Truman, David (1951). *The Governmental Process*. New York: Alfred Knopf.

Vig, Norman, and Kraft, Michael, eds. (1984). *Environmental Policy in the 1980s*. Washington, DC: Congressional Quarterly Press.

Wamsley, Gary (1983). "Policy Subsystems as a Unit of Analysis in Implementation Studies," Paper presented at Erasmus Univ., Rotterdam, June.

Warwick, Paul (1979). "The Durability of Coalition Governments in Parliamentary Democracies," *Comparative Political Studies* 11 (January): 465–498.

Waterman, Richard (1989). *Presidential Influence and the Administrative State*. Knoxville: Univ. of Tennessee Press.

Weiss, Carol (1977a). *Using Social Research in Public Policy Making*. Lexington: D.C. Heath.

Weiss, Carol (1977b). "Research for Policy's Sake: The Enlightenment Function of Social Research." *Policy Analysis* 3 (Fall): 531–545.

White, Lawrence J. (1982). *The Regulation of Air Pollutant Emissions from Motor Vehicles*. Washington, DC: American Enterprise Institute.

Wicklund, Robert, and Brehan, Jack (1976). *Perspectives on Cognitive Dissonance*. Hillsdale, NJ: Lawrence Erlbaum Assoc.

Wildavsky, Aaron, and Tenenbaum, Ellen (1981). *The Politics of Mistrust*. Beverly Hills: Sage.

Wilker, Harry, and Milbrath, Lester (1972). "Political Belief Systems and Political Behavior," in D. Nimmo and C. Bonjean, *Political Attitudes and Public Opinion*, pp. 41–57. New York: David McKay.

Wood, B. Dan (1988). "Principals, Bureaucrats, and Responsiveness in Clean Air Enforcements," *American Political Science Review* 82 (March): 213–234.

———. (1991). "Federalism and Policy Responsiveness: The Clean Air Case," *Journal of Politics* 53 (August): 851–859.

Zariski, Raphael (1964). "Coalition Formation in the Italian Regions," *Comparative Politics* 16 (July): 403–420.

CHAPTER 4

HEALTH POLICY: THE POLITICS OF HEALTH

Politics has often been described as the "art of the possible." It is politics and the political process that translate our ideas and values into public policy. Each edition of *The Nation's Health* has included articles or book chapters on the politics of health, beginning in the first edition with Douglass Cater's preface to Cater and Philip R. Lee's book, *Politics of Health* (1972). Cater's ideas grew out of his experience as a journalist in Washington, D.C., and as a senior staff member in President Lyndon Johnson's White House during a period when more health legislation was passed by two Congresses than by all the previous Congresses put together. He coined the phrase "subgovernment of health" to describe the actors and the processes that influence federal health policy.

Prior to the period of Great Society activism in the 1960s, political alignment on most health policy issues, except biomedical research, had been largely determined on a geographic (state-by-state) basis. For a long period the physician, particularly the American Medical Association (AMA), was the dominant voice in health policy and the politics of health. The role and influence of the medical profession are described by Mark Peterson in Article 1. The Burton-Hill program for hospital planning and construction was the best postwar example of a major public health program that provided federal funds through the states to build a modern hospital system throughout the United States. The traditional grant-in-aid programs (e.g., tuberculosis control, venereal disease control) of the Public Health Service (PHS) were virtually all granted to states for categorical health programs. The funding of biomedical research, through the National Institutes of Health (NIH), was the exception.

THE HEALTH POLICY COMMUNITY

Although interest groups of one kind or another have characterized politics in the United States since the founding of the republic, they did not emerge as important in health policy (with the exception of the AMA) until after World War II and particularly not until after the enactment of Medicare in 1965. However, as in other areas of public policy, an "iron triangle" emerged. In health policy, the iron triangle consisted of three elements. First were the private-sector interests, which included the medical profession, initially through the AMA, and then involving multiple specialties and the medical schools. Along with the medical profession were the hospitals, the health insurance industry (especially after World War II), and the pharmaceutical industry, which focused most of its attention on drug regulation and the Food and Drug Administration (FDA). Second were legislative committees and their staff. The third leg of the triangle was composed of the executive branch agencies, such as the FDA and NIH, involved in specific policy areas.

The health policy community is now referred to as a "network" or "advocacy coalition" instead of an "iron triangle" because it represents a large array of players and interests. It includes organizations of investigators; medical schools; academic health centers; the pharmaceutical, biotechnology, and medical device industries; voluntary health agencies (e.g., American Cancer Society); unions, particularly of women employed in hospitals or by other health care organizations; consumer organizations (e.g., American Association of Retired Persons, or AARP); and other groups. As such, health policy has become more and more complex, and the subgovernment of health has become larger, more heterogeneous, and more loosely structured. The process has taken place particularly at the federal and state levels, but has occurred at the local level as well. The role of pluralism and the role of special interests are described in Article 2, "Health Care and Health Care Policy in a Changing World" by Donald A. Barr, Philip R. Lee, and A. E. Benjamin, and in "Health Policy and the Politics of Health Care" (1993) by Lee and Benjamin (see the Recommended Reading).

Although the advocates of the pluralist perspective find little problem with the proliferation of interest groups, it is clear that some groups, usually representing businesses, have a far more powerful voice and resources than many nonprofit, voluntary agencies. Also, those who have a focused interest and greater stake in a particular policy (e.g., physicians regarding Medicare policies related to physician payment) tend to have more influence than those with a diffuse interest in the issue (e.g., taxpayers). Representatives of special interests are currently among the greatest stakeholders and, as such, mobilize significant resources to influence the formulation of policy. For instance, political action committees (PACs) pour hundreds of millions of dollars to directly support candidates for office at all levels of government and additional millions of "soft" money to organizations for which there is no public accountability. Recently, there has been increased national attention to the growing role of soft money, particularly as a result of the Enron scandal. Although Congress enacted legislation in 2002 to limit soft-money contributions and the influence of campaign contributions, many doubt how effective these reforms will be because of the rules made by the Federal Elections Commission.

IDEOLOGICAL SHIFTS

The 1990s, and particularly the period since the demise of President Clinton's Health Security Act and the election of Republican majorities in both the U.S. Senate and

House of Representatives in 1994, has witnessed major changes in the politics of health. The federal budget has increasingly been the focus of major policy actions, with significant consequences for health policies (e.g., Medicare). In "The New Politics of U.S. Health Policy," Hacker and Skocpol (1997) focus on both an ideological shift and the overriding importance of the federal budget (see Recommended Reading). The need to reduce the budget deficit, they argue, is among the predominant concerns presently influencing the politics of health. Another factor — the strong antigovernment sentiment expressed by the Republicans — also influences the politics of health. Altogether, Hacker and Skocpol describe the dramatic shift in the politics of health as a three-fold strategy by the Republicans to (1) reduce spending on existing programs and preclude future spending increases by large tax cuts; (2) transfer authority to the states for programs that formerly were joint federal/state programs (e.g., welfare); and (3) privatize public programs, which would permit beneficiaries of public services to purchase them from the private sector. The actions by the administration of George W. Bush clearly reflect these three strategies.

The federal budget has been a particularly powerful driver of federal policy, including health policies, since the massive deficit that developed in the Reagan and first Bush administrations. Despite President Clinton's commitment to health care reform, reducing the federal deficit was his first priority after he took office, and it continued to be a priority even as budget surpluses developed in the last few years of his second term. For years, the size of the deficit alone precluded major health policy initiatives, except those responding to the HIV/AIDS epidemic. Furthermore, the introduction of new restrictive budget procedures in 1990 made President Clinton's Health Security Act almost impossible to enact without difficult tax increases. Given the surplus, politics was governed by the Republicans' successful push for a large tax cut in the first year of the George W. Bush administration in 2001. Many Democrats voted for the tax cut, fearful of further losses at the polls as "tax and spend" Democrats if they opposed it. The result of the tax cut and the recession has been the return of large federal budget deficits as well as deficits in most state budgets. There are also severe constraints on domestic spending in health, except that related to bioterrorism and biomedical research.

AMERICAN PUBLIC'S ATTITUDE TOWARD GOVERNMENT AND HEALTH REFORM

In the past, Americans placed great trust in the professionals who provided their health care, in the insurance companies that paid for much of their care, and in the government that regulated, oversaw, and, to a great extent, financed the health care system. However, until the September 11, 2001, terrorist attacks on the World Trade Center and the Pentagon, there had been a sharp decline in the public's trust in government to address key health issues, as well as other large policy issues. The reaction to the demise of Clinton's Health Security Act is a key example of the American public's critique of the efficiency, effectiveness, and costs of their health care system. Through constant media exposure and personal experiences with a system rife with increasing costs and rationing and decreasing access, the magnitude of the growing dissatisfaction has been highlighted. As a result, Americans tend to be more critical of their health care system than are the citizens of Canada, the United Kingdom, Germany, or other industrialized countries.

Sherry Glied, in *Chronic Condition: Why Health Reform Fails* (1997), described a rapid shift in the public attitude toward health care reform between 1993 and 1994 (see Recommended Reading). Whereas health reform had been the key to election platforms in 1993, Glied noted that by "Clinton's second term, national health reform guaranteeing coverage to all Americans [was] a dead issue" (p. 2). One factor that affected the shift in the public's attitude was the huge investment by various interest groups (insurance industry, small business) in media campaigns and other activities designed to influence the public. How long the greater trust in government that developed after the September 11 attacks will endure has yet to be seen.

POLITICAL INFLUENCES ON HEALTH POLICY FORMULATION

This edition of *The Nation's Health* includes "Health Care and Health Policy in a Changing World," in which Barr, Lee, and Benjamin (1999) update their previous work (Lee and Benjamin, 1993) and identify and discuss the political influences on health policy formulation over the past two hundred years. The authors' documentation of the evolution of U.S. health policy indicates that although consensus has emerged about the nature of the problems confronting the system, there is by no means agreement on the solutions. This conclusion was reflected in the health care reform debates of the early 1990s. Even when the nation was engaged in a major debate on health system reform in 1993 and 1994, disagreements about how such reform was to be accomplished and the influence of interest groups produced a deadlock in the policy process. In their discussion of incrementalism as the principal means of health policy reform, the authors note the value of understanding the policy process, described by Kingdon (1995), Longest (1998), and Sabatier (1988) through a conceptual framework or model.

POLITICS OF LONG-TERM CARE

The politics of health has also been reflected in the politics of long-term care (LTC). Article 3, by Carroll L. Estes, Joshua M. Wiener, Sheryl C. Goldberg, and Susan M. Goldenson (1999), updates the developments in LTC policy and the politics of long-term care. LTC policy was a major issue discussed during the development of President Clinton's Health Security Act. The discussions focused on both the elderly disabled and the disabled younger than 65 years. Politically, the initiatives in long-term care did not generate the groundswell of support that the Clinton administration had hoped for. Nonetheless, one of the most important political developments was the coming together of advocates representing different interests to agree on a common agenda. Estes and colleagues discuss a number of lessons learned from the politics of long-term care reform. A return to incrementalism as the best means to advance health care policy and the LTC policy agenda is proposed (Estes et al., 1999; Barr, Lee, and Benjamin, 1999). Estes and colleagues also suggest that it may have been more prudent or strategic to push for LTC reform separately from comprehensive health proposals so that LTC, a "popular idea," would not be lost in the shuffle of larger and more controversial health care reform efforts.

Another important element of successful health care reform efforts requires an understanding of the role of the states in supporting or opposing federal legislation (see the Recommended Reading article by Thomas Oliver, "State Health Politics and Policies: Rhetoric, Reality, and the Challenges Ahead"). Other "political prerequisites" include gauging and garnering bipartisan support; securing a "policy entrepreneur," that is, an individual (or individuals) with voice and commitment to your policy agenda (Kingdon, 1995); and investing in strong public education to present the problem and policy solutions.

FOOD POLITICS

The story of the politics of health could also be told from the politics of tobacco control, prescription drugs, air pollution, automobile safety, abortion, or other areas. Limitations in space preclude these additions, but we have chosen to include Marion Nestle's recent book, *Food Politics, How the Food Industry Influences Nutrition and Health* (2002), in the Recommended Reading list. In the introduction, she notes, "This book is about how the food industry influences what we eat and therefore, our health" (p. 1). Later, she adds:

> To satisfy stockholders, food companies must convince people to eat more of their product or to eat their product instead of those of competitors. They do so through advertising and public relations, of course, but also by working tirelessly to convince government officials, nutrition professionals, and the media that their products promote health — or at least do no harm. Much of this work is a virtually invisible part of contemporary culture that attracts only occasional notice (p. 1).

This is indeed a fascinating story of the politics of health, told in rich and very disturbing detail. She does not exempt public officials from her critical analysis. She describes the potential conflict of interest when a government agency (in this case the United States Department of Agriculture, or USDA) is simultaneously responsible for advising the public on matters of nutrition and health as well as for regulating meat and poultry safety and promoting the sale of agricultural products. Dr. Nestle raises significant questions concerning the validity of the policy development process when the membership of both the authorizing and appropriations committees in Congress emphasize agricultural rather than consumer interests, and the USDA must function despite a clear conflict of interest. Ultimately, the health of the U.S. population can be affected when nutrition, food safety, and health information for the public is impeded because of structural arrangements that limit information dissemination to protect the financial interests of agribusiness.

Nestle's book also raises an important and recurring question in health policy: To what extent will the new politics of health further tilt public health functions in the direction of proprietary interests? This question is applicable to many areas of public health — from nutrition and food safety to prescription drugs, consumer products, occupational health and safety, and highway safety.

SUMMARY

Politics ultimately determines the struggle for financial resources and interest group control of various system components. Underneath the regulations and legislation are power struggles, the outcomes of which ultimately determine not only the availability, cost, and quality of health care services, but also food safety, tobacco control, the price of prescription drugs, the funding of biomedical research, and the allocation of resources to combat bioterrorism. They determine who will care for us, when, where, and how; the methods by which we will pay for care; how much we will pay; where hospitals will be located, and their size and scope. The outcomes of these perpetual struggles also significantly influence the education of the health professions. They thereby determine the scope and direction of health-related research and the investment in public health programs. Furthermore, whether the transformation in the politics of health will persist or whether a new balance will be struck is greatly influenced by all levels of government — local, state, and federal.

The politics of health and the health policy process, which it influences ultimately, allocate resources for the benefit of the population or special interests. Sometimes, both groups benefit. Because this process is, in the long run, driven by our values, what we say and what we do sometimes seem distant from one another.

REFERENCES

Barr, D. A., Lee, P. R., and Benjamin, A. E. (1999). Health care and health care policy in a changing world. In H. Wallace, G. Green, K. J. Jaros, L. L. Paine, and M. Story (Eds.), *Health and welfare for families in the 21st century* (pp. 13–29). Boston: Jones and Bartlett.

Cater, D., and Lee, P. R. (Eds.). (1972). *Politics of health.* New York: Medcome Press.

Estes, C. L., Weiner, J. M., Goldberg, S. C., and Goldenson, S. M. (1999). *The politics of long term care reform under the Clinton health plan: Lessons for the future.* Washington, D.C./San Francisco: Health Policy Center and Institute for Health and Aging.

Glied, S. (1997). *Chronic condition: Why health reform fails.* Cambridge, MA: Harvard University Press.

Hacker, J. S., and Skocpol, T. (1997). The new politics of U.S. health policy. *Journal of Health Politics, Policy and Law, 22*(2), 315–336.

Kingdon, J. W. (1995). *Agendas, alternatives, and public policies* (2nd ed.). New York: Addison-Wesley Educational Publishers.

Lee, P. R., and Benjamin, A. E. (1993). Health policy and the politics of health care. Abridged from S. J. Williams and P. R. Torrens (Eds.), *Introduction to health services* (4th ed.).

Longest, B. B. (1998). *Health policymaking in the United States* (2nd ed.). Chicago: Health Administration Press.

Nestle, M. (2002). *Food politics: How the food industry influences nutrition and health.* Berkeley: University of California Press.

Sabatier, P. (1988). An advocacy coalition framework of policy change and the role of policy-oriented learning therein. *Policy Sciences, 21*, 129–168.

ARTICLE 1

From Trust to Political Power

Interest Groups, Public Choice, and Health Care

Mark A. Peterson

In 1963 Kenneth Arrow offered a simple empirical observation that suggested a core impediment to the effective functioning of market arrangements in health care. "Because medical knowledge is so complicated," he noted, "the information possessed by the physician as to the consequences and possibilities of treatment is very much greater than that of the patient, or at least it is so believed by both parties" (951). According to Arrow, however, society found a way to manage this information asymmetry that would otherwise leave people vulnerable to suboptimal decision making and exploitation by the suppliers of medical services. "Delegation and trust are the social institutions designed to obviate the problem of informational inequality" (966).

According to this reasoning, we make efficacious choices by permitting our physicians to both define the choice set of the various treatment options and weight their expected values. We feel comfortable delegating a significant chunk of our decision-making sovereignty regarding medical care because of the trust we have in our physicians. But in Arrow's framework, why does this dyadic trust emerge in which we place such faith, given the lack of a formal instrument for insuring against a failure to benefit from medical care? Not primarily because as individuals our physicians are gracious, or benevolent, or even just plain smart, although those characteristics may be relevant. We trust our physicians in this dyadic relationship because of a collective or social attribute we recognize in them, that is, a "generalized belief in the ability of the physician" predicated on his or her formally prescribed, scientifically grounded professional training and license to practice medicine in accordance with the standards of the profession (965). Indeed, should someone fall ill, say, at a public gathering, the general call goes out for "a doctor" and the individuals who may be lending immediate comfort yield without question to the entirely unknown woman or man who appears and establishes this professional link by stating simply "I'm a doctor" and proceeds to treat the patient.

Other essays in this volume explore, and often question, the reliability of individuals granting such inclusive trust to physicians to guide their personal medical care, especially as we know more about what "the doctor" does not know while social and technological change have evened the informational scales at least a bit. I examine a broader consequence of physicians' claims of knowledge and trust that Arrow minimized in his analysis but that have had profound implications for the organization, financing, and delivery of health care services as they are experienced by the nation as a whole. Based on the same claims to science and knowledge that medicine has used to invite our dyadic trust in physicians at the individual level, the medical profession has long sought, and often obtained, broad-based social trust in its leadership of health care policy making by local, state, and federal governments. Organized medicine has sought to dominate the politics and policy of health care by arguing that only it as a profession has the understanding of science and practice necessary to construct optimal social arrangements for providing access to care. Until the legitimacy of this exclusive claim was successfully disputed, starting primarily in the 1970s, and other groups developed the organizational wherewithal and informational capacity to call into question the social trust that physicians had enjoyed, the medical profession, with the rhetoric of commitment to the public good, had employed its trust-based political leverage to extend and protect its economic self-interest. This essay is about the negative social consequences of trust in physicians, which Arrow did not adequately anticipate given his focus on the dyadic form of trust, and how the social role of physicians has changed in the ensuing decades.

TRUST AND DELEGATION AS POLITICAL POWER

Professions gain respect and their members garner both dyadic and social trust because they develop and inculcate among their ranks specialized knowledge that the average person, lacking the profession's formal training, cannot acquire or easily interpret. As captured by the old cliché, however, knowledge is power — not only power evident in the application of a profession's knowledge about particular decisions in its standard workplace, but influence over the entire social structure that defines and regulates the environment in which that work is accomplished.

One of the most preeminent sociologists studying the professions, Eliot Freidson (1986: 185–186), notes that "to gain insight into the full range of professional powers, we must move outside the workplace and into the broader political economy.... [and look at] those who are in a position to influence the policies of the state on which the special position of the profession depends." Professions, says Albert Dzur (forthcoming), "are political entities, not just when they form interest groups, but because in the intermediary realm of civil society professions possess the power to distract, encourage, limit, and inform public recognition of and deliberation over social problems." In this realm, stated simply by Phillip Elliott (1972: 147), "the profession claims unique responsibility for some aspect of the *public* good. It also claims to know how that good should be achieved" (italics added). That assertion by a profession is always made with calls to the public interest and implied confidence in the objectivity of the profession's stance. Jürgen Habermas (1971) reminds us, however, that these claims may be no more than a politically astute fig leaf covering up efforts to usurp decisions that otherwise would be rightly pursued in the full light of democratic policy making, taking them in a direction contrary to the interests and will of the public. Ultimately an appeal may be made to what Gary Belkin (1998) calls "the technocratic wish," the erroneous notion that issues of real and contentious politics can be answered or managed most effectively by redefining them as scientific, technical, objective — based, of course, on the presumption that the relevant profession can dominate the meaning and historical logic given to these terms (see also Freidson 1970, 1986; Morone and Belkin 1995).

It would be fair to say that medicine is, or more accurately was, the paragon of professional power. Just as Arrow located the individual's need to trust his or her physician in the perspective that "medical knowledge is so complicated" and asymmetrically possessed by the doctor, so too the "profession bases its claim for its position on the possession of a skill so esoteric or complex that nonmembers of the profession cannot perform the work safely or satisfactorily and cannot even evaluate the work properly.... They claim that their esoteric expertise is such that only they are able to determine what is wrong with humanity, how it may best be served, and at what price" (Freidson 1970: 45, 368; Starr 1982). "All features of medical service in any method of medical practice," stated a 1934 resolution adopted by the American Medical Association's House of Delegates, "should be under the control of the profession. No other body or individual is legally or educationally equipped to exercise such control" (quoted in Millenson 1997a: 188). In Steven Brint's (1994: 36) terms, medicine "combined civic-minded *moral* appeals and circumscribed *technical* appeals" to project "social trustee professionalism." What undergirds faith in our individual physicians thus empowers them collectively in issues that are as removed from explicit medical practice as taxation, allocative fairness, public administration, and political accountability — issues on which other legitimate interests and the population as a whole may in fact have quite different positions than those promulgated by medical practitioners themselves.

Just about twenty years after Arrow's seminal analysis, with trust posed as a societal response to fill a crucial gap in the market, Paul Starr won the 1984 Pulitzer Prize for his historical and sociological study of how American medicine waged a long-term battle to gain scientifically grounded legitimacy and establish its professional dominance over clinical practice (physician-patient dyadic engagement), medical organization (the structure and leadership of health care institutions), and health care financing (the sources and arrangements for paying medical costs) (1982). In this struggle physicians were neither predetermined victors nor simply serving, by societal "design" or structural-function adaptability of social institutions, the interests of the larger community (see Elliott 1972: 6). They had to successfully make exclusive claims to science and medical efficacy — liking to view themselves, notes Brint (1994: 59), as "applied scientists" — and do so at the expense of the range of competing practitioners they confronted at the end of the nineteenth century. Establishing its scientific roots (and disparaging those of others), organized medicine gained a legitimacy that allowed it to acquire what Starr (1982: 13) calls "cultural authority, ... [which]

entails the construction of reality through definitions of fact and value." In Freidson's (1970: 205–206) words, "in the course of obtaining a monopoly over its work, medicine has also obtained well-nigh exclusive jurisdiction over determining what illness is and therefore how people must act in order to be treated as ill.... by virtue of being the authority on what illness 'really' is, *medicine creates the social possibilities for acting sick*" (italics in original). Through this domination of both its work and the social meaning and consequences of illness, Starr argues that physicians sought to preserve two core domains of autonomy: economic (the size and circumstances of their incomes) and clinical (control over the nature of medical practice and treatment decisions). From those forms of autonomy derives the motive for and resources, material and intellectual, to demand considerable autonomy in setting health policy, nominally the responsibility of federal, state, and local governments that should be responsive to their entire constituencies.

Does, in fact, the professional power of medicine translate into political power for organized medicine? Paul Starr's analysis would seem to make this a question hardly worth asking. Economist Paul Feldstein, in his book, *Health Associations*, states categorically, "In the past, health legislation at both a state and a federal level has been strongly influenced by health interest groups. In many respects, the structure of our health care system is a result of the legislative activity of these groups.... The American Medical Association is the most influential of the health professional organizations" (1977: 2, 27).

These declarations, however, are offered devoid of any citations to explicit evidence of this power. As a general proposition, the demonstrated influence of organized interests is far more circumspect. Consider this summary judgment from Frank Baumgartner and Beth Leech (1998), who recently combed the political science literature on interest group efforts to affect the outcomes of policy making:

> Early interest-group studies shared the outlook of early subsystem studies. Interest groups were enormously powerful, and insider groups had the advantage.... Several important studies published in the 1960s helped challenge this view. Interest-group influence was ... benign.... The popular conclusion drawn from these studies was that interest groups did not exert pressure, indeed were not influential. If it were that simple, we could simply say that interest groups were once seen as all-powerful, but more recent studies have shown this to be wrong.... However, interest groups at times probably are weak and ineffectual, and at other times very effective at getting what they want.... Unfortunately, the accumulated mass of quantitative and qualitative studies of lobbying behavior has generated a great number of contradictions, with few consistent findings.... The studies reviewed ..., for all their contradictions, have in fact taught us something important: they allow us to stipulate at least occasional interest-group influence and to concentrate instead on the circumstances under which groups are influential. (125, 126, 127, 140, 146)

Briefly stated, having the capacity to shape public policy requires possessing the kinds of attributes that matter to and could influence elected officials, their advisers, and agency officials. A quick survey of the literature reveals a number of group characteristics that would be advantageous in the "political market"[1]:

- *Information*: Government officials who have policy-making authority and are accountable to election constituencies need information to overcome two types of uncertainty. The first involves the linkages between proposed policy actions and actual policy outcomes as experienced by the public. The second pertains to how one's own constituency is likely to see and interpret what government does and respond to it politically. Organizations representing knowledge-based, high-status individuals or institutions earn automatic recognition and have particular credibility in helping to resolve both kinds of uncertainty.
- *Recurrent interactions with policy makers*: The credibility of the information provided by organized interests to policy makers is tested through repeated interactions and the establishment of stable relationships. In the competition among groups, active participation in issues that are regularly on the government agenda gives an organization the opportunity to solidify impressions of its value as an information source.
- *Large and dispersed membership*: Because elected officials are so sensitive to the attitudes of the districts or states they represent, organizations have greater access and potential influence when they include a policy maker's constituents (and can make valid claims to actually speak on their behalf). Large and widely distributed memberships or clientele expand the number of elected officials with whom the interest will have a direct relationship. The effects are strengthened if an organization can stimulate grassroots mobilization. However, an interest with a large and dispersed base can also fall victim to the collective action and free-rider problems identified by Mancur Olson (1965) and thus need other attributes, such as an occupational connection and selective benefits, discussed by Olson (1965) and Walker (1991), to overcome this hurdle.
- *Quasi-unanimity*: Large organizations are also more prone to having disparate interests among their memberships, possibly yielding factionalization, threatening their ability to take expressed positions in issues of public policy. Effective organized interests have to possess enough cohesion and focus on shared core interests to project something representing a unified front on high-priority policy concerns.
- *Organizational resources*: Economic and status resources make it possible for an association to attract one of its most important organizational resources: a large, skilled, experienced, and professional staff. Staffs of this caliber have a better sense of how to frame issues, gather appropriate information and

1. One could cite an extensive literature, but the main themes that follow can be found in Arnold 1990; Bauer, Pool, and Dexter 1972; Baumgartner and Leech 1998: Browne 1995; Hansen 1991; Hayes 1981; Hojnacki 1997; Hula 1999; Kollman 1998; Krehbiel 1991; Olson 1965; Peterson 1993, 1995a, 1998a; Sabao 1984; Walker 1991; and Weissert and Weissert 1996.

conduct research, mobilize the membership, orchestrate media campaigns, and facilitate communications with policy makers.

- *Electoral resources*: Policy makers need both political intelligence about their constituencies and campaign funds to launch effective drives for election and reelection. At the national level, since the Federal Election Campaign Act of 1974, campaign contributions by organized interests have been primarily formalized through the establishment of associated political action committees (PACs). In addition to having a large, dispersed, unified membership, PAC money provides signals about an organization's political wherewithal, issue priorities, and constituency influence.
- *Policy niche and coalition leadership*: No group could hope to become a forceful and respected voice on all matters of public policy. Credibility, unity, and impact are enhanced when an organized interest is able to claim a comparative advantage in information and resources over other interests in a particular policy niche or domain, especially if the group's association is recognized and supported by other compatible interests as a coalition leader.

ORGANIZED MEDICINE AS AN ORGANIZED INTEREST, CIRCA 1963

Has organized medicine, as a profession and as formally represented by the American Medical Association (and other physician societies), had the attributes one would associate with being able to influence political agenda setting, debate, and policy making? Most organized interests at the national or state level at any given time do not possess any of these attributes, at least reliably. A relatively small proportion can lay claim to more than a couple, and they may even be in conflict with one another (for example, as noted earlier, a large membership can interfere with developing a unified policy position and establishing niche leadership). It is profoundly striking that at the time Arrow published his article, the American Medical Association — the primary organization representing physician interests — unquestionably possessed *all* of these attributes (see Campion 1984). It may have been the only organized interest in America for which that has ever been true. In addition, among the individual characteristics noted earlier, the AMA quite simply stood out among other interests. When Arrow was surveying the health care marketplace, organized medicine had almost no worthy competitors for providing policy makers with substantive information about medicine and its practice. The trust that individuals felt toward their personal physicians had its social complement in the general trust extended to organized medicine in matters of public policy. Other physician societies and health organizations, too, deferred to the AMA in this collective policy-making role. The entire health services research and health policy research enterprise, and the community of specialists in this domain who eventually challenged positions of the AMA, did not really begin until after 1965 and the passage of Medicare and took years to mature (Brown 1991).

In addition, too, few organizations could compete with the reach of organized medicine, with members in probably close to every single legislative district (state or federal) and certainly every state, responsive to requests for direct grassroots participation and able to expand the effects of their ranks by stimulating favorable reactions among their trusting patients. At the time, more than nine out of ten practicing physicians in the country belonged to the AMA as well as its state associations and county medical societies. The AMA has often spent more money than any other group represented in the nation's capital to influence government policy (Rayak 1967; Feldstein 1977). In AMPAC (the AMA Political Action Committee), the AMA also had the third oldest political action committee in the country (formed just before Arrow began to write his seminal essay); it is far and away the leading campaign contributor among health care organizations (Weissert and Weissert 1996). Certainly in 1963, when the Arrow article was published, the AMA was the undisputed leader of an alliance of physicians, hospitals, insurers, and employers that sought to shape state and federal public policies in accordance with its interest and perspectives (Peterson 1993). It is no wonder, therefore, that Carol Weissert and William Weissert (1996: 97), in their opening summary of health care interest groups, commented that "in 1965 the American Medical Association was the strongest health lobby and probably the most powerful lobby of any kind in the country."

What did organized medicine seek to accomplish with the repeated and sustained application of this political leverage? To use the terminology of Arrow's economist colleagues, a main objective was the acquisition of *rents*. In the public choice framework, physicians, as a rational, self-interested profession, sought to get the state to use its power and resources to their economic benefit. The foundation for this line of analysis, anticipated by Arrow, was laid in 1971 by George Stigler in his article on "The Theory of Economic Regulation." Stigler emphasized industry efforts to secure direct governmental subsidies, control entry, restrict substitutes and promote complements, and engage in price-fixing. These issues were later pursued in much greater detail, with a specific health care application, by Paul Feldstein (1977). He hypothesized that one would find organized medicine promoting "demand increasing policies," "preferred methods of reimbursement," "reductions in the price of complements to the production of physician services," "increases in the price of substitutes for physicians," and "restrictions in the supply of physicians" (chaps. 1 and 2). Like the sociologists Starr and Freidson, Feldstein identified a number of enacted state and federal policies — from constraints on the availability of medical education to required licensure, from public subsidies to expand hospitals to restrictions on the practice of chiropractic, and so forth — that comport with the rent-seeking interests of organized medicine. Cause and effect are not fully drawn by Feldstein, but the health policy parameters of the American state, starting with early in the twentieth century as organized medicine was consolidating its legitimacy, look a lot like those that physicians as a group desired.

Many of these provisions, such as limiting the number of training slots for new physicians and licensing according to the dictates of the AMA, were sold to the public and policy makers by organized medicine as important means for ensuring quality and preventing the practice of "quack" medicine. But, as Feldstein notes, that justification loses merit when one identifies how few policies have been put forward by organized medicine to ensure the quality of practice once physicians have entered the workforce and how resistant it has been to alternative approaches. In addition, organized medicine purports to endorse a number of public health initiatives in addition to the policies that facilitate the clinical and economic autonomy of physicians. Where, though, does it put its political dollars? AMPAC consistently directs campaign contributions to those members of Congress who vote in favor of physicians' economic and clinical interests, punishes those who do not, and ends up penalizing the very members of the House of Representatives and Senate who are most in tune with the AMA's publicly stated public health agenda (Gutermuth 1999; Sharfstein and Sharfstein 1994; Wilkerson and Carrell 1999). In the parlance of modern scandal prosecutions, "follow the money."

The rent-seeking activities of organized medicine were matched by its extensive efforts to veto proposed policies that, although perceived by the profession to run counter to physician interests, would have advanced societal objectives. They include expanding insurance coverage and access to medical care, enhancing the efficiency of health care organization and delivery, and constraining inflationary pressures in health care costs. U.S. doctors have not been the only ones in the world pursing this "negative" agenda, but the design of our governing and political institutions, fragmenting government power, have catered to the projection of their will (Maioni 1995; Immergut 1992; Peterson 1993). If one accepts the analyses at face value, President Franklin Delano Roosevelt dropped the study of health insurance coverage as part of Social Security and President Harry Truman could not even get a serious congressional hearing on compulsory health insurance due to the opposition, and widely accepted power, of the American Medical Association (Starr 1982; Poen 1979). The AMA spent most of the twentieth century fighting third-party coverage through private insurance, then public insurance, even retooling for the Medicare debates its rhetoric from the 1940s about socialism and the threat to the very fabric of America's cherished liberties (Starr 1982; Marmor 2000). There was no more stalwart an opponent to wresting control over medical care costs, expanding the range of treatment approaches available to the American public, or ensuring equitable access to even its own definition of medical care. Trust in physicians came with a steep price.

THE POLITICAL FALL OF ORGANIZED MEDICINE

Ironically, a few short years after Arrow had concluded that dyadic trust in physicians mitigated the market deficiencies created by information asymmetries though missed the increasingly clear evidence of the societal costs generated by social trust in physicians, the centrality of organized medicine in U.S. policy making began to wane. Physicians since then, to be sure, have remained a significant force in the United States. Individual "public physicians," if you will, such as Dr. C. Everett Koop, retain considerable authority and stature. Most people continue to report favorable encounters with their own physicians. And some political leverage lingers in specific policy domains. Few other interests, for example, effectively compete with physicians in designing public policies that affect academic medical centers or medical schools to which the public dollars continue to flow. Further, as illustrated by the relatively strong laws that several states have enacted to limit the use of selective contracting by managed care plans, physician organizations may still assert considerable influence in a number of state capitals (Marsteller et al. 1997).

Nonetheless, a number of both exogenous and endogenous factors began to converge in the 1960s that disrupted the old power relationships.[2] An emerging public consensus offered, first, more support for tending to the needs of those lacking health care coverage and other social services, and then later endorsed greater regulatory discipline of medical practice. Myriad groups often opposed to the AMA, including consumer organizations such as Citizen Action, Families USA, and the American Association of Retired Persons (AARP), were spawned or invigorated by the rise of social movements. The availability of supportive "patrons of political action," such as private foundations, government agencies, and wealthy individuals, provided the funding they needed for organizational development and maintenance (Walker 1991). With access to more government and foundation funding, the research community in universities, think tanks, government policy shops, nonprofit firms, and even research arms of traditional interest groups created a new cadre of health services and policy specialists who offered analytical perspectives and results contrary to those of organized medicine (Peterson 1995a). Eventually, employers and insurers (especially small business organizations such as the National Federation of Independent Business and representatives of commercial carriers such as the Health Insurance Association of America) joined together to transform the organizational principles of health care delivery and financing, reinvigorating the market model, and, with the American Association of Health Plans, promoted various versions of managed care leading the way (Peterson 1995b, 1998b). In the meantime, starting with the U.S. Supreme Court's *Goldfarb v. Virginia State Bar* (421 U.S. 773 [1975]) decision in 1975 that opened up "learned professions" to federal antitrust regulation, a series of state and federal judicial actions reduced the economic autonomy and leverage of organized medicine and thus improved the political position of its competitors.

Internally, the physician community began to split politically in response to these pressures, and by the late 1980s the old alliance that the AMA had led in opposition to major government initiatives had weakened considerably. Still invigorated by a number of the attributes that give interest groups perceived strength in the policymaking process, the AMA nonetheless saw its position diminished by erosion in its membership, the loss of "quasi-unanimity" within its ranks, the rise of both competing groups and new sources of information for policy makers, and the loss of its coalition leadership role in the health policy "niche." The concerted and perhaps

2. Heinz et al. 1993; Jacobs 1993; Peterson 1993, 1995b, 1998b, and unpublished; Starr 1982; Walker 1991; and Weissert and Weissert 1996.

increasingly explicit efforts of physicians as an organized interest group to protect their own economic interests, especially when other sources of information began to emerge, some far more objective, made it difficult for them to maintain social trust (Gutermuth 1999; Millenson 1997b; Wolinsky and Brune 1994; Sharfstein and Sharfstein 1994; Wilkerson and Carrell 1999).

As with other professions beginning in the 1960s, whose pretensions to serving social purposes came under closer scrutiny, medicine moved more to the image of "expert professionalism," which "emphasized the instrumental effectiveness of specialized, technically grounded knowledge, but included comparatively little concern with collegial organization, ethical standards, or service to the public interest" (Brint 1994: 37). In the process, although people continued to respect and trust their own physicians, albeit now armed with more information and an emerging aura of patient rights, organized medicine lost much of the social trust that had previously been built on those individual relationships and cemented its claims on policy making. Among the public, those expressing "a great deal of confidence in the leaders of medicine" dropped to 44 percent in 2000, down from 73 percent in 1966, and actually plummeted all the way to 22 percent when health care reform dominated the agenda in the early 1990s (Blendon and Benson 2001: 39).

The initial crack came about with the passage of the Medicare program. For the first time, a major government program was enacted over the objections of organized medicine, aided by the force of the extraordinary political circumstances engendered by the 1964 landslide elections (Marmor 2000). Even in "defeat," however, the physicians were influential enough to dictate, in Feldstein's terms, the method of reimbursement and administration under the program [and to] demand enhancing policies and subsidies and constraints on potentially competing providers (Jacobs 1993). The AMA may have opposed Medicare, but with the program's implementation, it compelled the institutionalization — for a time — of "usual, customary, and reasonable" (UCR) retrospective reimbursement that served physicians' economic self-interest well and fueled subsequent medical inflation. Next came a more profound challenge to physician dominance of health care decision making and policy. Under the National Health Planning and Resources Development Act of 1974, not only were competing health care providers and health policy specialists to share the decision-making stage with physicians, but also now even consumers themselves were to have equal status in community-level Health Systems Agencies responsible (unsuccessfully) for effective and coordinated state and federal health policy (Morone 1990).

By the late 1980s, the AMA was just another interest group (Heinz et al. 1993; Weissert and Weissert 1996). A vignette illustrates its decline in clout. In 1991, a young fellow recently hired by the AMA as a lobbyist noticed one of the most influential Democratic members of Congress in the hallway of the Capitol and, knowing that he chaired a crucial subcommittee, thought the occasion provided a good opportunity to introduce himself and begin building a relationship. When he approached the member of Congress, held out his hand, and cheerfully introduced himself and offered the upbeat line "I guess we'll be working together," the member of Congress looked with disdain at the extended hand and uttered simply, "Go f—— yourself."[3] A few years later, the AMA not only did not dominate the health care reform debate, it was hardly even a recognized player (Peterson 1995b). Representatives of small and large businesses, insurance plans, the pharmaceutical industry, consumer groups, and other citizen organizations played a far more significant role (Johnson and Broder 1996; Peterson 1998c; Skocpol 1996).

NEW CLAIMANTS ON SCIENTIFIC LEGITIMACY

In recent years physicians have suffered an additional form of competition with consequences for both Arrow's confidence in dyadic trust and the concomitant social trust nurtured by the profession. As I noted earlier from Starr's account, physicians originally achieved the cultural authority necessary to instill trust based on the profession's perceived direct and unique ties to the progress and application of medical science. Although the advances of medical science itself continue to generate awe among the public, policy specialists, and policy makers, physicians no longer enjoy a monopolist, or even a primary, claim to scientific legitimacy. Organized medicine began to weaken its own authority when the AMA, starting in the 1950s and 1960s, shifted the focus of its meetings and other activities from scientific exploration to more economic and political interests and avoided joining concerted efforts to measure and improve the quality of medical services (Millenson 1997a, 1997b). The discovery by health services research of wide variations in practice patterns (and costs) among physicians unassociated with patient conditions, mixed with physicians responding without collective restraint to the incentives of an unfettered fee-for-service system that produced dramatic increases in the cost of medical care not clearly correlated with improved quality, further eroded the favorable link to science (Dartmouth Medical School 1996; Millenson 1997b, 1998; Wolinsky and Brune 1994).

In response came, first, the development of physician peer review organizations under federal law and later more aggressive accreditation processes that imposed external evaluation of physician decision making. The most significant new claimants on scientific legitimacy, though, are managed care insurance plans, whose sway in the health care system expanded rapidly and dramatically thirty years after Arrow published his article, when Kaiser Permanente was about the only well-known example of what was then referred to as prepaid group practice. Managed care organizations argue, at least implicitly, that they now have the superior link to scientific progress and knowledge, garnered and tested in the application of evidenced-based medicine (Belkin 1998; *JHPPL* 2001). Armed with treatment protocols and guidelines predicated on the results of clinical trials, outcomes research, quality measures, and patient

3. This story was told to me by a congressional staff member soon after it happened; at the time I was a legislative assistant for health policy in the office of Senator Tom Daschle (D-SD).

satisfaction surveys, they have moved to supplant physicians as the primary arbiters of what works and does not work in medical practice.

The rise of managed care raises important and perhaps conflicting questions about Arrow's original judgment that trust in physicians serves as a protection against information asymmetry. On the one hand, one can imagine that managed care arrangements help overcome the practice and policy problems generated by placing excessive social trust in physicians. As both a countervailing power politically and a private regulator of medical practice through the use of research and incentives that limit rather than promote intense, often unnecessary utilization, managed care can stymie the rent-seeking behavior of physicians and constrain organized medicine's claims on public resources. In addition, focusing on Arrow's specific argument, health plans well attuned to the latest in biomedical research can help address the adverse consequences of information asymmetry by compelling physicians to treat their patients in accordance with the best practices, even if the patients themselves do not have the information necessary to identify those practices. Ideally, the aggregation of medical decision making in managed care plans erases information asymmetries overall and ensures that individual patients receive the most appropriate care.

On the other hand, there are reasons to question the veracity of this ideal image. First, managed care plans as a group are but one claimant to scientific legitimacy, among others, and their assertions of superiority are potentially as self-serving and politically motivated — including in support of rent-seeking behavior — as that of physicians (Belkin 1998). One has to develop trust in private insurers, much as Arrow identified trust in physicians, to be assured that the best interests of patients are being pursued rather than those of the managed care organization. But such organizations do not even have the professional foundation or personal characteristics that benefited physicians in this regard. Indeed, because most managed care insurance carriers are now for-profit entities and so many decisions by plans are seen by the public as motivated by economic instead of medical considerations, the idea of granting "delegation and trust" to insurance carriers similar to what Arrow suggested for physicians is highly problematic (*JHPPL* 1998, 1999). Following a sustained backlash against managed care, however justified, it comes as no surprise that in 2000 only 29 percent of the public believed that managed care companies were doing "a good job," just one percentage point above the assessment of the tobacco industry, the social nemesis of our era (Blendon and Benson 2001: 40).

Second, because evidence-based medicine with its clinical practice guidelines focuses on what is effective for the average patient presenting a specified set of conditions, it must ignore any idiosyncratic characteristics, histories, and needs of particular patients. Therefore, the physician is once again called to the fore as a mediator between the science of medicine, as encapsulated in managed care protocols, and the treatment of specific individuals (Tanenbaum 1994). Which returns us to trust in physicians. Vice President Albert Gore, in his speech accepting the Democratic party's nomination for president in 2000, captured the theme repeated by many: "It's time to take the medical decisions away from the HMOs and insurance companies — and give them back to the physicians, the nurses, and the health care professionals"

(*New York Times*, 18 August 2000, A21). But those health care professionals, including physicians, must make their decisions in the managed care context in which they are themselves deeply embedded. A physician has to choose as both a clinician, and perhaps a patient's advocate against the insurer, and as a "businessman" explicitly focused on costs and facing incentives defined by risk sharing and payment mechanisms that directly affect the physician's own bottom line (Stone 1998). If we should have been more circumspect about trust in physicians than Arrow was in 1963, it is difficult to make a case that we should be any less concerned today.

CONCLUSION

If Jamie Robinson in this volume is wrong and we are not about to witness "the end of asymmetrical information" as a result of various market transformations, or if Clark Havighurst is wrong and unfettered contract-based competitive markets cannot work well in health care, then other measures may be required to substitute for the trust on which Arrow relied — and one hopes with fewer pernicious social consequences. Arrow writing today in response to the empirical world he would see might well give more favor to governmental regulation or infusion of explicit protections for patients. Ah, but is that not a prescription for the same costly and distorting rent-seeking behavior associated with organized medicine in the past? Maybe. But today neither physicians nor the managed care industry has the political leverage that the AMA enjoyed in Washington, D.C., and state capitals for so much of this century. Managed care plans, and their American Association of Health Plans (AAHP), have never experienced the trust, status, membership scope, lack of informational and organizational competition, campaign resources, or coalition leadership that marked organized medicine in earlier times and allowed it to wield so much influence. They, too, are just another interest group.

REFERENCES

Arnold, R. Douglas. 1990. *The Logic of Congressional Action.* New Haven, CT: Yale University Press.

Arrow, Kenneth J. 1963. Uncertainty and the Welfare Economics of Medical Care. *American Economic Review* 53(5):941–973.

Bauer, Raymond A., Ithiel de Sola Pool, and Lewis Anthony Dexter. 1972. *American Business & Public Policy: The Politics of Foreign Trade.* Chicago: Aldine-Atherton.

Baumgartner, Frank R., and Beth L. Leech. 1998. *Basic Interests: The Importance of Groups in Politics and Political Science.* Princeton, NJ: Princeton University Press.

Belkin, Gary S. 1998. The Technocratic Wish: Making Sense and Finding Power in the "Managed" Medical Marketplace. In *Healthy Markets? The New Competition in Medicare Care,* ed. Mark A. Peterson. Durham, NC: Duke University Press.

Blendon, Robert J., and John M. Benson. 2001. Americans' Views on Health Policy: A Fifty-Year Perspective. *Health Affairs* 20(2):33–46.

Brint, Steven. 1994. *In an Age of Experts: The Changing Role of Professionals in Politics and Public Life.* Princeton, NJ: Princeton University Press.

Brown, Lawrence D. 1991. Knowledge and Power: Health Services Research as a Political Resource. In *Health Services Research: Key to Health Policy,* ed. Eli Ginzberg. Cambridge: Harvard University Press.

Browne, William P. 1995. *Cultivating Congress: Constituents, Issues, and Interests in Agricultural Policy Making.* Lawrence: University of Kansas Press.

Campion, Frank D. 1984. *The AMA and U.S. Health Policy Since 1940.* Chicago: Chicago Review Press.

Dartmouth Medical School. 1996. *The Dartmouth Atlas of Health Care.* Chicago: American Hospital Publishing.

Dzur, Albert W. Forthcoming. Democratizing the Hospital: Deliberative Democratic Bioethics. *Journal of Health Politics, Policy and Law* 27(2).

Elliott, Philip. 1972. *The Sociology of the Professions.* London: Macmillan.

Feldstein, Paul J. 1977. *Health Associations and the Demand for Legislation: The Political Economy of Health.* Cambridge, MA: Ballinger.

Freidson, Eliot. 1970. *Profession of Medicine: A Study of the Sociology of Applied Knowledge.* New York: Dodd, Mead.

———. 1986. *Professional Powers: A Study of the Institutionalization of Formal Knowledge.* Chicago: University of Chicago Press.

Gutermuth, Karen. 1999. The American Medical Political Action Committee: Which Senators Get the Money and Why? *Journal of Health Politics, Policy and Law* 24(2):357–382.

Habermas, Jürgen. 1971. *Toward a Rational Society.* Boston: Beacon.

Hansen, John Mark. 1991. *Gaining Access: Congress and the Farm Lobby, 1919–1981.* Chicago: University of Chicago Press.

Hayes, Michael T. 1981. *Lobbyists & Legislators: A Theory of Political Markets.* New Brunswick, NJ: Rutgers University Press.

Heinz, John P., Edward O. Laumann, Robert L. Nelson, and Robert H. Salisbury. 1993. *The Hollow Core: Private Interests in National Policy Making.* Cambridge: Harvard University Press.

Hojnacki, Marie E. 1997. Interest Groups' Decisions to Join Alliances or Work Alone. *American Journal of Political Science* 41(1):61–87.

Hula, Kevin W. 1999. *Lobbying Together: Interest Group Coalitions in Legislative Politics.* Washington, DC: Georgetown University Press.

Immergut, Ellen M. 1992. *Health Politics: Interests and Institutions in Western Europe.* New York: Cambridge University Press.

Jacobs, Lawrence R. 1993. *The Health of Nations: Public Opinion and the Making of American and British Health Policy.* Ithaca, NY: Cornell University Press.

Johnson, Haynes, and David S. Broder. 1996. *The System: The American Way of Politics at the Breaking Point.* Boston: Little, Brown.

JHPPL. 1998. Special Issue. Managed Care: Ethics, Trust, and Accountability. *Journal of Health Politics, Policy and Law* 23(4).

JHPPL. 1999. Special Issue. The Managed Care Backlash. *Journal of Health Politics, Policy and Law* 24(5).

JHPPL. 2001. Special Issue. Evidence: Its Meaning in Health Care and in Law. *Journal of Health Politics, Policy and Law* 26(2).

Kollman, Ken. 1998. *Outside Lobbying: Public Opinion & Interest Group Strategies.* Princeton, NJ: Princeton University Press.

Krehbiel, Keith. 1991. *Information and Legislative Organization.* Ann Arbor, MI: University of Michigan Press.

Maioni, Antonia. 1995. Nothing Succeeds Like the Right Kind of Failure: Postwar National Health Insurance Initiatives in Canada and the United States. *Journal of Health Politics, Policy and Law* 20(1):5–30.

Marmor, Theodore R. 2000. *The Politics of Medicare.* 2d ed. New York: Aldine de Gruyter.

Marsteller, Jill A., Randall R. Bovbjerg, Len M. Nichols, and Dianna K. Verrilli. 1997. The Resurgence of Selective Contracting Restrictions. *Journal of Health Politics, Policy and Law* 22(5):1133–1189.

Millenson, Michael L. 1997a. "Miracle and Wonder": The AMA Embraces Quality Measurement. *Health Affairs* 16(3):183–194.

———. 1997b. *Demanding Medical Excellence: Physicians and Accountability in the Information Age.* Chicago: University of Chicago Press.

———. 1998. What Physicians Don't Know. *Washington Monthly,* December, 8–12.

Morone, James A. 1990. *The Democratic Wish: Popular Participation and the Limits of American Government.* New York: Basic Books.

Morone, James A., and Gary S. Belkin. 1995. The Science Illusion and the Triumph of Medical Capitalism. Paper presented at the American Political Science Association annual meeting, Chicago, 2 September.

New York Times. 2000. Democrats: In His Own Words: Gore to Delegates and Nation: "My Focus Will Be on Working Families." *New York Times*, 18 August. 21A.

Olson, Mancur. 1965. *The Logic of Collective Action.* Cambridge: Harvard University Press.

Peterson, Mark A. 1993. Political Influence in the 1990s: From Iron Triangles to Policy Networks. *Journal of Health Politics, Policy and Law* 18(2):395–438.

———.1995a. How Health Policy Information Is Used in Congress. In *Intensive Care: How Congress Shapes Health Policy*, ed. Thomas E. Mann and Norman J. Ornstein. Washington, DC: American Enterprise Institute and Brookings Institution.

———. 1995b. Interest Groups as Allies and Antagonists: Their Role in the Politics of Health Care Reform. Paper prepared for delivery at the annual meeting of the Association for Health Services Research and Foundation for Health Services Research, Chicago.

———. 1998a. The Limits of Social Learning: Translating Analysis into Action. In *Healthy Markets? The New Competition in Medicare Care*, ed. Mark A. Peterson. Durham, NC: Duke University Press.

———. ed. 1998b. *Healthy Markets? The New Competition in Medicare Care.* Durham, NC: Duke University Press.

———. 1998c. The Politics of Health Care Policy: Overreaching in an Age of Polarization. In *The Social Divide: Political Parties and the Future of Activist Government*, ed. Margaret Weir. New York: Russell Sage Foundation.

———. Unpublished. Stalemate: Opportunities, Gambles, and Miscalculations in Health Policy Innovation. Book manuscript.

Poen, Monte M. 1979. *Harry S. Truman versus the Medical Lobby.* Columbia: University of Missouri Press.

Rayak, Elton. 1967. *Professional Power and American Medicine: The Economics of the American Medical Association.* Cleveland: World Publishing.

Sabato, Larry J. 1984. *PAC Power: Inside the World of Political Action Committees.* New York: Norton.

Sharfstein, Joshua M., and Steven S. Sharfstein. 1994. Campaign Contributions from the American Medical Political Action Committee to Members of Congress — for or against the Public Health? *New England Journal of Medicine* 330(1):32–37.

Skocpol, Theda. 1996. *Boomerang: Clinton's Health Security Effort and the Turn Against Government in U.S. Politics.* New York: Norton.

Starr, Paul. 1982. *The Social Transformation of American Medicine.* New York: Basic Books.

Stigler, George J. 1971. The Theory of Economic Regulation. *Bell Journal of Economics* 2(1):3–21.

Stone, Deborah A. 1998. The Doctor as Businessman: The Changing Politics of a Cultural Icon. In *Healthy Markets? The New Competition in Medicare Care*, ed. Mark A. Peterson. Durham, NC: Duke University Press.

Tanenbaum, Sandra J. 1994. "Knowing and Acting in Medical Practice: The Epistemological Politics of Outcomes Research." *Journal of Health Politics, Policy and Law* 19(1):27–44.

Walker, Jack L. 1991. *Mobilizing Interest Groups in America: Patrons, Professions, and Social Movements.* Ann Arbor, MI: University of Michigan Press.

Weissert, Carol S., and William G. Weissert. 1996. *Governing Health: The Politics of Health Policy.* Baltimore, MD: Johns Hopkins University Press.

Wilkerson, John D., and David Carrell. 1999. Money, Politics, and Medicine: The American Medical PAC's Strategy of Giving in U.S. House Races. *Journal of Health Politics, Policy and Law* 24(2):335–355.

Wolinsky, Howard, and Tom Brune. 1994. *The Serpent on the Staff: The Unhealthy Politics of the American Medical Association.* New York: Putnam.

ARTICLE 2

HEALTH CARE AND HEALTH CARE POLICY IN A CHANGING WORLD

Donald A. Barr, Philip R. Lee, and A. E. Benjamin

> The organization of medicine is not a thing apart which can be subjected to study in isolation. It is an aspect of culture, whose arrangements are inseparable from the general organization of society.[1]
> — Walter H. Hamilton

Understanding the structure of a health care system first requires understanding the society in which that system exists. The health care system that has evolved in the United States reflects not only the impact of science and technology but also the politics, cultural values, and priorities that have deep historical roots. In other texts, we have described five characteristics of American society and policy that have had powerful influences on the evolution of the health care system, including the American character (e.g., individualism), federalism, pluralism, and incrementalism.[2,3] We will briefly describe each of these and will then offer a historical perspective of how they have shaped health care policies over time and how each of them has contributed to the problems our health care system now faces.

THE AMERICAN CHARACTER

The concept of autonomy and the ethical principle of respect for autonomy has been one of the fundamental building blocks of public policy since the founding of the nation. The policies that established the nation were built on the strongly held view that the right of individuals to their own beliefs and values should be protected by government and protected from the government. To this day the principles of individual choice, confidentiality, and privacy are strongly held. In 1990, the Patient Self Determination Act (P.L. 101–508) translated the concept of autonomy into public health policy concerning the individual's right to make decisions with respect to his or her own medical care, to refuse treatment, and to prepare advanced directives regarding care.

Along with the concept of autonomy has been a deeply held distrust of government. Although the distrust of government waxes and wanes, it is ever present and is reflected in the limited role of government in dealing with such issues as the financing of health care. Distrust of government was one of the factors that resulted in the lack of action by the United States Congress on the health care reforms proposed by President Clinton in 1993. In 1993, the President raised the issue of health care reform to the top of the domestic policy agenda, but the United States Congress ended more than a year of deliberation without taking any action. In this case, it was in part the concentrated interests of those who opposed reform (insurance industry, small business) that tapped the broad distrust of government to sap public support and generate opposition to the proposed reforms. The creation of three branches of government by the founding fathers reflected in part the distrust of government and the need to create the necessary checks and balances to prevent the abuse of power by any branch of government or by the majority of the populace.

Throughout the history of the country there have been shifts toward a strong federal role, originally advocated by Alexander Hamilton, and away from such a role. During the 20th century, periods of public action (1900s, 1930s, and 1960s) were preceded and followed by periods of private action (1890s, 1920s, 1950s, and 1980s).

FEDERALISM AND THE ROLE OF GOVERNMENT IN HEALTH CARE

Government at all levels plays an important role in planning, financing, organization, and delivering health services in the United States. At the federal level, Medicare is the dominant program for financing health care for the elderly. The Departments of Veterans Affairs, Defense, and Health and Human Services all maintain large, complex health care delivery systems to meet the needs of veterans, the military and their dependents, and American Indians and Alaska Natives.

The federal government, particularly through the U.S. Public Health Service, funds a range of categorical public health and medical care programs, largely through grants-in-aid to states and local governments.

At the state level, Medicaid has become the largest medical care program, financed with federal, state, and, in some cases, local government matching funds. The states have historically had the major role in public health programs in the financing and provision of care for the chronically mentally ill and in substance abuse prevention and treatment.

Local governments, particularly in urban areas, have often been major providers of medical care for the indigent, largely through public hospitals and clinics.

Much of the modern infrastructure for health care has been funded or subsidized with public funds during the past 50 years, including the construction of public and most voluntary hospitals, the training of most of the health professions, and the bulk of basic biomedical research. Currently, approximately 40% of all health care expenditures are provided by the federal, states, and local governments.

Although government's role in financing health care is a major one, this role is not the result of a consistent or comprehensive plan for the organization of health care services, but an episodic response to market failures (e.g., Medicare). Over time, as the private sector has been unable or unwilling to meet the health care needs of specific segments of the population, government has stepped in to fill the gap. Initially, the needs were met largely by local government and voluntary efforts. Later, states stepped in to meet the needs of the mentally ill. The federal government played a limited role, except for specific beneficiary groups such as veterans and specific public health problems (e.g., venereal disease, tuberculosis), until the enactment of Medicare and Medicaid in 1965. The Balanced Budget Act of 1997 includes some of the most significant changes ever made in the Medicare and Medicaid programs, providing states with greater flexibility in the administration of Medicaid and individuals greater choice of competing plans in Medicare. The result of this piecemeal approach to the development of health policy has been a proliferation of federal categorical programs administered by more than a dozen government departments and agencies (e.g., Department of Health and Human Services, Transportation, Agriculture, Energy, and the Environmental Protection Agency).

The role of government, particularly the federal government, has been at the heart of this debate about the future of health care in the United States since President Truman proposed a program of federally financed national health insurance in 1947.

This evolving role of government in the financing, organization, and delivery of health care reflects the role of federalism in the United States. The concept of federalism, and the concomitant role of the federal government in social policy, has evolved in the 200 years since the American Revolution and the drafting of the U.S. Constitution. After the failure of the Articles of Confederation, the drafters of the Constitution saw a need for a central government with clear but delineated authority in areas of common concern such as national defense and foreign policy. Functions such as education, police protection, and health care were left under state and local authority. The lines between federal and state authority were clearly drawn. It was not until after the Civil War, however, that state governments began to play a significant role in health care and public health policy.

This arrangement worked well so long as two conditions were met:

1. There was consistency between the levels of administrative authority and financial accountability.
2. The various levels of government involved had the appropriate resources and other capacities to carry out their responsibilities.

In health care, it is clear that these conditions have not been consistently maintained. The result often has been an increase in federal responsibility for health care, particularly in the financing of care. In some areas, such as Medicare, the shift to federal responsibility has included both administrative authority and financial accountability. In others, such as Medicaid and family planning, the disjunction between authority (i.e., federal) and accountability (i.e., states) has led to dysfunctional outcomes, including funding cutbacks, eligibility restrictions, low levels of payment to providers of care, and programmatic restrictions. The success of the federalist system depends on maintaining this balance between administrative authority and financial responsibility and between federal, state, and local responsibility.

There have been a number of reasons why state and local governments were not able to maintain their historical authority over social policy, not the least of which has been the lack of political will to extend government authority into new or controversial areas (e.g., civil rights). In parallel with the variation among states in the political will to assume responsibility for social needs have been variations in the ability of states to generate sufficient revenue through taxation and in the capacity to plan and administer complex programs. An important pattern has emerged as to how states respond to health programs that are initiated by the federal government for vulnerable populations but left to states to establish local eligibility and funding criteria: states will vary widely around a median level of benefits. Any federal attempt to guarantee a basic level of benefits using this decentralized approach will succeed for only a certain segment of the intended population.

One final consequence of the approach to health policy that decentralizes responsibility over health care programs has been the vulnerability of local governments and agencies to state funding cutbacks. These local entities are important providers of many health services, particularly hospital, outpatient, and emergency services for the poor; mental health and substance abuse services; and a variety of public health services. When local governments are mandated to provide these services (either by regulation or court order) but are not provided the supplemental resources to do so, both the quality of the local programs and the fiscal health of the local agency can be compromised. Although this does not usually occur during periods of sustained economic growth and low unemployment, quality of programs can vary strikingly from one community to another during economic downturns.

PLURALISM AND THE ROLE OF SPECIAL INTERESTS

In addition to establishing a central government with delineated authority, the founders of this country established a legislative and regulatory system based on pluralism in order to protect the individual from the power of government. Decision-making power in a pluralistic society is spread among many groups so that no one group gains excessive power. Over time, pluralism has become not only a mechanism for making decisions but also an ideology that shapes our perceptions of the proper role of government. In order for their voices to be heard, individuals have increasingly organized into groups with interests as broad as the political parties and as narrow as single issues (e.g., abortion). These groups not only are allowed to influence the legislation process, they are encouraged to do so. During the first half of this century, the groups that dominated the health policy process were characterized as an iron triangle, including legislative committees, executive branch agencies, and private interest groups (e.g., the American Medical Association [AMA]). More recently, the process has become more complex and the iron triangles replaced by policy networks. Peterson has observed that the health policy community today "is heterogeneous and loosely structured, creating a network whose broad boundaries are defined by shared attentiveness of participants to the same issues in the policy domain."[4]

The influence of special interests as a manifestation of our pluralistic system is clearly seen throughout the health policy process. In this century, the American Medical Association has exerted a powerful influence on health policy, although its influence has diminished significantly since the enactment of Medicare. Other influential interests have been the hospitals, the insurance industry, and the pharmaceutical companies. Although groups representing patients (e.g., American Association of Retired Persons, organized labor) have exerted influence over specific programs, it has been these four general groups that have tended to shape health policy in the period after World War II. More recently, business interest groups (e.g., Business Group on Health) have begun to be more influential.

Since the late 1960s, as the cost of health care has become a predominant issue, power over health policy has shifted from the providers to the purchasers (e.g., large employers). Regardless of this realignment of power among interest groups, the power of special interests over the process of establishing and implementing health policy has remained intact. The effectiveness of many of these interest groups (e.g., small businesses, insurance) was very evident in President Clinton's ill-fated attempt at health care reform. It is extremely difficult to achieve broad consensus or to implement broad health policy — or even to convince Congress to make minor changes in policy — in the face of the power of special interests. This inhibition inherent in the pluralistic system in the United States has shaped and continues to shape the health policy process.

INCREMENTALISM AS THE PRINCIPAL MEANS OF HEALTH POLICY REFORM

Kingdon[5] and more recently Longest[6] have provided a model for understanding how policy decisions are made. In Longest's model, the process includes policy formulation and policy implementation phases, with both influenced by a policy modification phase. It is very clear that although President Clinton played the key role in placing national health insurance on the policy agenda in 1993, he did not control the process after that. When a policy issue rises to the top of the agenda, two other factors must then be present for successful reform to take place: a policy solution that is broadly seen as successfully addressing the issue, and political circumstances that allow for reform to take place. When all three (agenda, solution, political circumstances) are present simultaneously, a "window of opportunity" exists for significant policy reform. If any one of the three is absent, the potential for significant reform is diminished substantially. A number of analysts have suggested that such a window for major health care reform existed in the early Clinton years, but his policy solution proved unacceptable to a majority in Congress and later the success of the "Republican Revolution" in 1994 fundamentally altered the political circumstances, thus removing one of the factors and dooming any efforts at major health care reform.

Once a policy has been enacted, a second process of implementation takes place, usually involving the executive branch agency responsible for establishing the necessary guidelines and regulations. In the case of Medicare, this is the Health Care Financing Administration (HCFA), Department of Health and Human Services (HHS). The HCFA also has a major role in approving state Medicaid regulations. For many categorical public health programs, although the authority is ultimately vested in the Secretary of HHS, the implementation is provided by the agencies (e.g., National Institutes of Health, Food and Drug Administration, Centers for Disease Control and Prevention). In addition to having the potential to influence all phases of the policy formulating phase, special interest groups can also play an important role in guiding policy implementation. Through ongoing relationships with the implementing agencies, they are able to influence the rules by which policy programs will operate. The AMA, for example, works closely with HCFA to influence Medicare regulations.

A third phase of the policy process as it affects health care — policy modification — has also been described by Longest.[6] Part of the responsibility of the legislative process is in oversight of the implementation of programs in achieving their intended goals. Oversight will become increasingly important in the future in view of the strict limits set on discretionary spending and in Medicare and Medicaid spending during the next five years. Although oversight has always been important in ensuring implementation, it is now being pursued vigorously because the Congress is in Republican hands and the Executive branch is controlled by the Democrats.

When policies either do not have clear goals by which to measure them or have not been successful in attaining their stated goals, they often enter back into the legislative process for further modification. From this perspective, the policy process becomes cyclical: policy formation leads to implementation, which leads to modification, which feeds back into the formation phase. In fact, many key health policies have been modifications to previously existing policies. For example, Medicare and Medicaid were amendments to the Social Security Act and were actually extensions of earlier programs (the Old Age, Survivors' and Disability Insurance program and the Kerr-Mills program to provide medical care for the elderly poor). Medicare, in turn, was shaped by major amendments affecting hospital payments (1983) and physician payments (1989), largely because of the rising costs of health care. The Balanced Budget Act of 1997 represented yet another major shift in Medicare policy, following years of oversight hearings.

The complexity of the policy-setting process, the susceptibility of policy implementation to outside influence, and the cyclical nature of policy modification all have led to a phenomenon that is characteristic of the United States government: the incremental approach to decision-making. Whether for health care or any other social issue, policy is usually made in this country in small steps (increments). An exception was welfare reform, which did call for sweeping changes. One of the reasons for the failure of Clinton's health care reform plan was that it did not propose an incremental approach to change.

Incrementalism has come to be understood by most of the players as the way things are to be done. There is a general hesitance to take anything but a small bite out of a major policy issue, both because of a general comfort with the status quo and because of the risk of unforeseen and unintended consequences of major policy modifications. It appears that only at times of crisis, when there is broad consensus that the need for major action overshadows the risk of unintended outcomes, is our governmental system able to adopt major policy reform. (It should be pointed out that the failed Clinton health care reforms were followed by incremental health insurance reform in the Kennedy-Kassebaum bill and the incremental expansion of health insurance coverage to a portion of uninsured children.)

HISTORICAL DEVELOPMENT OF AMERICAN HEALTH POLICY

Throughout most of the nation's history, the federal government played a minor role in health policy; most of the policy interventions in public health were at the state and local levels, and most of medical care was left to the private sector. At times of crisis, such as the Civil War, the Great Depression, or, more recently, the Civil Rights Movement, quantum shifts in authority from the state level to the federal level or from the private sector to the public sector take place.

In a series of earlier books,[1,2,7] we have reviewed the historical development of health policy in the United States. Others, including Rosemary Stevens[8,9] and Paul Starr,[10] have dealt with the sweeping changes in Medicare and medical care, and Mullen[11] has provided a history of the U.S. Public Health Service.

We have described four distinct periods in the evolution of health policy:

1. A limited role for the federal government (1798–1862)
2. The emergence of a larger federal role (1862–1932)
3. The expansion of the federal role (1935–1969)
4. New federalism (1969–present)

In the early years of the republic, the Elizabethan poor laws of England were the foundation of most policies for the poor, the aged, and the infirm. In 1798, Congress passed the Act for the Relief of Sick and Disabled Seamen, imposing a twenty cent per month tax on seamen's wages to pay for their medical care. This legislation represented the first step in establishing the U.S. Public Health Service.[11]

After the Civil War, the development of the germ theory of disease by Pasteur was the most powerful force affecting both public health and medical care. In public health, progress was more rapid than in medical care, with policies related to environmental sanitation, clean water, the pasteurization of milk, and expanded programs of quarantine grounded largely in the police power of state and local governments. The first federal law directly related to public health broadly was the Biologies Control Act of 1902 (P.L. 57–244), followed by the Pure Food and Drug Act (P.L. 59–384) in 1906.

In addition to the gradual increase in federal authority during this period, significant shifts were taking place in the private sector's role in health care.

During the latter half of the 19th century, there was a rapid growth in the number and in the role of hospitals. During this period, there was also the establishment of proprietary medical schools (replacing apprenticeship training) and the development of state and local public health agencies. The fragmentation of the hospitals' governance and management began with the growing number of voluntary, nonprofit, often religious hospitals in addition to local public hospitals and the proliferation of proprietary hospitals, usually owned by physicians. As medicine began to be rooted in science, and physicians gained more respect, physicians began to replace the hospital trustees in determining who was and who was not admitted to the hospital.

Late in the 19th century and early in the 20th century, hospitals gradually shifted from places for the poor to come to die to centers of medical, but particularly surgical, care for the general public. Two general types of hospitals emerged: public hospitals financed largely at the local level, and private, community-based, nonprofit hospitals, many of them operated by religious institutions. Both the proprietary, hospital-based medical schools and physician-owned proprietary hospitals gradually disappeared in the early decades of the 20th century, largely due to the efforts of the American Medical Association, stimulated by the Flexner Report in 1910.[12]

It was also during this time that state governments, at the urging of state medical societies, became involved in licensing practitioners and supporting medical education. Thus, while government was becoming increasingly involved in guiding health policy during this period, most of this activity was at the state and local rather than the federal level, and the public role in health policy was still quite limited compared with that of the private sector.

Substitution of Public Services and Financing for Private Efforts (1935–1969)

The crisis presented by the Great Depression brought action by the federal government in areas that previously had been left to state and local control. From banking regulation to support for small businesses, from public employment to old age security, there was a broadly held perception that the federal government should do what state governments had been unable or unwilling to do to respond to the crisis. Over the span of a few years, the role of the federal government vis-à-vis the states changed fundamentally. American federalism evolved from a pattern of limited federal responsibility for domestic policy to a cooperative relationship between federal and state governments with a strong, often leading role for the federal government.

This new relationship is seen nowhere more clearly than in the Social Security Act. Included within the Act was the new principle of federal aid to the states for public health and welfare assistance, including grants for maternal and child health and crippled children's services (Title V) and for general public health programs (Title VI). The Old Age, Survivors' and Disability Insurance (OASDI) program included in the original Act provided the philosophical and fiscal basis for the Medicare program enacted 30 years later.

During this period of transformation, the National Cancer Institute was established (1938); the authority of the Food and Drug Administration (FDA) was greatly strengthened, requiring approval of drugs for safety before marketing (1938); and the Nurse Training Act was passed (1941), providing schools of nursing with direct federal aid to permit them to increase their enrollments and improve their physical facilities.

After World War II, there was a growing federal role in the support of medical research, mental health research and treatment programs, and the construction of community hospitals (Burton-Hill Act of 1946). The establishment of the Department of Health, Education, and Welfare in 1953 (now the Department of Health and Human Services), including the U.S. Public Health Service, the then separate FDA, and the Social Security Administration, firmly established the federal government's role in the nation's health care system. This new role was not, however, the result of any comprehensive or coordinated plan to develop a national health care policy. Rather, it was the amalgamation of a variety of incremental steps taken for a variety of reasons at a variety of times.

In the 1960s, there was further expansion of this new federal role in health policy. Through the "creative federalism" followed by the Kennedy and Johnson Administrations, the federal government became increasingly involved in a number of areas, including environmental health (e.g., air pollution control), community mental health centers, neighborhood health centers, health professions training, family planning, and other efforts to improve health care delivery to underserved communities. Many of these programs were financed through direct federal support for local governments and local nonprofit agencies. One of the most important laws enacted in the 1960s was the Civil Rights Act of 1964, later used as the means to desegregate the hospitals in the south. A further extension of the federal government's direct regulatory authority came with the 1962 amendments to the Food, Drug, and Cosmetics Act, which specified that manufacturers must demonstrate that a drug is both safe and effective before marketing it. Congress, between 1965 and 1967, enacted more new health legislation than all the previous congresses in the nation's 175 years.

The most dramatic expansion of federal authority in health policy was through the Social Security Amendments of 1965, establishing the Medicare and Medicaid programs to finance health care for all people older than 65 and all people receiving cash welfare assistance. These policies marked one of the first times that major health care programs were enacted over the objection of the American Medical Association, fundamentally altering the power relationship between physicians and the federal government. Never again was the medical profession able to exercise veto authority over federal health policy.

These programs of the Kennedy and Johnson years had a profound effect on intergovernmental relationships and on federal expenditures for domestic social programs. The combination of direct federal payments for Medicare and Medicaid and federal grants-in-aid helped lead to a ballooning of the federal budget, which, in the face of the strain on the domestic economy caused by the Vietnam War, created a new crisis and a dramatic shift in the role of the federal government.

The trend away from community involvement in health care was temporarily reversed with an effort in the Great Society era to base health care for vulnerable, underserved populations in community-controlled programs (e.g., neighborhood health centers, community mental health centers). Other efforts to strengthen the communities' role in the 1970s include health planning and the beginning of the "health cities" movement. Market forces, which began to play an increasingly important role in health care in the 1970s and 1980s, can have either a positive or negative impact on the role of the community, but their initial impact has been to shift control away from communities.

Entering the Era of Limited Resources: The "New Federalism" (1969–1997)

First coined by President Nixon, the term *New Federalism* described a movement to reverse the swing of government power to the federal government, transferring authority over policy and programs to the states. The Nixon and Ford administrations favored block grants to the states for the support of local policy initiatives, with relatively little federal oversight. Congress resisted this move, favoring instead the continued use of categorical grants requiring detailed provisions regulating the type and level of services to be provided.

While Congress and the President argued over the issue of block versus categorical grants in the 1970s, the federal government confronted the problem of skyrocketing health care costs, largely a result of the Medicare and Medicaid programs. Federal and state governments had become third parties that underwrote the costs of a fee-for-service-based health care system that included few if any mechanisms to constrain costs. Coupled with a growing physician work force and increasing specialization, the explosion of new technology catalyzed by the enactment of the Medicare and Medicaid systems and the rapid expansion of biomedical research funded by the National Institutes of Health helped lead to a rapid upward spiral in health care costs and thus in federal expenditures.

The federal response to rapidly rising health care expenditures assumed a variety of forms, ranging from the elimination of federal subsidies for hospital construction and health professions education to price controls for a limited period and more permanent limits on hospital and physician payments by Medicare.

Additionally, in a step that was to have profound effects on the direction later market-based reforms would take, the federal government stimulated the development and expansion of health maintenance organizations (HMOs) through the Health Maintenance Organization Act of 1972. Historically an anathema to most physicians and especially to the American Medical Association, HMOs had grown very slowly.

The movement away from federal responsibility for domestic social policy accelerated when Ronald Reagan was elected President in 1980. The most prominent changes enacted by the Reagan administration that directly affected health care included (1) a sharp reduction in federal expenditures for social programs, including elimination of the revenue-sharing program initiated by President Nixon; (2) decentralization of regulatory and programmatic authority to the states, particularly through the use or block grants that came with few strings attached; (3) an increasing reliance on market forces and private institutions to stimulate needed reforms and control rising costs; and (4) through across-the-board federal tax reductions, a substantial decline in the ability of the federal government to fund new health programs. Contrary to the "deregulatory" philosophy of the administration, it established the means to regulate hospital costs, using prospective payment through the diagnosis-related group (DRG) system as an alternative to Medicare's cost-based reimbursement for hospital costs.

No longer was the federal government to be the unquestioning payer for health services. No longer did the federal government have the capacity, even if the political will were present, to fund new health care programs. The rising budget deficit, not health care, became foremost on the national agenda. The Bush Administration followed in 1989 with its support for a congressionally initiated Medicare fee schedule, to be set by the government, to control Medicare payments to physicians specified in the Omnibus Budget Reconciliation Act of 1989 (P.L. 101–239).

At the state level, increasing policy authority brought with it increasing financial burdens. As states became more responsible for establishing and implementing their own programs, they also became increasingly responsible for the costs of those programs. In the area of health care, the spiral of rising costs of Medicaid continued largely unabated, leading to increasing strain on state budgets. Once again a situation was created in which there was a mismatch between authority over a policy program and the capacity to finance that program.

A number of states turned to the private market and to market-based competition as a means of holding down costs, both the costs of publicly financed programs and the costs of health care overall. An initial change that was to have profound effects on our system of health care was an increasing reliance on for-profit corporations to operate within the health care system. Traditionally functioning as nonprofit, community-based institutions, many hospitals were taken over by for-profit chains financed through the sale of stock. A number of organizations involved in the direct provision of care, such as home health agencies and kidney dialysis centers, shifted from community control or nonprofit status to a for-profit basis. The requirement that HMOs operate on a nonprofit basis, included in the original HMO Act, was removed, opening the market to for-profit companies to become directly involved in the financing and provision of care. A number of states chose to rely on private HMOs to provide care to Medicaid beneficiaries, leaving it to the HMO to determine what constitutes "medically necessary" care.

The continued increase in health care costs seen in the late 1980s coupled with the growing role of private markets in providing access to health care services led to a new awareness of what is really an old problem: the rising number of uninsured individuals and families. Currently as many as 44 million Americans have no insurance to pay for needed health care. The number of uninsured is increasing about 1 million per year despite the growing economy with its low levels of unemployment.

The dilemma that confronted the Clinton Administration when it took office in 1992 was that Americans want to have their health care cake and eat it too. They want health care made more available to the uninsured, and they want the cost of health care to come under control, but only if these actions don't diminish the ability of the average American to get whatever treatment he or she perceives to be necessary or appropriate in a timely manner. This perhaps is the fundamental American health policy dilemma. President Clinton and the Congress in 1993 faced conflicting needs and expectations with neither a mechanism to establish a broad-based consensus on how to reconcile them nor a mechanism to enact that consensus if it was achieved. President Clinton had campaigned on the need for the federal government to reassert itself in the area of health policy. With the broad goals of expanding coverage to the uninsured while simultaneously controlling health care costs, the Clinton health reform plan would have given broad new authority to the federal government to regulate the market for health insurance, while maintaining a reliance on market-based competition. It sought a new balance between the market-based delivery of care and a broad umbrella of federal oversight. The idea was an attempt to redefine the role of federalism in health policy, but it was seriously out of synch with the continued movement in the evolution of federal authority. As pointed out by Theda Skocpol,[13] the ebbing tide of federal authority over social policy had not yet run its course. With an irony that has not yet been fully appreciated, the country was ready for one part of the Clinton proposal but not the other. Although Congress rejected an increased role for the federal government in regulating the market for health insurance, the deliberations surrounding the Clinton proposal nevertheless opened the door even more widely for market-based competition among health plans to become the principal paradigm for American health care at the end of the 20th century. Although it is happening in some areas of the country more rapidly than others, there has been a clear shift to the evolving concept of managed care for the financing, provision, and oversight of health care to most Americans. The shift comes, however, without any organized system of oversight or regulation and with an increasing role for for-profit companies. As a reaction, many states are now proposing a variety of "consumer protective" laws (more than 400 bills introduced in state legislatures in 1997) to begin to place some limits on private sector managed care plans, and the President has proposed a "Consumer Bill of Rights." At the same time, states are increasingly mandating the enrollment of Medicaid beneficiaries (e.g., mothers and children) in managed care plans, and Medicare is poised to significantly expand the role of managed care plans.

Reductions in care, financial incentives that pit physicians' needs against those of patients, and a disavowal of responsibility for caring for the uninsured all are characteristics of this new American system of health care. In the words of one of the more vigorous advocates of for-profit health care plans,

> Investor-owned health plans are a driving force behind this transformation [of the health care delivery system in America], and nonprofit health plans, in my view, are a byproduct of the past . . . There is an appropriate role for nonprofit plans, but it is not in the operation of competitive health plans.[14]

Was this the health care system that the American public intended to have? Did the United States get here as a result of a well-thought-out policy deliberation? As with much of the history of American health policy, the answer to both questions is "no." Once again the separation of the authority over health policy and the financial responsibility for it has led to an outcome that was unintended and, as many believe, is not in the best interest of the American people.

While the private sector was moving rapidly, without adequate federal or state ground rules to "level the playing field," there was paralysis of health policy making at the federal level after the failure of President Clinton's health care reform proposals in 1993–1994. The situation only grew worse after the Republicans captured both the Senate and the House of Representatives in 1994. What followed was 2 years of ideological debate with a standoff between the President and the Congress. After President Clinton's reelection in 1996 and the continued control of Congress by the Republicans, the Congress and the Clinton Administration began to work together to produce potentially constructive changes in the Medicare program. The result was the Balanced Budget Act of 1997, signed by President Clinton in August 1997.

The basic Medicare provisions, including a 5-year spending reduction of $115 billion below Congressional Budget Office (CBO) projections based on existing policies, were

- Coordinated care plans, including HMOs, preferred provider organizations (PPOs), plans offered by provider sponsored organizations (PSOs), and point-of-service plans (POSs)
- Private fee-for-service
- On a demonstration basis, high deductible plans with medical savings account

The Balanced Budget Act of 1997 reflected a political consensus that had arisen from the ashes of the rancorous stalemate of 1995–1996 that followed the Republican capture of the Congress. The Medicare reform process reversed almost every aspect of the failed partisan debates of the previous 2 years. The Medicare reform process in 1997 was similar to the successful Medicare hospital and physician payment reform of 1983 and 1989 and the expansion of Medicaid eligibility for children in poverty in the early 1990s.

The direction for health care in the 21st century, at least in its early years, may well have been set by the Balanced Budget Act of 1997, just as it was set in the past 30 years by the Social Security Amendment of 1965, which established Medicare and Medicaid as public programs that bought into and reinforced the then dominant fee-for-service system. Times have changed and health care will change as well.

REFERENCES

1. Hamilton, W. H. *Medical care for the American people: The final report of the Committee on the Cost of Medical Care.* Adopted October 31, 1932. Chicago: University of Chicago Press, 1932.

2. Lee, P. R., and Benjamin, A. E. Health policy and the politics of health care. In S. J. Williams and P. R. Torrens (eds). *Introduction to health services.* 4th ed. Albany: Delmar Publishers, 1993.

3. Lee, P. R., Benjamin, A. E., and Weber, M. A. Policies and strategies for health care in the United States. In *Oxford Textbook of Public Health.* 3rd ed. Oxford: Oxford University Press, 1996.

4. Peterson, M. A. Political influence in the 1990s: From iron triangle to policy network. *Journal of Health Politics, Policy and Law.* Summer, 1993;18:395–438.

5. Kingdon, J. W. *Agendas, alternatives, and public policies.* Boston: Little, Brown, 1993.

6. Longest, B. *Health policymaking in the United States.* Ann Arbor, MI: Health Administration Press, 1994.

7. Lee, P. R., and Silver, G. A. Health planning — A view from the top with specific reference to the U.S.A. In J. Fry and W. A. J. Farndale (eds). *International medical care.* Oxford: MTP Medical and Technical Publishing, 1972.

8. Stevens, R. *American medicine and the public interest.* New York: Basic Books, 1971.

9. Stevens, R. *In sickness and in wealth: American hospitals in the twentieth century.* New York: Basic Books, 1989.

10. Starr, P. *Social transformation of American medicine: The rise of the sovereign profession and the making of a vast industry.* New York: Basic Books, 1982.

11. Mullen, F. *Plague and politics.* New York: Basic Books, 1989.

12. Flexner, A. *Medical education in the United States and Canada.* New York: Carnegie Foundation for the Advancement of Teaching, 1910.

13. Skocpol, T. *Boomerang: Clinton's health security effort and the turn against government in U.S. politics.* New York: W. W. Norton, 1996.

14. Hassan, M. Let's end the nonprofit charade. *New England Journal of Medicine.* 1996;334:1055–1057.

ARTICLE 3

THE POLITICS OF LONG-TERM CARE REFORM UNDER THE CLINTON HEALTH PLAN

LESSONS FOR THE FUTURE

Carroll L. Estes, Joshua M. Wiener, Sheryl C. Goldberg, and Susan M. Goldenson

During 1993 and 1994, the United States debated but did not enact major health care reform. Although the primary focus of reform proposals was on providing health coverage for the uninsured and controlling acute care costs, many proposals included long-term care. President Clinton proposed a long-term care plan comprised of four key elements: 1) a large new home care program for the severely disabled of all ages and all income groups, to be administered with a lot of flexibility by the states, 2) a slight liberalization of the financial eligibility rules for the Medicaid nursing home benefit, 3) favorable tax clarification and tougher regulation of private long-term care insurance, and 4) tax credits for the long-term care expenses of the nonelderly disabled workers in order to permit the younger disabled to work without loss of coverage. Significantly, the President's plan was a major departure from the current Medicaid-dominated financing system for long-term care in that it was not based on low income eligibility (i.e., means-tested), yet it was designed as a public program to be offered by the states. As proposed, the Clinton long-term care plan was not an individual entitlement, but rather was described as an *entitlement to the states* to offer the program, and it was one that was "capped" in terms of federal funding.

While a lot has been written on what happened to health reform involving acute care during the early days of President Clinton's first term, the long-term care component of the debate has been largely ignored (Johnson and Broder, 1996; Skocpol,

This chapter is adapted and excerpted from Joshua M. Wiener, Carroll L. Estes, Susan M. Goldenson, and Sheryl C. Goldberg, *What Happened to Long Term Care in the Health Reform Debate of 1993–1994? Lessons for the Future.* Urban Institute, Washington D.C. and Institute for Health & Aging, University of California, San Francisco, 1999. Funded by the AARP/Andrus Foundation and The Commonwealth Fund. The authors acknowledge the assistance of reviewers at the Commonwealth Fund and AARP. The authors assume full responsibility for the interpretation of the data.

1997; Aaron, 1996). The aim of this chapter is to describe some of the lessons learned from the long-term care component of the Clinton health reform debate.

Long-term care was on the health policy agenda in 1993 and 1994 largely as a result of efforts of advocates for older people and the younger disabled and as part of the political calculus of the Clinton Administration to increase both the popularity and likely passage of the overall health reform package. The inclusion of long-term care in the larger health reform effort also was plausible because of the extremely comprehensive nature of the Clinton reform initiative and the personal backgrounds and experiences of President Clinton as a former state governor and those of his major health advisors.

As the Clinton Administration prepared its proposal, the high costs of a major long-term care initiative threatened, but in the end, did not thwart its inclusion. The long-term care plan contained a new home care proposal that represented a notable break from previous plans since it relied heavily on the states for the *design* as well as the administration of the program, it included younger people as well as older people with disabilities, and it allowed coverage of an extremely broad range rather than a limited number of specific services. Indeed, while designers started with a traditional notion of social insurance, the commitment to a very wide array of services within budget limits eventually forced the elimination of the concepts of a defined benefit and an individual entitlement. The long-term care proposal was transformed from one linked to traditional notions of social insurance, to one linked to social insurance only by the nonmeans-tested eligibility criteria.

Politically, while the long-term care plan was generally supported by consumer advocacy groups, it did not generate the groundswell of enthusiasm for which the Clinton Administration had hoped. Support for health reform from the largest aging organization, the American Association of Retired Persons (AARP), was focused on many elements of the plan and the education of its membership in preparation for what it hoped would develop into a bipartisan proposal that the organization could fully endorse. AARP's strategy was interpreted by the media and politicians as granting only "tepid" support for both the President's larger health reform and the long-term care reform. Nevertheless, as health reform worked its way through Congress and efforts were made to reduce the costs of the package, long-term care succeeded in remaining a significant component of most of the Democratic plans, although generally on a smaller scale.

THEMES AND LESSONS FOR THE FUTURE

Participants in the long-term care reform process were generally cautious in drawing lessons from the experience of 1993–1994 for future long-term care reform. According to a member of the Executive Branch, "long-term care was never seriously discussed. It was there, but it never was real." Others, however, contended that long-term care (LTC) was the most positive part of the Clinton reform package, as shown below.

Nonetheless, there are at least seven major themes, lessons, or cautionary tales that can inform future action.

First, long-term care reform is a popular idea and did not cause the demise of health reform. In fact, long-term care was often described as one of the initiatives (although relatively neglected) that helped sustain commitment to health reform, although not a lot. One elderly advocacy organization representative contended that, "the fact that we got long-term care into the final package helped to obtain support for the final package." Among long-term care activists, there was a consistent belief that "there was always more public support for long-term care than for larger health reform." The fact that a public program for long-term care would not displace existing private sector insurance gave it a certain advantage over acute care.

Second, being part of a very large, comprehensive proposal for health reform does not necessarily aid long-term care reform. Although long-term care reform "tried to get on the big train," it got lost in the shuffle of the larger health care reform effort. Virtually all of the interest group representatives, including elderly and disability advocates, agreed that "long-term care went down with the larger ship" and the "battle was not won or lost on long-term care." One elderly advocate put it this way, "You have to be careful what you hitch your wagon to. The big broad health reform approach is unlikely to happen." The lesson learned may be that the reform of long-term care needs to go its own way and not be part of health, Medicare, or Social Security reform.

Third, although inclusion of long-term care in the reform package had a clear political goal of increasing public enthusiasm for health reform, several key decisions in the design of the long-term care program and the inclusion of substantial Medicare cuts were thought to undercut its political support, although there was little unanimity on these points. The states were concerned about their potential financial liability in long-term care and did not receive fiscal relief for state nursing home care costs under Medicaid in the Clinton proposal. States were afraid of being "left holding the bag" for what some described as an "under-financed state level program that easily could be misunderstood as an individual entitlement." For elderly advocacy organizations, key problems were "the lack of a defined benefit and entitlement" for individuals, which made it difficult to explain to the public "what people were going to get." Also, support both for the president's long term care plan and larger health reform was diluted by the fact that there were substantial Medicare cuts on the table at the same time. According to the Clinton Administration, these cuts were needed to generate funds to pay for the proposed reforms for the elderly. Similarly, the proposed Medicare cuts in home health splintered the industry, leading some home care groups to actually oppose the president's Health Security Act.

Fourth, health reform generally, including long-term care, neglected certain political prerequisites. The expectation that major reform could be passed without significant bipartisan support in Congress was not realistic. An elderly advocate recounts that, "really we did not work with the Republicans at all; the sense was that we could do it without them. Hindsight is 20-20; it wasn't a very good idea." Further, for long-term care, there is the need for a spokesperson for whom this is *the* issue: "When our strongest Congressional advocate, Representative Claude Pepper, died we lost the voice. For years, we tried to find someone with the voice and commitment, but we never identified a true successor." In addition, stronger public education is needed to present the problem and policy solutions.

> We have to make people understand better the shortcomings of the current system. Ultimately, in the case of health insurance, most of us are covered. *In the case of long-term care, almost nobody is covered and they do not know it.* If we could get that point across, broaden the constituency, and sharpen the problem, long-term care would be much higher on the political agenda.

Fifth, long-term care policy is largely about money, i.e., how much are we willing to spend? While long-term care was in many ways politically popular, it was also expensive and added substantially to the costs of health reform, which some felt helped to drag down support for the reform package. Many participants in the process observed that the long-term care needs are so great and the current system so inadequate that to do any significant reform requires spending billions of dollars. They pointed out that the first Clinton plan, which would only have covered home care for persons with severe disabilities, was projected to cost an additional $36 billion a year when fully implemented (Office of the Assistant Secretary for Planning and Evaluation, DHHS, 1994).

Sixth, a major outcome of the failed health reform effort in 1994 is the begrudging acceptance of incremental rather than comprehensive change as the most feasible (if not the only) way to achieve policy reform in health and long-term care. The recent trend towards incremental health care reforms has generated significant debate within the long-term care policy community. Advocates of long-term care reform note ruefully the difficulty, if not the impossibility, of achieving success with any reforms that are seen as "big governmental programs." A Congressional staffer states bluntly, "We learned that a comprehensive proposal will not fly. You need to introduce incremental pieces to get anything accomplished." Another state official observes:

> We should never do such a big plan again. We should deal with health reform incrementally. You cannot fundamentally change 14 percent of the U.S. economy with a single piece of legislation . . . As a social movement emerges, there is piling on — with everyone trying to deal with everything at once. The problem is — especially if you are Democrats — that you have so many constituencies who feel they need their piece of the pie to be dealt with. They think there is only one shot to get at something. You always live for another day. I strongly believe in incremental policy development.

The pervasive effect of this new incremental thinking has reached far and wide. Even the Long-Term Care Campaign, an intergenerational coalition of more than 100 organizations initially founded in 1988 to promote universal entitlement to social insurance for long-term care, has altered its approach to policy. A decade later (1998), the LTC Campaign endorsed something far short of its initial goals, as reflected in its

Policy Blueprint (LTC Campaign, 1998). No longer promoting "a social insurance program like Social Security or Medicare, paid for by all ages" or using such explicit words as calling for "a comprehensive national solution" (LTC Campaign, 1994), the LTC Campaign now reaches for "appropriate, affordable solutions."

Five years after the defeat of health and long-term care reform, President Clinton raised the political profile on long-term care by proposing a modest set of initiatives including a $1,000 tax credit for severely disabled individuals and their caregivers, unsubsidized private long-term care insurance to federal employees, limited funds for respite care, and an educational program for older people about the limits of Medicare and Medicaid long-term care coverage. These proposals sparked legislation to provide additional tax incentives for the purchase of private long-term care insurance, which were included in the 1999 tax bill passed by Congress and vetoed by President Clinton.[1]

Paradoxically, even the advocates of small scale improvements acknowledge the difficulty of doing anything meaningful incrementally in long-term care. One aging advocate notes, "long-term care is such a big issue in terms of what you have to deal with. In an era when incrementalism is how people think about health policy, it is hard to think what to do in long-term care without spending some big dollars." Even President Clinton's 1999 proposed tax credit for long-term care, as limited as it was, would have cost $1 billion a year in lost revenue, not a trivial amount even in Washington, D.C. Nevertheless, others, such as writer Robert Kuttner in *The Washington Post*, vehemently reject such incremental proposals as inadequate and cling to the hope of comprehensive reform (Kuttner, 1999). An Executive branch official scornfully confesses that "the incremental approaches in health reform of the last five years haven't gotten us much. The President's proposal for a tax credit for caregivers is less than one-half of a drop in the bucket."

The initiatives proposed by President Clinton and the Congress subsequent to the failed comprehensive health reform of 1994 illustrate the lesson that most participants enunciated: They are incremental in character and they use tax incentives rather than direct spending. For example, the President's 1999 long-term care plan would have cost a little more than $1 billion a year, a mere shadow of the $36 billion a year price tag that was envisioned in the 1993–1994 proposal. Demonstrating the case of dramatically reduced expectations, most elderly and disability groups supported the President's 1999 proposal, even though in the past they would have dismissed it as hopelessly inadequate. The advocacy groups' self-described explanation for currently supporting such small steps in long-term care policy is that the President's tax credit proposal "puts something on the agenda."

Seventh, there has been a profound shift in the framing of the options that is consistent with the recent acceptance of the "small steps, incremental approach." Traditional

1. The Republican tax bill would have allowed an "above the line" deduction for individual spending for private long-term care insurance, making its costs completely tax deductible within limits. However, note that even President Clinton's proposal would serve to promote private long-term care insurance.

"social insurance" for long-term care in the mold of Medicare and Social Security is no longer actively debated as it was in the late 1980s. This is a result of at least two factors: a more conservative Congress, and the unintentional "deconstruction" of the concept of social insurance through the design process of the long-term care component of the Clinton health plan, which replaced social insurance with a capped entitlement to the states for long term care. Under the Clinton plan, it was the states and not individuals that were to become entitled to having long term care programs.

Eighth, as incrementalism dominates current efforts to promote policy change in long term care and there is a dearth of major federal initiatives, there also has been the time and space for private sector interests and initiatives to develop. Members of the long-term care workgroup, advocates, provider groups, and Congressional members and staff concur that there are now increased interests working toward meeting long-term care needs through private insurance and other market mechanisms. One states that "private long-term care insurance has become the primary policy where most of the work has been done."

Two additional lessons are that: 1) the President's long-term care proposal may have actually lost support because it was not a real social insurance program, which diluted the investment in it by the elderly and, perhaps, even by the states; and 2) the fact that there was no proposed dedicated revenue source for the long term care provisions made it hard to give assurances of needed federal funding for the program proposed.

PROSPECTS FOR LONG-TERM CARE REFORM

So what are the prospects for long-term care reform in the near term and in the more distant future? For the more distant future, few observers doubt that when the baby boom generation needs long-term care, it will be a major domestic policy issue. If nursing home utilization rates remain constant on an age-specific basis, there will be nearly three times as many people in nursing homes as there were in 1990—5.7 million people in institutions in 2040 compared to 1.6 million in 1990 (U.S. Bureau of the Census, 1996). Whatever stage in life the baby boomers are, many argue that they tend to set the policy agenda.

For the near term, the political salience of long-term care is less certain. The changing demographic profile of the United States is expected to increase awareness of the long-term care issue. While the baby boom generation is not yet using long-term care, many of their parents are. A Congressional staffer adds,

> Because the baby boomers are now caring for their parents, they are going to drive an interest in this issue in a way that hasn't been the focus before and they will also think about the need for long-term care for themselves. There will be a great demand for the government to address part of the problem.

Another provider commented, "The soccer moms are eight years older; now they are concerned with long-term care for their parents. Their needs are different." In contrast, there is also pessimism about the possibility for progress relating to long-term care due to its public or private cost, the desire for tax cuts, the funding and financing problems currently evident with Medicare and Social Security, and the lack of consensus in the policy community.

Finally, in what may be an important development for the future, a new Washington, DC, coalition was formed in 1999 to put long-term care reform on the national agenda again. Chaired by former Senator David Durenberger (R–MN), Citizens for Long-Term Care (CLTC) is composed of organizations from all segments of the long-term care and political spectrum, including consumer groups, providers organizations, insurers, unions, women's groups, and business interests. Its goal is to educate the public by raising awareness of the issue of long-term care financing within the year 2000 presidential election. While this new coalition will function as a "clearinghouse of solutions," it will not endorse any particular proposal.

FINAL THOUGHTS

During long-term care reform efforts in 1993–1994, an important alliance between the elderly and disability populations emerged and was solidified. The result is that "aging groups in town are now better educated, especially about younger people with disability." The inter-generational solidarity and working relationships between the elder and disabled lobbies have endured throughout the 1990s. There is increased activism of the younger people with disabilities that continues to energize the now-ongoing coalition of the elderly and disability communities.

Another legacy of the long-term care reform of 1994 is significant change in the way long-term care is conceptualized. A major change has been the united commitment of the elderly and the younger disabled to the idea of intergenerational (cross-age) and cross-disability solutions to the long-term care problem. This new political alignment has been sustained in the post-reform period and aided in the successful defense against a proposed Medicaid block grant in the mid 1990s. Other significant changes are that the long-term care reform process and work between 1992 and 1994 contributed to a new paradigm that sought to counterbalance the bias and limits of 1) categorical thinking that previously allowed only specified medical and supportive services, and 2) institutional thinking in which the predominant public financing has been for nursing home care rather than for home and community care. Other elements of the strategy that also gained favor during the construction of the Clinton long-term care plan sought to promote independent living and self-directed care models that challenge what has been described as the "over-professionalization" and the "over-medicalization" of long-term care.

The final approach contained in the 1993–1994 reform met the bottom-line requirement of many advocates that there be no means-testing in long-term care. In so doing, the design of President Clinton's long-term care reform plan finessed some of the most difficult stumbling blocks that could easily have set off unwanted opposition from the states and consumer groups to the proposed reform. For elder and disabled activists, the Clinton long-term care plan met the test of incorporating eligibility that was based solely on functional capacity and "looked like a social insurance program." For the states, the carrots were flexibility, no new individual entitlement, and sufficient "fiscal and political cover" for them to "buy in." The final plan strengthened and continued the state's primary role in long-term care, while — on the negative side — also ensuring the continuing unevenness and differences in long-term care benefits across the states.

The casualties of the health reform experience — almost all of which were previously non-negotiable by most elderly advocates at the outset of the Clinton Presidency — are the abandonment of the somewhat hallowed concepts of individual entitlement and a "defined benefit." Also lost under the long-term care plan was the idea that long-term care must be a uniform "universal national program," and, with it, the imperative of a traditional "social insurance" approach to the problem.

As we enter the next millennium, it appears that long-term care is coming back onto the national political agenda, albeit in a radically altered form.

NOTE ON METHODS

Data for this article were collected primarily from interviews with 38 federal executive branch officials, health reform task force staff and members, representatives of nursing home, home care, elderly and disability organizations, state officials, legislators, Congressional staff, and researchers. Supplementary information was obtained from newspaper and other media accounts of health reform and government documents relating to the long-term care component of health reform. In addition, one of the authors was a member of the long-term care workgroup of the White House's Task Force on National Health Reform and provided his recollections of the process and lessons for the future.

REFERENCES

Aaron, Henry J. (editor). 1996. *The Problem That Won't Go Away: Reforming Health Care Financing.* Washington, D.C.: The Brookings Institution.

Johnson, Haynes and David S. Broder. 1996. *The System: The American Way of Politics at the Breaking Point.* Boston: Little, Brown & Co., 1996.

Kuttner, Robert. 1999. "Taking Exception" *Washington Post,* January 8, 1999.

LTC Campaign. 1998. *A Policy Blueprint.* Washington, D.C.: LTC Campaign.

LTC Campaign. 1994. *What Is the Long Term Care Campaign?* Washington, D.C.: LTC Campaign.

Skocpol, Theda. 1997. *Boomerang: Health Care Reform and the Turn Against Government.* New York: W.W. Norton & Co., 1997.

Part III

Identifying, Understanding, and Addressing Population Health Problems

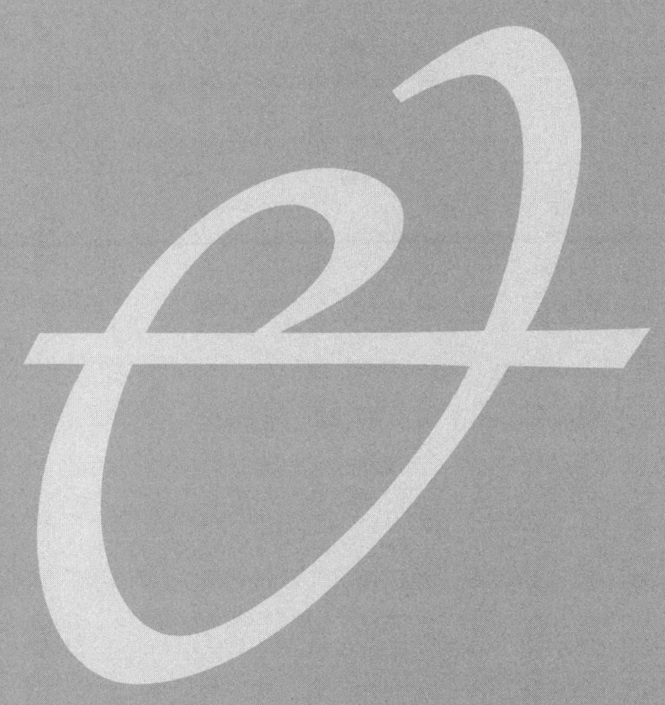

CHAPTER 5

PUBLIC HEALTH AND COMMUNITY PROBLEM SOLVING

This chapter introduction begins by highlighting the important role of the public health sector in identifying, understanding, and addressing population health problems. In the 1988 Institute of Medicine (IOM) report, *The Future of Public Health*, the broad mission of public health was described as follows: "Public health is what we, as a society, do collectively to assure the conditions in which people can be healthy" (p. 1). This introduction also describes the early progress in public health in identifying and combating infectious diseases; the development of public health at the federal, state, and local levels; the issues faced because of the rise in chronic diseases that followed the relative effectiveness in controlling infectious diseases; and, finally, the current challenges facing public health. The 1988 Institute of Medicine Report; three articles in the *Annual Review of Public Health* by Breslow (1990), Lee and Paxman (1997), and Fielding (1999); and the monograph *Medicine and Public Health: The Power of Collaboration* (1997) by Roz D. Lasker and the Committee on Medicine and Public Health provide more detail and are included in the Recommended Reading.

SCIENTIFIC DISCOVERIES AND SOCIAL EXPERIMENTS IN PUBLIC HEALTH

Public health measures, beginning with the sanitary revolution in the United Kingdom and the United States more than 150 years ago, contributed significantly to the improvements in the health status of the population, particularly the decline in mortality from infectious diseases, described in Chapter 1. Although the problem was identified as largely related to the filthy environment and actions were taken to correct this, the scientific basis for these measures had not been identified. The critical role played by public health in Great Britain between 1850 and 1914 has been reviewed by Szreter (see Recommended Reading), in other European countries by Samuel Preston (1975), and in the United States by Duffy (1990), Breslow (1990),

Fee (1991), Lee (1995), and Lasker and the Committee on Medicine and Public Health (1997). The picture in the 19th and early 20th centuries was described clearly by Lasker and colleagues in *Medicine & Public Health: The Power of Collaboration* (1997):

> During this period, the nation's most pressing health problems were infectious diseases. Tuberculosis was "captain of the men of death." Influenza, pneumonia, streptococcal infections, and other airborne diseases struck the population with great force, mainly during the winter months. Infants died routinely as a result of acute communicable respiratory and diarrheal diseases. Measles and chicken pox were a "natural" part of childhood. It was not unusual for women giving birth to succumb to perinatal infections. Smallpox epidemics, with their considerable mortality, struck communities from time to time. Typhoid fever occurred on a small scale, spread within and between families, and occasionally erupted in outbreaks. Cholera epidemics created alarm and were a major cause of death in American ports (p. 12).

In the 1850s, the sanitary revolution began in the United States with the first organized community efforts to deal with unsanitary conditions in the environment: contamination of water supplies due to human and animal wastes, primitive methods of waste disposal, and miserable, overcrowded housing in the cities. The initial focus on environmental sanitation produced dramatic benefits for the health of the population, most notably a reduction in mortality from diarrheal diseases and cholera epidemics. Although smallpox vaccination was begun by Edward Jenner in England in the late 18th century, it did not become widespread until almost a century later. Tuberculosis began to decline even before the pioneering studies by Robert Koch in the late 1800s that identified the tubercle bacillus as the cause of the disease. Despite this progress, tuberculosis was still the nation's leading cause of death in 1900, particularly among young adults.

The application of Louis Pasteur's and Robert Koch's bacteriological research, Pasteur's germ theory of disease, and Koch's postulates began to bear fruit after the turn of the 20th century. Specifically, the contributions of these two scientists were most noted in the development of bacteriological laboratories to identify specific bacterial causes of disease, and in such practical public health applications as the pasteurization of milk. The New York City Health Department led the nation in its development of milk stations to distribute safe milk to poor infants. These efforts, as well as the chlorination of water supplies and the development of sewer systems, which included indoor plumbing and waste treatment facilities, dramatically reduced mortality from communicable diseases prior to the influenza pandemic of 1918 to 1919. The impact was most dramatic on infant mortality, especially from the early 1900s until the early 1950s (see Article 3, Chapter 1).

From the late 1950s to the mid-1960s, little progress was made in reducing infant mortality or increasing life expectancy in the United States. However, beginning in the mid-1960s and continuing into the 1990s, America's health improved. Infant mortality began to decline again in the late 1960s. Major developments, including the implementation of federal health policies and programs, contributed to this improvement. From the 1960s to the mid 1970s, there was a rapid expansion of federal health programs — from Medicare (1965) and Medicaid (1965) to family planning, community health centers, maternal and infant care, and safety and environmental health programs. The nation's hospitals were desegregated in early 1966 due to rigorous enforcement of the Civil Rights Act of 1964, using the power of Medicare dollars. In a very short period of time, a major transformation in health care was initiated. Soon thereafter, health professional education was changed dramatically, and action occurred on many other fronts. The Department of Agriculture's Women, Infants, and Children (WIC) Program, providing milk and other essential foods to poor women and children, expanded. Rapid improvements in neonatal intensive care also occurred during this period. Infant deaths gradually dropped to about one half the 1965 level. The life expectancy of those born in 1979 rose more than three years over those born in 1965. Progress has continued, although many challenges remain.

The *Flexner Report* in 1910 (Flexner, 1960) gave a strong impetus to the transformation of medical education from a fly-by-night proprietary operation to a university-based enterprise soundly based in science. This was to have a profound impact on medical education and later on medical care. Early in the 20th century, scientists began to identify the specific causes of such classic vitamin deficiency diseases as scurvy, beri beri, and pellegra. Although these diseases were known to be associated with diet in some way, specific vitamin deficiencies had not been identified until the 20th century. These discoveries led to actions by the United States Department of Agriculture (USDA) to educate parents and the public in general about micronutrients, including vitamins and minerals.

Research was also advancing in other areas, particularly endocrinology, but the advances did not have a major impact on medical care until the discovery of insulin by Banting and Best in Canada in the 1920s. The introduction of the sulfonamides in the 1930s to treat streptococcal and staphylococcal infections began the era of modern medical care with the development of a number of antimicrobial agents, particularly penicillin, streptomycin, and later a broad spectrum of antibiotics effective in treating a number of major infectious diseases, including tuberculosis. This resulted in a further fall in mortality from 1935 until the late 1950s. It was during this period that the effectiveness of medical care began to increase dramatically. Interestingly, as the role of medical care and the medical profession gained increasing influence and attention, the role of public health seemed less important.

STRUCTURE OF THE PUBLIC HEALTH SYSTEM

The first state health department was established in Massachusetts in 1889. By 1900, 40 states had health departments that focused primarily on sanitation and the applications of the rapidly developing advances in bacteriology. Perhaps the most important step at the local level was the establishment of the Metropolitan Board of Health in New York City in 1866. Major cities established boards of health well in advance of county health departments. The first county health department was established in Yakima, Washington in 1911. By 1920, 131 county health departments had been established. By 1931, the number grew to 599 county health departments, which provided services to a fifth of the nation. Local health departments and population services expanded rapidly, numbering 865 by 1950. In 1993, there were 2,888 local health departments, including city, county, and special districts operating in 3,042 counties (CDC, 1999a, p. 1145). These developments were related primarily to the U.S. Public Health Service and are summarized in Article 1, "Changes in the Public Health System," prepared by the CDC.

Initially, the federal government had little engagement in health or long-term care policies, except with regard to foreign quarantine and medical care for merchant seamen, soldiers, and sailors (U.S. Navy). With the advent of the sanitary revolution, state and local governments began to establish departments of health or of public health to deal with communicable diseases. At the local level, medical care was mostly a private affair of little benefit to the greater community. Gradually, local governments assumed responsibility for the care of the indigent sick, including the elderly through municipal hospitals.

Although the Marine Hospital/Service was established in 1798, it was almost 90 years before the first elements of the modern U.S. Public Health Service were established in 1912. It began with the creation of the Hygienic Laboratory in the Marine Hospital on Staten Island in 1887, which moved to Washington, D.C., in 1900 and grew to become the National Institutes of Health (NIH) in 1930. The Food and Drug Administration (FDA), which became part of the U.S. Public Health Service in 1968, traces its origins to the Biologics Control Act of 1902 and the Pure Food and Drug Act of 1906. The FDA was part of the Department of Agriculture until 1938, when it became part of the Federal Security Agency. In 1953, it became part of the Department of Health, Education, and Welfare, as did the U.S. Public Health Service. The programs of the Indian Health Service (IHS) were first authorized in 1921. These were transferred to the U.S. Public Health Service from the Department of the Interior (DOI) in 1955.

The multiple categorical grant-in-aid programs for public health and those that made provisions for maternal and child health had their origins in the Social Security Act of 1935. Soon tuberculosis control and venereal disease control programs were added to the public health grant-in-aid programs for states in the late 1930s and early 1940s. These categorical programs grew gradually after World War II. There was a proliferation of categorical public health programs in the 1960s and 1970s. During this time, a major emphasis was placed on rapidly expanding support for biomedical research through the NIH. Programs to treat mental illness were first authorized by Congress in 1948, but it was not until the 1970s that major public health programs were launched to deal with substance abuse. In 1944, the Program for Malarial Control in War Zones became the Communicable Disease Control Program and later the Centers for Disease Control and Prevention. A number of environmental health programs, such as air and water pollution control, which began in the U.S. Public Health Service, were transferred to other agencies and departments in the 1960s and 1970s, including the Environmental Protection Agency (EPA). The nation's Highway Safety Administration (Department of Transportation) and the Occupational Safety and Health Administration (Department of Labor) became the base for highway safety and occupational safety and health programs in the late 1960s and early 1970s. It was not until 1965, when Medicare and Medicaid joined the range of federal health programs respectively, that substantial federal health spending was first directed toward medical care for the elderly and poor. However, they were soon to consume the bulk of federal dollars devoted to the nation's health.

The public health system is, of necessity, large and complex because of the variety of problems to be addressed and the fact that responsibility for addressing these issues is split between public health and non-public health agencies. A range of issues exists related to the relationship of the federal government to state and local health agencies. There are problems at all levels related to the management and coordination of health programs in many different agencies and departments. Many of the problems confronting the U.S. Department of Health and Human Services and the agencies (e.g., NIH, FDA) that compose the U.S. Public Health Service were addressed by Boufford and Lee (2001). Some of these, such as the control of sexually transmitted diseases and immunizations, are in the U.S. Public Health Service and in traditional health departments at the state and local level. Others, such as occupational health and safety, are in the federal Department of Labor and comparable state agencies. Air and water pollution are most often the domain of the federal Environmental Protection Agency but may be addressed by separate agencies at the state, regional, or local level. Mental health and substance abuse prevention and treatment services may be in separate agencies at the state and local level or may be included within a public health agency. In addition, medical care for indigent populations may be provided by local health departments or by separate counties or municipal public hospital systems. This issue is in the greatest state of flux given the medical care cost crisis and the reduction in charity care by hospitals, physicians, and other providers, raising the question of who exactly is responsible for assuring the availability of these basic services.

The early development of the public health system in the United States has been described by Fee (1991) and Duffy (1990), with summaries particularly related to recent developments by Breslow (1990), Lee and Paxman (1997), Fielding (1999), and Lasker and colleagues (1997). Breslow noted that in response to the threats posed by infectious diseases, "many states and local jurisdictions developed health departments to protect people against these severe threats to health" (1990, p. 1).

MOMENTUM FROM THE INSTITUTE OF MEDICINE (IOM) REPORT

In 1988, the IOM's critically important report, *The Future of Public Health*, reviewed the health problems facing the nation and proposed a conceptual framework for public health. The IOM argued that the three broad functions of public health include assessment, policy development, and ensuring that policies are implemented and achieved.

Two leaders in public health, Abdelmonem A. Afifi and Lester Breslow, added to the IOM's description of public health. They defined the core disciplines of public health as epidemiology and biostatistics (composing the "diagnostic tools"), followed by health behaviors, environmental health, and personal health services (the "treatment tools" of public health). In addition, they noted that public health practice "embraces all those activities that are directed to assessment of health and disease problems of the population; the formulation of policies for dealing with such problems; and the assurance of environmental, behavioral and medical services designed to accelerate favorable health trends and reduce the unfavorable" (Afifi and Breslow, 1994, p. 232).

After the 1988 IOM report, further discussions about the role and future of public health took place in many settings, and a great deal of action was generated, particularly in the public health community. The IOM established a public health roundtable, funded by the U.S. Public Health Service and several major private foundations, to conduct major studies of prevalent public health problems. A number of key functions of public health agencies were identified, including preventing epidemics and the spread of disease, protecting against environmental threats, preventing injuries, promoting and encouraging healthy behaviors, responding to disasters and assisting communities in recovery; and ensuring the quality and accessibility of health services (see Lee & Paxman, 1997). Local, state, and federal governments, as well as professional associations such as the American Public Health Association (APHA), state and territorial health officers, and the American Medical Association (AMA), moved to address the issues identified in the IOM report.

The Robert Wood Johnson and the Kellogg Foundations launched a major public health initiative to strengthen state and local public health departments. President Clinton's Health Security Act of 1993 included a $6 billion public health initiative; however, only $1.5 billion was earmarked for the support of core public activities such as immunization, protection of the environment, housing, food and water safety, investigation and control of disease and injuries, and health-related data collection and outcomes monitoring. Although not enacted, the Health Security Act nonetheless identified a number of public health components, such as food safety and immunization, which later received significantly increased funding.

CHALLENGES FACING OUR PUBLIC HEALTH SYSTEM

Breslow (1990) identified five major issues facing public health in the final decade of the 20th century: (1) the reconstitution of public health, (2) the setting of objectives for public health, (3) a shift in focus from disease control to health promotion, (4) an effort to redress continuing social inequities and their impacts on health, and (5) the health implications of accelerating developments in technology. These issues were further addressed by Afifi and Breslow in 1994, and by Lee and Paxman in 1997. Breslow revisited the issue in 1999. As these articles would seem to indicate, the foundations of public health remain in a precarious state at the beginning of the 21st century, as they were when the 1988 IOM report described them as being in "disarray." Therefore, focusing national attention on the critical role of population-based public health functions may or may not result in a stabilization, or even a strengthening, of the public health infrastructure.

Despite aggressive measures, the current challenges to medicine and public health are many. Our nation has a public health infrastructure that is sorely lacking and a medical care system that despite its high costs provides a very uneven level of service. Our public-private system of financing leaves 40 million people uninsured and dependent on public hospitals and other safety net providers for care. The health sector also faces a wide range of health problems. Foremost are tobacco use, HIV/AIDS and other newly emerging or reemerging infections, current dietary patterns, sedentary lifestyles, and alcohol and illicit drug abuse. Injuries (including those due to violence), recurring adolescent health problems such as unintended pregnancies, and vaccine-preventable illnesses in children (e.g., pertussis, meningitis) and adults (e.g., pneumonia, influenza) are of primary significance. Finally, an even greater number of chronic diseases, including heart disease, cancer, cerebrovascular disease, diabetes mellitus, and obesity, as well as a growing list of environmental hazards, require prompt attention. Moreover, the public health and medical care response to terrorism or the threat of terrorism, be it nuclear, chemical, biological, or conventional (e.g., bombs), must be added to the list of public health responsibilities of the modern day.

PERFORMANCE MEASUREMENT AND PUBLIC HEALTH

Public health agencies at the federal, state, and local level are increasingly aware of "the need to formally and quantitatively assess and improve the quality of their programs" (Derose et al., 2002, p. 1). The challenges faced by local health departments in quantitatively assessing their programs, and the tools available to them to do so have recently been reviewed. Over the past 80 years, a number of assessment tools have been developed and utilized. Most recently, a new tool, Mobilizing for Action through Planning and Partnership (MAPP), was designed to help facilitate more effective partnerships at the community level (Derose et al., p. 12).

Healthy People 2010: Understanding and Improving Health lists ten leading health indicators (e.g., physical activity, overweight and obesity, tobacco use), that will be linked to the initiative's 467 objectives and will be used through national and state-level report cards to spotlight achievements and to identify challenges in the next decade.

NATIONAL HEALTH OBJECTIVES

In the late 1970s, a national focus was placed on achieving broad national health objectives. This movement had its roots in the 1964 report to Surgeon General Luther J. Terry on smoking and health. Similarly, Surgeon General Julius Richmond's *Report on Health Promotion and Disease Prevention* (1977) initiated a process to establish national health objectives for 1990. This process involved a wide array of organizations, including state governments, many private-sector organizations, and commercial and voluntary entities.

Based on the experience in the 1980s with the health objectives for 1990, the health objectives for the year 2000 were detailed in *Healthy People 2000: National Health Promotion and Disease Prevention Objectives* and launched in 1990. In the year 2000, the goals for 2010 were launched (see Article 5, Chapter 1). The two overall goals of Healthy People 2010 are to: (1) increase quality and years of healthy life and (2) eliminate health disparities. The content of Healthy People 2010 reflects the changing context for public health and health care.

OPPORTUNITIES FOR IMPROVEMENT THROUGH BROADLY PARTICIPATORY COMMUNITY PROBLEM SOLVING

The 1988 IOM report highlighted the need for collective action to improve population health. Recognizing that most population health objectives cannot be achieved by any single person, organization, or sector working alone, leaders in public health have been focusing considerable attention on engaging the community in core public health functions. As such, foundations and government agencies in the United States have invested hundreds of millions of dollars in health partnerships. Some of these partnerships focus on particular health problems such as asthma, substance abuse, obesity, or teen pregnancy. Others, like Turning Point and Partnerships for the Public's Health, use collaboration as the mechanism by which states and communities are transforming their public health systems.

The last article in this chapter, by Roz D. Lasker and Elisa S. Weiss, looks at collaboration from the perspective of community problem solving. Building on a large body of literature, the authors provide a compelling argument for involving a broad array of people and organizations in collaborative processes to identify, understand, and solve complex community health problems. Going further, they present a multidisciplinary model that explains how broadly participatory processes lead to more effective community problem solving and to improvements in community health. This model is important for two reasons. First, collaborative problem solving, although needed, is extremely difficult to do well. Only by understanding *how* collaboration works is it possible to identify the special kinds of leadership and management that *make* collaborative processes effective. It is interesting that when the authors compare their model with current practice, it appears that many people involved in the leadership and management of partnerships are compromising their own success by the way they are going about collaboration. The article provides valuable insights for strengthening these collaborative efforts and for engaging the community more effectively in new partnerships (e.g., partnerships that might be created to deal with emerging health threats, such as bioterrorism).

Second, in addition to explaining how broadly participatory processes strengthen the ability of communities to solve problems that have a direct impact on health, the model explains why these kinds of collaborations can be health promoting in and of themselves, even if they do not focus on health problems. This aspect of the model has important implications for the nation's health. It suggests that community collaboration can serve not only as a mechanism for solving complex health problems, but also as a strategy for countering the disempowerment and social isolation that have been shown to have negative effects on physical and mental health. It also suggests that population health might be improved by moving toward more participatory forms of democracy.

It is very clear from the work of Lasker and her colleagues, as well as the experience of a growing number of communities, that the old ways of practicing public health and clinical medicine cannot deal with the range of health problems facing communities throughout the country. From asthma in children to the HIV/AIDS epidemic and obesity and diabetes in an aging population, the issues facing our modern-day society require modern-day solutions, which are only beginning to be appreciated. The seminal paper by Lasker and Weiss provides an innovative approach to community health problem solving that we consider a major advance.

REFERENCES

Afifi, A., and Breslow, L. (1994). The maturing paradigm of public health. *Annual Review of Public Health, 15,* 223–235.

Boufford, and Lee. (2001). *Health Policies for the 21st Century: Challenges and Recommendations for the U.S. Department of Health and Human Services.* New York: Milbank Memorial Fund.

Breslow, L. (1990). The future of public health: Prospects in the United States for the 1990s. *Annual Review of Public Health, 11,* 1–28.

Breslow, L. (1999). From disease prevention to health promotion. *Journal of the American Medical Association, 281* (11), 1030–1033.

Centers for Disease Control and Prevention (1999a). Achievements in public health, 1900–1999: Changes in the public health system. *MMWR, 48* (50), 1141–1147.

Centers for Disease Control and Prevention (1999b). Achievements in public health, 1900–1999: Fluoridation of drinking water to prevent dental caries. *MMWR, 48* (41), 933–940.

Derose, S. F., Schuster, M. A., Fielding, J. E., and Asch, S. M. (2002). Public health quality measurement: Concepts and challenges. *Annual Review of Public Health, 23,* 1–21.

Duffy, J. (1990). *The sanitarians: A history of public health.* Chicago: University of Illinois Press.

Fee, E. (1991). The origins and development of public health in the United States. In W. Holland, R. Detels, and G. Knox (Eds.), *Oxford textbook of public health* (2nd ed.). New York: Oxford Medical Publications.

Fielding, J. E. (1999). Public health in the twentieth century: Advances and challenges. *Annual Review of Public Health, 20,* xiii–xxx.

Flexner, A. (1960). *The Flexner report on medical education in the United States and Canada 1910.* Washington, DC: Science and Health Publications.

Institute of Medicine. (1988). *The future of public health: Summary and recommendations.* Washington, DC: National Academy Press.

Lasker, R. D., and the Committee on Medicine and Public Health. (1997). *Medicine and public health: The power of collaboration.* Chicago: Health Administration Press.

Lasker, R. D., and Weiss, E. S. (2003). Broadening participation in community problem solving: A multidisciplinary model to support collaborative practice and research. *Journal of Urban Health* 80(1).

Lee, P. R. (1995). Keynote address. *Bulletin of the New York Academy of Medicine, 72* (Suppl. 2), 552–569.

Lee, P. R., and Paxman, D. (1997). Reinventing public health. *Annual Review of Public Health, 18,* 1–35.

Preston, S. H. (1975). The changing relation between mortality and level of economic development. *Population Studies,* 231–248.

U.S. Department of Health and Human Services. (2000). *Healthy People 2010: Understanding and Improving Health.* Washington, DC: Government Printing Office.

ARTICLE 1

ACHIEVEMENTS IN PUBLIC HEALTH, 1900–1999

CHANGES IN THE PUBLIC HEALTH SYSTEM

The Centers for Disease Control and Prevention

The 10 public health achievements highlighted in this *MMWR* series (see Table 1) reflect the successful response of public health to the major causes of morbidity and mortality of the 20th century (1–11). In addition, these achievements demonstrate the ability of public health to meet an increasingly diverse array of public health challenges. This report highlights critical changes in the U.S. public health system this century.

In the early 1900s in the United States, many major health threats were infectious diseases associated with poor hygiene and poor sanitation (e.g., typhoid), diseases associated with poor nutrition (e.g., pellagra and goiter), poor maternal and infant health, and diseases or injuries associated with unsafe workplaces or hazardous occupations (4, 5, 7, 8). The success of the early public health system to incorporate biomedical advances (e.g., vaccinations and antibiotics) and to develop interventions such as health education programs resulted in decreases in the impact in these diseases. However, as the incidence of these diseases decreased, chronic diseases (e.g., cardiovascular disease and cancer) increased (6, 10). In the last half of the century, public health identified the risk factors for many chronic diseases and intervened to reduce mortality. Public efforts also led to reduced deaths attributed to a new technology, the motor vehicle (3). These successes demonstrated the value of community action to address public health issues and have fostered public support for the growth of institutions that are components of the public health infrastructure.* The focus of public health research and programs shifted to respond to the effects of chronic diseases on the public's health (12–17). While continuing to develop and refine interventions, enhanced morbidity and mortality surveillance helped to maintain these

* The government, community, professional, voluntary, and academic institutions and organizations that support or conduct public health research or programs.

TABLE 1

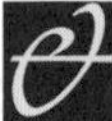

TEN GREAT PUBLIC HEALTH ACHIEVEMENTS—UNITED STATES, 1900–1999

- Vaccination
- Motor-vehicle safety
- Safer workplaces
- Control of infectious diseases
- Decline in deaths from coronary heart disease and stroke
- Safer and healthier foods
- Healthier mothers and babies
- Family planning
- Fluoridation of drinking water
- Recognition of tobacco use as a health hazard

earlier successes. The shift in focus led to improved capacity of epidemiology and to changes in public health training and programs.

QUANTITATIVE ANALYTIC TECHNIQUES

Epidemiology, the population-based study of disease and an important part of the scientific foundation of public health, acquired greater quantitative capacity during the 20th century. Improvements occurred in both study design and periodic standardized health surveys (12, 18–21). Methods of data collection evolved from simple measures of disease prevalence (e.g., field surveys) to complex studies of precise analyses (e.g., cohort studies, case-control studies, and randomized clinical trials) (12). The first well-developed, longitudinal cohort study was conducted in 1947 among the 28,000 residents of Framingham, Massachusetts, many of whom volunteered to be followed over time to determine incidence of heart disease (12). The Framingham Heart Study served as the model for other longitudinal cohort studies and for the concept that biologic, environmental, and behavioral risk factors exist for disease (6, 12).

In 1948, modern clinical trials began with publication of a clinical trial of streptomycin therapy for tuberculosis, which employed randomization, selection criteria, predetermined evaluation criteria, and ethical considerations (19, 21). In 1950, the case-control study gained prominence when this method provided the first solidly scientific evidence of an association between lung cancer and cigarette smoking (22). Subsequently, high-powered statistical tests and analytic computer programs enabled multiple variables collected in large-scale studies to be measured and to the development of tools for mathematical modeling. Advances in epidemiology permitted elucidation of risk factors for heart disease and other chronic diseases and the development of effective interventions.

PERIODIC STANDARDIZED HEALTH SURVEYS

In 1921, periodic standardized health surveys began in Hagerstown, Maryland (12). In 1935, the first national health survey was conducted among U.S. residents (12, 23). In 1956, these efforts resulted in the National Health Survey, a population-based survey that evolved from focusing on chronic disease to estimating disease prevalence for major causes of death, measuring the burden of infectious diseases, assessing exposure to environmental toxicants, and measuring the population's vaccination coverage. Other population-based surveys (e.g., Behavioral Risk Factor Surveillance System, Youth Risk Behavior Survey, and the National Survey of Family Growth) were developed to assess risk factors for chronic diseases and other conditions (24–26). Methods developed by social scientists and statisticians to address issues such as sampling and interviewing techniques have enhanced survey methods used in epidemiologic studies (12).

MORBIDITY AND MORTALITY SURVEILLANCE

National disease monitoring was first conducted in the United States in 1850, when mortality statistics based on death registrations were first published by the federal government (23, 27). During 1878–1902, Congress authorized the collection of morbidity reports on cholera, smallpox, plague, and yellow fever for use in quarantine measures, to provide funds to collect and disseminate these data, to expand authority for weekly reporting from states and municipal authorities, and to provide forms for collecting data and publishing reports (15, 23, 27). The first annual summary of *The Notifiable Diseases* in 1912 included reports of 10 diseases from 19 states, the District of Columbia, and Hawaii. By 1928, all states, the District of Columbia, Hawaii, and Puerto Rico were participating in the national reporting of 29 diseases. In 1950, state and territorial health officers authorized the Council of State and Territorial Epidemiologists (CSTE) to determine which diseases should be reported to the U.S. Public Health Service (PHS) (27). In 1961, the Centers for Disease Control and Prevention (CDC) assumed responsibility for collecting and publishing nationally notifiable diseases data. As of January 1, 1998, 52 infectious diseases were notifiable at the national level.

In the early 1900s, efforts at surveillance focused on tracking persons with disease; by mid-century, the focus had changed to tracking trends in disease occurrence (28, 29). In 1947, Alexander Langmuir at the newly formed Communicable Disease Center, the early name for CDC, began the first disease surveillance system (27). In 1955, surveillance data helped to determine the cause of poliomyelitis among children recently vaccinated with an inactivated vaccine (28). After the first polio cases were recognized, data from the national polio surveillance program confirmed that the cases were linked to one brand of vaccine contaminated with live wild poliovirus. The national vaccine program continued by using supplies from other polio vaccine manufacturers (28). Since these initial disease surveillance efforts, morbidity tracking has become a standard feature of public health infectious disease control (29).

PUBLIC HEALTH TRAINING

In 1916, with the support of the Rockefeller Foundation, the Johns Hopkins School of Hygiene and Public Health was started (30, 31). By 1922, Columbia, Harvard, and Yale universities had established schools of public health. In 1969, the number of schools of public health had increased to 12, and in 1999, 29 accredited schools of public health enrolled approximately 15,000 students (31, 32). Besides the increase in the number of schools and students, the types of student in public health schools changed. Traditionally, students in public health training already had obtained a medical degree. However, increasing numbers of students entered public health training to obtain a primary postgraduate degree. In 1978, 3753 (69%) public health students enrolled with only baccalaureates. The proportion of students who were physicians declined from 35% in 1944–1945 to 11% in 1978 (28, 31). Thus, public health training evolved from a second degree for medical professionals to a primary health discipline (33). Schools of public health initially emphasized the study of hygiene and sanitation; subsequently, the study of public health has expanded into five core disciplines: biostatistics, epidemiology, health services administration, health education/ behavioral science, and environmental science (30, 34).

Programs also were started to provide field training in epidemiology and public health. In 1948, a board was established to certify training of physicians in public health administration, and by 1951, approximately 40 local health departments had accredited preventive medicine and public residency programs. In 1951, CDC developed the Epidemic Intelligence Service (EIS) to guard against domestic acts of biologic warfare during the Korean conflict and to address common public health threats. Since 1951, more than 2000 EIS officers have responded to requests for epidemiologic assistance within the United States and throughout the world. In 1999, 149 EIS officers are on duty.

NONGOVERNMENT AND GOVERNMENT ORGANIZATIONS

At the beginning of the century, many public health initiatives were started and supported by nongovernment organizations. However, as federal, state, and local public health infrastructure expanded, governments' role increased and assumed more responsibility for public health research and programs. Today, public health represents the work of both government and nongovernment organizations.

Nongovernment Organizations

The Rockefeller Sanitary Committee's Hookworm Eradication Project conducted during 1910–1920 was one of the earliest voluntary efforts to engage in a campaign for a specific disease (35). During 1914–1933, the Rockefeller Foundation also provided $2.6 million to support county health departments and sponsored medical education reform. Other early efforts to promote community health include the National

Tuberculosis Association work for TB treatment and prevention, the National Consumers League's support of maternal and infant health in the 1920s, the American Red Cross' sponsorship of nutrition programs in the 1930s, and the March of Dimes' support of research in the 1940s and 1950s that led to a successful polio vaccine. Mothers Against Drunk Driving was started in 1980 by a group of women in California after a girl was killed by an intoxicated driver, and grew into a national campaign for stronger laws against drunk driving.

Professional organizations and labor unions also worked to promote public health. The American Medical Association advocated better vital statistics and safer foods and drugs (17). The American Dental Association endorsed water fluoridation despite the economic consequences to its members (9). Labor organizations worked for safer workplaces in industry (4). In the 1990s, nongovernment organizations sponsor diverse public health research projects and programs (e.g., family planning, human immunodeficiency virus prevention, vaccine development, and heart disease and cancer prevention).

State Health Departments

The 1850 Report of the Sanitary Commission of Massachusetts, authored by Lemuel Shattuck (13, 14), outlined many elements of the modern public health infrastructure including a recommendation for establishing state and local health boards. Massachusetts formed the first state health department in 1889. By 1900, 40 states had health departments that made advances in sanitation and microbial sciences available to the public. Later, states also provided other public health interventions: personal health services (e.g., disabled children and maternal and child health care, and sexually transmitted disease treatment), environmental health (e.g., waste management and radiation control), and health resources (e.g., health planning, regulation of health care and emergency services, and health statistics). All states have public health laboratories that provide direct services and oversight functions (36).

County Health Departments

Although some cities had local public health boards in the early 1900s, no county health departments existed (33). During 1910–1911, the success of a county sanitation campaign to control a severe typhoid epidemic in Yakima County, Washington, created public support for a permanent health service, and a local health department was organized on July 1, 1911 (33). Concurrently, the Rockefeller Sanitary Commission began supporting county hookworm eradication efforts (17, 35). By 1920, 131 county health departments had been established; by 1931, 599 county health departments were providing services to one fifth of the U.S. population (33); in 1950, 86% of the U.S. population was served by a local health department, and 34,895 persons were employed full-time in public health agencies (37).

Local Health Departments

In 1945, the American Public Health Association proposed six minimum functions of local health departments (38). In 1988, the Institute of Medicine defined these functions as assessment, policy development, and assurance, and PHS has proposed 10 organizational practices to implement the three core functions (39, 40). The national health objectives for 2000, released in 1990, provided a framework to monitor the progress of local health departments (41). In 1993, 2888 local health departments,[†] representing county, city, and district health organizations, operated in 3042 U.S. counties. Of the 2079 local health departments surveyed in 1993, nearly all provided vaccination services (96%) and tuberculosis treatment (86%); fewer provided family planning (68%) and cancer prevention programs (54%) (42).

Federal Government

In 1798, the federal government established the Marine Hospital Service to provide health services to seamen (15). To recognize its expanding quarantine duties, in 1902, Congress changed the service's name to the Public Health and Marine Hospital Service and, in 1912, to the Public Health Service. In 1917, PHS support of state and local public health activities began with a small grant to study rural health (35). During World War I, PHS received resources from Congress to assist states in treating venereal diseases. The Social Security Act of 1935, which authorized health grants to states, and a second Federal Venereal Diseases Control Act in 1938 (13, 14), expanded the federal government's role in public health (15, 35). In 1939, PHS and other health, education, and welfare agencies were combined in the Federal Security Agency, forerunner of the Department of Health and Human Services. In the 1930s, the federal government began to provide resources for specific conditions, beginning with care for crippled children. After World War II, the federal role in public health continued to expand with the Hospital Services and Construction Act (Burton-Hill) of 1946[§] (15). In 1930, Congress established the National Institutes of Health [formerly the Hygiene Laboratories of the Public Health Service] and the Food and Drug Administration. CDC was established in 1946 (29). Legislation to form Medicare and Medicaid was enacted in 1965, and the Occupational Safety and Health Administration and the Environmental Protection Agency were organized in 1970.

Although federal, state, and local health agencies and services have increased throughout the century, public health resources represent a small proportion of overall health-care costs. In 1933, federal, state, and local health agencies spent an estimated $14.4 billion on core public health functions, 1%–2% of the $903 billion in total health-care expenditure (43).

[†] A local health department is an administrative or service unit of local or state government responsible for the health of a jurisdiction smaller than the state.

[§] T = P.L. 79-725

CONCLUSION

The public health infrastructure changed to provide the elements necessary for successful public health interventions: organized and systematic observations through morbidity and mortality surveillance, well-designed epidemiologic studies and other data to facilitate the decision-making process, and individuals and organizations to advocate for resources and to ensure that effective policies and programs were implemented and conducted properly. In 1999, public health is a complex partnership among federal agencies, state and local governments, nongovernment organizations, academia, and community members. In the 21st century, the success of the U.S. public health system will depend on its ability to change to meet new threats to the public's health.

REFERENCES

1. CDC. Ten great public health achievements — United States, 1900–1999. *MMWR* 1999;48:241–3.
2. CDC. Impact of vaccines universally recommended for children — United States, 1990–1998. *MMWR* 1999;48:243–8.
3. CDC. Motor-vehicle safety: a 20th century public health achievement. *MMWR* 1999;48:369–74.
4. CDC. Improvements in workplace safety — United States, 1900–1999. *MMWR* 1999;48:461–9.
5. CDC. Control of infectious diseases. *MMWR* 1999;48:621–9.
6. CDC. Decline in deaths from heart disease and stroke — United States, 1900–1999. *MMWR* 1999;48:649–56.
7. CDC. Healthier mothers and babies. *MMWR* 1999;48:849–57.
8. CDC. Safer and healthier foods. *MMWR* 1999;48:905–13.
9. CDC. Fluoridation of drinking water to prevent dental caries. *MMWR* 1999; 48:933–40.
10. CDC. Tobacco use — United States, 1900–1999. *MMWR* 1999;48:986–93.
11. CDC. Family planning. *MMWR* 1999;48:1073–80.
12. Susser M. Epidemiology in the United States after World War II: the evolution of technique. *Epid Reviews* 1985;7:147–77.
13. Turnock BJ. The organization of public health in the United States. In: Turnock BJ, ed. Public health: What it is and how it works. Gaithersburg, Maryland: Aspen Publications, 1997:1121–68.
14. Last JM. Scope and method of prevention. In: Last JM, Wallace RB, eds. Maxcy-Rosenau-Last Public health and preventive medicine. 13th ed. Norwalk, Connecticut: Appleton & Lange, 1992:11–39.
15. Hanlon JJ, Pickett GE. Public health: administration and practice. 8th ed. St. Louis, Missouri: Times Mirror/Mosby College Publishing, 1984:22–44.

16. Koplan JP, Thacker SB, Lezin NA. Epidemiology in the 21st century: calculation, communication, and intervention. *Am J Public Health* 1999;89:1153–5.
17. Terris M. Evolution of public health and preventive medicine in the United States. *Am J Public Health* 1975;65:161–9.
18. Vandenbroucke JP. Clinical investigation in the 20th century: the ascendency of numerical reasoning. *Lancet* 1998;352(suppl 2):12–6.
19. Vandenbroucke JP. A short note on the history of the randomized controlled trial. *J Chronic Dis* 1987;40:985–6.
20. Doll R. Clinical trials: retrospect and prospect. *Statistics in Medicine* 1982; 1:337–44.
21. Armitage P. The role of randomization in clinical trials. *Statistics in Medicine* 1982;1:345–52.
22. Doll R, Hill AB. Smoking and carcinoma of the lung. *Br Med J* 1950;2:740–8.
23. Teutsch SM, Churchill RE, eds. Principles and practice of public health surveillance. New York: Oxford University Press, 1994.
24. Remington PL, Smith MY, Williamson DF, Anda RF, Gentry EM, Hogelin GC. Design, characteristics and usefulness of state-based behavioral risk factor surveillance, 1981–87. *Public Health Rep* 1988;103:366–75.
25. Kann L, Kinchen SA, Williams BI, et al. Youth risk behavior surveillance — United States, 1997. In: CDC surveillance summaries (August 14). *MMWR 47* (no. SS-3).
26. Mosher WD. Design and operation of the 1995 national survey of family growth. *Fam Plann Perspect* 1998;43–6.
27. CDC. Summary of notifiable diseases, United States, 1997. *MMWR* 1997; 46(no. SS-54).
28. Langmuir AD. The surveillance of communicable diseases of national importance. *N Engl J Med* 1963;268:182–92.
29. CDC. History perspectives: history of CDC. *MMWR* 1996;45:526–8.
30. Roemer MI. Preparing public health leaders for the 1990s. *Public Health Rep* 1988;103:443–51.
31. Winkelstein W, French FE. The training of epidemiologists in schools of public health in the United States: a historical note. *Int J Epidemiol* 1973;2:415–6.
32. Association of Schools of Public Health. Enrollment of U.S. schools of public health 1987–1997. Available at http://www.asph.org/webstud1.gif. Accessed December 14, 1999.
33. Crawford BL. Graduate students in U.S. schools of public health: Comparison of 3 academic years. *Public Health Rep* 1979;94:67–72.
34. Association of Schools of Public Health. Ten most frequently asked questions by perspective students. Available at http://www.asph.org/10quest.htm. Accessed December 14, 1999.
35. US Treasury Department/Public Health Service. History of county health organizations in the United States 1908–1933. In: *Public health bulletin* (No. 222). Washington, DC: Public Health Service, 1936.
36. Altman D, Morgan DH. The role of state and local government in health. *Health Affairs* 1983;2:7–31.

37. Mountin JW, Flook E. Guide to health organization in the United States, 1951. Washington, DC: Public Health Service, Federal Security Agency, Bureau of State Services, 1951; PHS publication no. 196.
38. Emerson H, Luginbuhl M. 1200 local public school departments for the United States. *Am J Public Health* 1945;35:898–904.
39. Dyal WW. Ten organizational practices of public health: a historical perspective. *Am J Prev Med* 1995;11(suppl 2):6–8.
40. Institute of Medicine. The future of public health. Washington, DC: National Academy Press, 1988.
41. Public Health Service. *Healthy People 2000: national health promotion and disease prevention objectives* — full report, with commentary. Washington, DC: US Department of Health and Human Services, Public Health Service, 1991; DHHS publication no. (PHS)91-50212.
42. CDC. Selected characteristics of local health departments — United States, 1992–1993. *MMWR* 1994;43:839–43.
43. CDC. Estimated expenditures for core public health functions — selected states, October 1992–September 1993. *MMWR* 1995;44:421,427–9.

ARTICLE 2

BROADENING PARTICIPATION IN COMMUNITY PROBLEM SOLVING

A MULTIDISCIPLINARY MODEL TO SUPPORT COLLABORATIVE PRACTICE AND RESEARCH*

Roz D. Lasker and Elisa S. Weiss

ABSTRACT

Over the last 40 years, thousands of communities — in the United States and internationally — have been working to broaden the involvement of people and organizations in addressing community-level problems related to health and other areas. Yet, in spite of this experience, many communities are having substantial difficulty achieving their collaborative objective, and many funders of community partnerships and participation initiatives are looking for ways to get more out of their investment. One of the reasons we are in this predicament is that the practitioners and researchers who are interested in community collaboration come from a variety of contexts, initiatives, and academic disciplines, and few of them have integrated their work with experiences or literatures beyond their own domain. In this paper, we seek to overcome some of this fragmentation of effort by presenting a multidisciplinary model that lays out the pathways by which broadly participatory processes lead to more effective community problem solving and to improvements in community health. The model, which builds on a broad array of practical experience, as well as conceptual and empirical work in multiple fields, is an outgrowth of a joint-learning workgroup that was organized to support nine communities in the Turning Point initiative. Following a detailed explication of the model, the paper focuses on the implications of the model for research, practice, and policy. It describes how the model can help researchers answer the fundamental effectiveness and "how to" questions related to community collaboration. In addition, the paper explores differences between the model and current practice, suggesting strategies that can help the participants in, and funders of, community collaborations strengthen their efforts.

* From the *Journal of Urban Health*, March 2003 80(1). Published with permission from Oxford University Press.

INTRODUCTION

There are compelling reasons to promote broad community participation in addressing community health problems. From a philosophical perspective, people living in democratic societies have a right to a direct and meaningful voice about issues and services that affect them.[1–3] At a practical level, many of the problems that affect the health and well-being of people in communities — such as substance abuse, poverty, environmental hazards, obesity, inadequate access to care, and terrorism — cannot be solved by any person, organization, or sector working alone.[4–9] These problems are complex and interrelated, defying easy answers. They affect diverse populations and occur in many different kinds of local contexts. The local context, in turn, is dependent on decisions made at state, national, and international levels. Only by combining the knowledge, skills, and resources of a broad array of people and organizations can communities understand the underlying nature of these problems and develop effective and locally feasible solutions to address them.[10–13]

Responding to the promising potential of collaboration to give voice to people in communities and to enhance the effectiveness and efficiency of achieving challenging health objectives, foundations and government agencies in the United States have invested hundreds of millions of dollars in community partnerships and participation initiatives.[8,9,12,14–18] Some examples of participatory initiatives focusing on community health and the delivery of health services, and community-based research for health include Community Health Centers, Target Cities, Ryan White, CSAP Community Partnerships, Healthy Cities and Healthy Communities, Community Care Networks, Healthy Start, Community-Based Public Health, Community Voices, Community Access Program, Urban Research Centers, Free to Grow, Turning Point, and Partnerships for the Public's Health.

The substantial interest and investment of funders in community collaboration have been matched by the passion of the people involved in collaborative efforts to make a real difference in their communities. Yet, for a number of reasons, the experience with community participation initiatives in the United States over the last forty years seems to have generated more frustration than results. The terminology associated with these initiatives has been one source of frustration. Terms like "community engagement," "partnership," and "collaboration" mean different things to different people. Because of this ambiguity, expectations about the purpose and nature of community involvement vary substantially among participants and often are not met.[19] Another challenge has been translating the rhetoric and abstract principles of community participation into practice. Engaging a broad array of people and organizations in a successful collaborative process is extremely difficult. On the front lines, many collaborations are struggling — often unsuccessfully — to find ways to recruit and retain community participants, to run a process that enables diverse participants to work together productively, and to sustain their collaborative efforts over time.[17,20–22] An additional source of frustration relates to effectiveness. Thus far, it has been very difficult to document that broad participation and collaboration actually strengthen the ability of communities to improve the health and well-being of their residents.[17,22–26]

Without evidence showing that community engagement works — or for what kinds of problems it works — participatory approaches to civic problem solving have not been taken seriously by many policy makers.[2,27–28]

Why are we in this predicament? For one, many efforts to broaden participation in community-level problem solving have been too short-term or thinly resourced to reach a level where their impacts can be fairly evaluated.[19] Moreover, the evaluations of these initiatives have focused more on their ultimate goals than on the impact of the collaborative process in achieving those goals. This focus on distal outcomes relates to several factors: broad-based collaborative processes are not scientifically designed interventions; by nature, these processes are interactive and evolving; and there are no standard benchmarks by which to evaluate the effectiveness of the process.[29,30] As a result, broad-based collaborative processes have not been considered to be amenable to the "gold standard" of evaluation: the randomized controlled trial.[30] When process evaluations are conducted, most tend to be anecdotal and not comparative, which limits their generalizability.[31–32]

Another factor contributing to the current predicament is the multidisciplinary scope of this work. Community participation initiatives have been established to address not only physical and mental health issues, but also many other problems as well, in areas such as child welfare, economic development, education, the environment, housing, jobs, safety, community building, civic democracy, and urban planning.[2,19,32–41] Compounding this diversity, the researchers and theoreticians who are interested in community engagement, collaboration, and civic problem solving come from a variety of fields, including not only the health professions but also sociology, community psychology, political science, public administration, social work, education, business, and philosophy. Although the practical and methodological knowledge base about community collaboration should be strengthened by such a broad array of experience and expertise, fragmentation of effort has prevented much of this from happening. Very few of the people involved in this work have drawn on the literature or experiences outside their specific focus or discipline, and most of them have not worked together. Consequently, as they attempt to deal with the challenges they face, it is difficult for anyone involved in community partnerships and participation initiatives to know or fully benefit from what others have learned.[32]

Two years ago, the Center for the Advancement of Collaborative Strategies in Health at the New York Academy of Medicine organized a joint-learning workgroup to enable nine community partnerships in the Turning Point initiative to learn not only from each other but also from the broader experience. These geographically and sociodemographically diverse partnerships — located in Chautauqua County, New York; Cherokee County, Oklahoma; Decatur, Illinois; New Orleans, Louisiana; New York City, New York; North Central Nebraska; Prince William, Virginia; Sitka, Alaska; and Twin Rivers, New Hampshire — are a subset of the 41 local grantees that were funded by the W. K. Kellogg Foundation in 1997 to use collaboration to transform and strengthen the public health infrastructure.[42–45] The nine partnerships were brought together because they all sought to achieve the goal of Turning Point in a similar way — by establishing locally tailored processes that enable a broad array of people and organizations to work together on an ongoing basis to (1) talk to each other about community health; (2) define and assess the health of the community; (3) identify and understand the nature of problems that affect community health; and (4) leverage their complementary strengths and capabilities to solve community health problems. The workgroup calls this kind of broadly participatory collaborative process "community health governance" (CHG).*

To provide the community partnerships with technical assistance, and to broaden their knowledge base, the workgroup has involved a number of "resource participants" with experience in other kinds of community participation initiatives and with expertise in a variety of disciplines.† Over the last two years, as the workgroup's characterization of CHG has become increasingly clear, the objectives and challenges of the sites were used as a lens with which to identify relevant literatures. By combining the aspirations and experiences of the sites with the knowledge of the resource participants and with information gleaned from an extensive review of these literatures, the workgroup developed a model that explains how broadly participatory collaborative processes, like CHG, strengthen community problem solving. This model, which synthesizes a number of previously disparate ideas, defines — operationally— what a successful collaborative problem-solving process is. Although the model has been very useful to the participants in the workgroup, its applicability appears to be considerably broader. By providing a pathway to explain *how* broad-based community collaborations work, the model makes it easier to determine *whether* they work, and to identify the particular *characteristics* these collaborative processes need to have in order to strengthen community problem solving.

The purpose of this paper is to share the CHG model with other interested parties and, by doing so, to stimulate discourse about broad-based community collaboration across contexts, initiatives, and fields. The paper begins with an explication of the model, which includes a review of conceptual and empirical work in multiple literatures. We then focus on the implications of the model for research, practice, and policy. In this concluding section we discuss how the model can help researchers answer the fundamental effectiveness and "how to" questions related to community

---

* In the term "community health governance," "community" is defined geographically, "health" is defined as a broad, positive concept (consistent with the World Health Organization definition, see ref. 46), and "governance" is defined as the means by which communities make decisions (see ref. 49).

† The workgroup's resource participants have included Quinton Baker (Consultant, Community Health, Leadership, and Development), Anne Barry (Minnesota Department of Finance), Barbara Blum (National Center for Children in Poverty), Charles Bruner (Child and Family Policy Center), Phyllis Brunson (Center for the Study of Social Policy), Moses Carey, Jr. (Piedmont Health Services, Inc.), Robert Chaskin (Chapin Hall Center for Children, University of Chicago), David Chrislip (Skillful Means), Otis Johnson (Savannah State University; Chatham-Savannah Youth Futures Authority), Roz Lasker (The New York Academy of Medicine), Alonzo Plough (Seattle-King County Department of Public Health), Keith Provan (School of Public Administration and Policy, University of Arizona), Trish Riley (National Academy for State Health Policy), Barbara Sabol (W. K. Kellogg Foundation), James Schowalter (Minnesota Department of Finance), Steven Rathgeb Smith (University of Washington), and Norman Zimlich (Zimlich & Associates, Inc.).

collaboration. We also compare the model with current practice, identifying strategies that can help the participants in, and funders of, community collaborations strengthen their efforts.

THE MODEL OF COMMUNITY HEALTH GOVERNANCE

The model of community health governance is a road map that lays out the pathways by which broadly participatory collaborative processes lead to more effective community problem solving and to improvements in community health (Figure 1). It hypothesizes that in order to strengthen their capacity to solve problems that affect the health and well-being of their residents, communities need collaborative processes that achieve three proximal outcomes: individual empowerment, bridging social ties, and synergy. The model hypothesizes that all three of these proximal outcomes are needed to strengthen community problem solving, and that these proximal outcomes improve community health directly as well as by enhancing the capacity of the collaborative process to solve health problems. Going further, the model hypothesizes that a collaborative process needs to have certain characteristics in order to achieve these proximal outcomes, and that special kinds of leadership and management are required to achieve these characteristics.

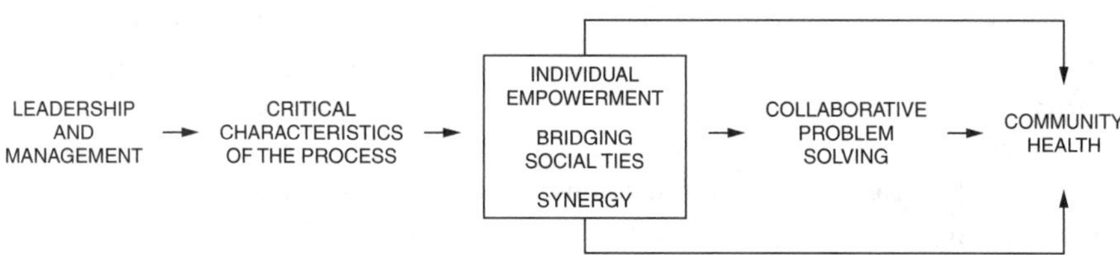

Figure 1 Model of community health governance.

Below, we explicate the model by walking through it from right to left. First, we focus on why collaborative problem solving is needed to improve community health. Next, we identify shortcomings that are undermining the ability of people and organizations in communities to work together effectively to solve problems. We then discuss the three proximal outcomes in the model, describing how they reinforce each other in addressing current shortcomings with community problem solving and how they directly impact health. We continue by elucidating the particular characteristics that enable a collaborative process to achieve these proximal outcomes and, thus, to effectively engage a broad array of people and organizations in solving complex problems. Finally, we discuss the implications of these process characteristics for leadership and management.

The Need for Collaborative Problem Solving to Improve Community Health

Consistent with the World Health Organization, the partnerships in the CHG workgroup define community health broadly — as a positive concept, encompassing all of the environmental, social, and economic resources as well as the emotional and physical capacities that enable people in a geographic area to realize their aspirations and satisfy their needs.[46] But even if health is conceptualized more narrowly, as the absence of disease, many of the problems that impair the health of people in communities are daunting, and communities cannot improve the health of their residents or eliminate current disparities in health unless these problems are effectively addressed.

The growing interest in using collaboration to deal with problems that affect community health stems from the fact that many of these problems are complex; consequently, they go beyond the capacity, resources, or jurisdiction of any single person, program, organization, or sector to change or control.[4–9] Without sufficiently broad-based collaboration, it has been difficult for communities to understand the underlying nature of these kinds of problems or to develop effective and locally feasible solutions to address them. For example, strategies that focus on the services or programs of one kind of professional or organization have not been adequate to solve problems like low birth weight, substance abuse, depression, teen pregnancy, asthma, and inadequate access to care because these problems are interrelated and depend on a broad array of social, economic, environmental, political, emotional, and biologic determinants.[47–50] Problems that require comprehensive actions have been difficult to solve when needed participants have not been involved or when programs, organizations, and/or policies work at cross-purposes with each other.[51] The tremendous diversity in the populations affected by health problems, and in the local contexts in which these problems occur, have limited the effectiveness of top down, "one size fits all" solutions.[13,29,37,49] The lack of community involvement in, and ownership of, solutions, has made it difficult to sustain strategies to improve health.[20,51,52] When effective solutions depend on the actions of people and organizations at regional, state, national, and/or international levels, communities have been at a disadvantage working on their own.[13,53]

Reflecting the complexity of problems that affect community health and well-being, and the need for broad-based collaboration to deal with these kinds of problems, the concept of collaboration has been embedded in the way people think about effective community problem solving. Cottrell, whose work has influenced recent approaches to health promotion and health education, coined the term "community competence" to refer to the ability of community members to "collaborate effectively in identifying problems and needs, to reach consensus on goals and strategies, to agree on ways and means to implement their agreed-upon goals, and to collaborate effectively in the required actions."[54] He defines a competent community as one that is able to cope with the problems of its collective life. At a more general level — going beyond health — the National Civic League and others involved in civic problem solving have used the term "civic infrastructure" to refer to the formal and informal processes and networks by which communities make decisions and solve problems.[38,55] They refer to the capacity of people and organizations to work together constructively to solve problems as "civic health."[28,38]

Current Shortcomings with Community Problem Solving

Although collaborative problem solving appears to have an important role to play in improving community health, there is substantial and growing concern about the ability of people in communities to work together effectively to solve problems.[32,34,38,49,55] This concern is more than academic. Many communities attempting to address a particular health problem have noted that they cannot do so unless they also fix the problem-solving process *per se*.[22,32,34,54,57] Communities in the CHG workgroup have been spurred to strengthen their collaborative problem solving capacity for a number of reasons — to identify important problems and assets that are currently being overlooked, to get a better understanding of the root causes of complex problems, to find effective ways to deal with problems that have been intractable, and to be able to take action to address problems that people in the community care about without waiting for external players, like the federal and state government or national foundations, to develop programs and initiatives.

At a practical level, what does it mean to strengthen community problem solving? The participants in the CHG workgroup recognized that in order to figure out how to achieve this goal, they first had to clarify what needs to be fixed. Below, we discuss shortcomings that have been cited as undermining collaborative problem solving in communities in the United States. These shortcomings include the politics of interest groups, the eroding sense of community, and the limited involvement of community residents in civic problem solving.

Politics of Interest Groups. Despite the importance of the political process in identifying and solving problems in democratic societies, increasing dissatisfaction with politics in the United States has led the National Civic League to state that "America's democracy is in need of repair."[38] As everyone is aware, there have been numerous scandals and breaches of trust.[38,56] Many people have little or no voice in the political process or perceive the process to be controlled by powerful interest groups; they feel that "public life is beyond their control, that their own values and interests are not reflected in the policies that shape the larger society."[38,56] As people feel cut out and unheard, some have opted out of the traditional political process.[34,56] Others have looked to confrontation and advocacy to influence the forces that affect their lives.[58]

Advocacy gives people a way to draw attention to issues that would otherwise be ignored. But when the politics of interest groups goes too far it can hinder, rather than strengthen, community problem solving.[34,58,59] For example, ideological debates look at problems in isolation rather than in relation to each other or to the broader community context.[32,54,55] The sound bites and slogans of most of these debates lack substance, and public hearings — in which representatives of different interest groups speak *at* each other — do not promote the broad and open discourse that is needed to understand and solve complex problems.[58,60] Moreover, when one solution is advocated over another, in a zero-sum fight with different interests choosing sides, winning the fight and beating opponents become more important than developing solutions.[22,38,55,59] In this environment, "shouting, confrontation, name-calling, and obfuscating nondiscussion" weaken the capacity of people to listen to each other and think critically.[54] Often, the end result is rancor, gridlock, abandoned programs, and fragmented, short-sighted, and reactive policy making.[47,55,59,61]

Eroding Sense of Community. Putnam's treatise *Bowling Alone*, which spurred much of the current interest in community building, resonated with many people's perceptions that civic life in the United States is deteriorating.[62,63] This eroding sense of community has been attributed to several factors. Confrontational politics and the growing diversity of the American population have both been cited as contributing to the polarization of people and organizations.[55,64] In addition, the new business orientation of government, which sees citizens as customers, encourages people to focus on their own self-interest rather than the public good.[2,3] The net result of this diminished sense of connectedness is a frayed social fabric in which ties within groups may be strong, but people from different backgrounds, organizations, sectors, and jurisdictions do not know each other and trust each other enough to work together to solve problems. As Cottrell bemoaned twenty-five years ago — in a statement that still seems to be true — this frayed social fabric is leading to "such a welter of institutional rivalries, jurisdictional disputes, doctrinal differences, and lack of communication that effective joint action seems well beyond practical possibility."[54]

Limited Involvement of Community Residents. Many people want to be directly and actively involved in addressing community-level problems that affect their lives. Yet, they are rarely treated as peers or resources in problem solving.[2,3,34] In both the public and private sectors, community residents are usually treated as customers, clients, "objects of concern," sources of data, or targets of problem-solving efforts.[39,54,61] Because people treated in these ways have little or nothing to do or say concerning setting policy or making decisions, these approaches devalue and discredit their contributions and breed feelings of helplessness and dependency.[2,39,54,65] Equally important, when decisions are left to experts, the community lacks the information and resources it needs to come up with effective solutions to problems.[21,40,66–67]

Expertise and statistical data are important, but experts are limited in their own foresight and capability, and statistical data alone do not yield the whole answer to complex problems.[21,40] Moreover, when experts or service providers "run the show," problems tend to be viewed narrowly within professional boundaries, and the knowledge, skills, and resources of people and organizations in the community are often not utilized.[23,65] Without these community assets, it is difficult for a problem-solving process to identify what residents actually want and need, to frame issues in ways that make sense to people in the community, to identify the underlying causes of problems, or to develop and implement solutions that are likely to work in the local environment.[21,40,66,67] Without the commitment that comes from having community members involved in the design of solutions, initiatives are often disbanded after external funding ends.[21,30,51,52,61]

The Proximal Outcomes

The three proximal outcomes in the model explain what we think a collaborative process needs to accomplish, in the short term, in order to be effective in solving community-level problems and improving community health. Put simply, the model hypothesizes that in order to address current shortcomings in community problem solving, communities need collaborative processes that:

- *empower individuals* by getting them directly and actively involved in addressing problems that affect their lives
- create *bridging social ties* that bring people together across society's dividing lines, build trust and a sense of community, and enable people to provide each other with various kinds of support
- create *synergy* — the breakthroughs in thinking and action that are produced when a collaborative process successfully combines the knowledge, skills, and resources of a group of diverse participants

One can think of the proximal outcomes in the model as the mechanisms by which successful collaborative processes address the shortcomings in community problem solving that we discussed above. Each of these mechanisms operates at a different level: empowerment is experienced by individuals; bridging social ties are created dyadically, between people; and synergy is the product of a group. The model hypothesizes that *all three* of these proximal outcomes are needed to strengthen community problem solving. It also hypothesizes that two of the proximal outcomes — individual empowerment and bridging social ties — improve community health *directly* as well as by enhancing the capacity of collaborative processes to solve health problems. Below, we discuss the proximal outcomes in turn.

Individual Empowerment. The CHG model draws on the rich literature on empowerment, which has identified empowerment as a link between community participation and health, both conceptually and in practice.[23] Yet, it is important to clarify how this concept is used in the model. Because the literature on empowerment spans multiple disciplines — including community psychology, health education, community organizing, social work, and education — the term "empowerment" has different meanings for different groups.[47,48,68] For example, it has been used to connote both an outcome and a process, and it has been applied at individual and community levels.[23,48,69–72]

In the CHG model, different aspects of empowerment are incorporated in different parts of the pathway. *Individual* empowerment appears as a proximal outcome in the model. The notion of *community* empowerment is embedded in a distal outcome in the model: effective community problem solving. A community can be said to be empowered when it has the capacity to solve problems, identifying its own problems and solutions.[73] This definition is closely related to Cottrell's concept of community competency, which we use to define effective community problem solving. The notion of empowerment as a *process* is incorporated in earlier components of the model: leadership/management and process characteristics (discussed later in the paper).

By distinguishing these process aspects of empowerment, the model can build on them to explain how empowerment outcomes are achieved.

Why are we focusing on individual-level empowerment as a proximal outcome in the model? The reason is straightforward — the empowerment of individuals appears to be an important mechanism for addressing current shortcomings in community problem solving and for improving community health. Considered as an individual-level outcome, empowerment has been defined as the ability of people to make decisions and have control over forces that affect their lives.[48] According to Zimmerman, individual empowerment has three dimensions. People are empowered when they (1) believe they have the ability to exert control over forces that affect their lives; (2) have the knowledge, skills, and resources to do so; and (3) are actually involved in making decisions and taking actions.[71] These dimensions of individual empowerment resonate closely with the basic tenets of participatory democracy.[1,56,74–76] By actively taking part in making decisions and by determining the results of decisions, people in democratic societies gain control over their lives.

The literature suggests that individual empowerment has a direct affect on health, independent of problem solving. A number of studies have shown that both physical and mental health are significantly affected by the extent to which people perceive that they have control over their lives. For example, nursing home residents with more choice and decision making power have been shown to have better mental and physical health.[77,78] The risk of coronary heart disease has been associated with the degree to which employees have control over their work environment.[79,80] The lack of individual control has been associated with alienation, devaluation of self, passivity, apathy, and a loss of sense of significance, which compromise people's mental health.[54] At a biological level, the most likely explanation for these findings is that the perception of control directly affects the nervous, endocrine, and immune systems, reducing autonomic reactivity and levels of stress hormones, which have been a negative impact on health, and improving immunologic responsiveness.[77,78]

In addition to its direct affect on health, individual empowerment also appears to be a prerequisite for strengthening the capacity of communities to solve complex health problems. As the discussion in the previous section suggests, a much broader array of community members needs to be empowered in order to address shortcomings in community problem solving. Currently, many people whose lives are affected by community-level decisions and actions are excluded from community problem-solving activities. When people are disempowered in this way, they have no opportunity to use their knowledge, skills, and resources to influence forces that affect their lives.[81] At the same time, the community lacks the knowledge, skills, and resources that it needs to identify, understand, and solve complex problems.

Collaborative processes that lead to the empowerment of a broad array of community members can strengthen problem solving by giving the community access to valuable knowledge, skills, and resources that it otherwise would not have.*

---

* It is important to point out that, in the CHG model, individual empowerment is a product of the collaborative process. It is *not* something that powerful participants give to other participants.

For example, local people understand the needs, opportunities, priorities, history, and dynamics of the community in ways that professional nonresidents do not.[67] Users of services have perspectives and experiences that the community needs to develop services that will actually be useful to them, and people directly affected by problems have important insights about the root causes of problems and ways to address problems.[21,40] Actively involving these community members in problem solving can lead to more effective, feasible, and responsive solutions, prevent the repetition of ill-advised decisions, and enhance the acceptance and legitimacy of decisions.[66,67]

It is important to point out that solving a problem that affects the health and well-being of a person is not the same as empowering that person. People who are not directly involved in a community problem-solving process can benefit from the results that are achieved without being empowered. Equally important, people can be empowered by a collaborative process that is not effective in solving problems. The reason this can happen is that empowerment is necessary for effective problem solving, but it is *not sufficient* by itself. The concept of individual empowerment relates to "being involved" and "the ability to exert control" rather than to the quality of any decisions that are made or actions that are taken.[82] Consequently, just because people are empowered does not mean that they are making the kinds of decisions and taking the kinds of actions that can actually solve problems.

Bridging Social Ties. The CHG model hypothesizes that, in addition to empowering people, collaborative problem-solving processes also need to create social relationships that bridge many sectors and levels. The inclusion of this proximal outcome in the model is supported by literatures that have linked social ties — both conceptually and empirically — to community problem-solving capacity and to the physical and mental health of people in communities. This work suggests that bridging social ties, as distinct from the bonding ties that undergird ethnic and interest groups, are needed to address the factors that are currently undermining community problem solving.

While the literature relating social ties to community problem solving is not as robust as the literature relating social ties to health, a number of studies have documented such an association. For example, Putnam's classic study of civic traditions in Italy related the performance of local governments, including their ability to identify and solve problems, to the density of associations among community members and the vibrancy of associational life.[83] In the context of community-level health interventions, the intentional development of social networks has been associated with an enhanced capacity to solve problems.[84,85] The importance of *bridging* social ties in community problem solving has also been highlighted in the literature. Chrislip, for instance, has noted that solving complex problems — in ways that further the public interest — requires not only connections among like-minded people who advocate particular causes, but also connections that bring people together across society's dividing lines.[58] The National Civic League has emphasized that strengthening the way communities solve problems requires collaborative relationships that cross many sectors and initiatives.[38,49] Referring to social capital — the networks and norms of reciprocity and trustworthiness that arise from social ties — Putnam states that in order to address our biggest collective problems, we need ties of the most broad and bridging kind.[62]

Why are bridging social ties needed to solve community-level problems? The reasons become apparent when social ties are considered in terms of the shortcomings in problem solving that many communities are experiencing today. To go beyond the adversarial politics of competing interests — so that problems can be viewed in relation to each other and to broader community concerns — people in communities need to establish relationships that extend further than their own immediate networks. To repair the frayed social fabric that impedes cooperation for mutual benefit, connections need to be established between people who are currently polarized and skeptical of each others' motivations. To obtain the full range of knowledge, skills, and resources that the community needs to identify, understand, and solve complex problems, ties need to be created between people and organizations from a broad range of backgrounds, disciplines, and sectors — including ties between community residents directly affected by problems and people with various kinds of professional expertise. Finally, to address problems that depend on actions at regional, state, national, or international levels, relationships need to be established that go beyond the local community. The importance of these cross-level ties has been emphasized in efforts to improve economic opportunities in inner-city neighborhoods.[53,63]

The literature suggests a number of mechanisms by which bridging social ties strengthen community problem solving. For one, social relationships play an important role in promoting the development of trust. Indeed, as Durkheim noted over one hundred years ago, decreased civic trust is one of the serious consequences of a fragmented social fabric.[86] Social relationships also foster a sense of social identity; people with a network of social relationships feel they are part of a community.[86,87] Going further, social ties and networks provide a way for people to provide each other with various kinds of support, such as (1) information, advice, and guidance; (2) tangible aid and assistance; (3) emotional affirmation; and (4) encouragement and motivation.[57] As Heany and Israel point out, the exchange of social support increases a community's ability to garner the resources it needs to solve problems.[57]

As with empowerment, the development of social ties and the exchange of social support appears to improve health directly as well as by fostering more effective problem solving. In fact, there is an extensive body of evidence relating the physical and mental health of individuals to the number, strength, and reciprocity of their social relationships.[88–90] The lack of social relationships has been shown to be a major risk factor for health; House et al. note that this risk rivals "the effects of well-established risk factors, such as smoking, hypertension, obesity, and inactivity."[87] On the other hand, when people have strong and supportive social relationships, they are significantly healthier.[91,92] According to Berkman, social support enhances health by meeting basic human needs for companionship, intimacy, and reassurance of a person's own self-worth.[93] Other beneficial effects of social relationships have been attributed to a sense of meaning and coherence, which decreases reactivity to stress, and to a sense of belonging and social identity, which promote psychological well-being.[70,86,87,94] Taken together, the literature suggests that a collaborative process that empowers individuals and builds social relationships between people can be health promoting in and of itself — even if it does not solve any community health problems.

Synergy. Empowerment and bridging social ties are important, but even together they do not explain how a collaborative process enables people and organizations in a community to work together constructively to identify, understand, and solve complex problems. Consequently, the CHG model hypothesizes that in addition to getting people directly and actively involved in addressing problems that affect them, and creating relationships that enable them to trust each other and provide each other with support, a collaborative process also needs to achieve another proximal outcome — it needs to create synergy.

Synergy can be defined as the breakthroughs in thinking and action that are produced when a collaborative process successfully combines the complementary knowledge, skills, and resources of a group of participants.[95; see also 10,11,13,96] In contrast to empowerment, which focuses on individuals, and social ties, which focus on dyadic relationships, synergy is the product of a group. It is created when a group of people and organizations combine their resources rather than dyadically exchange them.[97,98] In a collaborative process that creates synergy, the group, as a whole, has an advantage over its separate participants.[95]

Although the literature on collaboration is rich with allusions to synergy, very little empirical work has been done in this area. Nonetheless, recent conceptual work on synergy by Lasker and colleagues helps explain how the active involvement of a broad array of people and organizations strengthens community problem solving.[95,99] Often, it is difficult for individuals, organizations, or interest groups to make good decisions on their own because they have imperfect or incomplete information. For example, they see only part of a problem, consider an issue from only one perspective, or make incorrect assumptions about what other people think. But when a collaborative process combines the complementary knowledge of different kinds of people — such as professionals in various fields, service providers, people who use services, and residents who are directly affected by health problems — the group as a whole can overcome these individual limitations and improve the information and thinking that undergird community problem solving.[8,10,11,13,36,49,95,96,100–103] Working together in this way, a broad array of participants can:

- obtain more accurate information (e.g., about the concerns and priorities of people in the community and the trade-offs they are willing to make)
- see the "big picture" (e.g., look at issues in relation to each other and the broader community context; appreciate how different services, programs, and policies in the community relate to each other and to the problems the community is trying to address)
- break new ground (e.g., challenge ideologies and the "accepted wisdom" to understand the root causes of problems and discover innovative solutions to problems)

- understand the local context (e.g., appreciate the values, politics, assets, and history of the local environment and use this information to identify strategies that are most likely to work in that environment)

Synergy is manifested not only in the way a community thinks about problems, but also in the actions it takes to address these problems.[7,10–13,20,95,102] By combining the skills and resources of diverse participants, a community has the potential to take actions that go beyond the capacity of any single person, organization, or sector. Working together, people and organizations in a community can take actions that:

- build on community assets
- are tailored to local conditions
- connect multiple services, programs, policies, and sectors
- attack a problem from multiple vantage points simultaneously

Finally, synergy can strengthen community problem solving by promoting a special kind of consensus or collective purpose. Rather than agreeing to a position or solution that a person, organization, or interest group advocated at the start, a group of people who create synergy develops consensus around ideas and strategies they generate together. In this kind of process, consensus does not require anyone to "give in" or "give up." Instead, participants contribute to the development of something new and feasible that many people can support.[95,97,98] When a broad group of participants develop and "own" a solution that makes sense to them, implementation is more likely to go smoothly and is more likely to be sustained.[21,39,51,52]

Critical Characteristics of the Process

Having gone through the proximal and distal outcomes in the model, we are now in a position to look at the collaborative process itself. The CHG model hypothesizes that a collaborative process needs to have certain characteristics in order to achieve the three proximal outcomes — individual empowerment, bridging social ties, and synergy — and, thus, to effectively engage a broad array of people and organizations in solving complex problems and improving community health. These process characteristics, which relate to *who* is involved, *how* they are involved, and the *scope* of the process, build on the literatures related to the proximal and distal outcomes in the model as well as the practical experiences of the sites in the CHG workgroup. Below we discuss the critical characteristics of the process, explaining how they enable a collaborative process to achieve the three proximal outcomes.

Who Is Involved. Engaging a *broad array of people and organizations* is central to the work of many community partnerships and participation initiatives. The partnerships in the CHG workgroup, for example, have involved people and organizations from many different backgrounds, disciplines, sectors, and levels — including not only various kinds of service providers, but also people directly affected by health problems, formal and informal community leaders, academics, government agencies, schools, businesses, and faith-based organizations. Some of these participants, particularly youth and low-income residents, had not previously been involved in community-level processes to identify and solve health problems.

While there are strong philosophical reasons to involve diverse people and organizations in collaborative endeavors, the CHG model shows that broad engagement is more than an end in itself. It is needed to strengthen the capacity of the community to identify, understand, and solve complex problems and improve community health.[34,49,61,104] To achieve the three proximal outcomes, and thus rectify current shortcomings in community problem solving, the model hypothesizes that collaborative processes need to involve more than the "usual suspects." Broader participation is required in order to (1) empower people who have not been involved in community-level problem solving before; (2) create relationships between people from various backgrounds, disciplines, sectors, and levels; and (3) bring together people and organizations with a sufficient range of knowledge, skills, and resources so the group, as a whole, can achieve the breakthroughs in thinking and action that are needed to understand and solve complex problems. Indeed, recent research on partnership synergy by Weiss and colleagues has documented the value of broad and diverse involvement in collaborative endeavors. They found that the ability of partnerships to achieve a high level of synergy is related to the sufficiency of the partnership's nonfinancial resources (i.e., knowledge, skills, and expertise; perceptual, observational, and statistical information; connections to people, organizations, and groups; legitimacy and credibility; convening power).[105] Partnerships with many different kinds of participants have a greater variety of nonfinancial resources with which to create synergy than partnerships with a few homogeneous partners.

Ultimately, everything that comes out of a collaborative process depends on the people and organizations who participate in it. While the optimal mix of participants in a collaborative process is likely to vary according to the phase of the process, the scope of the process, and the particular problems it is addressing, the CHG model provides a structured way to identify people and organizations who ought to be involved. For example, one might consider the following kinds of questions when thinking about participation in relation to the three proximal outcomes in the model.

- *Individual empowerment:* Who has been left out of community problem solving before? Whose voice has not been heard? Of these people, who can help the group identify important community problems and community assets? Who has knowledge, skills, and resources that the group needs to understand and develop effective and locally feasible solutions to problems? Whose health and well-being is affected by the problem(s) the process is trying to address?
- *Bridging social ties:* Of the people and organizations who need to work together to identify, understand, and/or solve the problem(s) the collaborative process is trying to address, who doesn't know each other? Who doesn't

understand each other? Who doesn't respect each other? Who doesn't trust each other?

- *Synergy:* Which people and organizations need to be brought together to enable the group, as a whole, to obtain complete and accurate information, to see the full picture, to challenge the conventional wisdom, to understand and appreciate the local environment, and to carry out comprehensive strategies? Are there people and organizations not currently involved in the process who have knowledge, skills, or resources that can help the group identify the concerns and priorities of people in the community, understand the root causes and context of the problem(s) it is trying to address, develop effective and locally feasible solutions, and/or take action to implement solutions?

How Participants Are Involved. Just because a collaborative process includes the "right" mix of people and organizations does not mean that it will automatically achieve the three proximal outcomes in the model or be effective in solving problems or improving health. In fact, the CHG model hypothesizes that participants need to be involved in special ways in order to achieve these outcomes — ways that the workgroup sites find to be very different from the "usual way of doing business." Below, we discuss participant involvement in collaborative problem solving by focusing on process characteristics related to (1) feasibility, (2) influence and control, and (3) group dynamics.

Feasibility. The CHG model hypothesizes that a collaborative problem-solving process needs to be structured so that it is feasible for a broad array of people to be involved. The rationale for this process characteristic is simple. People cannot be involved if they are not aware of the opportunity to participate in the process or if they face logistical barriers that make participation difficult.[106] People who are not involved for these reasons cannot be empowered through the process, develop relationships with other participants, or strengthen the ability of the group to create synergy.

Influence and Control. The CHG model also hypothesizes that the participants need to have real influence in, and control over, the collaborative process. Consistent with work on "empowering processes," this means that the collaborative process needs to be designed and run by its diverse participants rather than by any single stakeholder and that, together, the participants need to determine how their collective work gets done.[48] The model's call for such a community-driven process reflects not only the experiences of the sites in the CHG workgroup, but also numerous concerns raised in the literature about the control of community collaborations by experts and specialists and the domination of such endeavors by the agenda of powerful stakeholders.[3,22,23,31,54,65,104,107]

The proximal outcomes in the model help to clarify the importance of broad-based community influence and control. People are not fully empowered when their participation in a collaborative process is limited to providing a lead agency with input or advice or to helping a lead agency obtain additional resources and community "buy-in" to carry out a predetermined program. Moreover, the participants in a collaborative process cannot challenge the conventional wisdom and achieve the significant breakthroughs in thinking and action that are required to understand and solve complex problems (i.e., create synergy) if the process is constrained by the agenda or paradigm of a dominant stakeholder.

Operationally, the literature suggests that to achieve broad-based influence and control, everyone in the process needs to *participate on an equal footing* — as peers — regardless of their position in the social hierarchy.[23,31,34,69] In addition, if the community is to have real influence in the ultimate outcome of the process, a broad array of people and organizations needs to be actively involved in *all phases* of community problem solving — identifying and framing problems, understanding the causes of problems and the context in which they occur, developing strategies to address problems, taking collective actions to solve problems, and refining these actions over time.[99] In a health-oriented process like CHG, this means that broad and diverse groups of participants are involved in determining the geographic area(s) that make sense in dealing with community health issues, how community health is defined, how it is assessed, how problems affecting community health are identified and prioritized, which problems are addressed, and how these problems are understood and addressed.

Group Dynamics. The model hypothesizes that in order to empower people, build bridging social relationships, and create synergy, a collaborative process needs to enable a group of diverse participants to talk to, learn from, and work with each other over an extended period of time. The CHG workgroup has operationalized such a group process as follows. The process brings a group (or groups) of people together to talk to each other on a regular basis. It promotes meaningful discourse — i.e., it enables diverse participants to talk *with* each other rather than *at* each other — by valuing listening as well as speaking, by honoring and respecting different kinds of knowledge and points of view, and by fostering the development of a jargon-free language that is widely understood. It creates an environment in which participants feel comfortable raising questions, expressing different opinions, and voicing new ideas. In addition to giving people voice, the process also combines the complementary knowledge, skills, and resources of participants so they can create new ideas and strategies together. When that happens, the way the group thinks about problems and the way it addresses problems are often very different from where any of the participants started out.

By explaining the need for this kind of group process to achieve the three proximal outcomes, the model provides further justification for certain process characteristics that have been highlighted in a variety of literatures. Theorists and practitioners interested in such diverse fields as participatory democracy, empowerment education, and health promotion have repeatedly emphasized the importance of meaningful discourse in their work. Unlike sound bites and adversarial confrontations — such as hearings and debates — open, inclusive, and ongoing discussions enable people to discover shared values about what is good for the community and to work out their personal interests in the context of community concerns.[1,8,22,23,38,54,60,62,69,108–110] A key objective of group dialogue is to promote critical thinking — to help people develop a healthy skepticism, skills in weighing information, and a sensitivity to fresh ideas and perspectives.[54,69] Consequently, this kind of dialogue has been cited as having a role to play in every stage of a problem-solving or policy-making process.[75] As in the CHG model, listening, empathy, and a common language have been highlighted as critical characteristics of group discourse.[54,69,75] Participants in a group dialogue need to be able to listen as well as talk, and, as Friere notes, this listening is not the same as conducting a needs assessment.[69] Instead, it is a participatory and ongoing interaction that uncovers issues of emotional and social significance to those involved and enables participants to see a situation from each others' perspectives.[54,69] This level of understanding is only possible if the group develops common meanings so that they are all speaking the same language.[54,111]

The Scope of the Process. While the process characteristics described above are applicable to many different kinds of partnerships and community participation initiatives — including those focusing on a particular problem — the CHG model hypothesizes that communities need collaborative processes that are broad in scope in order to fully achieve the three proximal outcomes and thus rectify the shortcomings that are currently undermining community problem solving. Consistent with the literature on civic problem solving, the model hypothesizes that communities need collaborative processes — like CHG — that are *ongoing and iterative*, include *agenda-setting as well as planning and action*, and focus on *multiple issues and problems*.[22,28,32,38,49,50]

Again, the proximal outcomes in the model help to explain why these particular process characteristics are important. Collaborative processes with an agenda-setting capacity have a greater potential to empower people than partnerships that focus on a predetermined problem because they enable participants to identify, and draw attention to, additional problems they care about that might otherwise be overlooked. A multi-issue focus also promotes empowerment because it enables participants in a collaborative process to leverage the relationships and skills they develop in addressing one problem toward the solution of others.

The scope of a collaborative process has implications for synergy as well as empowerment. For example, the participants in a process like CHG — which deals with multiple factors and problems related to community health — are able to see a "bigger picture" and take more comprehensive actions than the participants in a categorical partnership. Rather than considering environmental, social, economic, and medical problems in isolation, they can appreciate how policies, programs, and services in these different areas relate to each other, and can reinforce each other, in efforts to improve community health.

Leadership and Management

Ultimately, the success of any community collaboration depends on the way it is run. The CHG model is illuminating in this regard because it hypothesizes that leadership and management influence the success of a community collaboration by determining who is involved in the process, how participants are involved, and the scope of the process. These process characteristics, in turn, determine the extent to which a collaboration can achieve the three proximal outcomes in the model — individual empowerment, bridging social ties, and synergy — and thus strengthen community problem solving and community health. Leadership and management have been linked, conceptually, to all of the proximal and distal outcomes in the model.[26,95,112] In empirical work, leadership and certain aspects of management have been shown to be closely correlated with the ability of collaborations to create synergy and to solve community-level problems.[105,112] The process characteristics in the model explain *how* leadership and management affect these outcomes. Moreover, they provide a useful lens for *identifying important attributes* of leadership and management.

Building on the growing body of literature on collaborative leadership and democratic management, as well as the experiences of the sites in the CHG workgroup, the model hypothesizes that special kinds of leadership and management are required to achieve the critical characteristics of a collaborative problem-solving process. This type of leadership and management is very different than what is needed to coordinate services or to run a program or organization. One difference relates to the number and mind-set of the people involved. Rather than having one person "run the show," successful community collaborations often involve a variety of people in the provision of leadership, in both formal and informal capacities.[105,112] Going further, the people who seem to be most successful do not function as traditional leaders and administrators — who tend to have a narrow range of expertise, are used to being in control, have their own vision of what should be done, and relate to the people they work with as subordinates rather than as peers. Instead, community collaborations appear to benefit from having leaders and staff who believe deeply in the capacity of diverse people and organizations to work together to identify, understand, and solve community problems. These kinds of individuals understand and appreciate different perspectives, are able to bridge diverse cultures, and are comfortable sharing ideas, resources, and power.[95,112–115]

Another difference relates to what the leadership and management of a community collaboration need to do. The CHG model hypothesizes that in order to achieve the critical characteristics of a collaborative process, the leaders and staff of a community collaboration need to play certain roles and carry out certain functions. Below, we operationalize this aspect of the model by describing the particular roles and functions that appear to be required to (1) promote broad and active participation, (2) assure broad-based influence and control, (3) facilitate productive group dynamics, and (4) extend the scope of the process.

Promote Broad and Active Participation. The CHG model hypothesizes that community collaborations need a diverse group of leaders who come from the community and that a key role of these leaders is to build broad-based involvement in the process.[58,112] To accomplish this objective, the leaders need to continually get out into the community to see how people perceive the process, to establish new relationships, and to identify and engage new and diverse participants. Rather than convincing people in the community to support or "buy into" the process, the purpose of this outreach is to make people aware of the process and to be sure that the process is a valuable resource for them. Equally important, the leaders need to work with current participants to identify and modify attitudes that lead to "filtering" — the intentional or unintentional exclusion of certain kinds of people or organizations from the process. For example, the training and socialization of some professionals involved in the collaboration may create "blinders" that make it difficult for them to appreciate the limitations of their own expertise or the value of combining that expertise with the knowledge and skills of other people in the community.[99]

The model also hypothesizes that the management of a collaborative process has important roles to play in promoting broad and active involvement. For example, to make it feasible for people to be involved, the collaboration needs to provide orientation and mentoring for new participants and minimize the logistical barriers that some people face. In workgroup sites, this objective has been achieved by offering participants a variety of ways to be involved, by holding meetings at convenient places and times, by providing transportation and child care, by serving meals and refreshments, and by encouraging organizational partners to make participation part of their representatives' job descriptions.

Another function of management is to optimize the way participants are involved. At a practical level, this means recognizing and making use of the assets that each participant brings to the collaboration, matching the roles and responsibilities of participants to their particular interests and skills, and running the collaboration in a way that makes good use of participants' financial and in-kind resources and time.[95,102,116,117] It also means paying attention to the relative benefits and drawbacks that each participant experiences.[113,118–120] Management strategies that workgroup sites have used in this regard include asking participants what they want and need from the process, trying to realize the particular benefits that participants seek, minimizing the drawbacks associated with the process, and giving participants credit for the collaboration's accomplishments. To optimize the involvement of organizational participants, relationships often need to be established at multiple levels, for example, by entering into agreements with the board of the organization, by involving chief executives in making organizational commitments, and by involving organizational staff in the collaboration's activities and projects.

Assure Broad-Based Influence and Control. Experience suggests that broad-based community influence and control is the most critical characteristic of a collaborative problem-solving process and the one that is most difficult to achieve. The potential for domination is a continual and challenging issue for community collaborations because while powerful people and organizations *need* to be involved in the process, they often have their own agenda and are used to being in control.[23,40,48,56] The CHG model hypothesizes that the leadership and management of a collaboration need to play critical roles to prevent these powerful participants from having undue influence that compromises the integrity of the collaborative process.

To assure that everyone involved in the process participates on an equal footing, the leadership of a collaboration needs to treat powerful participants — including staff and content experts — like everyone else and use norms, discussion, and peer pressure to prevent powerful participants from taking control. To help participants in different tiers of the social hierarchy see each other as peers, the leaders needs to continually highlight the value of different kinds of knowledge and contributions.

The model hypothesizes that a democratic approach to management plays an important role in preventing domination.[48,121] A key management strategy in this regard is to involve a broad and diverse array of participants in all decision making. Another is to make all of the leaders, staff, lead agencies, and fiscal agents formally accountable to the decision-making body of the collaboration rather than to their own employer or board. A democratically managed collaboration diffuses power among participants by having different organizational partners assume fiscal responsibility for different project grants. It also uses a variety of strategies to prevent powerful participants from dominating meetings and activities — for example, by making sure all participants are kept up to date and receive information at the same time, by involving a broadly representative group of participants in creating meeting agendas, by making sure that the minutes of meetings provide a complete and accurate record of what transpired, and by not allowing any small group of participants to reinterpret and refine decisions that the full group has already made. Another, and critically important, role of management is to help the collaboration develop a diversified resource base, including commitments of both in-kind and financial resources from a broad array of participants. When a collaborative process is not dependent on one or a few organizations for all or most of its support, it is much less of a "set-up" for domination.

Facilitate Productive Group Dynamics. The CHG model hypothesizes that community collaborations need strong "facilitative leadership" to enable their diverse participants to engage in meaningful discourse and combine their knowledge, skills, and resources.[58] The more successful a collaboration is in engaging a broad and diverse array of participants — who often do not know each other and are skeptical of each others' motivations — the more this kind of leadership is required.

The leadership of a collaboration fosters a meaningful and productive group process by creating an environment that values listening as well as speaking, honors and respects different kinds of knowledge and points of view, promotes the development of a jargon-free language, makes participants feel comfortable expressing their ideas, and combines what different people know. While little empirical work has been done to identify exactly what the leaders of community collaborations need to do in order to create such an environment, a number of practical ideas have come out of the experiences of sites in the CHG workgroup and other collaborations.

The model hypothesizes that one role — of both leadership and management — is to make sure that enough time is allotted for the group process. It is very difficult, if not impossible, to create a robust group dynamic if participants meet only for an hour or two, three or four times per year. In addition, the leadership needs to help diverse participants get to know each other in both formal and informal ways. What participants learn in these encounters often runs counter to their previous assumptions. Leaders can use this new knowledge to help participants acknowledge their past history and relationships so they can move beyond them.

Another important role of leadership is to give meaningful voice to participants. Through the use of structured exercises, for example, leaders help participants appreciate the value of listening and give them practice doing so. Variants of the nominal group process can be used to assure that everyone has an opportunity to speak. By welcoming new ideas and by responding to ideas in nonjudgmental ways, leaders encourage reticent participants to join in the discussion. To help the group develop a language that everyone understands, leaders make participants aware of when they are using jargon and ask them to define the meaning of terms that are unclear to others or seem to be contributing to disagreements. Leaders also foster voice by encouraging participants to communicate their ideas in ways that are most comfortable for them — for example, through story telling, drawings, and photography.

Going beyond giving people voice, the model hypothesizes that leaders need to stimulate the people involved in a community collaboration to be creative and look at things differently. In addition, a key leadership role is to relate and synthesize the knowledge of diverse participants so the group can create new ideas and understanding — that no single participant had before — and combine their complementary skills and resources to carry out effective and feasible actions. Enabling a diverse group of participants to bring their knowledge, skills, and resources together in this way may be one of the most difficult roles that leaders of collaborations need to play.

Extend the Scope of the Process. Communities need collaborative processes that are broad in scope in order to fully rectify current shortcomings in problem solving. The CHG model hypothesizes that the roles of leadership and management become more complex when a collaborative process includes agenda setting as well as planning and action and when it focuses on multiple issues and problems.

Extending the scope of the process is challenging for the leadership of a collaboration because the group of participants that needs to be engaged and work together is more diverse, the "picture" these participants need to see is bigger, the interrelationships they need to appreciate are more complex, and the strategies they need to develop and implement are more comprehensive. From a management perspective, collaborations that are broader in scope are more challenging because they have more group processes to support and more projects and programs to run.

Due to the paucity of empirical and conceptual work in this area, it is difficult to identify exactly what the leadership and management of a collaboration need to do to broaden the scope of a collaborative process. Nonetheless, the model makes some hypotheses based on the experiences of the sites in the CHG workgroup. For one, the leadership should extend the scope of a collaborative problem-solving process incrementally — building on, and connecting, what the collaboration has already done. Second, to support agenda setting, as well as planning and action, group processes often need to be established at multiple levels (for example, in neighborhoods and boroughs as well as the city-wide level). Third, to help participants appreciate and benefit from interrelationships, the management needs to create functional connections that not only link the various group processes to each other, but also link the action projects that come out of these group processes to the community-wide problem-solving effort. In workgroup sites this objective has been accomplished by creating project task teams that are headed by members of the community-wide collaborative process and that report back to it, by inviting participants in local problem-solving processes to become members of the community-wide process, and by using community-wide meetings to explore how local and community-wide efforts can support each other. Finally, to build local and community-wide capacity for broad-based problem solving, the management needs to provide current and potential participants with training and technical assistance.

IMPLICATIONS FOR RESEARCH, PRACTICE, AND POLICY

The CHG model brings together a broad array of practical experience, as well as conceptual and empirical work from multiple fields, and it organizes this information in a new and coherent way. The product is a theoretical road map that lays out the pathways by which broadly participatory processes lead to more effective community problem solving and to improvements in community health. The explication of these pathways provides an operational definition of collaborative problem solving (Table 1). The CHG model is unique in that it represents the first time that empowerment, social ties, and synergy have been considered together in the context of collaborative problem solving. Moreover, prior to the development of this model, neither the characteristics of the collaborative process nor the leadership and management that undergird these characteristics had been considered in relation to all three of these proximal outcomes.

Although the model was developed to explain a particular kind of collaborative problem-solving process — CHG — its applicability is considerably broader. The purpose of CHG is to enable diverse people and organizations to work together on an ongoing basis to identify, understand, and solve multiple problems that have an impact on community health. While the model hypothesizes that multi-issue collaborations with an agenda-setting capacity are needed to fully rectify current shortcomings with community problem solving, most aspects of the model are relevant to collaborations with a narrower scope, such as time-limited partnerships dealing with a particular problem. Because the pathways are general in nature, the model is not limited to collaborations that are dealing with health issues. Indeed, the model explains a common observation of people involved in community participation initiatives — that a broadly participatory collaborative process can be health-promoting in itself, even if the collaboration is not focusing on community health problems.[54] In addition, since the critical characteristics of the process can be realized in many different ways, depending on the unique circumstances of the local environment, the model is not limited to any particular kind of community context. This geographic and sociodemographic applicability has been demonstrated in the communities in the CHG workgroup. Coming from all parts of the country, these communities include cities of various sizes, suburban "bedroom" communities, rural areas, and frontier regions, and they are inhabited by different population groups. The model not only resonates with these diverse communities; it provides them with a framework for identifying and dealing with the particular challenges they face and for establishing locally tailored structures to support their collaborative processes.

TABLE 1

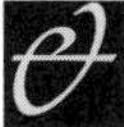

EXPLICATION OF THE MODEL OF COMMUNITY HEALTH GOVERNANCE

COMMUNITY HEALTH

The extent to which people in a community are able to realize their aspirations, satisfy their needs, and cope with their environment.

COLLABORATIVE PROBLEM SOLVING

The ability of people and organizations in the community to work together constructively to identify, understand, and solve complex community-level problems.

- *Current shortcomings in community problem solving*: (1) politics of interest groups; (2) eroding sense of community; (3) limited involvement of community residents

PROXIMAL OUTCOMES

What a collaborative process needs to accomplish, in the short term, in order to be effective in solving community-level problems and improving community health.

- *Individual empowerment*: the ability of people to make decisions and have control over forces that affect their lives
- *Bridging social ties*: relationships and networks that (1) bring people together across society's dividing lines; (2) build trust and a sense of community; and (3) enable people to provide each other with various kinds of support
- *Synergy*: the breakthroughs in thinking and action that are produced when a collaborative process successfully combines the complementary knowledge, skills, and resources of a group of participants

CRITICAL CHARACTERISTICS OF THE PROCESS

Attributes that a collaborative process needs to have in order to achieve the three proximal outcomes.

- *Who is involved*: a broad and diverse array of people and organizations, including people directly affected by problems
- *How participants are involved*: (1) participation is feasible; (2) the process is designed and run by its diverse participants; (3) a broad array of participants are actively involved on an equal footing in all phases of problem solving; (4) the process enables participants to talk to, learn from, and work with each other
- *The scope of the process*: (1) ongoing and iterative; (2) includes agenda-setting as well as planning and action; (3) focuses on multiple issues and problems

LEADERSHIP AND MANAGEMENT

What the *shared* leadership and management of a collaborative process need to do in order to achieve the critical characteristics of the process.

- *Promote broad and active participation*: (1) make the process a valuable resource for participants; (2) modify attitudes that lead to "filtering"; (3) provide orientation and mentoring; (4) address logistical barriers; (5) match roles/responsibilities to participants' interests/skills; (6) make good use of participants' resources and time; (7) maximize benefits/minimize drawbacks; (8) relate to organizational participants at multiple levels; (9) give participants credit for the collaboration's accomplishments

(*Continued*)

TABLE 1 (Continued)

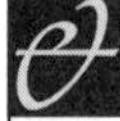

Explication of the Model of Community Health Governance

- *Assure broad-based influence and control*: (1) involve a broad and diverse array of participants in all decision making; (2) make all leaders, staff, lead agencies, and fiscal agents formally accountable to the decision-making body of the collaborative process; (3) develop a diversified resource-base, including commitments of financial and in-kind resources from many different participants; (4) prevent powerful participants from dominating meetings and activities; (5) highlight the value of different kinds of knowledge and contributions
- *Facilitate productive group dynamics*: (1) make sure there *is* a group process and that enough time is allotted for it; (2) provide a variety of ways for participants to get to know each other; (3) promote meaningful discourse by giving everyone an opportunity to speak, encouraging different ideas and points of view, helping participants appreciate the value of listening, helping the group develop a commonly understood language, and encouraging people to communicate their ideas in comfortable ways; (4) relate and synthesize the knowledge/skills/resources of different participants so the group, as a whole, can be creative and look at things differently and develop understanding/take actions that go beyond anyone's preconceived notions
- *Extend the scope of the process*: (1) build incrementally; (2) establish group processes at multiple levels; (3) make functional connections across levels and between planning and action projects; (4) provide training and technical assistance

The multidisciplinary scope of the CHG model, and its broad applicability, are important because these features are at the heart of the model's potential usefulness in addressing concerns and challenges related to broad-based community collaboration. As we mentioned at the beginning of this paper, thousands of communities — in the United States and internationally — are working to expand participation in some aspect of community decision making and problem solving. Yet, most of these communities are finding this objective very difficult to achieve, and many of the government agencies and foundations that support community partnerships and participation initiatives are looking for ways to get more out of their investment. The CHG model has the potential to overcome some of the fragmentation of effort that is currently compromising success by providing a platform that makes it easier for people from different contexts, content areas, academic disciplines, and initiatives to talk to, and learn from, each other. More specifically, the model can help the broad array of people interested in community collaboration answer the following policy questions:

- Does broad participation actually strengthen community problem solving? If so, for what kinds of problems is this approach best suited?
- What does it take to successfully involve a broad array of people and organizations in community problem solving? If communities, policy makers, and private foundations want to promote this kind of collaboration, what do they need to do to make it work?

Below, we describe how the CHG model can contribute to the research that is needed to answer both the basic effectiveness question and the applied "how to" question. We then compare the "how to" laid out in the model with current practice, exploring the implications of these differences for the people and organizations who participate in, and fund, community collaborations.

Using the Model to Strengthen Research

There is no doubt that some communities have solved problems — including [seemingly] intractable ones — using broad-based collaboration. Nonetheless, in spite of these successes, collaborative problem solving is not mainstream. In fact, as Norris has noted, this approach is "below the radar screen" for most pundits and policy makers.[28] Why is this so? For one, success does not necessarily mean that the community could not have solved the problem just as well using more traditional, noncollaborative approaches. Consequently, it is not clear that the additional time and effort involved in collaboration is warranted. Going further, many communities are not successful in their collaborative efforts. Yet, because it is so difficult to engage a broad array of people and organizations in a collaborative problem-solving process, it is hard to tell if the problem is with the collaborative approach, *per se*, or with the way the collaborative problem-solving process has been implemented.

These concerns reflect two important limitations of the current evidence. The first limitation is that most of the research that has been done on broad-based community collaboration has not been comparative. We are not aware of any studies that have compared the effectiveness of collaborative and noncollaborative approaches in solving similar kinds of problems, and very few studies have compared successful and unsuccessful endeavors. When studies look only at successful cases, as is commonly done, it is not possible to be sure that they are really identifying the attributes needed for success, because the same attributes could have been present in unsuccessful cases.

Another limitation with the current evidence is that most research studies have not been based on a comprehensive theory of change.* Much of the research has looked at collaborative problem solving from a limited perspective (focusing, for example, on leadership, empowerment, or synergy). Such studies may be missing important aspects of the collaborative process or what the process needs to accomplish in order to solve problems. In addition, no research study has tested a comprehensive, step-by-step pathway for collaborative problem solving. Without such a pathway, it is not possible to distinguish communities that are "on the right track" and would benefit from additional support from those that would not. Moreover, in unsuccessful cases, it is not possible to determine what caused the community's lack of success or what the community can do to rectify the situation.

---

* The terminology used to describe a causal model differs across disciplines; what we are calling a "theory of change" has also been called a "theory of action" or a "logic model."

The CHG model can help address these limitations in several ways. First, and perhaps most important, the multidisciplinary underpinnings of the model provide a platform for bringing an otherwise disparate group of researchers together to combine their complementary knowledge and methodologies. Second, the model provides these researchers with a comprehensive and testable theory of change to jump-start their discussion. The model's pathway explains the "how to" of collaborative problem solving — it describes what the leadership and management of a collaboration need to do to achieve the critical characteristics of the process, and it lays out the proximal outcomes that the collaborative process needs to achieve in order to be effective in solving problems. Building on a large body of work in numerous fields, this pathway incorporates a broad array of variables at multiple levels, and the importance of these variables is justified by the model's theory. The model also provides researchers with a strong foundation for measurement. Valid measures have already been developed for a number of the variables in the model, including aspects of leadership and management, individual empowerment, and synergy.[48,105] Widely used measures of social networks and social support provide a basis for the measurement of social ties.[122,123] The model facilitates the development of additional measures by clarifying and operationalizing certain concepts, and by providing a framework for identifying and leveraging relevant conceptual work.

A third way that the model can help address the limitations of current evidence is by supporting comparative research. The model is amenable to testing through a comparative case study design. For example, a longitudinal study of communities attempting to solve a similar problem in different ways could be used to test the degree to which successful problem solving is related to the achievement of the critical process characteristics and proximal outcomes in the model. The applicability of the model to various problems could be explored by comparing the ability of communities that have achieved these process characteristics and proximal outcomes to solve different kinds of problems. Of note, the model may also be amenable to testing through a randomized controlled trial. Building on the pathways in the model, it may be possible to develop an intervention that achieves specific process characteristics and proximal outcomes, yet respects the interactive and evolving nature of community collaboration.

Validating the model — or a variant of it — will help to answer the key policy questions related to broad-based community collaboration. The ability to distinguish communities that are, and are not, able to achieve the critical process characteristics and proximal outcomes in the model will make it easier to document the overall effectiveness of broad-based collaboration in solving community problems. A validated pathway will make a substantial contribution to the "how to" question and facilitate evaluation by demonstrating what a collaboration needs to do, and accomplish in the short term, in order to be successful in solving problems.[19,124] Because the pathway identifies markers of success that can be measured along the way (for example, the critical characteristics of the process reflect the effectiveness of leadership and management; the three proximal outcomes — individual empowerment, bridging social ties, and synergy — reflect the effectiveness of the collaborative process), it will support the development of evidence-based evaluation tools and practice guides that can help communities assess how well they are doing and take early and effective corrective action.

Comparing the Model with Current Practice

The need to conduct the research described above becomes even more compelling when one compares the "how to" laid out in the model with currently used approaches to community collaboration. The participants in the CHG workgroup have been struck by how different the model is from much of mainstream practice. Pending validation of the model, it is not possible to be sure what approach is best. Nonetheless, the CHG model warrants serious consideration because it is based on a lot of practical experience — both positive and negative — and some of the relationships in the model have been documented by empirical work. Moreover, current approaches do not seem to be working well in many communities; people directly involved in broad-based collaborations, and organizations that fund community partnerships and participation initiatives, are having substantial difficulty achieving the results they seek.

The differences between the model and current practice suggest that some people and organizations may be inadvertently compromising their own success by the way they are going about collaboration. Below, we illustrate this supposition by focusing on three important aspects of practice: (1) community engagement, (2) group discourse, and (3) the role of government in collaborative problem solving. The insights that the CHG model provides suggest specific ways that the participants and funders of community collaborations might be able to strengthen their efforts. Moving in this direction will not be easy, however. Communities in the CHG workgroup have identified a number of barriers to implementing the model, relating to the negative past experiences of community members with partnerships and participation initiatives; professional socialization and culture; constraining funding requirements; and insufficient incentives, technical assistance, and training. Ultimately, all of these issues will need to be addressed to realize the full potential of community collaboration to solve complex problems.

Community Engagement. One practical benefit of the CHG model is that it defines the otherwise ambiguous phrase "meaningful community engagement" in terms of who needs to be involved in a collaborative process, and how they need to be involved, in order to strengthen the ability of the community to solve complex problems. Broad-based influence is central to this definition. According to the model, if a collaborative process seeks to engage the community in a meaningful way, it needs to actively involve diverse people and organizations on an equal footing in all phases of problem solving — identifying and framing problems, understanding the causes of problems and the context in which they occur, and developing and carrying out strategies to address problems. The model hypothesizes that this degree of influence is a prerequisite for empowering community members, for creating the breakthroughs in thinking and action that are needed to solve complex problems, and for developing a sufficiently broad sense of community ownership and commitment to sustain collaborative efforts over time. The model also hypothesizes that broad-based influence facilitates the recruitment and retention of community members by making participation in the collaboration worthwhile.

In contrast to the model, both anecdotal experience and concerns raised in the literature suggest that community members do not currently have this kind of influence in many partnerships and participation initiatives.[23,48,125] As Robertson and Minkler note, when professionals take the lead, community members are often treated as objects of concern or sources of data rather than as peers in problem solving.[22] Moreover, professionals often determine the language that people use to discuss issues, the paradigm they use to frame and understand issues, and the "boundaries around the domain of issues that will be considered germane."[126]

One illustration of current practice — very common in the health arena — is a community partnership in which a lead agency is funded to carry out a predetermined program. In this kind of collaboration, virtually all of the thinking and planning are done by the funder and the lead agency, which is usually a local hospital, health department, academic center, or community-based organization. Typically, the funder identifies the problem that needs to be addressed, and the lead agency, following guidelines from the funder, develops an intervention to address the problem. While community residents and other community stakeholders are often asked to provide the lead agency with feedback and input about its plans (for example, advice about how to tailor a program to a particular neighborhood or group), their primary role is to help the lead agency obtain community "buy-in" and to provide the additional skills and resources that are needed to carry out the predetermined program. So, for instance, they are often engaged to provide the lead agency with access to a target audience it currently does not reach, greater credibility for its message and program, and/or cosponsorship of programs and events. In the context of the CHG model, it is not surprising that many of these partnership initiatives are not as successful as they would like to be in recruiting community members, solving problems, or sustaining interventions over time. The model suggests that it may not be possible to deal with these challenges unless the partnerships, and the organizations that fund them, make substantial changes in the way community members are engaged.

Group Discourse. The CHG model hypothesizes that in order to solve complex community problems, a collaborative process needs to promote ongoing, meaningful discourse among a diverse group (or groups) of people. This kind of discourse — in which participants from different backgrounds get together on a regular basis to listen to each other, talk with each other, and influence each other — is at the heart of collaborative problem solving. Without it, a collaborative process cannot achieve individual empowerment, bridging social ties, or synergy.

In spite of the importance of group discourse in the model, our experience suggests that many community partnerships around the country are not structured in a way that makes such discourse possible. Some of these partnerships do not have any group process at all. One common example is a partnership that is organized like the spokes of a wheel, with one person or organization at the hub. In this type of arrangement, the leader of the partnership talks to each of the other participants, but these participants do not engage in discourse with each other. In other partnerships, a group process exists, but it involves a small, and often homogeneous, group of people. The core group may use focus groups, surveys, and other forms of data collection to obtain other community perspectives. But this communication goes only one way, so there is no opportunity for the core group and the people who provide information to discuss issues with each other. The model suggests that while these kinds of partnerships may be able to coordinate services or carry out a predetermined program, they are unlikely to be able to understand and solve complex community problems.

Going beyond structural issues, many community collaborations appear to lack the leadership that is needed to promote meaningful discourse. The model hypothesizes that without the right kind of leadership, even collaborations that bring a diverse group of people and organizations together on an ongoing basis will not achieve meaningful group discourse. Along these lines, we are aware of numerous partnerships in which certain participants have a seat at the table, but have little or no voice. Even when all participants are given an opportunity to speak — and other participants listen to what they say — understanding is often compromised by preconceived notions or the use of jargon, and breakthroughs in thinking are often not achieved because the discourse is constrained by a narrow professional paradigm or because the knowledge and ideas of different participants are not connected. While this type of partnership may be successful in empowering its participants, it is unlikely to create the bridging social ties and synergy that are needed to solve complex problems.

Role of Government in Collaborative Problem Solving. Rectifying current shortcomings in community problem solving clearly requires broader, and more active, citizen involvement in the work of government. Toward that end, over the last 40 years, federal, state, and local government agencies have created a variety of initiatives to engage local residents and organizations in carrying out assessments, implementing government programs, reforming government services, and working collaboratively to address government-identified problems. Unfortunately, both community residents and government agencies have been dissatisfied with the experience and results of many of these initiatives.[1,2,35,106,127] Consequently, there have been repeated calls for new and better ways to engage the community in government activities.[1,2,3,35,38,104] While the insights discussed above — related to community engagement and group discourse — can help government agencies as well as private-sector organizations be more effective in structuring their community partnerships and participation initiatives, there is an even more fundamental implication of the CHG model for the role of government in collaborative problem solving. In addition to broadening community involvement in their own work, government agencies and elected officials need to participate in collaborative problem-solving processes that reside in civil society.

Although the CHG model does not address the roles of any particular group, organization, or sector *per se*, the critical characteristics of the collaborative process, coupled with the experiences of the workgroup sites, suggest that it may not be feasible or appropriate for a broad-based community problem-solving process like CHG to be housed in, or run by, government. One reason is that the CHG model is a very different approach to community collaboration than what most government agencies are used to. Instead of any single participant — such as a government agency — being in control, a broad array of people and organizations in the community decide what the process focuses on and how the work gets done. The broad scope of the process is another issue. The collaborative process delineated in the model is a comprehensive one that encompasses a wide range of problems, related to social and environmental policy, economic development, public health, and medical care. Addressing such problems goes beyond the jurisdiction or control of any single government agency. Even when a government agency *wants* to promote this kind of collaborative problem-solving process, it is difficult, if not impossible, for the agency to be viewed at the same level as other participants if it manages the process or is its dominant funder. Moreover, as Hollar points out, low-income residents are often intimidated by government; they have "an absolute fear of speaking out lest they lose all benefits."[106]

The need for "neutral" or "safe" spaces in civic society to support broad-based collaborative problem solving has been highlighted in the literature.[2,22,38] Yet, rather than duplicating or replacing the role of government in community problem solving, processes in civil society are seen as complementary.[38,49] By providing a venue in civil society where people can engage in discourse that goes beyond ideological debates, processes like CHG can function as a valuable resource for government. In one workgroup site, for example, the process contributed to the development of an innovative, broadly supported strategy for dealing with an intractable solid waste problem, which was subsequently enacted into law by the local legislature. In other sites, the process is enhancing the ability of local health departments to identify problems that people in the community care about, to connect and work with other government agencies and community-based organizations (so they can have more of an impact on the broad determinants of health), and to accomplish more than would otherwise be possible on their limited budgets. Although some local health departments have been concerned about the potential for a process like CHG to privatize public health, so far that has not happened. None of the local health departments in workgroup sites has given up any of its functions when it participates in CHG; in fact, in two of the sites, new regional governmental public health entities are being created.

Ultimately, it appears that two complementary forms of collaboration are required to strengthen the ability of communities to solve complex problems — one in which the community participates in the work of government and another in which government participates in community-driven processes in civil society. While we are far from knowing how these collaborative processes can best be implemented or aligned, there is a tremendous amount of experience and scholarly work to learn from. By providing a framework that synthesizes much of this knowledge, and by establishing a multidisciplinary platform for bringing diverse practitioners, scholars, and policy makers together, the CHG model can promote the kinds of coordinated efforts that are needed to move us forward.

ACKNOWLEDGMENTS

The authors are grateful to the W. K. Kellogg Foundation for its generous support of this work, and to Quinton Baker, Charles Bruner, David Chrislip, Barbara Israel, and Alonzo Plough, whose ideas and suggestions substantially strengthened the paper. In addition, we are indebted to the representatives of the Turning Point partnerships that have participated in the CHG workgroup — Robert Berke, Lynn Delevan, Joy Guarino, and Peggy Szczukowski from Chautauqua County, NY; Marvin Apple, Douglas Nelson, and Hickory Starr from Cherokee County, OK; Jerry Andrews and Shelith Hansbro from Decatur, IL; Michael Andry, Helen Kitzman, Shelia Webb, and Loyce Wright from New Orleans, LA; Eve Cagan, Sandra Page Cook, Hermansu Mangal, and Sandy Trujillo from New York City, NY; Jack Green, Melissa Janulewicz, and Roger Wiese from North Central Nebraska; Sherry Dunphy, Patrick Finnerty, Jared Florance, and Stephanie Franklin from Prince William, VA; Althea Buckingham, Nancy Cavanaugh, and Julia Smith from Sitka, AK; and Jane D'Ovidio, Richard Silverberg, and Larry Turns from Twin Rivers, NH. Their aspirations and experiences — both positive and negative — guided the literature review and provided the grounded basis for the CHG model.

REFERENCES

1. Box RC. *Citizen Governance: Leading American Communities into the 21st Century*. Thousand Oaks, CA: Sage Publications; 1998.
2. King CS, Stivers C. *Government Is Us: Public Administration in an Anti-government Era*. Thousand Oaks, CA: Sage Publications; 1998.
3. Denhardt RB, Denhardt JV. The new public service: Serving rather than steering. *Public Adm Rev.* 2000; 60:549–559.
4. McGinnis JM, Foege WH. Actual causes of death in the United States. *JAMA*. 1993;270:2207–2212.
5. Goodman RM, Wandersman A. FORECAST: A formative approach to evaluating community coalitions and community-based initiatives. *J Community Psychol.* 1994; CSAP Special Issue:6–25.
6. Butterfoss FD, Goodman RM, Wandersman A. Community coalitions for prevention and health promotion: Factors predicting satisfaction, participation, and planning. *Health Educ Q*. 1996;23:65–79.
7. Lasker RD, Committee on Medicine and Public Health. *Medicine and Public Health: The Power of Collaboration*. Chicago: Health Administration Press; 1997.
8. Israel BA, Schulz AJ, Parker EA, Becker AB. Review of community-based research: Assessing partnership approaches to improve public health. *Ann Rev Public Health*. 1998;19:173–202.
9. Mitchell SM, Shortell SM. The governance and management of effective community health partnerships: A typology for research, policy and practice. *Milbank Q*. 2000;78:241–289.

10. Gray B. *Collaborating: Finding Common Ground for Multiparty Problems*. 1st ed. San Francisco: Jossey-Bass; 1989.

11. Mattesich PW, Monsey BR. *Collaboration: What Makes It Work*? St. Paul, MN: Amherst H. Wilder Foundation; 1992.

12. Zuckerman HS, Kaluzny AD, Ricketts TC. Alliances in health care: What we know, what we think we know, and what we should know. *Health Care Manage Rev*. 1994;20:54–64.

13. Richardson WC, Allegrante JP. Shaping the future of health through global partnerships. In: Koop CE, Pearson CE, Schwarz MR, eds. *Critical Issues in Global Health*. San Francisco: Jossey-Bass; 2000:375–383.

14. Bazzoli GJ, Stein R, Alexander JA, Conrad DA, Sofaer A, Shortell S. Public-private collaboration in health and human service delivery: Evidence from community partnerships. *Milbank Q*. 1997;75:533–561.

15. Fawcett SB, Lewis RK, Paine-Andrews A, Francisco VT, Richter KP, Williams ED, Copple B. Evaluating community coalitions for prevention of substance abuse: The case of Project Freedom. *Health Educ Behav*. 1997;24:812–828.

16. Bruce TA, McKane SU, eds. *Community-Based Public Health: A Partnership Model*. Washington, DC: American Public Health Association; 2000.

17. Kreuter MW, Lezin NA, Young LA. Evaluating community-based collaborative mechanisms: Implications for practitioners. *Health Promotion Pract*. 2000;1:49–63.

18. Galea S, Factor SH, Bonner S, et al. Collaboration among community members, local health service providers, and researchers in an urban research center in Harlem, New York. *Pub Health Rep*. 2001;116:530–539.

19. Chaskin RJ. *Lessons Learned from the Implementation of the Neighborhood and Family Initiative: A Summary of Findings*. Chicago: Chapin Hall Center for Children; 2001.

20. Wandersman A, Goodman RM, Butterfoss RD. Understanding coalitions and how they operate. In: Minkler M, ed. *Community Organizing and Community Building for Health*. New Brunswick, NJ: Rutgers University Press; 1997: 261–277.

21. Okubo D, Weidman K. Engaging the community in core public health functions. *Natl Civ Rev*. 2000;89:309–325.

22. Swain D. Linking civic engagement and community improvement: A practitioner perspective on the communities movement. *Natl Civ Rev*. 2001;90:319–334.

23. Robertson A, Minkler M. New health promotion movement: A critical examination. *Health Educ Q*. 1994;21:295–312.

24. Kegler MC, Twiss JM, Look V. Assessing community change at multiple levels: The genesis of an evaluation framework for the California Healthy Cities Project. *Health Edu Behav*. 2000;27:760–779.

25. Roussos ST, Fawcett SB. A review of collaborative partnerships as a strategy for improving community health. *Ann Rev Public Health*. 2000;21:369–402.

26. Shortell SM, Zukoski AP, Alexander JA, et al. Evaluating partnerships for community health improvement: Tracking the footprints. *J Health Polit Policy Law*. 2002;27:49–91.

27. Kenney DS. *Arguing About Consensus: Examining the Case Against Western Watershed Initiatives and Other Collaborative Groups Active in Natural Resources Management*. Boulder, CO: Natural Resources Law Center; 2000.
28. Norris T. Civic gemstones: The emergent communities movement. *Natl Civ Rev*. 2001;90:307–318.
29. Aspen Institute Roundtable on Comprehensive Community Initiatives for Children and Families. *Voices from the Field: Learning from the Early Work of Comprehensive Community Initiatives*. Washington, DC: The Aspen Institute; 1997.
30. Bruner C, Greenberg M, Guy C, Little M, Schorr L, Weiss H. *Funding What Works: Exploring the Role of Research on Effective Programs and Practices in Government Decision-Making*. Des Moines, IA: National Center for Service Integration; 2001.
31. MacFarlane S, Racelis M, Muli-Musiime F. Public health in developing countries. *Lancet*. 2000;356:841–846.
32. Kesler JT, O'Connor D. The American communities movement. *Natl Civ Rev*. 2001;90:295–306.
33. Chang H. *Drawing Strength from Diversity: Effective Services for Children, Youth, and Families*. Oakland, CA: California Tomorrow; 1994.
34. Chrislip DD. American renewal: Reconnecting citizens with public life. *Natl Civ Rev*. 1994;83:26–31.
35. Thomson K, Berry JM, Portney KE. *Kernels of Democracy*. Boston: Lincoln Filene Center at Tufts University; 1994.
36. Chaskin RJ, Garg S. *The Issue of Governance in Neighborhood-Based Initiatives*. Chicago: Chapin Hall Center for Children at the University of Chicago; 1997.
37. Center for the Study of Social Policy. *Creating a Community Agenda: How Governance Partnerships Can Improve Results for Children, Youth, and Families*. Washington, DC: Center for the Study of Social Policy; 1998.
38. National Civic League. *The Civic Index: Measuring Your Community's Civic Health*. 2nd ed. Denver, CO: National Civic League; 1999.
39. Bruner C. *Social Services Systems Reform in Poor Neighborhoods: What We Know and What We Need to Find Out*. Des Moines, IA: National Center for Service Integration; 2000.
40. Fung A. Accountable autonomy: Toward empowered deliberation in Chicago schools and policing. *Polit Soc*. 2001; 29(1).
41. Kato L, Riccio J. *Building New Partnerships for Employment: Collaboration Among Agencies and Public Housing Residents in the JOBS-PLUS Demonstration*. Manpower Demonstration Research Corporation; 2001.
42. Baxter RJ. *What Turning Point Tells Us: Implications for National Policy*. Battle Creek, MI: The W. K. Kellogg Foundation; 2001.
43. Center for the Advancement of Collaborative Strategies in Health. *Turning Point Community Health Governance Workgroup: Creating Community-Driven Structures to Advance Community Health*. New York: The New York Academy of Medicine; 2001.

44. Nicola RM, Berkowitz B, Lafronza V. A turning point for public health. *J Public Health Manag Pract*. 2002;8:4–7.
45. Sabol B. Innovations in collaboration for the public's health through the Turning Point initiative: The W. K. Kellogg Foundation perspective. *J Public Health Manag Pract*. 2002;8:6–12.
46. World Health Organization. A discussion document on the concept and principles of health promotion. *Health Promotion*. 1986;1:73–78.
47. Eisen A. Survey of neighborhood-based, comprehensive community empowerment initiatives. *Health Edu Q*. 1994;21:235–252.
48. Israel BA, Checkoway B, Schulz A, Zimmerman M. Health education and community empowerment: Conceptualizing and measuring perceptions of individual, organizational, and community control. *Health Educ Q*. 1994;21: 149–170.
49. Potapchuk WR, Crocker JP, Schechter WH. The transformative power of governance. *Natl Civ Rev*. 1999;88:217–247.
50. Wilcox R, Knapp A. Building communities that create health. *Public Health Rep*. 2000;115:139–143.
51. Clark NM, Baker EA, Chawla A, Maru M. Sustaining collaborative problem solving: strategies from a study in six Asian countries. *Health Educ Res*. 1993;8:385–402.
52. Dearing JW, Larson SR, Randall LM, Pope RS. Local reinvention of the CDC HIV prevention community planning initiative. *J Community Health*. 1998;23:113–126.
53. Wallis A, Crocker JP, Schechter B. Social capital and community building: Part one. *Natl Civ Rev.* 1998;87:253–271.
54. Cottrell CS. The competent community. In: Kaplan BH, Wilson RN, Leighton AH, eds. *Further Explorations in Social Psychiatry*. New York: Basic Books; 1976: 195–209.
55. O'Connor D, Gates CT. Toward a healthy democracy. *Public Health Rep*. 2000; 115:157–160.
56. Berry JM, Portney KE, Thomson K. *The Rebirth of Urban Democracy*. Washington, DC: The Brookings Institution; 1993.
57. Heaney CA, Israel BA. Social networks and social support. In: Glanz K., Lewis FM, Rimer BK, eds. *Health Behavior and Health Education*. 3rd ed. San Francisco: Jossey-Bass; 2002:185–209.
58. Chrislip DD. *The Collaborative Leadership Fieldbook*. San Francisco: Jossey-Bass; 2002.
59. Chrislip DD. Collaboration: The new leadership. *Health Forum J*. 1995;38(6).
60. Miller H. Reasoning together: Any chance? Paper presented at the annual meeting of the Public Administration Theory Network, University of Leiden, The Netherlands, June 21–23, 2000.
61. McKnight JL. Health and empowerment. *Canadian J Public Health*. 1985; 76:37–38.
62. Putnam RD. *Bowling Alone*. New York: Simon & Schuster; 2000.

63. Macinko J, Starfield B. The utility of social capital in research on health determinants. *Milbank Q*. 2001;79:387–427.
64. Blackwell AG, Colmenar R. Community-building: From local wisdom to public policy. *Public Health Rep*. 2000;115:161–166.
65. McKnight JL, Kretzmann JP. *Mapping Community Capacity*. Evanston, IL: Center for Urban Affairs and Policy Research, Northwestern University; 1992.
66. Thomas J. *Public Participation in Public Decisions*. San Francisco: Jossey-Bass; 1995.
67. Chaskin RJ, Peters C. *Decision Making and Action at the Neighborhood Level: An Exploration of Mechanisms and Processes*. Chicago: Chapin Hall Center for Children; 2000.
68. Rissel C. Empowerment: The holy grail of health promotion? *Health Promot International*. 1994;9:39–47.
69. Freire P. *Education for Critical Consciousness*. New York: Seabury Press; 1973.
70. Wallerstein N. Powerlessness, empowerment, and health: Implications for health promotion programs. *AJHP*. 1992;6:197–206.
71. Zimmerman MA. Psychological empowerment: Issues and illustrations. *Am J Community Psychol*. 1995;23:581–599.
72. Cornell Empowerment Group. Empowerment and family support. *Networking Bulletin*. 1989;1:1–23.
73. Minkler M, Wallerstein N. Improving health through community organization and community building. In: Glanz K, Lewis FM, Rimer BK, eds. *Health Behavior and Health Education: Theory, Research, and Practice*. 2nd ed. San Francisco: Jossey-Bass; 1997:241–269.
74. Rousseau JJ. *The Social Contract* [1762]. Harmondsworth, UK: Penguin; 1968.
75. Barber B. *Strong Democracy: Participatory Politics for a New Age*. Berkeley and Los Angeles: University of California Press; 1984.
76. Morone J. *The Democratic Wish: Popular Participation and the Limits of American Government*. New York: Basic Books; 1990.
77. Schultz R. Aging and control. In: Garber J, Seligman M, eds. *Human Helplessness: Theory and Applications*. New York: Academic Press; 1980:261–277.
78. Rodin J. Aging and health: Effects of the sense of control. *Science*. 1986;233: 1271–1276.
79. Karasek R, Baker D, Marxer F, Ahlbom A, Theorell T. Job decision latitude, job demands, and cardiovascular disease: A prospective study of Swedish men. *Am J Public Health*. 1981;71:694–705.
80. Alfredsson L, Karasek R, Theorell T. Myocardial infarction risk and psychological work environment: An analysis of the male Swedish working force. *Soc Sci Med*. 1982;16:463–476.
81. Heller K. The return to community. *Am J Community Psychol*. 1989;17:1–15.
82. Zimmerman MA. Empowerment theory. In: Rappaport J, Seidman E, eds. *Handbook of Community Psychology*. New York: Kluwer Academic/Plenum Publishers; 2000:43–63.

83. Putnam RD, Leonardi R, Nanetti R. *Making Democracy Work: Civic Traditions in Modern Italy*. Princeton, NJ: Princeton University Press; 1993.
84. Minkler M. Building supportive ties and sense of community among the inner-city elderly: The Tenderloin senior outreach project. *Health Educ Q*. 1985;12: 303–314.
85. Eng E, Parker E. Measuring community competence in the Mississippi delta: The interface between program evaluation and empowerment. *Health Educ Q*. 1994; 21:199–220.
86. Durkheim E. *Suicide* [1897]. New York: The Free Press; 1951.
87. House JS, Landis KR, Umberson D. Social relationships and health. In: Conrad P, Kerns R, eds. *The Sociology of Health and Illness: Critical Perspectives*. 3rd ed. New York: St. Martins Press; 1990:85–94.
88. House JS, Kahn RL. Measures and concepts of social support. In: Cohen S, Syme SL, eds. *Social Support and Health*. Orlando, FL: Academic Press; 1985: 83–108.
89. Israel BA, Rounds KA. Social networks and social support: A synthesis for health educators. *Adv Health Educ Promotion*. 1987;2:311–351.
90. Turner RJ, Turner JB. Social integration and support. In: Aneshensel CS, Phelan JC, eds. *Handbook of the Sociology of Mental Health*. New York: Plenum Publishers; 1999:301–319.
91. Berkman LF. The role of social relations in health promotion. *Psychosom Med*. 1995;57:245–254.
92. Thoits PA. Stress, coping, and social support processes: Where are we? What next? *J Health Soc Behav*. 1995; Extra Issue:53–79.
93. Berkman LF. Assessing the physical health effects of social networks and social support. *Ann Rev Public Health*. 1984;5:413–432.
94. Lin N, Ye X, Ensel WM. Social support and depressed mood: A structural analysis. *J Health Soc Behav*. 1999;40:344–359.
95. Lasker RD, Weiss ES, Miller R. Partnership synergy: A practical framework for studying and strengthening the collaborative advantage. *Milbank Q*. 2001;79: 179–206.
96. Fried BJ, Rundall TG. Managing groups and teams. In: Shortell SM, Kaluzny AD, eds. *Health Care Management: Organization, Design, and Behavior*. 1994; 137–163.
97. Shannon VJ. Partnerships: The foundation for future success. *Canadian J Nurs Adm*. 1998;11:61–76.
98. Taylor-Powell E, Rossing B, Geran J. *Evaluating Collaboratives: Reaching the Potential*. Madison: University of Wisconsin-Extension, Cooperative Extension; 1998.
99. Lasker RD, Weiss ES. Creating partnership synergy: The critical role of community stakeholders. *J Health Human Serv Adm*. In press; 2003.
100. Farmer JD. *The Language of Public Administration*. Tuscaloosa: University of Alabama Press; 1995.
101. McSwite OC. *Legitimacy in Public Administration*. Thousand Oaks, CA: Sage Publications; 1997.

102. Jewiss J, Hasazi S. *Advancing Community Well-Being: A Developmental Perspective of Two Community Partnerships in Vermont*. Burlington: University of Vermont; 1999.
103. Silka L. Paradoxes of partnerships: Reflections on university-community collaborations. In: Kleniewski N, ed. *Research in Politics and Society*. Greenwich, CT: JAI Press; 1999;7:335–359.
104. CDC/ATSDR Committee on Community Engagement. *Principles of Community Engagement*. Atlanta, GA: Centers for Disease Control and Prevention, Public Health Practice Program Office; 1997.
105. Weiss ES, Anderson R, Lasker RD. Making the most of collaboration: Exploring the relationship between partnership synergy and partnership functioning. *Health Edu Behav*. In press; 2002.
106. Hollar D. Challenges of community engagement: Conversations with people in low-income communities in Mississippi. Paper presented at the National Conference of the American Society for Public Administration; 2001.
107. Kingsley GT, McNeely JB, Gibson JO. *Community Building Coming of Age*. Washington, DC: The Urban Institute; 1999.
108. Reich R. *The Power of Public Ideas*. Cambridge, MA: Harvard University Press; 1988.
109. Mansbridge J. Public spirit in political systems. In: Aaron H, ed. *Values and Public Policy*. Washington, DC: Brookings Institution; 1994.
110. Kesler JT. Healthy communities and civil discourse: A leadership opportunity for public health professionals. *Public Health Rep*. 2000;115:238–242.
111. Miles-Polka B. Investment-based business plans for human service delivery: A new model takes shape in Des Moines, Iowa. *Natl Civ Rev*. 2001;90:335–346.
112. Chrislip DD, Larson CE. *Collaborative Leadership*. San Francisco: Jossey-Bass; 1994.
113. Alter C, Hage J. *Organizations Working Together*. Newbury Park, CA: Sage Publications; 1993.
114. McKinney MM, Morrissey JP, Kaluzny AD. Interorganizational exchanges as performance markers in a community cancer network. *Health Serv Res*. 1993;28: 518–539.
115. Weiner BJ, Alexander JA. The challenges of governing public-private community health partnerships. *Health Care Manage Rev*. 1998;23:39–55.
116. Winer M, Ray K. *Collaboration Handbook: Creating, Sustaining, and Enjoying the Journey*. Saint Paul, MN: Amherst H. Wilder Foundation; 1994.
117. Huxham C. Collaboration and collaborative advantage. In: Huxham C, ed. *Creating Collaborative Advantage*. London: Sage Publications; 1996:1–18.
118. Wandersman A, Florin PF, Meier R. Who participates, who does not and why? An analysis of voluntary neighborhood associations in the United States and Israel. *Social Forum*. 1987;2:534–555.
119. Chinman MJ, Anderson CM, Imm PS, Wandersman A, Goodman RM. The perceptions of costs and benefits of high active groups versus low active groups in

community coalitions at different stages in coalition development. *J Community Psychol.* 1996;24:263–274.

120. Goodman RM, Speers MA, McLeroy K, et al. Identifying and defining the dimensions of community capacity to provide a basis for measurement. *Health Educ Behav.* 1998;25:258–278.

121. Minkler M, Thompson M, Bell J, Rose K. Contribution of community involvement to organizational-level empowerment: The federal Healthy Start experience. *Health Educ Behav.* 2001;28:783–807.

122. Heitzmann CA, Kaplan RM. Assessment of methods for measuring social support. *Health Psychol.* 1998;79:75–109.

123. Barrera A. Social support research in community psychology. In: Rappaport J, Seidman E, eds. *Handbook of Community Psychology.* New York: Kluwer Academic/Plenum Publishers; 2000.

124. Gambone MA. Challenges of measurement on community change initiatives. In: Fulbright-Anderson K, Kubish AC, Connell JP, eds. *New Approaches to Evaluating Community Initiatives: Theory, Measurement, and Analysis.* Washington, DC: Aspen Institute; 1999.

125. Sigmond RM. Back to the future: partnerships and coordination for community health. *Front Health Serv Manage.* 1995;11:5–36.

126. Simon BL. Rethinking empowerment. *J. Progressive Hum Services.* 1990;1: 27–39.

127. Arnstein SR. A ladder of citizen participation. *J American Inst Planners.* 1969; 35:216–224.

PART IV

PREPARING FOR TERRORISM: A PUBLIC HEALTH RESPONSE

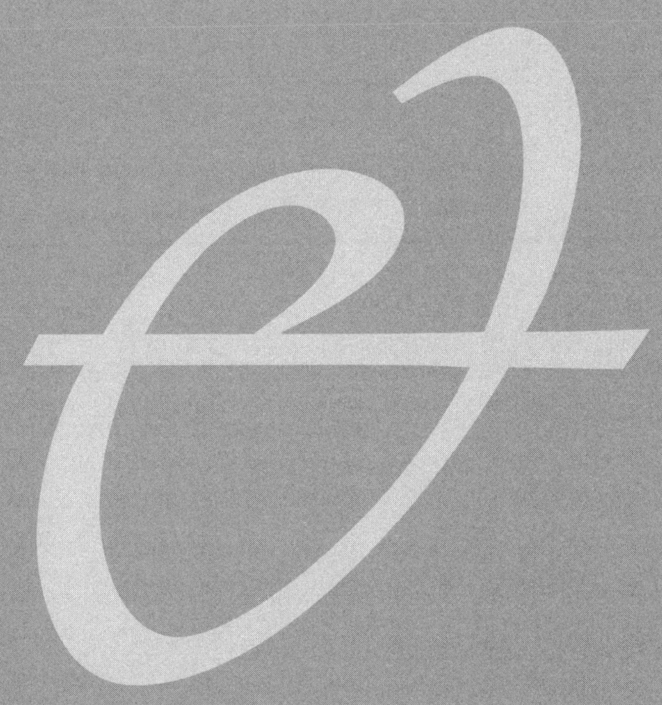

CHAPTER 6

COORDINATING AN EFFECTIVE PUBLIC HEALTH RESPONSE

Terrorism has been a known threat to the nation's health for decades. Recent events have revealed the vulnerability of the U.S. population to terrorist attacks and the improvements needed in our public health infrastructure to best respond to future threats. The September 11, 2001, attack on the World Trade Center and the Pentagon and the subsequent anthrax mailings were events that not only caused a tremendous loss of lives but also had lasting psychological effects on individuals affected by the tragedies. This chapter examines the rising role and responsibilities of federal, state, and local public health systems in preparing for and responding to terrorist attacks to protect the nation's health.

Terrorism is defined by the U.S. Federal Bureau of Investigation (FBI) as "the unlawful use of force and violence against persons or property to intimidate or coerce a government, the civilian population, or any segment thereof, in furtherance of political or social objectives" (Code of Federal Regulations Title 28). Terrorist attacks can originate from international or domestic threats and through the use of biological, chemical, or radiological weapons. Thus, terrorism presents both a national security and a public health threat. Bioterrorism agents are of particular concern for public health because infectious agents can spread rapidly and covertly through a population. Evans and colleagues (see Recommended Reading) describe the six most likely agents for a biological attack, which have been identified and categorized by the United States Army Medical Research Institute of Infectious Disease (USAMRIID). USAMRIID divides the agents into three categories based on the likelihood that each will be used for an attack: Category 1 agents include anthrax and smallpox; category 2 agents cause plague and tularemia; and category 3 agents include botulinum toxin and those causing viral hemorrhagic fevers (Evans et al., 2002, p. 294). Means of transmitting bioterrorism agents include the spread of contagious diseases, airborne dissemination of infectious agents, or contamination of food or water (Hodge, 2002).

TERRORISM AND PUBLIC HEALTH

Public health officials and medical providers must respond to attacks by communicating accurate information such that the public trusts their capabilities and complies with their efforts. As Hyams, Murphy, and Wessley (2002) state in their article "Responding to Chemical, Biological, or Nuclear Terrorism" (included as Article 1), "Terrorism is not simply about killing people; it is also about destroying our sense of well-being and trust in government" (p. 286). Collaboration of health care providers and local, state, and federal public health agencies in responding to terrorism is critical because unlike other health threats such as heart disease or diabetes, terrorist attacks can affect civilians of all ages, health status, and geographic locations. As such, the role of public health agencies includes prevention, preparation, and response to the threat of terrorist attacks. As Christopher F. Chyba (2002) describes in his article "Toward Biological Security," recent attacks exposed our nation's lack of a comprehensive strategy for biological security to protect people and agriculture from disease threats presented by both biological weapons and natural outbreaks (see Recommended Reading).

The West Nile virus outbreak during the summer of 2002, which occurred in multiple southern and midwestern states, as well as New York, tested the surveillance and prevention capabilities of local, state, and federal agencies. Although the outbreak of West Nile virus was not caused by a terrorist attack, it tested the system in ways that resemble a bioterrorism event because it required effective surveillance, prompt laboratory confirmation of the causative agent, preventive measures (e.g., mosquito abatement), care to those afflicted, and clear communication with the public. After an act of bioterrorism, environmental health agencies will also play a leading role in the surveillance and monitoring of agents that persist or may recur in the environment.

In the wake of September 11, 2001, the rising need for a partnership of local, state, and federal agencies in preparing for terrorism in the future became clearer than ever. Clarifying the respective roles and primary responsibilities of these actors will strengthen response capabilities and allow efforts to be coordinated more effectively in the event of an attack. Hodge (2002) states that:

> A large-scale bioterrorism event will accentuate existing uncertainties in the distribution of public health powers. It may also prove to be a catalyst for redefining roles for the future. The critical choice for public health authorities is not to decide where the power to protect public health lies or which level of government has the primary power to act, but rather where the leadership to respond to a bioterrorism event will derive. If leadership capacity is properly developed, public health authorities can use their respective powers to bring about desired goals (p. 257).

FEDERAL SUPPORT FOR STATE AND LOCAL PUBLIC HEALTH RESPONSE

The federal government will provide critical support to state and local government responses. While the decentralization and devolution of government power in recent decades has emphasized a primary responsibility of the states in public health, the recent terrorist attacks have shown the prominent role that federal agencies must play, including the Centers for Disease Control and Prevention (CDC) and the FBI. The centers and institutes of the CDC that are involved in developing a strategic plan of response to biological and chemical terrorism include the National Center for Infectious Diseases, the National Center for Environmental Health, the Public Health Practice Program Office, the Epidemiology Program Office, the National Institute for Occupational Safety and Health, the Office of Health and Safety, the National Immunization Program, and the National Center for Injury Prevention and Control. In 2000, the CDC identified five areas as the focus of training and research: (1) preparedness and prevention, (2) detection and surveillance, (3) diagnosis and characterization of biological and chemical agents, (4) response, and (5) communication (see Recommended Reading).

The federal government has the financial resources to stockpile antibiotics and vaccines. Thus, in the event of an attack, the federal government will be responsible for allocating scarce resources and supplies and ensuring their prompt delivery to the area of a terrorist attack. The federal government must also ensure that domestic security preparedness keeps pace with scientific and technological advances.

MODEL STATE EMERGENCY HEALTH POWERS ACT

The 2001 terrorist attacks have precipitated a reexamination of state laws, including the power of states to quarantine and vaccinate citizens involuntarily in public health emergencies to protect the health of the population. Given the decentralization and devolution of federal government powers over the decades, states now have considerably more responsibility and flexibility in their power to protect the public's health. The scope of state powers are described in the Model State Emergency Health Powers Act and individual state statutes, which have undergone revisions since the September 11 event. According to a recent review of the Model State Emergency Health Powers Act by Gostin and colleagues (2002),

> The Model Act is structured to reflect five basic public health functions to be facilitated by law: (1) *preparedness*, comprehensive planning for a public health emergency; (2) *surveillance*, measures to detect and track public health emergencies; (3) *management of property*, ensuring adequate availability of vaccines, pharmaceuticals, and hospitals, as well as providing power to abate hazards to the public's health; (4) *protection of persons*, powers to compel vaccination, testing, treatment, isolation, and quarantine when clearly necessary; and (5) *communication*, providing clear and authoritative information to the public (p. 622).

Although state public health laws were contested in the 19th century for infringing upon civil rights (e.g., *Morris v. City of Columbus, Boston Beer Co. v. Massachusetts*), the outcomes of these cases tended to reinforce the common-law maxim *salus populi suprema lex* — the safety of the people is the supreme law (Parmet, 2002). George Annas's paper (2002) is included as Article 4, which examines the extent to which there is a necessary trade-off between individual liberties and protection of public health.

CRITICAL ROLE OF COMMUNITY-LEVEL MEDICAL RESPONDERS

At the community level, emergency medicine, primary care physicians, and other health workers will be the first to see patients affected by agents of terrorist attacks. Article 2 by Julie Gerberding, James M. Hughes, and Jeffrey P. Koplan (2002) describes the first-responder role of clinicians in recognizing and reporting cases. Many of the initial symptoms caused by bioterrorism agents are flulike, and professional educational programs can help in training clinicians to identify uncommon conditions caused by bioterrorism agents in the differential diagnosis.

Clinicians will also play a critical role in soothing the fears of patients and instilling health practices that can help protect community health in the event of an attack. As Gerberding and colleagues note regarding the anthrax mailings, "Frontline clinicians faced a challenge that often was even more difficult than diagnosis of anthrax — that of excluding the diagnosis among the many worried patients with concerns about potential exposure or among those who sought care for rashes or illnesses suggestive of the diagnosis" (p. 899). The anthrax mailings set off a wave of demand for the potent antibiotic ciprofloxican by individuals wanting to stockpile or take the antibiotic as prophylaxis. Clinicians will need to educate patients to ensure the continued, prudent use of antibiotics, thereby preserving the efficacy of these drugs for future use for those who have been exposed to agents or who have other bacterial infections.

Clinicians and public health officials may also be asked to provide statements for press releases or media. These communications are a vital source for helping the community to understand the ongoing collaborative response to an attack and what they can do to assist in the response and to protect their health. In a national survey of stress reactions after the September 11 attacks, Schuster and colleagues (2001) found that American adults and children, even in locations far away from the attack site, showed trauma-related symptoms of stress in the week following, which were related to the hours of television coverage of the attack viewed. Indeed, the media coverage of a terrorist attack can have a significant impact on the psychological well-being of citizens, both in heightening fear and confusion and in helping individuals to cope with an attack.

The effective partnership of local, state, and federal agencies in responding to terrorism and other threats to population health is crucial. In the wake of a terrorist attack, all eyes focus on preparing for and improving response capability to a future attack. At the same time, we must not forget the challenges in addition to terrorism facing our nation's health and health care system, including caring for the aging population, addressing disparities in health access and outcome, and the prevalence of chronic, degenerative diseases.

REFERENCES

Annas, G. J. (2002). Bioterrorism, public health, and civil liberties. *New England Journal of Medicine, 346* (17), 1337–1341.

Chyba, C. F. (2002). Toward biological security. *Foreign Affairs, 81* (3), 122–136.

Code of Federal Regulations Title 28. Judicial administration, Chapter I — Department of Justice, Part 0, Subpart P — Federal Bureau of Investigation, Section 0.85, general functions.

Evans, R. G., Crutcher, J. M., Shadel, B., Clements, B., and Bronze, M. (2002). Terrorism from a public health perspective. *American Journal of the Medical Sciences, 323* (6), 291–297.

Gerberding, J. L., Hughes, J. M., and Koplan, J. P. (2002). Bioterrorism preparedness and response: Clinicians and public health agencies as essential partners. *Journal of the American Medical Association, 287* (7), 898–900.

Gostin, L. O., Sapsin, J. W., Teret, S. P., Burris, S., Mair, J. S., Hodge, J. G., and Vernick, J. S. (2002). The Model State Emergency Health Powers Act: Planning for and response to bioterrorism and naturally occurring infectious diseases. *Journal of the American Medical Association, 288* (5), 622–628.

Hodge, J. G. (2002). Bioterrorism law and policy: Critical choices in public health. *Journal of Law, Medicine and Ethics, 30* (2), 254–260.

Hyams, K. C., Murphy, F. M., and Wessely, S. (2002). Responding to chemical, biological, or nuclear terrorism: The indirect and long-term health effects may present the greatest challenge. *Journal of Health Politics, Policy and Law, 27* (2), 273–286.

Parmet, W. E. (2002). After September 11: Rethinking public health federalism. *Journal of Law, Medicine and Ethics, 30* (2), 201–211.

Schuster, M. A., Stein, B. D., Jaycox, L. H., Collins, R. L., Marshall, G. N., Elliott, M. N., Zhou, A. J., Kanouse, D. E., Morrison, J. L., and Berry, S. H. (2001). A national survey of stress reactions after the September 11, 2001, terrorist attacks. *New England Journal of Medicine, 345* (20), 1507–1512.

ARTICLE 1

RESPONDING TO CHEMICAL, BIOLOGICAL, OR NUCLEAR TERRORISM

THE INDIRECT AND LONG-TERM HEALTH EFFECTS MAY PRESENT THE GREATEST CHALLENGE

Kenneth C. Hyams, Frances M. Murphy, and Simon Wessely

Now that a deadly biological weapon, anthrax spores, has been spread through the mail, attention has focused on the possibility that future terrorism using chemical, biological, or nuclear/radiological (CBN) materials could cause mass numbers of casualties (Falkenrath 1998; Franz et al. 1997). For example, it has been estimated that 100,000 deaths could result from an airborne release of anthrax spores over a large urban area (Inglesby et al. 1999). As a consequence, considerable funding, resources, and training are being devoted to the rapid detection and containment of a CBN attack and to the provision of emergency health care (Brennan et al. 1999; *New York Times* 2001).

Although a catastrophic attack is conceivable, it is more likely that limited casualties would result from direct exposure to CBN agents because of technical difficulties in using these weapons against civilian populations (Betts 1998). Nevertheless, the confusion, fear, and long-term health consequences still may be severe. As demonstrated by recent events involving letters containing anthrax spores, even a small-scale incident with CBN materials can have a profound impact on the health of a community and a nation's sense of well-being (Guillemin 1999:245; Okie 2001) and lead to protracted social and economic problems (Falkenrath 1998). Why are terrorist attacks using CBN materials so devastating? Mainly because terrorism already is frightful, but the use of unconventional weapons is even more so. CBN agents are terrifying because

---

The following article was written over one year prior to the September 2001 terrorist attacks on the World Trade Center and the Pentagon and the mailing of anthrax spores to news organizations and political leaders. Sadly, some of the concerns raised in the original manuscript about the acute health effects of a terrorist attack have come to pass. What we underestimated in our original analysis was the impact that a terrorist attack would have on every segment of society, not just the targeted community but also the general population and its leaders. As a consequence, we have revised the original manuscript to reflect these recent developments.

they cause injury and death in strange and prolonged ways (Franz et al. 1997). In addition, we feel more vulnerable to these weapons than conventional explosives because they can harm large numbers of ordinary citizens in places generally considered safe, such as in the workplace and residential neighborhoods.

Other characteristics of CBN weapons place them in the category of health hazards that are likely to cause both public fear and heightened anxiety (Renn 1997). A large body of research has indicated that the following features of a health threat are associated with prolonged effects: (1) involuntary threats that occur without warning (as opposed to personal choices like cigarette smoking), (2) manufactured threats versus natural disasters ("acts of God"), (3) unfamiliar threats with unknown health effects, and (4) threats that pose a danger to children and future generations (Bennett 1999a; Smith et al. 1986). It is clear that CBN weapons fulfill all of the criteria for creating a major catastrophe. Not only are these weapons intended to cause death and terror, but a CBN incident also has the characteristics of disasters that induce lingering medical, psychological, and social reactions.

In order to combat acts of mass terror, contingency planning has to involve more than just emergency response. An effective strategy will have to consider a broader array of immediate and long-term consequences, which will arise regardless of the type of toxic exposure or number of casualties (Holloway et al. 1997; Institute of Medicine 1999).

IMMEDIATE HARM

The first casualties of a terrorist attack result from the direct effects of the CBN agent. Emergency response training is ongoing for this eventuality. This aspect of medical care may appear clear cut but could cause immediate controversy. Prophylactic measures that have been used to protect against biological and chemical warfare agents — like the anthrax vaccine and pyridostigmine bromide pills — have been postulated to cause chronic medical problems (Presidential Advisory Committee 1996: 114, 117; Institute of Medicine 2000). Attempts to use these problematic drugs and vaccines fuel controversy and add to a traumatized community's health concerns (Rosen 2000; Weiss 2001).

In addition to direct harm from a CBN agent, the impact on those not exposed may be almost as traumatic, as amply demonstrated since the terrorist attacks on the World Trade Center and Pentagon. In the immediate aftermath of a large-scale CBN attack, there is fear and bewilderment (Holloway et al. 1997). Everyone involved worries about his or her family and friends. Accidents can occur from people fleeing the disaster area (Erikson 1990). Essential hospital employees may be incapacitated by secondary exposure to the CBN agent or leave work out of personal concerns (Guillemin 1999:54). The normal reaction to an unfamiliar, life-threatening event — fear, confusion, and flight — could cause greater damage than the attack itself (Bleich et al. 1991).

Until the nature of the CBN exposure is clearly determined, uncertainty and fear will be present even among skilled rescue and medical personnel (Holloway et al. 1997).

Although prophylactic drugs and vaccines and the use of gas masks and protective clothing help alleviate anxiety among "first responders," dramatic and hurried activities of rescue workers frighten residents of the disaster area (Barker and Selvey 1992). The perceptions of a much larger population can be affected by television and newspaper reports of emergency medical care and decontamination efforts (Jones et al. 2000). Media images of spacesuit-clad investigators unsettled a worldwide audience during recent anthrax scares (Dobbs 2001). With uncertainty about the identity of the perpetrators and the extent of anthrax contamination, no person is certain that he or she will not be involved in a terrorist attack.

Following reports of a CBN attack, health care facilities can become quickly overrun by both medical and psychological casualties and concerned citizens (Falkenrath 1998). For example, after recent anthrax deaths, it has not been possible to satisfy public demand for ciprofloxacin, an antibiotic approved for the treatment of anthrax; patients have inundated emergency rooms seeking reassurance; and the public health system has been stretched to the limit trying to screen populations that may have been exposed to contaminated letters (Firestone 2001; Prial 2001). For another example, after the incident in Goiânia, Brazil, in which accidental exposure to a medical radiation source led to several hundred casualties and four deaths, 10 percent of the population (more than 100,000 people) sought medical checks (Collins and Carvalho 1993; Petterson 1988).

Urgent questions can be expected about the causes of common physical (somatic) complaints because nonspecific symptoms are often the first manifestation of injury from CBN agents (Bleich et al. 1992; Rosen 2000). However, somatic symptoms are frequently reported in healthy populations of adults and become even more prominent under stressful circumstances (Barsky and Borus 1999; Schwartz, White, and Hughes 1985). There already have been reports of increased complaints of pain, sleeplessness, headaches, palpitations, and other somatic symptoms since the 11 September 2001 terrorist attacks in the United States (Morin 2001; Goldstein 2001). Common flu-like symptoms, such as cough and fever, are particularly frightening after an attack with anthrax spores. Symptoms that arise from normal fear and uncertainty in a chaotic emergency, like headaches and difficulty concentrating, are indistinguishable from the early effects of nerve gas exposure (Bleich et al. 1991). The nonspecificity of these symptoms and the resulting difficulty in rapidly determining their causes can misdirect and deplete emergency medical care and containment resources.

Even though there has been acknowledgment that the indirect consequences of a CBN incident will be substantial (Falkenrath 1998), official planning may nevertheless underestimate the potential scale of the response. With uncertainty about who was exposed and whether further exposures were occurring, large numbers of both endangered and unaffected residents will present to medical care providers with health concerns, as occurred after the release of sarin in a Tokyo subway (Woodall 1997) and more recently following potential exposure to anthrax spores (Prial 2001). Additionally, stress, fear, worry, and grief can exacerbate existing medical and psychological problems in the entire community.

As one example of indirect outcomes, a widely reported CBN incident could act as a powerful trigger for outbreaks of "mass sociogenic illness" (DiGiovanni 1991). In fact, several outbreaks have occurred in the aftermath of recent terrorist attacks (Wessely, Hyams, and Bartholomew 2001). These episodes of physical symptoms suggestive of acute injury, which have been misleadingly called mass hysteria, can be set off by toxic exposures, unusual odors, or even rumors of contamination (Boss 1997). The immediate response to multiple casualties, such as the arrival of emergency workers wearing decontamination clothing and television cameras, accelerates the spread of this illness (Krug 1992; Selden 1989). It is important to realize that, given the appropriate circumstances of stress, fear, and confusion (Boss 1997), mass sociogenic illness can effect any population. Because there is limited understanding of this phenomenon, symptoms of mass sociogenic illness frequently are medicalized rather than treated with education and reassurance, which subsequently leads to protracted controversy in affected communities.

In addition to increased demands for health care after a CBN attack, immediate changes in reproductive behavior may occur. Following the Chernobyl radiation disaster there was a decrease in the birth rate across Western Europe and an increase in induced abortions (Bertollini et al. 1990; Knudsen 1991). More recently, abortions and delayed pregnancy became an issue in the Balkans during aerial bombing of chemical plants (Fineman 1999). Similar fears about birth defects were expressed by victims of the 1995 Tokyo sarin attack (Watts 1999). Whether recent terrorist attacks will affect reproductive behavior is not yet known, but numerous anthrax hoaxes were perpetrated against abortion clinics in the United States immediately following reports that anthrax spores were being spread through the mail (Booth 2001).

For the emergency response to a major CBN event, planning therefore has to take into account two different health care scenarios. The first relates to managing the deaths and injuries caused directly by the attack. The second involves dealing with the fears, health concerns, and psychological reactions that normally arise in disasters. Because enormous numbers of people will feel at risk before the extent of exposure can be determined, these indirect consequences may pose the greater challenge to authority, acute health care, and public confidence. After the emergency response, many of these initial health problems may have prolonged consequences.

LONG-TERM CONSEQUENCES

As natural and manufactured disasters have shown, the long-term effects can be substantial. Experience indicates that following a CBN attack there would be four major health concerns: (1) chronic injuries and diseases directly caused by the toxic agent, (2) questions about adverse reproductive outcomes, (3) psychological effects, and (4) increased levels of somatic symptoms (David and Wessely 1995; Schwartz, White, and Hughes 1985; Nakajima et al. 1999). Acute injuries caused by a particular CBN exposure are manageable because they can be identified and treated according to established guidelines.

As during the emergency response, more difficulties may result over the longer term from harder to prove or disprove health outcomes. For instance, cancer, birth defects, and various neurological, rheumatic, and immunological diseases are increasingly being attributed to diverse types of chemical and radiation exposures (Neutra, Lipscomb, and Satin 1991). There are many social, historical, and cultural reasons why these health concerns would be prevalent after a CBN attack. Everyone has been sensitized by the AIDS epidemic, mad cow disease, and numerous environmental tragedies. The scientific debate over the health effects of pesticides, genetically modified food, electrical power lines, and cellular telephones also has influenced public perceptions. The result is a heightened sensitivity over environmental exposures. A terrorist attack not only would create new fears but would surely amplify existing concerns about the safety of our food, water, and air. For instance, residents downwind of an anthrax-contaminated building in Florida were concerned about the possibility of infection (Firestone 2001).

The current scientific uncertainty over the chronic health effects of low-level exposure to toxic agents will further increase anxiety in the affected communities (Brown and Brix 1998). Because health officials cannot give blanket assurances that no harm will result from brief or nonsymptom-producing exposure to chemical, biological, or radiological materials (Institute of Medicine 2000), distrust of medical experts and government officials may result (Birchard 1999). Furthermore, unconfirmed and controversial hypotheses about the health effects of exposure to CBN materials can become contentious scientific and legal issues (Birchard 1998).

One contemporary example demonstrates the potential long-term impact of environmental concerns. Residents in a market town in the west of England have blamed a variety of health problems on "germ warfare experiments" that involved aerial spraying of bacteria thirty years ago during the Cold War (Townsend 1997). What is noteworthy is the wide range of conditions attributed to the experiments: cancers, cerebral palsy, Down syndrome, miscarriages, learning difficulties, autism, and skin ulcers, to name a few. The result has been "an entire Dorset village torn apart." Similar health fears can be anticipated on a larger scale following recent deaths from exposure to anthrax-contaminated letters.

The long-term psychological consequences of a CBN incident also can be substantial. Posttraumatic stress disorder (PTSD), which is characterized by reexperience of traumatic events, affects victims, witnesses, and rescue workers most directly involved in the initial exposure (Holloway et al. 1997). Recent estimates are that one-third of those who were most closely involved with the World Trade Center tragedy may suffer from the condition. However, PTSD will be only one of the mental health problems facing a community, as demonstrated in Japan following two terrorist attacks with the chemical nerve agent sarin (Ohbu et al. 1997; Watts 1999). And as we have recently witnessed, routine activities that once felt familiar and safe, like visiting the post office, can now seem threatening and strange (Whoriskey and Jenkins 2001). The general level of fear and anxiety can remain high for years, exacerbating preexisting psychiatric disorders and posing a challenge to the entire public mental health system. In the case of the recent World Trade Center events, thousands of children were left without a parent or orphaned, and even more witnessed the tragedy both directly and on television (Davidson, Baum, and Collins 1982; Prince-Embury and Rooney 1988; Stepp 2001).

Although we have considerable information about high background levels of physical symptoms in adult populations (Hannay 1978; Mayou 1991), there is less understanding of the causes of more complex symptoms and of the factors that effect the experience and reporting of distress (Roht et al. 1985; Shusterman et al. 1991). As a consequence, when clusters of unexplained symptoms have been observed following toxic exposures (Hyams, Wignall, and Roswell 1996; Reuters 1999), there is often heated debate over the role of psychological stress in causing or contributing to reported health problems (Joseph et al. 1998; Stiehm 1992; Presidential Advisory Committee 1996:123–125). These controversies are difficult to resolve because stress is an inevitable aspect of any life-threatening experience. A population exposed to a terrorist attack experiences both direct injuries and numerous physical symptoms due to prolonged stress, muscular tension, and sleep deprivation (Bravo et al. 1990; Nakano 1995).

As noted in the discussion of emergency medical care, public concern can arise from well-intended health care decisions. The nonstandard, off-label, and even investigational drugs and vaccines that may help save lives in a CBN attack can become protracted health and legal issues. In particular, therapeutic agents that have not received official approval, like licensing from the U.S. Food and Drug Administration (FDA), are distrusted (Berezuk and McCarty 1992). Increased symptoms and illnesses reported long after a terrorist attack may be attributed to side effects of medical interventions (Institute of Medicine 2000).

It has been difficult to obtain FDA approval for many potentially useful therapeutic and prophylactic measures because CBN materials are too toxic to expose human volunteers in required efficacy studies (Institute of Medicine 1999:110–164). To address this problem, the FDA is considering a different standard — the use of animal studies — for the approval of new vaccines and pharmaceutical products to counter chemical and biological warfare agents (Zoon 1999). These rule changes will directly impact the development of a new generation of vaccines for anthrax and smallpox because it is not ethically feasible to expose study subjects to these deadly diseases in order to demonstrate protection.

Controversy over the health effects of hazardous exposures and therapeutic interventions may impede other aspects of the recovery effort. As in any disaster, government assistance will be required to rebuild communities and restore the local economy. However, the issue of compensation for personal injuries could have a damaging effect on public faith in government (David and Wessely 1995). The reason is that many health claims will be hard to prove or to relate to the CBN incident (Huber 1992:92–110). The fear of cover-up may surface, and litigation will lead to an adversarial relationship between the public and the government. Assigning blame and legal liability could become the focus of acrimonious public and political debate, which hinders public health efforts.

The nature of the particular terrorist weapon also has a consequential impact on recovery efforts. For example, chemical nerve agents dissipate rapidly and do not pose a long-term health risk (Institute of Medicine 1999:174–183). In contrast, anthrax spores and radiological material can persist in the environment for decades; this would make decontamination efforts problematic and lead to persistent health concerns.

The demographic and cultural characteristics of an affected community, as well as the availability of public transportation and medical and social services, further influence recovery efforts (Nakano 1995). Less well-off communities need greater medical, social, and economic assistance. In wealthy communities, however, it is difficult to monitor the health impact of the attack because residents have greater mobility and access to a diversity of health care services. The economy of a community may be permanently harmed because of fears that locally produced agricultural and manufacturing products may be contaminated with harmful CBN agents (Petterson 1988). For the same reason, the value of individual homes and commercial property could drop precipitously, which will engender feelings of hopelessness in the community (ibid.).

RECOMMENDATIONS

A community attacked with a CBN weapon will need both emergency intervention and long-term health care, extensive medical and risk assessment information, and economic support. Also, multiple challenges to the credibility of governmental and scientific authority could hamper recovery efforts. The following recommendations are made for dealing with these consequences.

Health Care

Emergency response teams already train for acute medical care of mass casualties. What remains to be decided is how long health care should be provided and whether health care should be comprehensive or restricted to the probable toxic effects of the CBN agent. These are critical questions in countries like the United States, which does not have universal health care. In the event of a large-scale CBN attack, there are compelling reasons for offering comprehensive health care over an extended period of time. For one, readily available clinical care would ensure that an affected community's health care needs are met, which is arguably a prime responsibility of the government after a disaster. In addition, provision of medical care represents one of many tangible indications that the government is committed to recovery and as such helps restore confidence in public institutions (Watts 1999).

If health care is offered, who should provide the care? In the United States, health care would have to be furnished by private physicians and health maintenance organizations or by the two major federal health care systems in the Department of Veterans Affairs (VA), which maintains hospitals in every state, and the Department of Defense (DOD). The VA and DOD already are involved in the emergency response under the Federal Response Plan but would require appropriate authority and resources to provide health care for a longer period (Montello and Ames 1998).

Several arguments can be made for centralizing health care in local medical facilities. For one, this approach would ensure access to health care. Second, a smaller number of health care providers could be more intensively educated on relevant health issues and new scientific findings. Finally, a consistent set of providers would be more likely to detect the development of new or worsening health problems in the affected population.

The need for readily available health care and specially trained providers cannot be underestimated. The Gulf War syndrome controversy demonstrates how complex health issues can become after a possible CBN attack and how important it is for health care providers to have up-to-date information (Murphy et al. 1999). When a traumatized population cannot obtain answers to health questions from knowledgeable providers, misinformation fills the void and concerns multiply. Moreover, specially trained providers could maintain standardized medical records, which are important for scientific and medical-legal purposes.

Although it can be argued that freely available health care will foster the sick role and prolong disability, properly trained health care providers can help patients work through their health problems and grief, with restoration of function as the primary goal of treatment. Although offering mental health care after an act of mass terror is important, immediate grief counseling or psychological debriefing may not be the most effective approach (Raphael, Meldrum, and McFarlane 1995; Wessely, Bisson, and Rose 1999).

Risk Communication and Management

A concerted risk communication and management effort is critical after a CBN attack in order to keep the public informed and to promote recovery (Bennett, Coles, and McDonald 1999). In the immediate aftermath of a terrorist attack, the primary method for rapidly disseminating information is through the popular news media. Accordingly, public officials and scientific experts have to be as open, clear, and forthcoming as possible with the press and avoid the development of an adversarial relationship. After a community's sense of well-being has been shattered, there is a tendency for information and reassurance to be met with disbelief and anger (Brewin 1994; David and Wessely 1995). A frustrated press corps only makes communicating with the public harder.

To enlist the help of the press, health officials have to provide the press with the best available information. It is important for crisis managers to work cooperatively with the press to discourage the reporting of false rumors and inaccurate information, while at the same time not providing false reassurance (Modan et al. 1983). The press also has to educate itself about a new health threat in order to accurately report the news, as exemplified recently by early media reports that did not distinguish between anthrax exposure and infection. Over time, diverse methods have to be developed for communicating with the affected population (Neutra 1985). These include mass mailings, use of the Internet, and especially community meetings. Open meetings help disseminate useful information and involve the public in the recovery process, which speeds recovery and increases confidence in governmental actions (Holloway et al. 1997). Effective risk communication is a long-term process that requires a two-way exchange of information with the affected population. Public concerns should also be addressed by working closely with community leaders (Coote and Franklin 1999).

Maintaining credibility over the long term will be one of the most difficult challenges for government institutions. Precipitous decisions made in a crisis to care for casualties and to prevent further injury will be judged later in a deliberative manner using more complete and accurate information. Mistakes will be identified. The government should take responsibility for its mistakes and clearly explain the reasons for critical decisions in order to maintain trust.

An noted, unsupported health claims could become a problem. There will be nonorthodox views and hypotheses on events and scientific issues (Glassner 1999; Presidential Advisory Committee 1996:90–91). These ideas cannot be ignored, but public health policy and medical care cannot be based on unsubstantiated opinion. A successful risk communication strategy has to deal fairly and openly with unproven assertions and new hypotheses, not least because the existence of dissident views appeals to the popular media's commitment to balanced reporting (Singer and Endreny 1993).

For recovery to work, risk management efforts have to prevent demoralization and ensure that members of the affected population are ultimately characterized as survivors rather than as victims. A shift in thinking from vulnerability and dependency to pride in overcoming adversity will do more to overcome long-term health problems in both the targeted community and the nation at large than any other health measure (Giel 1991; Summerfield 2000). Even after a devastating disaster, communities display substantial resilience when not rendered helpless and passive in the recovery process (Bravo et al. 1990). Additionally, rapid financial assistance and the rebuilding of the community's economy provide substantial health benefits (Summerfield 1999).

Surveillance and Research

An extensive surveillance and research effort is important following a major CBN attack. The identification of persons injured or killed by a CBN weapon will be a priority during the emergency response. Accurate detection requires the establishment of a case definition of affected individuals (Brennan et al. 1999). This case definition should be based primarily on the objective characteristics of the injury caused by the particular CBN exposure (Franz et al. 1997; Pavlin 1999). Diagnostic criteria should not rely on nonspecific symptoms that become prominent in a highly stressful situation and may be related to mass sociogenic illness (Jones et al. 2000). Misclassification of unaffected communities as exposed to a deadly CBN agent will not only misdirect emergency efforts, but will also confuse the public and result in protracted scientific and legal disputes about who was injured. The recent confusion over who may have been exposed to anthrax spores from contact with contaminated mail could easily lead to prolonged controversy.

After a major CBN attack, longitudinal surveillance studies should be initiated. Evidence-based answers have to be available for questions that will arise after a toxic exposure about increased rates of various diseases, birth defects, physical and mental symptoms, and psychiatric disorders. Failure to conduct epidemiological surveillance is likely to lead to accusations of government insensitivity, incompetence, and cover-up (Schwartz, White, and Hughes 1985). Delaying sound research also opens the door to unsubstantiated claims and may eventually preclude the initiation of definitive research studies because accurate data become less accessible over time (Institute of Medicine 2000).

Although a concerted research effort may be misinterpreted as evidence of more widespread harm than officially acknowledged (Jones et al. 2000), it is better for the responsible authorities to initiate scientific investigations rather than to be pushed into them by public and media criticism (David and Wessely 1995). By being able to respond to the public's legitimate need for answers, fear and anxiety can be lessened and credibility of responsible authorities improved. Research is necessary, not only to answer pressing health questions but as part of the risk-management process itself.

To implement the preceding set of recommendations, a high degree of communication, coordination, and cooperation is required among governmental and social institutions. To organize an effective response is difficult given the many different groups involved, such as the civilian government agencies at the local, state, and national level; law enforcement; the military; emergency response teams; community health care providers; social services; local business interests; the court system; and the news media (Tucker 1997). Because most of these organizations are not accustomed to working together and have different priorities, conflicts arise. Therefore, clear lines of authority are essential to guide an effective response and recovery effort (Centers for Disease Control and Prevention 2000).

In the United States, lead responsibility for the initial operational response to acts of terrorism ("crisis management") has been assigned to the Federal Bureau of Investigation (PDD-39, 1995). The U.S. attorney general can subsequently transfer lead responsibility to the Federal Emergency Management Agency (FEMA) for "consequent management," that is, measures to protect public health and safety, restore essential government services, and provide emergency relief to governments, businesses, and individuals affected by the consequences of terrorism. The establishment in the United States of the new Office of Homeland Security should lead to greater coordination in the government's response to acts of terrorism (Pianin 2001).

CONCLUSION

Because of the success of recent terrorist attacks, concrete steps have to be taken now to better prepare for further threats. Along with efforts to prevent acts of mass terrorism and to mount an effective emergency response, greater discussion and awareness are needed about the potential for indirect and long-term consequences. Without a comprehensive plan of action that considers all eventualities, government agencies are more likely to respond ineffectually or to overreact, creating unnecessary panic and infringing on basic civil liberties (Stern 1999; Guillemin 1999:248; Lancaster 2001). Thorough preparedness could also aid deterrence efforts. In the future, terrorists may be dissuaded from attempting to use these technically demanding and unpredictable agents if they think the responses will minimize widespread injury and fear.

Responding to an actual CBN attack is an even more daunting task because many of the issues involved — eligibility for health care, the effects of low-level chemical and radiation exposure, stress-related illnesses, unlicensed therapeutics, financial compensation — are complex and controversial. Only government institutions that maintain credibility with the public will be capable of dealing effectively with the broad range of problems that evolve after a terrorist attack.

A successful recovery effort must provide for long-term health care, risk communication, and surveillance. Although advanced technologies help in the emergency response, there is a greater need for a general plan of action, central coordination, and basic education (Pincus 1999; Sharp et al. 1998). Not just the medical community but government officials, the press, and the general public have to be more fully informed about the nature of this threat. Moreover, additional research is necessary concerning the best methods of risk management and communication (Bennett 1999b).

Future chemical, biological, or nuclear terrorism should be anticipated. In preparing for these attacks, we have to walk a fine line between lack of preparedness and creating undue fear in our daily lives (Shalala 1999). Terrorism is not simply about killing people; it is also about destroying our sense of well-being and trust in government. This outcome cannot be allowed to happen either before or after a terrorist attack.

REFERENCES

Barker, P., and D. Selvey. 1992. Malathion-Induced Epidemic Hysteria in an Elementary School. *Veterinary and Human Toxicology* 34:156–160.

Barsky, A., and J. Borus. 1999. Functional Somatic Syndromes. *Annals of Internal Medicine* 130:910–921.

Bennett, P. 1999a. Understanding Responses to Risk: Some Basic Findings. In *Risk Communication and Public Health*, ed. P. Bennett and K. Calman. Oxford: Oxford University Press.

———. 1999b. Research Priorities. In *Risk Communication and Public Health*, ed. P. Bennett and K. Calman. Oxford: Oxford University Press.

Bennett, P., D. Coles, and A. McDonald. 1999. Risk Communication as a Decision Process. In *Risk Communication and Public Health*, ed. P. Bennett and K. Calman. Oxford: Oxford University Press.

Berezuk, G., and G. McCarty. 1992. Investigational Drugs and Vaccines Fielded in Support of Operation Desert Storm. *Military Medicine* 157:404–406.

Bertollini, R., D. DiLallo, P. Mastroiacovo, and C. Perucci. 1990. Reduction of Births in Italy after the Chernobyl Accident. *Scandinavian Journal of Work, Environment, and Health* 16:96–101.

Betts, R. 1998. The New Threat of Mass Destruction. *Foreign Affairs* 77:26–41.

Birchard, K. 1998. Does Iraq's Depleted Uranium Pose a Health Risk? *Lancet* 351:657.

———. 1999. Experts Still Arguing over Radiation Doses. *Lancet* 354:400.

Bleich, A., A. Dycian, M. Koslowsky, Z. Solomon, and M. Wiener. 1992. Psychiatric Implications of Missile Attacks on a Civilian Population: Israeli Lessons from the Persian Gulf War. *Journal of the American Medical Association* 268:613–615.

Bleich, A., S. Kron, C. Margalit, G. Inbar, Z. Kaplan, S. Cooper, and Z. Solomon. 1991. Israeli Psychological Casualties of the Persian Gulf War: Characteristics, Therapy, and Selected Issues. *Israel Journal of Medical Sciences* 27:673–676.

Booth, William. 2001. Bioterror Takes on Another Face. *Washington Post,* 21 October, A8.

Boss, L. 1997. Epidemic Hysteria: A Review of the Published Literature. *Epidemiologic Reviews* 19:233–243.

Bravo, M., M. Rubio-Stipec, G. Canino, M. Woodbury, and J. Ribera. 1990. The Psychological Sequelae of Disaster Stress Prospectively and Retrospectively Evaluated. *American Journal of Community Psychology* 18:661–680.

Brennan, R., J. Waeckerle, T. Sharp, and S. Lillibridge. 1999. Chemical Warfare Agents: Emergency Medical and Emergency Public Health Issues. *Annals of Emergency Medicine* 34:191–204.

Brewin, T. 1994. Chernobyl and the Media. *British Medical Journal* 309:208–209.

Brown, M., and K. Brix. 1998. Review of Health Consequences from High, Intermediate, and Low-Level Exposure to Organophosphorus Nerve Agents. *Journal of Applied Toxicology* 18:393–408.

Centers for Disease Control and Prevention. 2000. Biological and Chemical Terrorism: Strategic Plan for Preparedness and Response. *Morbidity and Mortality Weekly Report*, 12 April:1–14.

Collins, D., and Carvalho A. 1993. Chronic Stress from the Goiânia 137 Cs Radiation Accident. *Behavioral Medicine* 18:149–157.

Coote A., and J. Franklin. 1999. Negotiating Risks to Public Health — Models for Participation. In *Risk Communication and Public Health*, ed. P. Bennett and K. Calman. Oxford: Oxford University Press.

David, A., and S. Wessely. 1995. The Legend of Camelford: Medical Consequences of a Water Pollution Accident. *Journal of Psychosomatic Research* 39:1–10.

Davidson, L., A. Baum, and D. Collins. 1982. Stress and Control-Related Problems at Three-Mile Island. *Journal of Applied Social Psychology* 12:349–359.

DiGiovanni, C. 1999. Domestic Terrorism with Chemical or Biological Agents. *American Journal of Psychiatry* 156:1500–1505.

Dobbs, Michael. 2001. Anthrax Scare Spreads around the World. *Washington Post*, 18 October, A15.

Erikson, K. 1990. Toxic Reckoning: Business. *Harvard Business Review*, January–February, 118–126.

Falkenrath, R. 1998. Confronting Nuclear, Biological, and Chemical Terrorism. *Survival* 40:43–65.

Fineman, M. 1999. Yugoslav City Battling Toxic Enemies. *Los Angeles Times*, 6 July, A1.

Firestone, David. 2001. In Florida, an Outbreak of Anthrax Turns the Air into a Terror Suspect. *New York Times*, 12 October, 9.

Franz, D., P. Jahrling, A. Friedlander, D. McClain, D. Hoover, and W. Bryne. 1997. Clinical Recognition and Management of Patients Exposed to Biological Warfare Agents. *Journal of the American Medical Association* 278:399–411.

Giel, R. 1991. The Psychosocial Aftermath of Two Major Disasters in the Soviet Union. *Journal of Traumatic Stress* 4:381–393.

Glassner, B. 1999. *In the Culture of Fear: Why Americans Are Afraid of the Wrong Things*. New York: Basic Books.

Goldstein, Avram. 2001. Terrorism Tied to Jump in Pain Problems. *Washington Post*, 1 October, A1.

Guillemin, J. 1999. *Anthrax: The Investigation of a Deadly Outbreak*. Berkeley: University of California Press.

Hannay, D. 1978. Symptom Prevalence in the Community. *Journal of the Royal College of General Practitioners* 28:492–499.

Holloway, H., A. Norwood, C. Fullerton, C. Engel, and R. Ursano. 1997. The Threat of Biological Weapons: Prophylaxis and Mitigation of Psychological and Social Consequences. *Journal of the American Medical Association* 278:425–427.

Huber, P. 1992. *Galileo's Revenge: Junk Science in the Courtroom*. New York: Basic Books.

Hyams, K., F. Wignall, and R. Roswell. 1996. War Syndromes and Their Evaluation: From the U.S. Civil War to the Persian Gulf War. *Annals of Internal Medicine* 125:398–405.

Inglesby, T., D. Henderson, J. Barlett, M. Ascher, E. Eitzen, A. Friedlander, J. Hauer, J. McDade, M. Osterholm, T. O'Toole, G. Parker, T. Perl, P. Russell, K. Tonat, and the Working Group on Civilian Biodefense. 1999. Anthrax as a Biological Weapon: Medical and Public Health Management. *Journal of the American Medical Association* 281:1735–1745.

Institute of Medicine. 1999. *Chemical and Biological Terrorism: Research and Development to Improve Civilian Medical Response*. Washington, DC: National Academy Press.

———. 2000. *Gulf War and Health: Volume 1. Depleted Uranium, Sarin, Pyridostigmine Bromide, Vaccines*. Washington, DC: National Academy Press.

Jones, T., A. Craig, D. Hoy, E. Gunter, D. Ashley, D. Barr, J. Brock, and W. Schaffner. 2000. Mass Psychogenic Illness Attributed to Toxic Exposure at a High School. *New England Journal of Medicine* 342:96–100.

Joseph, S., K. Hyams, G. Gackstetter, E. Mathews, and R. Patterson. 1998. Persian Gulf War Health Issues. In *Environmental and Occupational Medicine*, 3d ed., ed. W. Rom. Philadelphia: Lippincott-Raven.

Knudsen, L. 1991. Legally-Induced Abortions in Denmark after Chernobyl. *Biomedicine and Pharmacotheraphy* 45:229–232.

Krug, S. 1992. Mass Illness at an Intermediate School: Toxic Fumes or Epidemic Hysteria? *Pediatric Emergency Care* 8:280–282.

Lancaster, John. 2001. House Approves Terrorism Measure. *Washington Post*, 25 October, A1.

Mayou, R. 1991. Medically Unexplained Physical Symptoms. *British Medical Journal* 303:534–535.

Modan, B., M. Tirosh, E. Weissenberg, C. Costin, T. A. Swartz, A. Donagi, C. Acker, M. Revach, and G. Vettorazzi. 1983. The Arjenyattah Epidemic — A Mass Phenomenon: Spread and Triggering Factors. *Lancet* 2:1472–1475.

Montello, M., and T. Ames. 1998. The Federal Disaster Response Plan. *Federal Practitioner,* December, 48–50.

Morin, Richard. 2001. Poll: National Pride, Confidence Soar. *Washington Post,* 25 October, A7.

Murphy, F., R. Allen, H. Kang, S. Mather, N. Dalager, K. Kizer, and K. Lee. 1999. The Health Status of Gulf War Veterans: Lessons Learned from the Department of Veterans Affairs Health Registry. *Military Medicine* 164:327–331.

Nakajima, T., S. Ohta, Y. Fukushima, and N. Yanagisawa. 1999. Sequelae of Sarin Toxicity at One and Three Years after Exposure in Matsumoto, Japan. *Journal of Epidemiology* 9:337–343.

Nakano, K. 1995. The Tokyo Sarin Gas Attack: Victims' Isolation and Post-Traumatic Stress Disorders. *Cross-Cultural Psychology Bulletin* 29:12–15.

Neutra, R. 1985. Epidemiology for and with a Distrustful Community. *Environmental Health Perspectives* 62:393–397.

Neutra, R., J. Lipscomb, and K. Satin. 1991. Hypotheses to Explain the Higher Symptom Rates Observed around Hazardous Waste Sites. *Environmental Health Perspectives* 94:31–38.

New York Times. 2001. Editorial: Responding to the Anthrax Threat. *New York Times,* 25 October, 20.

Ohbu, S., A. Yamashina, N. Takasu, T. Yamaguchi, T. Murai, and K. Nakano. 1997. Sarin Poisoning on Tokyo Subway. *Southern Medical Journal* 90:587–593.

Okie, Susan. 2001. Use of Anti-Anxiety Drugs Jumps in U.S. *Washington Post*, 14 October, A8.

Pavlin, J. 1999. Epidemiology of Bioterrorism. *Emerging Infectious Diseases* 5:528–530.

Petterson, J. 1988. Perception versus Reality of Radiological Impact: The Goiânia Model. *Nuclear News*, November, 84–90.

Pianin, Eric. 2001. Ridge Assumes Security Post amid Potential for New Attacks. *Washington Post*, 9 October, A6.

Pincus, W. 1999. U.S. Preparedness Faulted: Weapons of Mass Destruction Concern Panel. *Washington Post*, 9 July, A2.

Presidential Advisory Committee on Gulf War Veterans' Illnesses. 1996. Final Report. December. Washington, DC: U.S. Government Printing Office.

Presidential Decision Directive 39 (PDD-39). 1995. United States Policy on Counterterrorism. Available on-line at http://www.fema.gov/r-n-r/frp/frpterr.htm.

Prial, Dunstan. 2001. Mayor: Earlier Letter to News Anchor Tom Brokaw Contained Anthrax That Infected His Assistant. Associated Press wire story, 13 October.

Accessed on-line at www.nandotimes.com/healthscience/story/135560p-1375072c.html.

Prince-Embury, S., and J. Rooney. 1988. Psychological Symptoms of Residents in the Aftermath of the Three-Mile Island Nuclear Accident in the Aftermath of Technological Disaster. *Journal of Social Psychology* 128:779–790.

Raphael, B., L. Meldrum, and A. McFarlane. 1995. Does Debriefing after Psychological Trauma Work? *British Medical Journal* 310:1479–1480.

Renn, O. 1997. Mental Health, Stress, and Risk Perception: Insights from Psychological Research. In *Health Effects of Large Releases of Radionucleotides*, ed. G. Bock, G. Carden, and V. V. Lake. CIBA Foundation Symposium 203. New York: John Wiley.

Reuters. 1999. Dutch Crash Report Sees Health Link, Slams Government. Report broadcast on Cable Network News, 23 April.

Roht, L., S. Vernon, F. Weir, S. Pier, P. Sullivan, and L. Reed. 1985. Community Exposure to Hazardous Waste Disposal Sites: Assessing Reporting Bias. *American Journal of Epidemiology* 122:418–433.

Rosen, P. 2000. Coping with Bioterrorism Is Difficult, but May Help Us Respond to New Epidemics. *British Medical Journal* 320:71–72.

Schwartz, S., P. White, and R. Hughes. 1985. Environmental Threats, Communities, and Hysteria. *Journal of Public Health Policy* 6:58–77.

Selden, B. 1989. Adolescent Epidemic Hysteria Presenting as a Mass Casualty, Toxic Exposure Incident. *Annals of Emergency Medicine* 18:892–895.

Shalala, D. 1999. Bioterrorism: How Prepared Are We? *Emerging Infectious Diseases* 5:492–493.

Sharp, T., R. Brennan, M. Keim, R. Williams, E. Eitzen, and S. Lillibridge. 1998. Medical Preparedness for a Terrorist Incident Involving Chemical or Biological Agents during the 1996 Atlanta Olympic Games. *Annals of Emergency Medicine* 32:214–223.

Shusterman, D., J. Lipscomb, R. Neutra, and K. Satin. 1991. Symptom Prevalence and Odor-Worry Interaction near Hazardous Waste Sites. *Environmental Health Perspectives* 94:25–30.

Singer, E., and P. Endreny. 1993. *Reporting on Risk.* New York: Russell Sage Foundation.

Smith, E., L. Robins, T. Przybeck, E. Goldring, and S. Solomon. 1986. Psychosocial Consequences of a Disaster. In *Disaster Stress Studies: New Methods and Findings*, ed. J. Shore. Washington, DC: American Psychiatric Press.

Stepp, L. S. 2001. Children's Worries Take New Shape. Artwork Reveals the Effects of September 11. *Washington Post*, 2 November, C1.

Stern, J. 1999. The Prospect of Domestic Bioterrorism. *Emerging Infectious Diseases* 5:517–522.

Stiehm, E. 1992. The Psychologic Fallout from Chernobyl. *American Journal of Diseases of Children* 146:761–762.

Summerfield, D. 1999. A Critique of Seven Assumptions behind Psychological Trauma Programs in War-Affected Areas. *Social Science and Medicine* 48:1449–1462.

———. 2000. War and Mental Health: A Brief Overview. *British Medical Journal* 321:232–235.

Townsend, Mark. 1997. What Has Caused These Tragedies? *Western Morning News* [U.K.], 1 October, 16.

Tucker, J. 1997. National Health and Medical Services Response to Incidents of Chemical and Biological Terrorism. *Journal of the American Medical Association* 278:362–368.

Watts, J. 1999. Tokyo Terrorist Attack: Effects Still Felt 4 Years On. *Lancet* 353:569.

Wessely, S., J. Bisson, and S. Rose. 1999. A Systematic Review of Brief Psychological Interventions ("Debriefing") for the Treatment of Immediate Trauma Related Symptoms and the Prevention of Post Traumatic Stress Disorder. In *Depression, Anxiety and Neurosis Module of the Cochrane Database of Systematic Reviews, 1999*, ed. M. Oakley-Browne, R. Churchill, D. Gill, M. Trivedi, and S. Wessely. Oxford: Cochrane Collaboration, Issue 3, Update Software (updated quarterly).

Wessely, S., K. C. Hyams, and R. Bartholomew. 2001. Psychological Implications of Chemical and Biological Weapons. *British Medical Journal* 323:878–879.

Weiss, Rick. 2001. Demand Growing for Anthrax Vaccine. *Washington Post*, 29 September, A16.

Woodall, J. 1997. Tokyo Subway Gas Attack. *Lancet* 350:296.

Whoriskey, P., and C. L. Jenkins. 2001. Mailbox Trip Meets with Trepidation. *Washington Post*, 24 October, B1.

Zoon, K. 1999. Vaccines, Pharmaceutical Products, and Bioterrorism: Challenges for the U.S. Food and Drug Administration. *Emerging Infectious Diseases* 5:534–536.

ARTICLE 2

BIOTERRORISM PREPAREDNESS AND RESPONSE

CLINICIANS AND PUBLIC HEALTH AGENCIES AS ESSENTIAL PARTNERS

Julie Louise Gerberding, James M. Hughes, and Jeffrey P. Koplan

Beginning in mid-September 2001, the United States experienced unprecedented biological attacks involving the intentional distribution of *Bacillus anthracis* spores through the postal system.[1] The full impact of this bioterrorist activity has not been assessed, but already the toll is large. A total of 22 persons have developed anthrax and 5 have died as a direct result.[2–5] More than 10,000 persons were advised to take postexposure prophylactic treatment because they were at known or potential risk for inhalational anthrax; in addition, more than 20,000 others started such treatment until the investigation provided reassurance that exposure was unlikely and treatment could be stopped; thousands more were victims of hoaxes or false alarms, and still more were worried coworkers, friends, and family members of those directly affected.[6] The impact was not limited to the United States. Hoaxes involving threatening letters or powder-containing envelopes were reported from several countries; mail cross-contaminated with *B anthracis* was distributed to some US embassies, and persons in remote corners of the world were advised to take prophylactic antimicrobial treatment.

In this issue of the journal, three patients who acquired anthrax as a consequence of these attacks are described in detail.[7–9] They are unique from the other recent patients with anthrax in that their infection cannot be directly linked to an occupational exposure. At the time they first sought medical attention, none could provide a history suggestive of exposure to *B anthracis*, and other causes were considered more likely to explain their illnesses. In retrospect, the source of the infant's exposure was inferred when anthrax spores were found in his mother's workplace. For the other two patients, exposure to cross-contaminated mail remains a plausible but unproven hypothesis. Despite intensive investigations, the sources of their infections may never be known. These stories teach the important lesson that anyone — active elderly persons, healthy infants, and hard-working private citizens — could be infected during a bioterrorist event. Hence, the safety of all persons, regardless of age, health status, location, or occupation, must be addressed in bioterrorism preparedness and response programs.

From the public health perspective, recognition and response to the recent bioterrorist attacks has evolved in a series of overlapping phases at each location. The initial phase involved detection and then confirmation of a case of anthrax or a powder-containing envelope, followed by rapid deployment of public health and law enforcement personnel and other needed resources to the site. The second phase has been characterized by full-scale investigations as well as interventions to prevent additional cases. Longer-term consequence management, including follow-up of affected individuals and remediation of contaminated sites that could pose an occupational health risk, are major activities in the current phase. In all these phases, clinicians have proven to be essential partners, which is a lesson that must be incorporated into future bioterrorism preparedness and response efforts and professional education programs.

In most situations, alert clinicians actually initiated the first phase of the response by obtaining the appropriate laboratory tests, recognizing that a patient might have anthrax, and notifying health officials. Emergency physicians, outpatient primary care physicians and other practitioners, dermatologists, and pediatricians participated in the early recognition of infected patients, illustrating their critical role in surveillance for bioterrorism. Radiologists, infectious diseases specialists, pulmonologists, surgeons, hospitalists, critical care specialists, laboratorians, pathologists, and many other specialists also contributed to the diagnosis and management. Together, these clinicians have created a remarkably effective detection system for identifying and reporting cases. Their collective efforts provided an early warning to public health and law enforcement agencies that signaled the need for large-scale interventions to protect thousands of others at risk.

For this frontline surveillance system to function at its best, all clinicians, regardless of their specialty, must have enough basic information about the clinical manifestations of infections caused by the select agents of bioterrorism to raise their suspicion when they see a patient with a compatible illness. In addition, clinicians must know how to diagnose these conditions and when and how to report their suspicion to local public health and law enforcement officials. In the current response scenario, obtaining an accurate occupational history was vital in assessing anthrax risk; all clinicians need this skill to be prepared for similar scenarios in the future.

Enhancing the knowledge and skills of clinicians is not just a matter of one-time educational programs. Bioterrorism-related infections hopefully will remain rare events, and creative ongoing strategies will be required to sustain attention to potential new cases when the current phase of alarm and interest ebbs. Furthermore, better systems are needed for public health agencies to alert all clinicians when an attack is suspected or documented, facilitate real-time reporting, and disseminate credible information required for optimal exposure risk assessment, diagnosis, and treatment. Such efforts will simultaneously result in an improved capacity to detect and respond to naturally occurring emerging and reemerging infectious diseases.

Frontline clinicians faced a challenge that often was even more difficult than diagnosing anthrax — that of excluding the diagnosis among the many worried patients with concerns about potential exposure or among those who sought care for rashes or illnesses suggestive of the diagnosis. In the absence of clinical algorithms or rapid diagnostic tests, their clinical judgment helped reassure patients and avert the distraction that initiating unneeded response efforts would have otherwise entailed. For the future, developing clinical algorithms and laboratory testing protocols and reagents that rapidly and accurately identify all pathogens in the differential diagnosis of the suspicious illness, not just the select agents of bioterrorism, is important but will take time.

Primary care clinicians certainly have played a key role in managing postexposure prophylactic treatment interventions and their complications in the second phase of the response to the recent bioterrorist attacks. The initial distribution of antimicrobial drugs was usually coordinated through public health agencies, but often involved local clinicians as well. Those in outpatient settings have provided adherence counseling and advice about managing adverse events and other complications. Some clinicians also helped patients make decisions about their personal risk and the need for anthrax vaccine or additional days of antimicrobial prophylaxis. Patients with special concerns or underlying illnesses have solicited consultation about antimicrobial treatment from their obstetricians, pediatricians, and other medical specialists.

Many of the individualized preventive treatment decisions had to be made in the context of an inadequate or evolving evidence base. Input from clinicians directly involved in the affected areas and from professional medical societies and other organizations proved to be extremely useful for the development of the Centers for Disease Control and Prevention's interim treatment guidelines.[10–16] Clinicians also assisted many patients with decisions about anthrax vaccine treatment options, even though they had little advance warning or information about the program. Mechanisms to anticipate and more quickly respond to the needs of those caring for the diverse population of affected patients is another priority for enhancing bioterrorism response capacity as part of preparation for future events.

Clinicians are actively engaged in the current phase of the response (long-term consequence management and remediation) and are likely to be even more engaged in the future. The possibility of late onset of inhalational anthrax among exposed persons, even though considered unlikely by most experts, requires heightened concern about febrile illnesses, chest pain, sweats, profound fatigue, and other symptoms in persons who were exposed to *B anthracis.* Likewise, clinicians must be alert to the possibility of long-term adverse events attributable to antimicrobial treatment and vaccination. Prophylactic anitimicrobial treatment is not likely to cause frequent serious late-onset adverse events, but there is inadequate experience with 60 or more days of antimicrobial treatment and anthrax vaccine among the diverse populations represented in the treated group. During the next 24 months, the Centers for Disease Control and Prevention plans to survey the health status of the 10,000 people whose exposure history suggested a need for prolonged prophylactic antimicrobial treatment, but local clinicians will be the most important resource for detecting adverse events, recognizing their association with prophylactic treatment for anthrax, and reporting them to health officials and the Food and Drug Administration. Other occupational and mental health issues that will require the services of additional medical specialists may emerge among exposed persons over the next months to years.

Although it is tempting to respond as if the current anthrax threat is coming to an end, the criminal(s) who perpetrated these acts of bioterrorism has not been apprehended. The country remains at risk for additional exposures and infections with this deadly pathogen and perhaps with other agents. The importance of individual clinicians in bioterrorism preparedness and response was not fully appreciated by many until the current attacks occurred. Hopefully, the lessons learned during the past 4 months will motivate local health departments, health care organizations, and clinicians to engage in collaborative programs to enhance their communication and local preparedness and response capabilities. Knowledgeable clinicians, operating in the framework of a health care delivery system that is fully prepared to support the necessary diagnostic and treatment modalities to manage affected patients, and seamless linkages to local public health agencies will provide a strong foundation for detecting, responding to, and combating bioterrorism and other infectious disease threats to public health in the future.

REFERENCES

1. Recognition of illness associated with the intentional release of a biologic agent. *MMWR* 2001;50:893–897.

2. Jernigan JA, Stephens DS, Ashford DA, et al. Bioterrorism-related inhalational anthrax. *Emerg Infect Dis.* 2001;7:933–944.

3. Borio L, Frank D, Mani V, et al. Death due to bioterrorism-related inhalational anthrax: report of 2 patients. *JAMA.* 2001;286:2554–2559.

4. Mayer TA, Bersoff-Matcha S, Murphy C, et al. Clinical presentation of inhalational anthrax following bioterrorism exposure. *JAMA.* 2001;286:2549–2553.

5. Bush LM, Abrams BH, Beall A, Johnson CC. Index case of fatal inhalational anthrax due to bioterrorism in the United States. *N Engl J Med.* 2001;345:1607–1610.

6. Update; investigation of bioterrorism-related anthrax and adverse events from antimicrobial prophylaxis. *MMWR* 2001;50:973–976.

7. Mina B, Dym JP, Kuepper F, et al. Fatal inhalational anthrax with unknown source of exposure in a 61-year-old woman in New York City. *JAMA.* 2002;287: 858–862.

8. Freedman A, Afonja O, Chang MW, et al. Cutaneous anthrax associated with microangiopathic hemolytic anemia and coagulopathy in a 7-month-old infant. *JAMA.* 2002;287:869–874.

9. Barakat LA, Quentzel HL, Jernigan JA, et al. Fatal inhalational anthrax in a 94-year-old Connecticut woman. *JAMA.* 2002;287:863–868.

10. Update: investigation of anthrax associated with intentional exposure and interim public health guidelines, October 2001. *MMWR* 2001;50:889–893.

11. Update: investigation of bioterrorism-related anthrax and interim guidelines for exposure management and antimicrobial therapy, October 2001. *MMWR* 2001;50: 909–919.

12. Update: investigation of bioterrorism-related anthrax and interim guidelines for clinical evaluation of persons with possible anthrax. *MMWR* 2001;50:941–948.

13. Updated recommendations for antimicrobial prophylaxis among asymptomatic pregnant women after exposure to *Bacillus anthracis*. *MMWR* 2001;50:960.

14. Interim guidelines for investigation of and response to *Bacillus anthracis* exposures. *MMWR* 2001;50:987–990.

15. Update: interim recommendations for antimicrobial prophylaxis for children and breastfeeding mothers and treatment of children with anthrax. *MMWR* 2001;50: 1014–1016.

16. Bell DM, Kozarsky PE, Stephens DS. Meeting summary. *Emerg Infect Dis*. In press.

A R T I C L E 3

Bioterrorism Law and Policy

Critical Choices in Public Health

James G. Hodge, Jr.

There is perhaps no duty more fundamental to American government than the protection of the public's health, safety, and welfare.[1] On September 11, 2001, this governmental duty was severely tested through a series of terrorist acts. The destruction of the World Trade Towers in New York City and a portion of the Pentagon in Washington, D.C., presented many Americans with a new, visible reality of the potential harms that terrorists can cause. The staggering loss of lives (estimated from 2,600 to 2,900)[2] damaged the national psyche in ways far exceeding the physical scars to American institutions.

As horrific as the images of destruction and loss of human lives may be, events that unfolded after September 11 revealed another dreaded, and potentially more catastrophic, threat to Americans' sense of security and public health: *bioterrorism.* Unlike terrorists that use bombs, explosives, or other tools for mass destruction, a bioterrorist's weapon is an infectious agent. Bioterrorism involves the intentional use of an infectious agent (e.g., microorganism, virus, infectious substance, or biological product) to cause death or disease in humans or other organisms in order to negatively influence the conduct of government or intimidate a population.[3]

In the weeks that followed the terrorist attacks on September 11, public health and law enforcement officials discovered that some person or group had intentionally contaminated letters with potentially deadly anthrax spores. These letters were mailed to a variety of individuals in government and the media in three states and the District of Columbia. Dozens of persons that handled or received the tainted letters tested positive for anthrax exposure. To date, at least five persons have died. Many government officials predict the potential for additional bioterrorism attacks as the "war on terrorism" continues in Afghanistan and surrounding territories.

For state and local public health agencies that may find themselves on the frontline of defense to a bioterrorism event, prevention through preparation is essential.[4] Prior training exercises have demonstrated that preventing mass casualities or infections resulting from bioterrorism is difficult.[5] Public health authorities, medical practitioners, and hospitals[6] may lack the infrastructure,[7] resources, knowledge, or tools to effectively respond to mass exposure to diseases for which there are potentially inadequate detection[8] or tests,[9] no (or insufficient) vaccines, few treatments, or no cures. Prior to September 11, federal and state public health authorities had already allocated some resources and engaged in efforts to prevent a major bioterrorism event.[10] Congress authorized the spending of over $500 million in 2001 for bioterrorism preparedness through the Public Health Threats and Emergencies Act.[11] Additional commitments to improve surveillance of unusual diseases or clusters, train health-care workers, improve existing vaccination[12] and treatment supplies through increases of national stockpiles, and collaborate across jurisdictions are needed to improve the public health infrastructure.[13]

Public health authorities must also be legally empowered with the authority to respond to potential or actual bioterrorist threats.[14] Some states have legislatively (e.g., Colorado[15]) or administratively (e.g., Rhode Island[16]) developed public health response plans for a bioterrorism event. However, in many states, existing legal standards for response are absent, antiquated, or insufficient. Prior to September 11, many state health departments did not address bioterrorism in their emergency response plans.[17] Recently, public health lawyers and scholars at the Center for Law and the Public's Health at Georgetown and Johns Hopkins Universities were asked by the Centers for Disease Control and Prevention and a series of national partners (i.e., the National Governors Association, the National Conference of State Legislatures, the Association of State and Territorial Health Officials, the National Association of City and County Health Officers, the National Association of Attorneys General, and the Turning Point Public Health Statute Modernization National Collaborative) to develop a model act for states to respond to public health emergencies. The Model State Emergency Health Powers Act[18] gives state and local public health authorities a modern series of powers to track, prevent, and control disease threats resulting from bioterrorism or other public health emergencies. These powers include measures (e.g., isolation, quarantine, treatment, and vaccination requirements) that may temporarily compromise individual civil liberties (e.g., rights to due process, speech, assembly, travel, and privacy) to protect the public's health. To date, thirty-two states have introduced legislative bills based on the Model Act.[19]

Vesting state and local public health authorities with a modern series of public health powers is an important component of a national legal strategy to respond to bioterrorism events.[20] The Model Act, existing state laws, and other planning tools suggest the need for broad cooperation among all levels of government and the private sector. The consequences of a public health emergency, like many other emergencies, cannot be handled through the efforts of a single state or local agency. To ensure cooperation and better prepare for and respond to existing and future domestic bioterrorism attacks, federal, state, and local public health authorities must make a series of critical choices in law or policy based on the following questions:

- What is the extent of government's duty to protect the public's health in response to a bioterrorism event?

- When does a bioterrorism event justify the declaration of a "public health emergency"?
- What are the respective roles of federal, state, and local public health authorities?
- How should public health authorities coordinate with other governmental actors, specifically law enforcement authorities, to address criminal components of bioterrorism events?
- How can restrictive public health powers (e.g., isolation, quarantine, mandatory treatment, or vaccination) be balanced with individual civil liberties in responding to a public health emergency?
- How should scarce resources (e.g., vaccines, treatments, hospital beds, health-care personnel) be allocated during a public health emergency?

The section below presents an overview of the population-wide threats of bioterrorism to provide a context for addressing these questions. Making choices now about questions of governmental power, particularly from the perspective of state and local public health agencies that may be the nation's first source of detection, may improve coordination and accountability among the various levels and branches of governments in their efforts to prevent or respond to a future bioterrorism event.

BIOTERRORISM: PAST AND PRESENT

Recent developments concerning the intentional spread of anthrax through the U.S. mails provide a modern example of bioterrorism activity in the United States. However, bioterrorism has long been a part of the nation's past. Numerous examples of attempted and actual bioterrorist activity (with varying degrees of success and impact) have been documented in American and world history. The Chemical and Biological Weapons Nonproliferation Project of the Monterrey Institute's Center for Nonproliferation Studies has catalogued more than 400 incidents of known bioterrorist activity worldwide between 1900 and 1999. In the United States, British and French troops exchanged dry goods intentionally contaminated with smallpox with Native American populations.[21] In 1972, several persons were arrested for possessing kilograms of Typhoid bacteria intended for the contamination of the water supply of several Midwestern cities.[22] In 1984, members of the Rajneeshee cult contaminated restaurant salad bars in Oregon with a form of salmonella, resulting in more than 700 cases of non-fatal food poisoning.[23] Each of the past several years, the Federal Bureau of Investigation (FBI) has investigated hundreds of claims of bioterrorism threats.

Historical accounts and modern risk assessments of bioterrorism activities provide the nation with some experience in handling future events. Public health and other authorities have also conducted numerous hypothetical and table-top exercises to better prepare for a modern bioterrorism event. The subject of many of these exercises became reality immediately following the tragedy of September 11. In late September, the media reported that an individual in a Florida office building was potentially exposed to anthrax, a biological agent that can be deadly when inhaled and left untreated. Within a month, numerous additional cases of exposure and infection were tracked by public health authorities in Connecticut, Florida, New York, Maryland, Nevada, New Jersey, and Washington, D.C. Law enforcement and public health officials determined that most exposures resulted from intentional efforts to spread the pathogen through contaminated letters delivered through the U.S. postal service. Some of the anthrax strains were the product of sophisticated manufacturing techniques designed to make the agent more virulent.[24]

Authorities quickly began warning the public through broadcasts and printed sources to be cautious about suspicious packages or powdery substances in the mail, although government warnings were mixed in their accuracy and tone.[25] Media coverage was dominated by images of people lining up for testing and health officials clad in plastic, biodefense suits collecting samples of anthrax from mailrooms, elevators, and trucks. Mail service in some places was suspended or significantly delayed. Federal institutions, including some members of Congress and the Supreme Court, were forced to temporarily relocate. At least five people died from exposure to anthrax. Dozens of others, including aids to prominent members of Congress and news anchors, tested positive.[26]

The anthrax attacks fueled apprehension among government officials[27] and the public about future bioterrorism attacks.[28] A recent national poll suggests that 70 percent of the public believes a subsequent biological or chemical attack on the United States will occur in the next year.[29] These fears of bioterrorism may be justified. A broad range of groups or individuals may have access to and use biological agents as weapons to inflict harm on a population-wide basis.[30] Multiple infectious agents, including genetically enhanced agents, may be used.[31] Diseases such as smallpox,[32] tularemia (a.k.a. rabbit fever),[33] plague,[34] and viral hemorrhagic fever may present far more serious dangers to the public's health than the non-contagious and largely treatable anthrax.

Bioterrorists may infect individuals through multiple routes: (1) intentional spread of contagious diseases through individual contact; (2) airborne dissemination of some infectious agents; or (3) contamination of water, food, controlled substances, or other widely distributed products. The equipment needed to manufacture biological weapons is easy to obtain and conceal. Prior doubts about the potential or ability for an individual or group to intentionally unleash these agents on an innocent population have been nullified by the brazenness of recent terrorist events.[35]

BIOTERRORISM AND PUBLIC HEALTH LAW: THE CRITICAL CHOICES

Given the nation's current level of preparedness for bioterrorism, a large-scale bioterrorist attack would be unprecedented in its impact on morbidity and mortality in the U.S. population. The limited, intentional spread of anthrax has shown that public health (and other) authorities are not fully prepared to handle a large-scale bioterrorism event.[36]

Preparing for a bioterrorism event should become a central mission of federal, state, and local public health, law enforcement, and emergency authorities. As part of this mission, the public health community, law- and policymakers, and society in general must address a series of critical choices.

Understanding the Duty of Government to Protect the Public Health

Perhaps the most important choice is also the most difficult to make: What is the government's duty to protect the public health in response to a bioterrorism event? Few discount the responsibility of government to respond to a bioterrorism event, but what is the extent of this response? Consistent with the traditional police powers of state governments to protect the health, safety, and general welfare, government's duty to protect the public's health may be viewed as comprehensive and extensive.[37] This includes virtually any governmental action needed to control the threat in the population. Thus, to fulfill its responsibility to ensure the public's health, state public health authorities could (as they have in the past) temporarily constrain certain civil liberties, require private sector participation in public health objectives, shut down potentially harmful industries, destroy contaminated property, deport or prevent the entry of individuals who may infect others, ration supplies, and control the flow of information.

Do governmental duties to protect the public's health allow public health authorities to go further? Bioterrorism experts suggest that the intentional release of smallpox through just a few outlets could quickly spread the disease and leave hundreds of thousands of unvaccinated Americans dead in a few months.[38] At the apex of this type of human tragedy, can authorities temporarily ignore constitutional principles that respect individual liberties (e.g., rights to due process, travel, assembly, or privacy) or maintain the structure of government (e.g., federalism or separation of powers)? Concerning the latter powers, for example, can federal health authorities, who lack broad police powers, command state public health authorities to participate in a federal, national response to a bioterrorism event that is limited to one state (and thus not seen as an interstate matter or a threat to national security)? The federal government may lack the constitutional power to do this under existing interpretations of federal commerce powers consistent with principles of federalism.[39] Can we choose to ignore such legal interpretations to accomplish public health objectives? In reality, it is unlikely that any bioterrorism event, even one that is initially localized to one state, would be viewed solely as a state matter when it is highly predictable that the bioterrorism agent will spread to other states.

Declaring a Public Health Emergency

Responding to a bioterrorism event may require public health authorities to exercise broader powers than they traditionally employ. Who should choose when to declare a public health emergency and under what criteria? Many state legislatures presently fail to specify whether a bioterrorism event may justify a state of emergency status, leaving this decision to executive authorities. Though state executive authorities need some discretion, statutory laws must better define the conditions for declaring public health emergencies. Otherwise, a state of emergency may be called unjustifiably.

The Model State Emergency Health Powers Act gives public health authorities the ability to exercise enhanced powers to protect individuals and manage property upon the declaration of a public health emergency by the state governor. The Model Act broadly defines a "public health emergency" as:

> an occurrence or imminent threat of an illness or health condition that: (1) is believed to be caused by bioterrorism or the appearance of a novel or previously controlled or eradicated infectious agent or biological toxin; and (2) poses a high probability of any of the following harms: (a) a large number of deaths in the affected population; (b) a large number of incidents of serious permanent or long-term disability in the affected population; or (c) widespread exposure to an infectious or toxic agent that poses a significant risk of substantial future harm to a large number of people in the affected population.[40]

Thus, under this definition, the declaration of a public health emergency may follow (1) the occurrence or imminent threat of an illness or health condition, (2) caused by bioterrorism or the appearance of novel or previously controlled diseases through any means, (3) that poses a high probability of a significant number of current or future deaths or disabilities. These criteria serve as guides, but may allow for the declaration of a public health emergency for bioterrorism events that do not justify restrictive public health controls. Consider, for example, the definition of "bioterrorism" used in the Model Act:

> the intentional use of any microorganism, virus, infectious substance, or biological product that may be engineered as a result of biotechnology, or any naturally occurring or bioengineered component of any such microorganism, virus, infectious substance, or biological product, to cause death, disease, or other biological malfunction in a human, an animal, a plant, or another living organism in order to influence the conduct of government or to intimidate or coerce a civilian population.[41]

On its face, this definition might include the actions of persons who have recently attempted to infect others with anthrax through the mail. This may be unlikely, however, because their actions may not pose "a high probability" of a large number of human deaths or incidents of serious permanent or long-term disability, as defined under "public health emergency." From a public health perspective, this limited interpretation of the criteria for declaring a public health emergency may be preferable. It would be unwise to declare a public health emergency for an event that involves an infectious agent, but does not otherwise pose a significant risk to the public's health.

Consider, for example, an individual with HIV who intentionally tries to spread the virus to dozens of others through his own risky behavior (e.g., unprotected sex, unsafe sharing of needles for injecting drugs). Numerous individuals have attempted to intentionally infect others with HIV in documented cases across the United States.[42] Their activities probably were not motivated by an intent to "influence the conduct of government." Yet, depending on how a governor, or a court reviewing the governor's authority, may define what it means to "intimidate" or "coerce," or what constitutes a "population" (is it the population of a state, a county, a city, or a neighborhood?), the individual with HIV may be said to be engaging in bioterrorism. Depending on whether there is a high probability of a large number of human deaths or disabilities as a result, a governor could declare a state of public health emergency pursuant to the Model Act. This is problematic because (1) public health and law enforcement authorities have not traditionally viewed such persons as bioterrorists, but rather as mere criminals; and (2) declaring a public health emergency in these cases is an extreme response to a limited public health threat.

Additional refinement of the criteria for responding to a bioterrorism event through the declaring of a public health emergency is important where infringements of civil liberties and the legitimacy of public health activities are at stake. The criteria may be strengthened by employing more restrictive measures during a public health emergency depending on the severity of the disease threat.

Defining the Roles of Federal, State, and Local Public Health Authorities

There is no central public health system in the United States. Instead, a collaborative workforce of federal, state, and local authorities work in conjunction with other inter-level agencies (e.g., environmental protection agencies; departments of housing, labor, or civil rights) to accomplish public health outcomes. In this system, public health roles and responsibilities of the federal, state, and local levels of government are complex and unclear. As stated above, state public health authorities act pursuant to broad police powers that authorize the government to act in the interests of protecting or promoting the health, safety, or general welfare of the population. Some public health functions are delegated by states to local governments. A federal agency's power to act in the interest of public health is, comparably, more limited in the use of authorized powers. It must rely on its delegated authority pursuant to Congress's powers to protect national security, regulate interstate commerce, tax and spend, or promote the constitutional principles of the Fourteenth Amendment (e.g., due process, equal protection).[43]

A large-scale bioterrorism event will accentuate existing uncertainties in the distribution of public health powers.[44] It may also prove to be a catalyst for redefining roles for the future. The critical choice for public health authorities is not to decide where the power to protect the public health lies or which level of government has the primary power to act, but rather where the leadership to respond to a bioterrorism event will derive. If leadership capacity is properly developed, public health authorities can use their respective powers to bring about desired goals.

Through agencies such as the Department of Health and Human Services (DHHS), its subsidiary Centers for Disease Control and Prevention (CDC), and the newly created Office of Homeland Security, the federal government has taken a leadership role in response to existing and future bioterrorism threats.[45] There are many reasons state and local public health authorities might defer to this leadership initiative. First, the federal government has greater financial resources at its disposal to respond to a bioterrorism threat.[46] Second, it may be in a better position to negotiate the price of needed vaccines, drugs, or supplies, or to suspend the patent rights of high-demand medications. These techniques were recently used by President George Bush and DHHS in negotiations with the German drug company Bayer, concerning the sale of Cipro, the antibiotic used to treat anthrax.[47] Third, most significant bioterrorism threats will exceed the boundaries of any single state, thus requiring a national, coordinated response. Fourth, the federal government may be better able to rapidly develop personnel and institutional expertise in monitoring and identifying the existence of new or emerging infectious pathogens. Fifth, bioterrorism may also constitute a threat to national security (the protection of which is specifically a federal responsibility).[48] Finally, imminent warnings of bioterrorism activity may come through national intelligence or federal law enforcement agencies that can coordinate public health responses through federal agencies.

Choosing to assign a primary leadership role to the federal government for responding to bioterrorism threats does have its drawbacks. Federal public health authorities may be slowed by inter-organizational or bureaucratic problems.[49] As well, they are not well positioned to serve on the frontline of defense to a bioterrorist attack. State and local public health authorities, in conjunction with private sector health-care workers, will in most cases be the first to detect potential bioterrorism activity through effective surveillance. Federal authorities may facilitate detection by sharing resources or intelligence data. However, detection of a potential bioterrorism threat through state and local public health authorities is distinct from the response functions of the federal government. Clarifying these roles will improve response capabilities and public accountability over time.

Investigating Bioterrorism from the Public Health or Criminal Perspectives

Beyond setting roles and responsibilities among the various levels of government is the need for public health authorities to choose how to coordinate with law enforcement and national security authorities. Unlike the spread of naturally occurring diseases that can be monitored and controlled exclusively through public health authorities, a bioterrorism event always features an unlawful element. Bioterrorism, by definition, is the product of criminal activity. Existing and newly passed federal antiterrorism laws, for example, criminalize the mere possession of certain biological agents.[50] Every bioterrorism event thus involves a criminal investigation that is outside the purview of public health authorities. How should public health and criminal authorities choose to collaborate? Should they collaborate at all?

From either side's perspective, clearly they should collaborate. Public health and criminal authorities need to know of potential or actual health threats to the population in order to take steps to prevent or mitigate threats. Each can learn from the other about these threats without jeopardizing their differing central missions, provided that the exchange of information is confidential, accomplished through high-ranking personnel, and consistent with existing federal intelligence laws and federal or state privacy laws that may limit the sharing of some data.

Second, after a bioterrorism event has materialized, should public health authorities assist criminal investigators at the federal, state, or local level? Prevailing public health practice suggests they should not. Public health authorities resist participating in criminal investigations primarily because there is the potential that public health authorities could be seen by community members as health police. Yet, prevailing public health practice does not typically involve the spread of disease through criminal activity. In some cases where criminal activity has been at the source of potential infection (e.g., intentional spread of HIV, intentional contamination or pollution of air or water), public health authorities have worked with criminal investigators in limited ways to stymie a public health threat.[51] Bioterrorism events may justify a greater working relationship between criminal and public health authorities that the public may not only understand, but support.

If public health and criminal authorities must work in collaboration to control a bioterrorism event, who takes primary jurisdiction over an investigation, given an outbreak? In many of the places where anthrax exposures recently occurred, criminal authorities quickly asserted their jurisdiction over exposure sites to gather evidence and any other facts needed for their investigations. The potential for public health and criminal authorities to clash in executing their responsibilities is evident, especially where the primary criminal or intelligence authorities may be federal (e.g., the FBI, the Central Intelligence Agency), and the responding public health officials are primarily state or local. The only choice for public health officials in these circumstances may be to defer to law enforcement or intelligence authorities for a period of time as the investigation proceeds, but to encourage collaborative sharing of data to allow both sets of authorities to accomplish their respective goals.

Restricting Individuals for the Sake of Public Health

During a bioterrorism attack that involves the potential for mass casualties or disabilities, public health authorities may need to employ powers that restrict individual activities and behaviors. The Model Act, for example, allows public health authorities to quarantine or isolate persons believed to be exposed to or infected with a contagious disease during a public health emergency.[52] In addition, authorities can encourage persons to be vaccinated or treated where necessary to prevent the spread of a contagious disease. Persons who refuse to be vaccinated or treated may, if needed, be quarantined or isolated.[53]

Such measures have traditionally been used by public health authorities to control the spread of contagious disease. Few question their potential value in accomplishing the same, despite their potential to infringe on human rights. The critical choice for public health authorities during a bioterrorism emergency is how to balance these restrictive measures with civil liberties.[54] There may be strong legislative and public support for the use of highly restrictive powers during a bioterrorism crisis. Yet, constitutional principles and public health practices emphasizing an ethic of voluntarism intimate that not every restrictive measure can be taken. Professor Lawrence O. Gostin has summarized the modern constitutional criteria for exercising confining public health powers:[55]

- *A compelling state interest in confinement.* Public health authorities must have a compelling interest that is substantially furthered by civil confinement. Only persons who are truly dangerous (i.e., pose a significant risk of transmission) can be confined.
- *A "well-targeted" intervention.* Interventions that confine individuals must be well-targeted to accomplishing public health objectives. Thus, interventions that are over- or underinclusive may be constitutionally impermissible if they deprive individuals of liberty or equal protection without justification. For example, the quarantine of every person within a geographic area is overinclusive if some members would not transmit infection. Underinclusive interventions would restrain some, but not all, potentially contagious persons, and thus be open to criticisms of being arbitrary or purposefully discriminatory.
- *The least restrictive alternative.* Public health authorities should not resort to civil confinement if they can achieve their objectives through less drastic means (although it is not likely that they have to use extreme or unduly expensive means to avoid confinement).
- *Procedural due process.* Persons subject to confinement for public health purposes are entitled to some form of procedural due process depending on the nature and duration of the restraint. The Model Act requires a court order prior to the isolation or quarantine of any individual, unless emergency circumstances demand otherwise. In all cases, individuals have the right to a hearing and counsel to contest their confinement.[56]

Allocating Scarce Resources

In virtually any widespread and rapidly developing bioterrorism event, available public health resources will quickly be taxed. Scarce resources may include physical goods (e.g., vaccines, medical treatments and supplies, hospital beds, isolation or quarantine facilities), personnel (e.g., physicians, nurses, other health-care workers, epidemiologists, lab technicians), and services (e.g., laboratory testing, mental health counseling). Attempts to hoard existing supplies or personnel by competing governmental units or private sector groups may be expected. The private sector may be disinclined to donate its facilities for public health goals, or participate in the vaccination, treatment, or confinement of exposed or infected individuals. Concerning these issues, the Model Act allows state executive authorities to confiscate hoarded supplies, take possession of facilities or other property for public health purposes, and seek the assistance of medical personnel during a public health emergency.

A critical and unresolved choice for public health authorities is how to allocate scarce resources. There is no uniform, central proposal governing the distribution of limited resources during a public health emergency. In fact, such a proposal may be ill-advised. Public health authorities may need the discretion, depending on the circumstances of the specific bioterrorism event, to decide how best to allocate limited resources. *Ad hoc* allocation decisions, of course, leave open the possibility of egregious, unfair, or discriminatory distributions of limited resources. Is it predictable that: (1) wealthier individuals (or nations) will have access to potentially life-saving treatments over persons of lesser wealth; (2) persons in the military will be vaccinated before civilians; or (3) public health investigators will attend to health threats to legislators over other governmental workers?[57] Each of these choices, which are based on actual decisions made during the recent anthrax exposures in the United States, may be supported or contested on various legal, political, and ethical grounds.

Public health and other governmental authorities must be guided by a fair set of principles in making their allocation decisions. These principles include:

- *Promoting the public's health.* Any decision relating to allocating scarce resources during a public health emergency should be principally motivated by the need to promote the public's health to the highest extent possible, and not by outside political or social pressures.
- *Providing incentives to help.* To provide incentives to individuals to participate in public health efforts, certain resources may be allocated to protect the health of public health personnel or health-care workers (and their families) working to control the spread of disease or treat infected individuals.
- *Respecting each individual.* Distribution of limited resources may naturally tend to favor persons in government or those with sufficient wealth or stature in the community. Public health authorities need to determine a method of distributing resources evenly across at-risk populations to protect the public's health. Specific care should be taken to avoid making decisions that discriminate against equally situated individuals.
- *Prioritizing immediacy over potential.* The distribution of limited vaccines or treatments should be made with consideration of the immediate health consequences to affected populations rather than the potential impact on unaffected groups. Thus, for example, if a particular group of individuals living in one county of a state is presently susceptible to smallpox infection due to a localized outbreak, those persons should be vaccinated to the exclusion of other state residents who may be vulnerable in the future, provided such vaccinations are consistent with controlling the epidemic.

These principles will not resolve every difficult question, but they may provide some guidance as public health authorities struggle to decide how to allocate dwindling resources during an emergency.

CONCLUSION

Bioterrorism is a catalyst for change in public health practice. Preparing for existing and future bioterrorism events in the United States requires federal, state, and local public health authorities to collaborate in new ways with law enforcement, intelligence, and emergency personnel to strengthen the existing public health infrastructure. Working to improve public health detection, prevention, and response capabilities requires effective training, additional resources, use of existing and new technologies, and public health law reform. These and other tools for responding to existing and future bioterrorism events call for public health authorities, law- and policymakers, and society to make a series of critical choices.

The duty of government to protect the public's health must be understood within political, legal, and realistic limits. A central legal objective of the Model State Emergency Health Powers Act is to better define the criteria, powers, roles, and limits of governmental actions during a public health emergency. The leadership roles of federal, state, and local public health authorities must be distinguished between detection and response. Public health and law enforcement authorities need to share information and resources in the interest of protecting the public. Civil liberties must be respected, when possible, in the exercise of restrictive state public health powers. And limited resources must be allocated fairly according to a pre-determined set of principles. Addressing these critical choices may facilitate government's ability to effectively protect the public's health during the next, inevitable bioterrorism event.

REFERENCES

1. L.O. Gostin, *Public Health Law: Power, Duty, Restraint* (Berkeley: University of California Press, 2000): at 16.

2. E. Lipton, "Hard to Figure: A Difference in the Numbers," *New York Times,* October 25, 2001, at B1.

3. Model State Emergency Health Powers Act § 1-104(a) (December 21, 2001), *available at* <http://www.publichealthlaw.net/MSEHPA/MSEHPA2.pdf>.

4. D.E. Shalala, "Bioterrorism: How Prepared Are We?," *Emerging Infectious Diseases*, 5, no. 4(1999): 492–93, *available at* <http://www.cdc.gov/ncidod/EID/vol5no4/shalala.htm>.

5. T. Inglesby, R. Grossman, and T. O'Toole, "A Plague on Your City: Observations from TOPOFF," *Biodefense Quarterly*, 2 (2000): 1–10.

6. M. Freudenheim, "Few Hospitals Are Ready for a Surge of Bioterror Victims," *New York Times*, October 26, 2001, at B8.

7. S. Khan and D.A. Ashford, "Ready or Not — Preparedness for Bioterrorism," *N. Engl. J. Med.*, 345 (2001): 287–89.

8. D.E. Rosenbaum and S.G. Stolberg, "New Battlefield: Questions on Adequacy of Health System and Public Protection," *New York Times*, October 23, 2001, at A1.

9. R. Weiss, "Anthrax Testing Shaky," *Pittsburgh Post-Gazette*, October 16, 2001, at A4.

10. J. Fialka et al., "Are We Prepared for the Unthinkable?," *Wall Street Journal*, September 18, 2001, at B1.

11. Public Health Threats and Emergencies Act, Pub. L. No. 106–505, 114 Stat. 2314 (2000).

12. J. Miller and S.G. Stolberg, "Sept. 11 Attacks Led to Push for More Smallpox Vaccine," *New York Times*, October 22, 2001, at A1.

13. Shalala, *supra* note 4.

14. D.P. Fidler, "Legal Issues Surrounding Public Health Emergencies." Paper presented at the *Second Annual Symposium on Medical and Public Health Response to Bioterrorism*, Baltimore, November 28–29, 2000.

15. Colo. Rev. Stat. Ann. § 24-32-2103 (West 2001).

16. T. Bertrand et al., *The Emergence of Bioterrorism as a Public Health Concern in the 21st Century: Epidemiology and Surveillance, at* <http://www.healthri.org/environment/biot/article.htm> (last updated October 15, 2001).

17. Khan and Ashford, *supra* note 7.

18. Model State Emergency Health Powers Act (December 21, 2001).

19. These thirty-two states are Arizona, California, Connecticut, Delaware, Florida, Georgia, Hawaii, Idaho, Illinois, Kansas, Kentucky, Maine, Maryland, Massachusetts, Minnesota, Mississippi, Missouri, Nebraska, New Hampshire, New Jersey, New Mexico, New York, Oklahoma, Pennsylvania, Rhode Island, South Dakota, Tennessee, Utah, Vermont, Washington, Wisconsin, and Wyoming. Center for Law and the Public's Health, *Model State Emergency Health Powers Act State Legislative Activity* (April 8, 2002), *available at* <http://www.publichealthlaw.net/ MSEHPA/MSEHPA_Legis_Act.pdf>.

20. B. Kellman, "Biological Terrorism: Legal Measures for Preventing Catastrophe," *Harvard Journal of Law and Public Policy*, 24 (2001): 417–88.

21. R.S. Root-Bernstein, "Infectious Terrorism," *The Atlantic Monthly*, 267 (1991): 44–50.

22. Y. Alexander, "Terrorism in the Twenty-First Century: Threats and Responses," *DePaul Business Law Journal*, 12 (2000): 59–81.

23. J.B. Tucker, "Historical Trends Related to Bioterrorism: An Empirical Analysis," *Emerging Infectious Diseases*, 5, no. 4 (1999): 498–504, at 503, *available at* <http://www.cdc.gov/ncidod/eid/vol5no4/tucker.htm>.

24. C. Haberman, "New Legal Powers, Fresh Anthrax Worries, Resilient Taliban," *New York Times*, October 26, 2001, at B1.

25. J. Miller and S.G. Stolberg, "Wider Anthrax Monitoring; U.S. Officials Acknowledge Underestimating Mail Risks," *New York Times*, October 25, 2001, at A1.

26. J. Lancaster and S. Schmidt, "31 Exposed to Anthrax on Capitol Hill," *Washington Post*, October 18, 2001, at A1.

27. Fialka et al., *supra* note 10.

28. L. Parker, T. Watson, and K. Johnson, "Anthrax Incidents Create Growing Sense of Anxiety," *USA Today,* October 15, 2001, at A1.

29. "Snapshot," *USA Today,* October 25, 2001, at A1.

30. M.G. Kortepeter and G.W. Parker, "Potential Biological Weapons Threats," *Emerging Infectious Diseases*, 5 (1999): 523–27.
31. *Id.*
32. D.A. Henderson, "Smallpox: Clinical and Epidemiologic Features," *Emerging Infectious Diseases*, 5, no. 4 (1999): 537–39, *available at* <http://www.cdc.gov/ncidod/EID/vol5no4/henderson.htm>.
33. D.T. Dennis et al., "Tularemia as a Biological Weapon," *JAMA*, 285 (2001): 2763–73.
34. T. Inglesby et al., "Plague as a Biological Weapon," *JAMA*, 283 (2000): 2281–90.
35. Fialka et al., *supra* note 10.
36. L.K. Altman, "On Many Fronts, Experts Plan for the Unthinkable: Biowarfare," *New York Times*, October 23, 2001, at D4.
37. J.G. Hodge, "The Role of New Federalism and Public Health Law," *Journal of Law & Health*, 12 (1998): 309–57.
38. "Dark Winter," available online at <http://www.homelandsecurity.org/darkwinter/index.cfm>.
39. Hodge, *supra* note 37.
40. Model State Emergency Health Powers Act § 1-104(m) (December 21, 2001).
41. *Id.* § 1-104(a).
42. J.G. Hodge and L.O. Gostin, "Handling Cases of Willful Exposure Through HIV Partner Counseling and Referral Services," *Rutger's Women's Rights Law Reporter,* 22 (forthcoming 2002).
43. Gostin, *supra* note 1, at 34–46.
44. Letter from John J. Hamre, president and chief executive officer of the Center for Strategic and International Studies, dated July 26, 2001 (referring to findings from "Dark Winter" exercise in June, 2001).
45. Shalala, *supra* note 4.
46. C. Connolly and S. Gray, "Thompson Seeks $1.2 Billion to Expand Stockpile of Drugs," *Washington Post*, October 18, 2001, at A19.
47. E.L. Andrews, "Bayer Is a Bit Taken Aback by the Frenzy to Get Its Drug," *New York Times*, October 26, 2001, at B8.
48. V. Sutton, "Bioterrorism Preparation and Response Legislation — The Struggle to Protect States' Sovereignty While Preserving National Security," *Georgetown Public Policy Review*, 6 (2001): 92–103.
49. J. Lancaster and S. Schmidt, "31 Exposed to Anthrax on Capitol Hill," *Washington Post*, October 18, 2001, at A1.
50. R. Willing, "Anti-Terror Bill Extends Government's Reach," *USA Today*, October 25, 2001, at 7A.
51. Hodge and Gostin, *supra* note 42.
52. Model State Emergency Health Powers Act § 604 (December 21, 2001).
53. *Id.* § 603.
54. *Jacobson v. Massachusetts*, 197 U.S. 11 (1905).
55. Gostin, *supra* note 1, at 213–16.
56. Model State Emergency Health Powers Act § 604 (December 21, 2001).
57. Rosenbaum and Stolberg, *supra* note 8.

ARTICLE 4

BIOTERRORISM, PUBLIC HEALTH, AND CIVIL LIBERTIES

George J. Annas

The prospect of having to deal with a bioterrorist attack, especially one involving smallpox, has local, sate, and federal officials rightly concerned.[1,2] Before September 11, most procedures for dealing with a bioterrorist attack against the United States were based on fiction. Former President Bill Clinton became engaged in the bioterrorism issue in 1997, after reading Richard Preston's novel *The Cobra Event.*[3] In Tom Clancy's 1996 *Executive Orders*,[4] the United States is attacked by terrorists using a strain of Ebola virus that is transmissible through the air. To contain the epidemic, the President declares a state of emergency, orders that all nonessential businesses and places of public assembly be closed, and suspends all interstate travel by airplane, train, bus, and automobile. In defending the order, the fictional President makes a statement that is now often used to justify major changes in our criminal laws: "The Constitution is not a suicide pact."[4]

The anthrax attacks through the U.S. mail demonstrated that the federal government must provide better planning, coordination, and communication with the public, as well as better drugs and vaccines.[5,6] What remains more controversial is whether we must give up any civil liberties to deal with this "different kind of war." What steps should the government take to prepare for a bioterrorist attack involving the use of smallpox or another contagious agent, and which level of government, state or federal, should take the lead?

BIOTERRORISM AND PUBLIC HEALTH

The prospect of a bioterrorist attack and the actual attacks in Florida, the District of Columbia, New York, New Jersey, and Connecticut have changed public health in the United States. Since the founding of the country, public health has been considered primarily the business of the states. The reason is that when the former colonies delegated powers to the federal government in the U.S. Constitution, they retained the authority to protect the public's health and safety, usually referred to as the state's "police powers."[7,8] The federal government may, nonetheless, affect public health and safety through its constitutional authority to spend money, regulate interstate and foreign commerce, and provide for national defense. The Congress established the Public Health Service and the Centers for Disease Control and Prevention (CDC) with federal money and used its authority under the commerce clause of the Constitution to establish the Food and Drug Administration (FDA). The creation of these federal agencies, however, did not alter the states' responsibility for public health; the anthrax attacks did.

Bioterrorism — the deliberate release of a harmful biologic agent to intimidate civilians and their government — constitutes a threat to public health that differs from any other public health threat that our country has faced. An act of bioterrorism is both a state and a federal crime, and it can also be an act of war.[9] Because of our highly developed transportation system, communicable diseases can be spread widely in a short period of time. All these factors make it reasonable to view bioterrorism as an inherently federal matter under both the national-defense and commerce clauses of the Constitution. Thus, the Federal Bureau of Investigation (FBI) and the CDC took the lead in investigating all the anthrax mail attacks. Moreover, had the attacks originated outside the country, the U.S. military and the Central Intelligence Agency would have been called on to respond.

BUILDING A MODERN PUBLIC HEALTH SYSTEM

In the immediate aftermath of the September 11 attacks and the subsequent anthrax attacks through the U.S. mail, hospitals, cities, states, and federal officials began developing or revisiting protocols to deal with possible biologic attacks in the future. The federal response has so far emphasized the stockpiling of drugs and vaccines that could be used to respond to an attack, especially one involving smallpox.[10] Other proposals have included improving the public health infrastructure of the country (especially the ability to monitor diagnoses made in emergency departments and pharmacy sales of relevant drugs) and training emergency medical personnel to recognize and treat the diseases most likely to be caused by a bioterrorist attack (such as anthrax, smallpox, and plague).[11] Major efforts are also under way to improve coordination and communication among local, state, and federal officials who are responsible for responding to emergencies and to delineate more clearly the lines of authority involving "homeland security." All these measures are reasonable and responsible steps our government should take.

Properly worried that many state public health laws are outdated and perhaps inadequate to permit state officials to contain an epidemic caused by a bioterrorist attack, the CDC has advised all states to review the adequacy of their laws, with special attention to provisions for quarantining people in the event of a smallpox attack.[12] In addition, the CDC released a proposed model act for the states, the Model State Emergency Health Powers Act, on October 23, 2001.[12,13] The act was constructed by the Center for Law and the Public's Health at Georgetown University and Johns Hopkins University and was pieced together from a variety of existing state laws.

THE ORIGINAL MODEL STATE EMERGENCY HEALTH POWERS ACT

The original model act permits the governor to declare a "state of public health emergency," and this declaration, in turn, gives state public health officials the authority to take over all health care facilities in the state, order physicians to act in certain ways, and order citizens to submit to examinations and treatment, with those who refuse to do so subject to quarantine or criminal punishment. The model act specifies that public health officials and those working under their authority are immune from liability for their actions, including actions that cause permanent injury or death; the only exceptions are in cases of gross negligence and willful misconduct. A public health emergency (the condition that requires the governor to declare a state of public health emergency) is defined as "an occurrence or imminent threat of an illness or health condition, caused by bioterrorism, epidemic or pandemic disease, or [a] novel and highly fatal infectious agent or biological toxin, that poses a substantial risk of a significant number of human fatalities or incidents of permanent or long-term disability."[13]

The declaration of a state of public health emergency permits the governor to suspend state regulations, change the functions of state agencies, and mobilize the militia. Under the model act, all public health personnel will be issued special identification badges, to be worn "in plain view," that "shall indicate the authority of the bearer to exercise public health functions and emergency powers…."[13] Public health personnel may "compel a health care facility to provide services or the use of its facility if such services or use are reasonable and necessary for emergency response… [including] transferring the management and supervision of the health care facility to the public health authority."

According to the act's provisions, public health personnel have exceptionally broad powers, and failure of physicians and citizens to follow their orders is a crime. Section 502 of the act, which covers mandatory medical examinations and testing, states:

> Any person refusing to submit to the medical examination and/or testing is liable for a misdemeanor. If the public health authority is uncertain whether a person who refuses to undergo medical examination and/or testing may have been exposed to an infectious disease or otherwise poses a danger to public health, the public health authority may subject the individual to isolation or quarantine…. Any [health care provider] refusing to perform a medical examination or test as authorized herein shall be liable for a misdemeanor…. An order of the public health authority given to effectuate the purposes of this subsection shall be immediately enforceable by any peace officer.[13]

Section 504, on vaccination and treatment, states, "Individuals refusing to be vaccinated or treated shall be liable for a misdemeanor. If, by reason of refusal of vaccination or treatment, the person poses a danger to the public health, he or she may be subject to isolation or quarantine…. An order of the public health authority given to effectuate the purpose of this Section shall be immediately enforceable by any peace officer."[13]

THE NEED FOR NEW STATE LAWS ON BIOTERRORISM

Of course, state public health, police, fire, and emergency planners should be clear about their authority, and to the extent that it encourages states to review their emergency laws, the model act is constructive. On the other hand, many of the provisions of this act, especially those giving public health officials authority over physicians and hospitals, as well as authority to enforce a quarantine in the absence of meaningful standards, seem to be based on the assumption that neither physicians nor citizens are likely to cooperate with public health officials in the event of a bioterrorist attack. The assumption, in turn, seems to be based on the results of theoretical planning exercises involving simulated bioterrorist attacks, including the Top Officials 2000 (Top Off) and Dark Winter exercises.[12] Top Off was an exercise that simulated a bioterrorist attack on Denver that involved the use of aerosolized *Yersinia pestiss*, the bacteria that causes plague.[14] Dark Winter simulated a smallpox attack on Oklahoma City.[15] Using these simulated cases as a basis for legislation is unreasonable, given the extremely high level of voluntary cooperation on the part of the public, physicians, and hospitals after both the September 11 terrorist attacks and the subsequent anthrax attacks.

In my opinion, the model act poses several problems. First, proposed laws should respond to real problems. It is not at all clear what problem the model act is intended to solve, and this makes it extremely difficult to evaluate.

Second, the authority to respond to a bioterrorist attack or a new epidemic that the model act provides is much too broad, since it applies not just to real emergencies such as a smallpox attack but also to nonemergency conditions as diverse as annual influenza epidemics and the AIDS epidemic.[16,17]

Third, although it may make sense to put public health officials in charge of responding to a smallpox attack, it may not make sense to put them in charge of responding to every type of bioterrorist event. In the event of a bioterrorist attack, the state public health department has a major role in limiting the public's exposure to the agent. However, the tasks of identifying affected persons, reporting them, treating them, and taking preventive actions will be performed by physicians, nurses, emergency medical personnel, and hospitals. The primary role of public health authorities will usually be, as it was in the wake of the anthrax attacks, to provide guidance to the public and other government officials in identifying and dealing with the disease and to provide laboratory facilities where exposure can be evaluated and diagnoses definitively established.[5,6,18]

Fourth, there is no evidence from either the September 11 attacks or the anthrax attacks that physicians, nurses, or members of the public are reluctant to cooperate in the response to a bioterrorist attack or are reluctant to take drugs or vaccines recommended by public health or medical officials. In fact, medical personnel in the affected areas volunteered their time and expertise to help victims of the September 11 attacks, and the public lined up to be tested for anthrax and stockpiled ciprofloxacin.[19] The public demand for testing and treatment was so great that the CDC had to issue recommendations against both.

Of course, anthrax, unlike smallpox, is not spread from person to person. The situation might have been different if smallpox had been used as a biologic weapon or if thousands or ten of thousands of people had been infected with anthrax. Nonetheless, there is no empirical evidence that draconian provisions for quarantine, such as those outlined in the model act, are necessary or desirable. Persons with smallpox, for example, are most infectious only after fever and a rash have developed,[12] and then they are usually so sick that they are likely to accept whatever care is available. Moreover, according to Barbera et al., the "long incubation period (10–17 days) almost ensures that some persons who are infected in the [smallpox] attack will have traveled great distances from the site of the exposure before the disease is recognized or quarantine could be implemented."[14] The key to an effective public health response is identifying and helping those who have been exposed. Even with a sufficient supply of smallpox vaccine, a quarantine enforced by the police would probably not be effective in controlling an outbreak of smallpox.[12,14,20] This is a major reason for the current recommendation that smallpox vaccine be made available to the public on a voluntary basis.[21]

Finally, even if it is concluded that a quarantine law may be useful to respond to a bioterrorist attack (e.g., as a means of ensuring that the few unwilling Americans, if any, would be treated, vaccinated, or quarantined), it should be a federal law, not a state law. The reason is that bioterrorism is a matter of national security, not just of state police powers. The existing federal quarantine law is based on the commerce clause of the Constitution (with special provisions for cholera, plague, smallpox, typhus, and yellow fever), and Congress could examine and update it to deal with bioterrorism.[22,23] The governors of the states involved in the anthrax attacks all realized that bioterrorism is fundamentally a federal issue and quickly called for action from both the FBI and the CDC to deal with the attacks.

CIVIL LIBERTIES AND PUBLIC HEALTH EMERGENCIES

The model act is based on the belief that in public health emergencies, there must be a trade-off between the protection of civil rights and effective public health interventions. There is, of course, precedent for this belief, and the preamble to the model act cites the 1905 case of *Jacobson* v. *Massachusetts* in stating the proposition that "the whole people covenants with each citizen, and each citizen with the whole people, that all shall be governed by certain laws for the 'common good.'"[8,13] *Jacobson* v. *Massachusetts* involved a state statute that permitted local boards of health to require vaccination when they deemed it "necessary for the public health or safety." There were no provisions for quarantine in the statute, and refusal to be vaccinated was punishable by a $5 fine. Refusal was anticipated in the early 1900s because vaccination itself was controversial, there were no antibiotics, physicians were not widely trusted, science and medicine were in their infancy, and hospitals were primarily "pesthouses."[24] Trade-offs between civil liberties (the right to refuse treatment) and public health interventions (mandatory vaccination) seemed necessary in such circumstances.[25]

In *Jacobson* v. *Massachusetts*, the Supreme Court cited the military draft as the precedent for upholding the Massachusetts law. The point is not that the Constitution does not give the government wide latitude to respond in times of war and public health emergencies — it does. The point is that trade-offs between civil rights and public health measures are not always required and can be counterproductive. Just as we have been able to abolish the draft and rely on all-volunteer armed forces, so it seems reasonable to think that we can rely on Americans to follow the reasonable instructions of government officials for their own protection.

Today, almost 100 years after *Jacobson*, both medicine and constitutional law are radically different.[7] We now take constitutional rights much more seriously, including the right of a competent adult to refuse any medical treatment, even life-saving treatment.[26] Of course, we would still permit public health officials to quarantine persons with a serious communicable disease, such as infectious tuberculosis, but only if they could not or would not accept treatment and thus put others at risk for exposure.[27] Even then, however, we would require public officials to use the "least restrictive alternative" and resort to quarantine only after other interventions, such as directly observed therapy, had failed.[27] Provisions for quarantine are also accompanied by due-process rights, including the right to legal representation and the right to a hearing.[27]

The model act seems to have been drafted for a different age; it is more appropriate for the United States of the 19th century than for the United States of the 21st century. Today, all adults have the constitutional right to refuse examination and treatment, and such a refusal should not result in involuntary confinement simply on the whim of a public health official. At the very least, persons suspected of having a contagious disease should have the option of being examined by physicians of their own choice and, if isolation is necessary, of being isolated in their own homes.[27] The requirement that physicians treat patients against their will and against the physicians' medical judgment under penalty of criminal law has no precedent and makes no sense. Moreover, state governors already have broad emergency powers; there is no compelling reason to expand them.

Just as important as the constitutional questions posed by the model act is the pragmatic question of whether it is likely to undermine the public's trust in public health — trust that is absolutely essential for containing panic in a bioterrorist-induced epidemic. Unlike the situation at the turn of the last century, for example, we have televised news 24 hours a day, cell phones, and automobiles, making a large-scale quarantine impossible unless the public believes that it is absolutely necessary to prevent the spread of fatal disease and is fairly and safely administered. Enactment of a law that made it a crime to disobey a public health officer would rightly engender distrust, because it would suggest that public officials could not provide valid reasons for their actions.

The necessity of maintaining the public's trust also means that the argument that, in a public health emergency, there must be a trade-off between effective public health measures and civil rights is simply wrong. As the AIDS epidemic has demonstrated, the promotion of human rights can be essential for dealing effectively with an epidemic.[28]

Early in the course of the AIDS epidemic, public health officials recognized that mandatory screening for human immunodeficiency virus would simply help drive the epidemic underground, where it would spread faster and wider. Likewise, draconian quarantine measures would probably have the unintended effect of encouraging people to avoid public health officials and physicians rather than to seek them out. In this regard, the protection of civil liberties is a core ingredient in a successful response to a bioterrorist attack. Provisions that treat citizens as the enemy, with the use of the police for enforcement, are much more likely to cost lives than to save them. This is one reason why there has not been a large-scale quarantine in the United States for more than 80 years and why experts on bioterrorism doubt that such a quarantine would be effective.[14,20]

THE REVISED MODEL ACT

On December 21, 2001, in response to criticisms of the model act, including those I have summarized, a revised version was released.[29] No one any longer considers the act a "model." Instead, it is now labeled a "draft for discussion." The new version does "not represent the official policy, endorsement, or views" of anyone, including the authors themselves and the CDC.[29]

Although the revised act can be viewed as a modest improvement, all the fundamental problems remain. Failure to comply with the orders or public health officials for examination or treatment is no longer a crime but results in isolation or quarantine. Criminal penalties continue to apply to failure to follow isolation or quarantine "rules" that will be written at a future time. Physicians and other health care providers can still be required "to assist" public health officials, but cooperation is now coerced as "a condition of licensure" instead of a legal requirement with criminal penalties for noncompliance. The quarantine provisions have been improved, with a new requirement that quarantine or isolation be imposed by "the least restrictive means necessary" and stronger due-process protection, including hearings and legal representation for those actually quarantined.[29] Nonetheless, on the basis of a written directive by a public health official, a person can still be quarantined for 15 days before a hearing must be held, and the hearing itself can be for groups of quarantined persons rather than individuals.[29]

Some of the revised quarantine provisions seem even more arbitrary. A major criticism of the original version of the act was the extreme vagueness of its standard for quarantine, which invited the arbitrary use of force. According to the original version, quarantine can be ordered if a public health official is "uncertain whether a person who refuses to undergo medical examination or testing may have been exposed to an infectious disease or otherwise poses a danger to public health." In the revised version, the standard is even vaguer. Quarantine can be ordered when the person's refusal to be examined or tested "results in uncertainty regarding whether he or she has been exposed to or is infected with a contagious or possibly contagious disease or otherwise poses a danger to public health."[29] This is no standard at all; it simply permits public health authorities to quarantine anyone who refuses to be examined or treated, for whatever reason, since all refusals will result in uncertainty. If one were already certain, one would not order the test. At the hearing, if requested, the standard for a continued quarantine appears to be the finding that the person would "significantly jeopardize the public health authority's ability to prevent or limit the transmission of a contagious or possibly contagious disease to others." This standard also makes no sense because the public health focus, I think, should be on the person's condition and on the determination of whether it poses a danger to others, not on the public health authority's ability to function.

These vague standards are especially troublesome because the act's incredible immunity provision remains unchanged. Thus, all state public health officials and all private companies and persons operating under their authority are granted immunity from liability for their actions (except for gross negligence or willful misconduct), even in the case of death or permanent injury. Out-of-state emergency health care providers have even greater protection; they are given immunity from liability for everything but manslaughter. In my opinion, such immunity is something public health authorities should not want (even though it may have superficial appeal), because it means that they are not accountable for their actions, no matter how arbitrary. The immunity provision thus serves only to undermine the public's trust in public health authorities. Citizens should never be treated against their will by their government, but if they ever are, they should be fully compensated for injuries suffered as a result.

CONCLUSIONS

All sorts of proposals were floated in the wake of the September 11 attacks — some potentially useful, such as irradiation of mail at the facilities that had been targeted, and some potentially dangerous, such as the use of secret military tribunals and measures that would erode lawyer–client confidentiality, undermine our constitutional values, and make us less able to criticize authoritarian countries for similar behavior. I think the Model State Emergency Health Powers Act is one of the dangerous proposals.

Bioterrorism is primarily a federal, not a state, issue, and actions undertaken to prevent and respond to bioterrorism should be a federal priority.[30] Laws that provide funding for training in the recognition and treatment of diseases caused by pathogens that could be used as biologic weapons deserve support, as do laws that improve communication and coordination in response to such an attack. The Biological and Toxin Weapons Convention also deserves our support.[31] In my opinion, laws that treat Americans and their physicians as the enemy and grant broad, arbitrary powers to public health officials without making them accountable do not deserve support and distract us from important work that needs to be done. The fear and frenzy that prompted state legislatures to consider new antiterrorist laws after September 11 seem to have abated, and reason may yet prevail over panic.[32] Of course the Constitution is not a suicide pact, but we do not have to sacrifice civil liberties for an effective public health response to a bioterrorist attack.

REFERENCES

1. Tucker JB. Scourge: the once and future threat of smallpox. New York: Atlantic Monthly Press, 2001.
2. Gillis J, Connolly C. U.S. details response to smallpox: cities could be quarantined and public events banned. *Washington Post*. November 27, 2001:A1.
3. Preston R. The cobra event. New York: Random House, 1997.
4. Clancy T. Executive orders. New York: G.P. Putnam, 1996.
5. Lipton E, Johnson K. Tracking bioterror's tangled course. *New York Times*. December 26, 2001:A1.
6. Altman LK, Kolata G. Anthrax missteps offer guide to fight next bioterror battle. *New York Times*. January 6, 2002(Section 1):1.
7. Wing KR. The law and the public's health. 5th ed. Chicago: Health Administration Press, 1999.
8. Jacobson v. Massachusetts, 197 U.S. 11 (1905).
9. Fidler DP. The malevolent use of microbes and the rule of law: legal challenges presented by bioterrorism. *Clin Infect Dis* 2001;33:686–9.
10. Stolberg SG. Health secretary testifies about germ warfare defenses. *New York Times*. October 4, 2001:B7.
11. Miller J, Engelberg S, Broad W. Germs: biological weapons and America's secret war. New York: Simon & Schuster, 2001.
12. Interim smallpox response plan and guidelines, for distribution to state and local public health bioterrorism response planners, November 21, 2001 draft. Guide C: isolation and quarantine guidelines. Atlanta: Centers for Disease Control and Prevention, 2001.
13. The Model State Emergency Health Powers Act: as of October 23, 2001. Atlanta: Centers for Disease Control and Prevention, 2001. (Accessed April 5, 2002, at http://www.publichealthlaw.net/MSEHPA/MSEHPA.pdf.)
14. Barbera J, Macintyre A, Gostin L, et al. Large-scale quarantine following biological terrorism in the United States: scientific examination, logistic and legal limits, and possible consequences. *JAMA* 2001;286:2711–7.
15. Marlands L. Bioterror: all the rules change. *Christian Science Monitor*. December 17, 2001:1.
16. Mariner W. Bioterrorism act: the wrong response. *National Law Journal*. December 17, 2001:18.
17. Parmet WE, Mariner WK. A health act that jeopardizes public health. *Boston Globe*. December 1, 2001:A15.
18. Stolberg SG, Miller J. Bioterror role an uneasy fit for the C.D.C. *New York Times*. November 11, 2001:A1.
19. Martinez B, Harris G. Anxious patients plead with doctors for antibiotics. *Wall Street Journal*. October 15, 2001:B1.
20. Osterholm MT, Schwartz J. Living terrors: what America needs to know to survive the coming bio-terrorist catastrophe. New York: Delacorte Press, 2000.

21. Bicknell WJ. The case for voluntary smallpox vaccination. *N Engl J Med* 2002;346:1323–5.
22. Public Health Service Act, as amended, 42 U.S.C. 264 (1983).
23. Quarantine, inspection, licensing: interstate quarantine, 42 C.F.R. 70.1–8 (2000).
24. Rosenberg CE. The care of strangers: the rise of America's hospital system. New York: Basic Books, 1987.
25. Albert MR, Ostheimer KG, Breman JG. The last smallpox epidemic in Boston and the vaccination controversy, 1901–1903. *N Engl J Med* 2001;344:375–9.
26. Annas GJ. The bell tolls for a constitutional right to physician-assisted suicide. *N Engl J Med* 1997;337:1098–103.
27. *Idem.* Control of tuberculosis: the law and the public's health. *N Engl J Med* 1993;328:585–8.
28. Mann JM, Gostin L, Gruskin S, Brennan T, Lazzarini Z, Fineberg HV. Health and human rights. *Health Hum Rights* 1994;1:6–23.
29. The Model State Emergency Health Powers Act: as of December 21, 2001. Atlanta: Centers for Disease Control and Prevention, 2001. (Accessed April 5, 2002, at http://www.publichealthlaw.net/MSEHPA/MSEHPA2.pdf.)
30. Kellman B. Biological terrorism: legal measures for preventing a catastrophe. *Harv J Law Public Policy* 2001;24:417–85.
31. Scharf MP. Clear and present danger: enforcing the international ban on biological and chemical weapons through sanctions, use of force, and criminalization. *Mich J Int Law* 1999;20:477–521.
32. Gavin R. Frenzy to adopt terrorism laws starts to recede. *Wall Street Journal.* March 27, 2002:B1.

PART V

HEALTH CARE, HEALTH CARE ORGANIZATION, HEALTH CARE FINANCING, AND QUALITY OF CARE

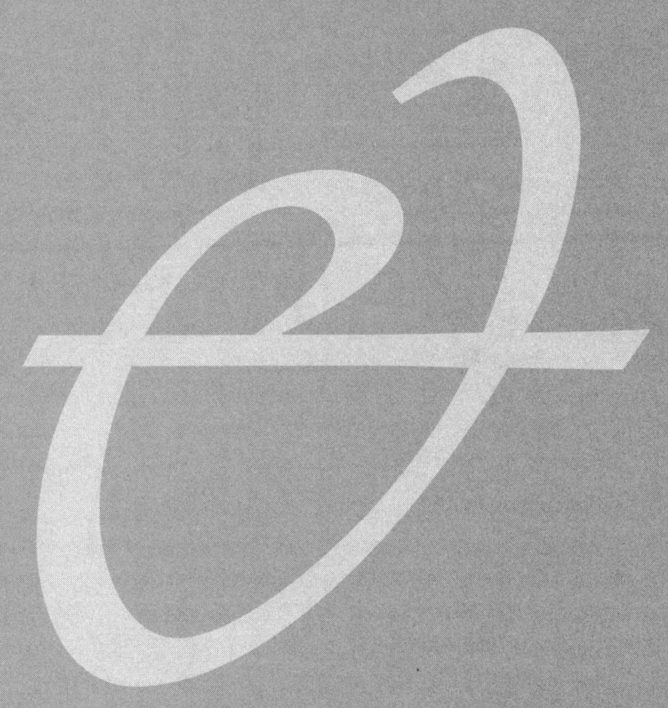

CHAPTER 7

HEALTH CARE, HEALTH INSURANCE, AND HEALTH CARE ORGANIZATION

It is impossible to describe the health care system in a few pages or a few selected articles from the literature. Therefore, to address such complexity, we have devoted Part V to health care, health insurance, and health care organization (Chapter 7); health care financing (Chapter 8); and quality of health care (Chapter 9).

HEALTH CARE IN A GLOBAL CONTEXT

Chapter 7 begins with an article by Robert W. Fogel and Chulhee Lee, "Who Gets Health Care?" (2002), that addresses disparities in health within a global context and presents the policy challenges of delivering "essential health care" services to the world. To answer the question of "who gets health care," Fogel and Lee begin their discussion by introducing U.S. and international examples of disparities in health. Disparities have been documented in countries such as the United States, Great Britain, and China, ranging from differences in the prevalence of illness, perinatal deaths, and low birth weight to differences in levels of health between urban and rural residents and treatment of cavities (p. 108). While socioeconomic differentials partially explain this phenomenon, other factors have also been proposed, including a shift to market-oriented health care delivery systems, which moves away from the principle of universal access, and rising income inequality (see Chapter 2, Article 2).

In their discussion, Fogel and Lee address the conundrum faced by policymakers. First, how does one define "essential" health care? Given the great variations in income and other conditions among the nations of the world, is it even appropriate to reach a consensus on a definition? The World Health Organization (WHO) and Organization for Economic Cooperation and Development (OECD) have "called on all countries to guarantee the delivery of high quality essential health care to all persons, defined mostly by criteria of effectiveness, cost, and social acceptability" (p. 110).

For most OECD countries, cost has been the determining factor, especially as the demand for health services has increased more rapidly than income, and the costs of operating government-run health and insurance systems have become prohibitive. Therefore, many countries have adopted strategies to control costs, including establishing priorities among health interventions and rationing health care services. In the United States, "cost control has focused more on setting limits in the individual medical encounter ('managing care') than on establishing budgetary limits for the entire sector" (Oberlander, 2002, p. 166). (See Chapter 7, Articles 2 and 4.)

To protect the poor under such stringent cost-control strategies, the WHO proposed three guiding principles:

> Health-care services should be prepaid (i.e., taxes for health care should be collected throughout the working life...); those who are healthy should subsidize those who are sick (which means that taxes should not be adjusted to reflect differential health risks, as policy rates often are under private insurance); and the rich should subsidize the poor (which means both that the rich should pay higher taxes than the poor, and that the quality of service in government-run programs should be no better or more comprehensive for privileged groups) (Fogel and Lee, 2002, pp. 110–111).

Inherent in these recommendations is the recognition that privately funded health programs and private insurance are integral to the nation's health care services. This raises a second question addressed by Fogel and Lee: What is the optimal mix of private and government components of health care services? Again, there are no set criteria to address this issue, and because of variations among countries, an "optimal" mix cannot be proposed. To elucidate this matter, Fogel and Lee point to the enormous range in annual per capita health expenditures — from $20 in Ethiopia, to $2,135 in France, to over $4,000 in the United States (Fogel and Lee, 2002; Kaiser Family Foundation, 2002a).

U.S. HEALTH CARE AND POSSIBLE PRIORITY AREAS

After examining these figures, one begins to wonder what Americans are buying with their health care dollars. Critical questions about the U.S. health care system are raised: Are Americans buying better health and longer lives, as compared with nations that spend significantly less per capita? Because increases in life expectancy have mostly been attributed to public health efforts and not medical care throughout the 20th century (see Chapter 1), and only a small proportion of health spending is directed at public health, what are U.S dollars really providing? Another important question asks whether we are investing our health care dollars in an efficient and prudent manner. Are we investing monies where we will reap the most health benefits (and during what part of the life course)? Is our U.S. health care system wasteful? Many of these questions are also addressed by Jonathan Oberlander in Article 2.

Based on their analysis, Fogel and Lee (2002, pp. 115–116) provide several policy recommendations, or priority areas, that can improve the U.S. health care system, particularly for the poor. These include the following:

1. An expansion of prenatal and postnatal care for young, single mothers
2. Improved health education and mentoring
3. A reintroduction of periodic health screening programs into public schools, particularly those in poor neighborhoods
4. The establishment of public health clinics in underserved poor neighborhoods that can supplement the emergency room use of regular hospitals

Intentionally, they exclude from their discussion an emphasis on expanding health insurance coverage or policies to cover the uninsured. According to Fogel and Lee, while health insurance may relieve "the pressure on the public purse, it will not guarantee better health care" (p. 116). As such, the other priority areas seem more appropriate, given their potential to improve the health of populations.

FROM THE 1990S TO THE PRESENT

Article 2, by Jonathan Oberlander (2002), offers a comprehensive analysis of major issues affecting health care and health care delivery from the 1990s to the present — the problems of the uninsured, the politics of health reform, incrementalism, and managed care.

Oberlander describes the U.S. health care system as a "paradox of excess and deprivation." The United States spends an exorbitant amount on medical services, more than any other nation, yet disparities in access to health care predominate. Well-insured Americans tend to have access to the latest in sophisticated technology and medical procedures. Rates of diffusion and availability of such resources are so widespread that many Americans receive too many medical services, thereby reflecting an excess (p. 163). However, at the other end of the spectrum are the deprived. Oberlander points to recent estimates that over 40 million Americans do not have insurance, making the United States the "only democratic country in the world with a substantial uninsured population" (p. 163).

Oberlander does not expect there to be much progress for the uninsured. Despite significant reductions in the number of uninsured during the 1960s and 1970s, resulting from the enactment of Medicare and Medicaid and the expansion of private health insurance and Medicaid and Medicare (including the distribution of Social Security to the disabled and to patients with end-stage renal disease), the number of uninsured has risen steadily since the 1980s. In 1980, it was 30 million; in 1990, 36 million; and in 1993, it was 41 million. A decline in Medicaid enrollment, in part related to welfare reform and lower levels of unemployment, has contributed to this pressing problem. Oberlander notes that "from 1990 to 1998, the number of uninsured people increased by nearly 10 million" (p. 164), and the future of the uninsured is not encouraging. In the United States, the 1990s was a decade with ideal conditions for an expansion of health insurance: "The economy (had) gone through an unprecedented era of sustained growth, the rates of general inflation and unemployment remained low, and the rate of health care inflation (had) moderated" (p. 164). Nonetheless, this period witnessed the failure of major health reform efforts, including Clinton's Health Security Act (see Chapter 4, Articles 2 and 3). Therefore, instead of attempts to revamp or restructure a system that is flailing and not serving all (or not serving all equally well), incrementalism has become the remaining strategy.

Interestingly, while the previous edition of *The Nation's Health* was being edited, there was a growing interest in the issue of the uninsured. On June 14, 1999, the six major medical organizations (American Medical Association, American College of Physicians, American Academy of Pediatrics, American College of Obstetricians and Gynecologists, and American Academy of Family Practice) issued a joint statement advocating universal coverage. Former Senator Bradley, a candidate for the Democratic Party's nomination for president, had proposed a plan to provide health insurance for at least 95% of the population, guaranteed by the federal government. The Institute of Medicine held a conference on the uninsured and planned a series of studies to help illuminate the issue. However, currently we find that the tide has changed, and there is little sustained momentum for universal health insurance, especially as the country prioritizes national security and terrorism preparedness over health reform.

HEALTH COVERAGE IN THE UNITED STATES

Article 3 presents a snapshot of health coverage in the United States based on the March 2001 Current Population Survey (CPS), which is conducted by the United States Census Bureau. Highlighted in this article from the *Current Population Reports* are changes in coverage from 1999 to 2000. Two key findings are that (1) the number of uninsured declined to 38.7 million (down by approximately 0.6 million from the previous year), and (2) the percentage of people covered by employment-based health insurance rose to 72.4% in 2000. (Also see Oberlander, Article 2, for his estimates.) It is important to point out that these figures depict a particular point in time, and rates may have changed as a result of the economic downturn facing America, which was influenced by many events, including September 11, 2001.

In this article, Robert Mills also presents data on key demographic factors that affect coverage rates: age, race and Hispanic origin, nativity, and educational attainment. Whereas 99.3% of persons aged 65 and over had health insurance in 2000, only 72.7% of persons aged 18 to 24 years had health insurance coverage. In 2000, a decline in the uninsured rate was observed for blacks (from 19.6% to 18.5%) and for white non-Hispanics (from 9.9% to 9.7%); however, Hispanics or Latinos continued to have the highest uninsured rates (32%) among all racial and ethnic groups. Also significant was a decline in the number of uninsured children (see Chapter 8 for a discussion of SCHIP and Medicaid). The March 2001 CPS also found that foreign-born persons were more than twice as likely to be without health coverage than those who were born in the United States. Educational attainment increased the likelihood of coverage among all adults, except the poor, whose rates did not vary across the education groups. Economic status, particularly income level, work experience, and firm size, also affected health care coverage. In addition, the likelihood of having health insurance increased with income, full-time workers were more likely to be covered by health insurance, and employer size influenced the availability of coverage.

Although health care insurance does not guarantee good health or access to care, serious medical and financial consequences often result from either a lack of health coverage or underinsurance. For instance,

> According to a recent report by the American College of Physicians and the American Society of Internal Medicine, uninsured persons are much more likely than insured persons to refrain from seeking needed care and to suffer the consequences of delayed or forgone care. For example, those without health insurance are more likely to have had hospitalizations that could have been prevented and to have received a diagnosis of cancer at an advanced stage (Schroeder, 2001).

Although much of the policy debate has centered on issues of the uninsured, a recent Henry J. Kaiser Family Foundation (KFF) fact sheet, *Underinsured in America: Is Health Coverage Adequate?* (2002b), highlights the problems faced by those who "have health insurance but face significant cost-sharing or limits on benefits that may affect its usefulness in accessing or paying for needed health services" (p. 1). The *Health Care Survey* conducted by National Public Radio, the Kaiser Family Foundation, and the Kennedy School of Government in May 2002 found that among the insured, 18% postponed seeking care, 15% had problems paying medical bills, 10% needed a prescription but did not get it, 8% were contacted by a collection agency about medical bills, and 6% needed medical care but did not get it (KFF, 2002b).

HEALTH CARE ORGANIZATION

In her book *Chronic Condition: Why Health Reform Fails* (1997), Sherry Glied discusses two very different sets of views about the nature of health care — health care as a market good or as a medically determined need. Each viewpoint influences the way health care is organized and delivered.

"*Marketists* see health care as just another good or service, not in any fundamental way different from other commodities bought and sold in the open market" (p. 17). As such, the value of health is based on the consumer's willingness to purchase the service, and "depends critically on [his or her] idiosyncratic preferences, income, and other opportunities" (p. 18). Glied adds that "marketists see no point in subsidizing health care for the poor or redistributing health care for the sick… Marketist reformers expect the private, competing insurers to solve allocation problems in the modern health care marketplace" (p. 21).

The view that health care is a social good implies philosophical differences regarding allocation of services and distribution principles. *Medicalists* do not see "medical care as a commodity. . . .[I]ts characteristics are scientifically determined and decisions must be entrusted exclusively to professionals" and not left to the marketplace (p. 26). Medical care is thus seen as a uniform right, with "equal access of all citizens to equivalent medical services" (p. 29).

The view that health care is a social good is widely accepted in other Western, industrialized democracies; however, in the United States, health care is considered a normal commodity or market good. In the United States, health care is supplied by competitive profit-maximizing firms and is ideally purchased by informed buyers, whose demand for health care is a function of the price of the services. As a result, there has been an outgrowth of managed care; for-profit health plans, hospitals, and health systems; and what has been described as the "medical industrial complex" (Glied, 1997; Starr, 1982; Salmon, 1995) (see Recommended Reading). The predominance of the idea within American society that health care is a market, and not a social, good has been dramatically illustrated in health care financing, organization, and delivery in the United States over the past 30 years.

More than 20 years ago, Starr (1982) described the evolution of the role of the medical profession and health care system in the 20th century as follows:

> In the 20th century not only did physicians become a powerful, prestigious and wealthy profession, but they succeeded in shaping the basic organization and financing structure of American medicine. More recently that system has begun to slip from their control, as power has moved away from the organized profession towards complexes of medical schools and hospitals, financing and regulatory agencies, health insurance companies, prepaid health plans, and other health care chains, conglomerates, holding companies, and other corporations (p. 8).

MANAGED CARE: A SOLUTION?

The rapid restructuring of the health care system, particularly the growth of managed care, has been attributed to a number of factors: (1) the explosion of health care costs in the 1970s and their continued increase in the 1980s; (2) the ability of large employers to self-insure due to the provisions of the 1974 Employment Retirement Income Security Act (ERISA); and (3) the preference of big employers for a competitive approach rather than a regulatory approach to health care cost containment that included managed care, limited employee choice (not consistent with a competitive model), and reduced employee benefits, particularly dependents' coverage.

The 1980s and 1990s saw a nationwide increase in the number and types of corporate for-profit providers and insurers, including managed care plans. The developments in managed care and organized delivery systems are described in detail by Gray (1991) and Salmon (1995) (see Recommended Reading). While these articles are comprehensive, they are now outdated. A number of the integrated systems reviewed have collapsed — both among for-profit as well as nonprofit models. In addition, there have been major conversions of nonprofit health entities to for-profit corporations, such as with Blue Cross of California, which have raised serious questions regarding the disposition and control of assets as well as access to care. This hotly debated phenomenon has resulted in the proprietary ownership of many hospitals, surgicenters, urgent care centers, clinical laboratories, and imaging facilities. Hospitals and other providers have become increasingly competitive, and, as a result, they have begun to operate more like businesses, using techniques such as advertising, marketing, specialization, and productivity monitoring. The effects of this trend are just beginning to be understood.

In view of the failure of Congress to enact the major health care reforms proposed by President Clinton in 1993, more and more people are looking for incremental reforms in health care policy at the federal level, and managed care is being pushed aggressively by employers and the health insurance industry as a means of controlling health care costs. Yet there are growing complaints about managed care, and the number of uninsured continues to increase. Moreover, health care costs have again begun to rise rapidly, even in the face of expanding managed care organizations. According to Oberlander (2002),

> health care spending rose at higher rates; insurance premiums increased by 8.3% in 2000, and even larger increases were expected for 2001. This suggests that the era of low medical care inflation is over and that managed care's ability to restrain spending has been exaggerated (p. 167).

Managed Care in Transition

Managed care is a dominant force in health care that affects the financing of health insurance and the way medicine is practiced in this country. According to R. Adams Dudley and Harold S. Luft (2001), "by 1999, only 8 percent of persons with employer-sponsored health insurance coverage had traditional indemnity insurance" (p. 1087). In recent years, there has also been a trend among public programs such as Medicaid and Medicare to deliver care within a prepaid managed care arrangement. However, enrollment of the elderly, poor, and disabled in such plans is "generally lower than for the employer-sponsored population" (Oberlander, 2002, p. 166).

In Article 4, Dudley and Luft describe the evolution of managed care, its effect on providers and patients, and responses from physicians and medical groups, employers, and government. They introduce the earliest models of managed care, the group- or staff-model health maintenance organizations (HMOs), such as Kaiser Permanente, that linked health insurance, hospitals, and physicians in what were capitated, prepaid group practice models, and other more loosely organized individual practice associations. In addition, they refer to California legislation, enacted in 1982, that altered the landscape in health care delivery. This legislation permitted Medicaid and private health insurance plans to contract selectively with hospitals; thereby, "insurers could exclude physicians who did not accept their rules and fee schedules" (Dudley and Luft, 2001, p. 1087). As a result, preferred provider organizations (or networks of individual physicians) emerged. Broader networks have also developed, including point-of-service (POS) plans, which include some coverage for services from providers outside of the network. In addition, insurers now offer "multitiered" plans that offer patients more options.

Managed care has had a great impact on physicians' practices. In 1999, managed care accounted for 48.9% of revenues received by all physicians, and almost all physicians had managed care contracts (Oberlander, 2002). Approximately one third of these contracts were for capitation, whereby physicians are prepaid on a per capita basis for an agreed list of services or for all services and drug costs (global capitation). Under this model, the financial risk is shifted from the insurer to the provider. As a result, many providers have faced financial difficulties, and some have terminated such contracts or restructured them (e.g., PacifiCare). To match the purchasing power of managed care organizations, physicians have banded together, and medical groups or independent practice associations (IPAs) emerged. In addition, larger systems such as physician-hospital organizations were created to "either accept global capitation or to ensure hospital admission" (Dudley and Luft, 2001, p. 1089). Employers have also united to negotiate discounts on health care, address problems of risk selection, and encourage health plans to improve quality of care. Given the public's concern about managed care and its cost-control practices, the government has also been more active in developing legislation on benefits packages, use of emergency room services, the physician-patient relationship, resolution of disputes, and liability issues in managed care. However, there has been deadlock, particularly regarding passage of a patient's bill of rights, because of issues involving the liability of health plans.

Although managed care has revolutionized the financing, structure, and delivery of medical care in the United States, many now realize that it is not the solution to the problems plaguing our health system. Costs continue to rise, the quality of care within managed care and other health delivery arrangements is being questioned, and the public's dissatisfaction with our current system is growing.

REFERENCES

Dudley, R. A., and Luft, H. A. (2001). Managed care in transition. *New England Journal of Medicine, 344* (14), 1087–1091.

Fogel, R. W., and Lee, C. (2002, Winter). Who gets health care? *Daedalus, 131,* 107–117.

Glied, S. (1997). *Chronic condition: Why health reform fails.* Cambridge, MA: Harvard University Press.

Kaiser Family Foundation. (2002a). *Underinsured in America: Is Health Coverage Adequate?* Menlo Park, CA: Kaiser Family Foundation.

Kaiser Family Foundation. (2002b). *Chartbook: Trends and indicators in the changing health care marketplace, 2002*. Menlo Park, CA: Kaiser Family Foundation.

Mills, R. J. (2001). Health insurance coverage: 2000. *Current Population Reports.* Washington, DC: U.S. Census Bureau (Department of Commerce).

Oberlander, J. 2002. The U.S. Health Care System: On a Road to Nowhere? *Canadian Medical Association Journal, 167* (2), 163–168.

Salmon, J. W. (1995). A perspective on the corporate transformation of health care. *International Journal of Health Services, 25* (1), 11–42.

Shroeder, S. A. (2001). Prospects for expanding health insurance coverage. *New England Journal of Medicine, 344* (11), 847–852.

Starr, P. (1982). *The social transformation of American medicine*. New York: Basic Books.

ARTICLE 1

WHO GETS HEALTH CARE?

Robert W. Fogel and Chulhee Lee

Around the world, as in the United States, concern is growing about who gets health care.[1] Individuals from different socioeconomic backgrounds face distressingly different prospects of living a healthy life. As numerous studies confirm, the disparities in various measures of health between the privileged and the deprived remain wide, even in rich countries, despite the long-term tendency toward a healthier society.

Some investigators believe that the disparities are actually increasing. They suggest that the shift in the heath-care system in advanced industrial countries from the principle of universal access to a more market-oriented system may be one cause of the growing disparities they observe; rising income inequality is another potential culprit.

Policymakers worldwide meanwhile speak of more efficiently delivering "essential" health care, but nobody is certain what this means in practice.

What counts as "essential" in health care? What is the optimal mix of private and government components of health-care services?

It is these questions that we wish to explore in more detail. After reviewing the economic and epidemiological literature on disparities in health and health-care systems, we will tackle directly the question of how to define "essential" health care — and then explore the policy implications of our analysis.

In the United States, substantial socioeconomic differences in illness and death rates have been documented by many researchers. These disparities not only vary widely by level of education but, as reported in 1993 in a paper published in *The New England Journal of Medicine*, the disparities increased between 1960 and 1986 for both men and women.[2]

Growing inequalities in well-being and access to health care have been reported for other nations, too. In Britain, recent studies by Russel Ecob and George Davey Smith, and also studies by Vani K. Borooah, have provided extensive evidence of socioeconomic disparities in the prevalence of illness, the probability of long-term limiting illness, perinatal deaths, low birth weight, and stillbirth risk. In Denmark, Finn Tüchsen and Lars A. Endahl found that illness and death due to cardiovascular disease was promoted by inequalities in income. Moreover, this disparity rapidly increased between the early 1980s and 1990s. In Rome, according to another recent study published in the *Journal of Epidemiology and Community Health*, socioeconomic differences in death rates rose during the early 1990s. In China, as Yuanli Liu, William C. Hsiao, and Karen Eggleston have shown, the gap in the levels of health between urban and rural residents also widened in the same period, despite rapid economic growth. Disparities have also increased in the treatment of less serious medical conditions. Thus, while overall oral health improved in Norway, the disparities in the treatment of cavities by socioeconomic group increased from 1983 to 1994.

Over the last decade, a number of studies have produced evidence that the extent of income inequality in a society is negatively associated with the health status of citizens, based on cross-sectional comparisons between and within countries.[3] These apparent empirical findings have provoked a debate over precisely how income inequality may affect individual health status. Some researchers have focused on the psychological stresses that may result from a perception of relative deprivation, or alienation from a highly unequal social order.[4] This hypothesis is bolstered by research showing that more egalitarian societies exhibit more cohesion, less violence, lower homicide rates, more trust, lower hostility scores, and more involvement in community life. Still other researchers have focused instead on material conditions, arguing that income inequality leaves the poor exposed to disease, while the state lowers its investment in education, housing, income, and public and private sanitation.[5]

At the same time, doubts have been raised about the validity of the empirical relationship between income inequality and health.[6] In a recent working paper on "Health, Inequality, and Economic Development," Angus Deaton argues that the evidence that income inequality affects individual health is not as strong as commonly assumed. According to him, previous studies based on international comparisons lack adequate data on health for some countries, and comparable data for others. The link between income inequality and health that is observed in cross-sectional U.S. data becomes insignificant once various effects of population composition, especially the effect of race, are considered. Deaton argues that it is the level of a country's income, rather than the degree of inequality, that is crucial.

Income inequality and levels of national income may not be the only factors that help to explain disparities in health: many researchers blame the rising inequality in access to health care for the trend toward a greater inequality in health. Jon Gabel, writing for *Health Affairs* in 1999, noted that the coverage of job-based health insurance in the United States declined between 1977 and 1998, particularly among low-skilled, marginal workers, because of the decline in real wages among low-skilled workers, a 2.6-fold real increase in the cost of health insurance, and a 3.5-fold nominal increase in the cost of health insurance. A survey published in May of 2000 in *The Journal of the American Medical Association* entitled "Inequality in Quality: Addressing the Socioeconomic, Racial, and Ethnic Disparities in Health Care" suggests that, even among those with health insurance, lower socioeconomic position is associated with receiving fewer mammograms, childhood and influenza immunizations, and diabetic eye examinations, later enrollment in prenatal care, and lower quality of ambulatory and hospital care.

In Britain, too, doctors serving poor populations reported significantly lower rates of utilization of more advanced technologies such as angiography and revascularization in coronary artery surgery.[7] In eight developing countries, including Burkina Faso, Guatemala, Kazakhstan, Kyrgyzstan, Paraguay, South Africa, Thailand, and Zambia, researchers found that richer groups were more likely to obtain care when sick, to be seen by a doctor, and to receive medicines when ill than poorer groups.[8] An interesting exception to these usual patterns of health-care disparities is New Zealand, where the poor were found to receive either an appropriate or a slightly excessive level of services given their estimated health needs. This may be explained by the effects of a continued restructuring of the New Zealand public-health system, which focuses on providing decent minimum care.

Some investigators believe that disparities in health delivery are increasing. Since the demand for health care has a relatively large income elasticity (defined as the percentage increase in health expenditures brought about by a 1 percent increase in income), a widening of the income gap between rich and poor would produce an even greater disparity in expenditure on health care. Additionally, a rise in income inequality in a locality may undermine primary health-care provisions, especially for its poorer residents.[9] Finally — and paradoxically — advances in medical technologies may help to produce more disparities in health and well-being. Because affluent and educated people tend to take care of themselves and know how to utilize the health-care system, according to the recent study "Understanding Health Disparities across Education Groups," by Dana Goldman and Darius Lakdawalla, reductions in the price of health care or expansions in the overall demand for health inputs may disproportionately benefit the well-educated.

As this review of the literature on health reveals, economists and epidemiologists are primarily focused on empirical issues: establishing the facts on differences in health and health care by socioeconomic status, and measuring the impact of inequality on health outcomes. Discussions of such normative issues as what proportion of national resources ought to be devoted to health care, or how these resources ought to be distributed within the population, are left largely to legislatures and to various specific-interest organizations and think tanks.

International organizations such as the World Health Organization (WHO) and the Organization for Economic Cooperation and Development (OECD) have called on all countries to guarantee delivery of "high-quality essential care to all persons, defined mostly by criteria of effectiveness, cost and social acceptability."[10] Cost has become a controlling issue since the health-care systems established in most OECD countries after World War II, which sought to guarantee complete health care for all through government-run health or insurance systems, have become too expensive and now threaten the fiscal stability of governments. As incomes have risen, the public demand for health services has increased much more rapidly than income (because of the high income elasticity of the demand for health care), making the cost of operating such systems unsustainable.

The new systems of "essential care," now in the course of construction in OECD countries, recognize the necessity of explicitly establishing priorities among health interventions (rather than unlimited coverage). As a result, it has become necessary to ration health-care services even more stringently than before. In order to guarantee that the health of the poor is not neglected under these circumstances, the WHO proposes three principles: health-care services should be prepaid (i.e., taxes for health care should be collected throughout the working life, even though the need for services is relatively low during young adult and middle ages); those who are healthy should subsidize those who are sick (which means that taxes should not be adjusted to reflect differential health risks, as policy rates often are under private insurance); and the rich should subsidize the poor (which means both that the rich should pay higher health taxes than the poor, and that the quality of service in government-run programs should be no better or more comprehensive for privileged groups).

This recommended standard explicitly recognizes that privately funded health programs and private insurance will need to provide a major part of a nation's health services. Since persons in the upper half of income distributions tend to spend more on health services than poorer people do, the distribution of health services is bound to be unequal. In fact, all OECD countries currently have mixed private and governmental systems, ranging from about 85 percent of total expenditures made by the government in Great Britain to about 45 percent in the United States. It is likely that the reforms now in progress will generally increase the private share of health-care services.

There is no clear agreement currently on the optimal mix of private and government components of health-care services. There is not much of a literature on this question, nor is there a consensus on the criteria that should be invoked to resolve the issue. Moreover, conditions vary so much from country to country that the optimal mix cannot be the same for all countries.

In very poor countries, where the need for health-care services is great, the average annual level of per capita expenditures from both private and government sources is shockingly low. In such countries as Ethiopia, Haiti, Indonesia, and Nepal, annual per capita expenditures range between $20 and $56 (using international dollars, which adjust exchange rates for the domestic purchasing power of a country's currency). In India, the figure is $84, and in China it is $74. By contrast, the figures for the five largest countries of Western Europe are: France $2,135, Germany $2,365, Italy $1,824, Spain $1,211, and the United Kingdom $1,193. Annual per capita expenditures on health care in the United States — $3,724 — are more than three times the British figure and more than 1.5 times the German figure. The spending on health care of the typical American in ten days exceeds the average *annual* expenditures of people living in countries with more than three-fifths of the world's population.

The fact that Europeans spend so much less on health care than Americans has led some critics to argue that the American system is wasteful. This contention is often buttressed by the fact that American disability-adjusted life expectancy (the average number of years expected before the onset of disabilities) at birth is less than that of

France, Spain, Italy, the United Kingdom, and Germany. If all those extra dollars spent by Americans are not buying better health and longer lives, what are they buying?

It is not yet possible to provide an adequate answer to that question. It is often assumed that the increase in longevity over the past two or three decades is due primarily to the increased amount and quality of health-care services. There is no doubt that medical interventions have saved many lives, especially in such areas as infectious diseases, cancer, and heart disease. However, we cannot yet say how much of the six or so years of increase in life expectancy since 1970 is due to medical interventions and how much is due to better levels of education, improvements in housing, and other factors that contribute to the increase in life expectancy.

Some recent findings suggest that most of the huge increase in life expectancy since 1900 is due to the large investment in public-health programs between 1880 and World War II that cleaned up the water and milk supplies, developed modern waste-disposal systems, reduced air pollution, and improved nutritional status. Of course, these public-health programs were made possible by advances in medical knowledge. But the research behind these public-health advances represents a relatively small part of what is included in the category of "health expenditures." In the United States, for example, medical research (not including R&D of drug companies and providers of medical equipment and supplies) adds up to just 1.7 percent of U.S. national health expenditures.

Since deaths due to infectious diseases are now a small proportion of total deaths, it might seem that environmental improvements that were so important in reducing health risks before 1950 have been exhausted. Such a conclusion is premature. A series of recent studies has reported a connection between exposure to stress (biological and social) in early life, including insults *in utero* and during infancy, with the onset of chronic diseases at middle and late ages, and with life expectancy.[11] The strongest evidence for such links that has emerged thus far is with respect to hypertension, coronary heart disease, and type II diabetes.[12] A review of the research dealing with the relationship between birth weight and hypertension showed a tendency for middle-aged blood pressure to increase as birth weight declined.[13] Evidence of a connection between birth size and later coronary heart disease has been found in England, Wales, Sweden, India, and Finland. The volume of studies confirming the impact of insults during developmental ages on health in later life has increased substantially since 1994.

One of the strongest recent confirmations of the impact of early life events on longevity is a study reporting a statistically significant relationship between longevity after age fifty and the week of birth for cohorts born between 1863 and 1918. In the northern hemisphere, average length of life is shortest for those born in the second quarter of the year and longest for those born in the fourth quarter. In Australia, a relationship between birth month and longevity exists, but the peak and trough are the mirror image of that in the northern hemisphere.[14] This result, which is apparently related to seasonal variations in nutritional status, has also been found in the Union Army data for cohorts born between 1820 and 1850.[15] Consequently, we cannot rule out the proposition that one of the biggest factors influencing the prevalence rates of chronic diseases among the elderly in 2001 (and which accounts for a huge slice of national medical expenditures) was their exposure to environmental insults half a century, or more, ago.

These new scientific findings are directly relevant to the problem of how to define "essential" health care and how to divide the national budget for health (regardless of how it is financed) among competing needs. It may well be that a very large increase in expenditures on antenatal care and pediatric care in infancy and early childhood is the most effective way to improve health over the entire life cycle, by delaying the onset of chronic diseases, alleviating their severity if they do occur, and increasing longevity.

Whatever the virtues of such a strategy, it raises the issue of intergenerational bias. This strategy gives a preference to the unborn and the very young over the immediate needs of the elderly. It is a kind of double blow to the elderly, who are now suffering from the early onset of chronic conditions and premature disability because of environmental insults they incurred *in utero* and during early childhood. Yet under a strategy that emphasizes antenatal and early childhood care, in order to make new generations better off throughout their life cycles, the elderly of today will be asked to restrain their demand for relief.

It is much easier to define "essential care" in the impoverished nations of the world because their alternatives are so stark. They are still suffering from deadly killers and cripplers, virtually eliminated from OECD nations, that can be vanquished at quite modest costs compared to the expensive procedures routinely used to deal with more modest complaints in rich countries. As the WHO reported in 2001, the prospects of the poorest billion in the Third World can be "radically improved by targeting a relatively small set of diseases and conditions."

Urgent needs include the distribution of drugs to combat tuberculosis, malaria, and acute gastrointestinal and respiratory infections; the widespread provision of vaccines to prevent measles, tetanus, and diphtheria; and improved nutrition in order to revitalize immune systems, reduce perinatal deaths, lower death rates from a wide range of infectious diseases, and improve the functioning of the central nervous system. The Commission on Macroeconomics and Health (CMH) of the World Health Organization has estimated that 87 percent of deaths among children under age five, 71 percent of deaths between ages five and twenty-nine, and 47 percent of deaths between ages thirty and sixty-nine can be avoided by making use of available drugs and vaccines, by the delivery of vital nutrients, and by public-health programs aimed at producing safe water supplies and improved sanitation and health education. CMH estimates that donations from private and public sources in OECD countries, amounting to just 0.14 percent of their combined GDP, will be enough to realize these opportunities rapidly.

Defining "essential care" for the United States is more problematic, because the technologies needed for rapid and dramatic improvements in health and longevity are still on the drawing board, in contrast to poor countries where the problem is how effectively to deliver food and existing drugs and vaccines. To clarify the issue of "essential care" in a country where per capita expenditures on health exceed those of poor nations by 50 to 150 times, it is necessary to consider exactly what it is that our luxurious (even by European standards) expenditures are buying.

Saving lives, as important as it is, and as effective at it as modern medicine has become, is not the main activity of physicians and other health professionals. As we have already indicated, it is likely that past public-health reforms, improvements in nutrition and other living standards, and the democratization of education have done much more to increase longevity than has clinical medicine. The main thing that physicians do is to make life more bearable: to relieve pain, to reduce the severity of chronic conditions, to postpone disabilities or even overcome some of them, to mend broken limbs, to prescribe drugs, and to reduce anxiety, overcome depression, and instruct individuals on how to take care of themselves.

Europeans are much more willing than Americans to stint on "unnecessary" services, on procedures that are "optional" rather than "vital," on conveniences rather than necessities, on small rather than large reductions in risk. Rather than insisting on wide choice, they will settle for limited choice or no choice at all (take it or leave it). Consider the issue of queuing, one of the principal devices employed by public-health systems in Europe to keep demand from exceeding politically negotiated budgets. Americans are unwilling to wait two years or more for a hernia operation, as is now the case in Britain, but demand that such a service be available quickly, in a few weeks in most cases. Americans chafe at another favorite European device to control costs: rationing. They do not want to be told that they are too old or too fit or not fit enough to be eligible for some course of treatment. Nor are they willing to have their access to specialists sharply curtailed, and so the ratio of specialists to primary-care physicians is much higher in the United States than elsewhere. They also resist hasty impersonal examinations and denial of access to inpatient hospital care. And the rich insist on being allowed to spend as much on health care as they desire, even if some of these expenditures are wasteful.

And so the United States has some 6,000 hospitals, while Britain's National Health Service has only 430 very large hospitals (beds per capita are similar in both countries). Every substantial suburban community in the United States demands its own facility with a wide range of services. In America today, not just research hospitals but many community hospitals have on staff physicians who specialize in heart bypass surgery and other high-tech procedures. Since Americans like to save a buck as much as Europeans, they are willing to join HMOs, but HMOs have found that to be competitive they have to offer numerous options on copayments, access to physicians outside of the primary network, and self-referral to specialists. Americans also demand the option to change health plans if they are dissatisfied. Such options cost money, among other things because they increase the cost of administration, even if they do not improve health outcomes.

The American passion for such individually tailored health services may be attributed to the country's wide-open spaces, evangelical religion, and longstanding hostility to government. But it also reflects income. The average American, after all, is 50 percent richer than the average British person. Hence, it is not strange that they are willing to consume services that are too expensive for poorer people. Americans are no more self-indulgent in their purchases of health care than they are in their purchases of appliances or cars.

And so, what is viewed as "essential" health care in the United States includes services that in other cultures would be regarded as wasteful luxuries.

This situation puts into fresh perspective the common lament that 15 percent of Americans are "uncovered" by health insurance. "Uncovered" does not mean that they are untreated. The uninsured see doctors almost as frequently as the insured. Nor is it clear that the effectiveness of their care is always less than those who have insurance. The uninsured are treated in public clinics and in emergency rooms, which (although they lack the conveniences of insured care and may have long queues) provide competent services, both standard and high-tech.[16]

Although access to health care matters, insurance does not guarantee adequate access. Moreover, while some of the uninsured in the U.S. system are in poorer health than the insured, others are in prime ages, have relatively good health, and prefer to self-insure. An important but poorly addressed issue is how different attitudes toward risk influence the insured and the uninsured in deciding when and where to seek health care. This issue is important when considering solutions to those who are underserved in health care, since underservice of the poor also exists in countries with universal health insurance. If the poor and the young are willing to accept higher health risks than are the rich and the elderly, merely extending entitlements may not be adequate. An aggressive outreach program, targeted at those who fail to take advantage of entitlements, may be required.

Our analysis has a variety of policy implications, both for health care in the United States and also for the world as a whole.

We believe that the most effective way to improve the U.S. health system for the poor is by identifying their most urgent needs and designing an effective way of ministering to those specific needs. This goal will not be met merely by equalizing the annual number of visits to doctors (since the rich often waste medical services) or the annual expenditures on drugs (since the rich often overmedicate). Focusing on the specific needs of the poor may not save money, but it will ensure that whatever is spent is properly targeted.

In this spirit, the number-one priority ought to be an expansion of prenatal and postnatal care targeted particularly at young single mothers. The priority is suggested by the new evidence that proper nutrition, including supplements of such key nutrients as folate and iron, can reduce perinatal deaths and birth defects, including damage to the central nervous system. It is also necessary to counsel pregnant women on the dangers to the fetus from smoking and consumption of alcohol, on the benefits from proper diets, regular and early examinations, and exposing the fetus to a stimulating environment (music and conversation). A focus on young, single mothers makes sense not only because they are among the most needy, but also because there is now persuasive evidence that insults *in utero* that reduce birth weight and length, as well as inadequate weight gains in infancy, greatly increase health risks throughout the life cycle.

A second priority is improved health education and mentoring to enable poorly educated people, both young and old, to identify their health problems, to be able to follow instructions for health care, to properly use medication, and to become involved in social networks conducive to good health. It is not enough to wait for such individuals to seek out available service. Outreach programs need to be developed to identify the needy individuals. Hence, support should be extended to organizations already experienced in outreach, such as the Girls Clubs of America and community churches, so that they can include health screening and counseling among their services. Systems for monitoring the effectiveness of such community organizations also need to be established.

Another priority is the reintroduction into public schools, particularly those in poor neighborhoods, from nursery school through the twelfth grade, of periodic health-screening programs, using nurses and physicians on a contract basis. Personnel should also be employed to ensure that parents understand the nature of their children's problems and to direct the parents to public-health facilities that can provide appropriate services.

A fourth initiative is the establishment of public-health clinics in underserved poor neighborhoods that can supplement the emergency rooms of regular hospitals, which are a frequent source of routine health-care services for the poor and near poor. Convenient access is a key issue, because even individuals with insurance, such as those on Medicaid, may fail to take advantage of available facilities if they are inconvenient. Time is a cost to the poor as well as the rich, and lack of convenient facilities may cause individuals to accept higher health risks than they would otherwise choose. The mission of community clinics should include health education in addition to treatment. Community clinics need to be regularly monitored to ensure their effectiveness. Basements of churches and space in public schools after normal teaching hours can be good locations for community clinics, both because they help to stretch available funds and because they provide familiar settings.

Readers may be surprised that we have not emphasized the extension of health-insurance policies to the 15 percent of the population not currently insured. The flap in the United States over insurance has more to do with taxation than with health services. Keep in mind that the poor are already entitled to health care under Medicaid, and that the near poor often receive free health care through county or city hospitals and emergency rooms. What they do not do is pay taxes for those services. Most proposals for health insurance imply the taxation of their wages for services they already receive. Such insurance may relieve the pressure on the public purse, but it will not guarantee better health care. We believe that health screening in schools and community clinics has a better chance at success than unexercised theoretical entitlements.

Last but not least, any consideration of how to improve health care must take into account the world as a whole, since a great many diseases are more easily transmitted than ever across national frontiers.

We believe that America has an obligation to increase its contribution to the international campaign to bring vaccines and other products to children and adults whose lives can be saved, if there is the international will to do so. The lack of access to such products in the poorest fifty or so countries is the most glaring instance of inequality in the global health system and a lingering threat to the health of those in rich countries.

The large advances in life expectancy in China and other emerging economies show that it is not necessary to wait for industrialization to be completed before making major advances in health and longevity. Modern methods of sanitation and other public-health programs can be introduced at modest cost. Cleaning up the water supply, improving the distribution of basic nutrients, draining swamps and otherwise disrupting vectors of disease, and making improvements in waste disposal can be achieved quickly and cheaply, as has been demonstrated by China, Indonesia, and Malaysia. OECD nations can help speed up the process in countries still lagging behind by training public-health officials and helping to supply food supplements, antibiotics, and other vital drugs and vaccines to needy nations.

A particularly urgent issue is posed by the worldwide pandemic of HIV/AIDS. Although death rates from AIDS have recently declined in the United States and other OECD nations, AIDS is ravaging Africa. Of the three million individuals worldwide who died of AIDS in 2000, more than two million lived in sub-Saharan Africa. Although rates of infection are still relatively low in India and China, there is a risk of a rapid escalation in the spread of the infection. Public campaigns to inform the populations of these countries of the threat of this disease, of means of reducing the odds of infection, and of available treatment for those already infected are urgently needed.

The OECD and other international agencies can provide both money and skilled personnel to confront AIDS and other deadly infectious diseases, and to help provide vaccines and other drug therapies to those who need them. One important way to help is by increasing the money spent in OECD nations on understanding diseases that afflict the poor countries of the world. It is not only morality but also self-interest that argues for these measures. There is always a risk that epidemics in the Third World may spread to OECD nations.

REFERENCES

1. We have benefited from the insightful suggestions of Bernard Harris and David Meltzer. Parts of the research for this paper were supported by a grant from the National Institute of Aging. A more fully documented version of this essay is available as a National Bureau of Economic Research (NBER) Working Paper at <http://www.nber.org>.

2. Gregory Pappas, Susan Queen, Wilbur Hadden, and Gail Fisher, "The Increasing Disparity in Mortality between Socioeconomic Groups in the United States, 1960 and 1986," *The New England Journal of Medicine* 329 (2) (8 July 1993): 103–109.

3. R. G. Wilkinson, "Income Distribution and Life-Expectancy," *British Medical Journal* 304 (6820) (18 January 1992): 165–168; I. Kawachi and B. P. Kennedy, "The Relationship of Income Inequality to Mortality: Does the Choice of Indicator Matter?" *Social Science & Medicine* 45 (7) (October 1997): 1121–1127.

4. R. G. Wilkinson, *Unhealthy Societies* (London: Routledge, 1996); Wilkinson, *Mind the Gap: Hierarchies, Health, and Human Evolution* (London: Weidenfeld and Nicolson, 2000).

5. John W. Lynch, George Davey-Smith, George A. Kaplan, and James S. House, "Income Inequality and Mortality: Importance to Health of Individual Income, Psychological Environment, or Material Conditions," *British Medical Journal* 320 (7243) (29 April 2000): 1200–1204.
6. K. Fiscella and P. Franks, "Poverty or Income Inequality as a Predictor of Mortality," *British Medical Journal* 314 (7096) (14 June 1997): 1724–1728; H. Gravelle, "How Much of the Relation between Population Mortality and Unequal Distribution of Income Is a Statistical Artefact?" *British Medical Journal* 316 (7128) (31 January 1998): 382–385.
7. Julia Hippisley-Cox, "Inequality in Access to Coronary Angiography and Revascularisation: The Association of Deprivation and Location of Primary Care Services," *British Journal of General Practice* 50 (455) (June 2000): 449–454.
8. M. Makinen et al., "Inequalities in Health Care Use and Expenditures," *Bulletin of the World Health Organization* 78 (1) (2000): 55–65.
9. Leiyu Shi, Barbara Starfield, Bruce Kennedy, and Ichiro Kawachi, "Income Inequality, Primary Care, and Health Indicators," *Journal of Family Practice* 48 (4) (April 1999): 275–284.
10. World Health Organization, *The World Health Report 2000: Health Systems: Improving Performance* (Geneva: World Health Organization, 2000), xiii.
11. D. J. P. Barker, *Mothers, Babies, and Health in Later Life*, 2d ed. (Edinburgh and New York: Churchill Livingstone, 1998).
12. Nevin S. Scrimshaw, "More Evidence that Foetal Nutrition Contributes to Chronic Disease in Later Life," *British Medical Journal* 315 (7112) (4 October 1997): 825–826.
13. Catherine M. Law and Alistair W. Shiell, "Is Blood Pressure Inversely Related to Birth Weight? The Strength of Evidence from a Systematic Review of the Literature," *Journal of Hypertension* 14 (8) (August 1996): 935–941.
14. Gabriele Doblhammer and James W. Vaupel, "Life Span Depends on Month of Birth," *Science* 98 (5) (27 February 2001): 2934–2939.
15. Tayatat Kanjanapipatkul, "The Effect of Month of Birth on Life Span of Union Veterans," typescript, Center for Population Economics, University of Chicago, 2001.
16. Marc L. Berk and Claudia L. Schur, "Access to Care: How Much Difference Does Medicare Make?" *Health Affairs* 17 (30) (May–June 1998): 169–180.

ARTICLE 2

THE US HEALTH CARE SYSTEM
ON A ROAD TO NOWHERE?

Jonathan Oberlander

The health care system in the United States remains a "paradox of excess and deprivation."[1] The United States spends more on medical services than any other nation, and US physicians earn more than their counterparts in Canada, Europe and Japan. Americans with insurance have access to the latest in sophisticated medical technology and innovative medical procedures; rates of diffusion for many medical technologies, such as magnetic resonance imaging, are generally higher in the United States than in other industrialized democracies.[2] Indeed, the availability of these resources is so widespread that some analysts believe that well-insured Americans are receiving too many medical services. At the same time, millions of Americans receive too little medical care.[3] Over 40 million Americans do not have health insurance,[4] which makes the United States the only democratic country in the world with a substantial uninsured population.

The 1990s was a decade of reform and change in US health care. After the 1994 failure of then President Bill Clinton's effort to enact a government-sponsored system of universal health care insurance, the private market emerged as the engine of health reform. US medicine moved toward "managed care" arrangements, with rising enrolment in health maintenance organizations (HMOs) and the growth of for-profit health plans. Market-based health reform was viewed by proponents as a solution to health care cost inflation and an opportunity to enhance both quality of care and patient choice. However, by the end of the decade a widespread backlash against managed care had developed.

What is the state of the US health care system after a decade of turbulence? What has been the impact of managed care? And what is the outlook for health care reform? This article reviews the current status and future prospects of the US health care system. In particular, I focus on the persistent problem of the uninsured, efforts at cost control and the role of managed care.

LITTLE PROGRESS FOR THE UNINSURED

The US health care system is often erroneously labelled a private health care system. In fact, the United States has a mixed system of public and private insurance, though the word "system" connotes much more organization and logic than is actually at work. Most working-age Americans receive health insurance through their employers. Medicare, a federal government program similar in structure to Canada's single-payer medicare insurance, provides health insurance to all Americans over 65 years of age as well as to persons with disabilities or end-stage renal disease. Medicaid, a jointly funded federal–state program, covers low-income Americans (it reaches about 40% of the poor), including seniors who "spend down" their incomes and assets to a level that qualifies them for Medicaid-funded nursing-home care. In between those covered by this hodgepodge of private and public plans, however, lies a substantial population without any health insurance at all (Table 1).[5]

In 2000, 14% of Americans lacked health insurance.[5] About 80% of the uninsured are either workers or live in families with workers. They typically have low-wage jobs or work in small businesses in which the employer does not offer health insurance or, if it is offered, they cannot afford to purchase it.[6] The uninsured are disproportionately of low income. In 2000, one-third of the poor were uninsured, and two-thirds of uninsured adults had incomes less than 200% of the federal poverty line, or US$26,580 (Can$39,498) for a family of 3.[6] Substantially more black (18.5%) and Hispanic (32%) than white (13%) Americans were uninsured in 2000.[5]

Many Americans mistakenly believe that the uninsured obtain adequate care from hospital emergency rooms and other charity sources. Studies have consistently found, however, that the uninsured receive significantly less medical care than the insured.[7] Nearly 25% of uninsured children and 40% of uninsured adults have no

TABLE 1

Sources of Health Insurance Coverage in the United States, 2000

Type of Coverage	*Population Covered, %**
Any private plan	72.4
Employer-based plan	64.1
Government plan	24.2
Medicare	13.4
Medicaid	10.4
Military plan	3.0
None	14.0

Note: Source of data is the US Census Bureau.[5]
*Total is not 100%, because some people have multiple sources of insurance.

regular source of medical care.[6] The uninsured are much more likely to delay or forgo needed treatment, have their conditions diagnosed at a later stage and be admitted to hospital for avoidable conditions.[6] Moreover, inadequate insurance coverage carries with it financial as well as medical risks: the costs of medical treatment are a leading cause of bankruptcy in the United States.[8] Indeed, about half of all bankruptcies in the United States "involve a medical reason or large medical debt."[9]

The number of uninsured individuals actually declined from 1998 to 1999, from 44.3 to 42.6 million, and in 2000 fell again to 38.7 million (though this latter drop was mainly due to statistical adjustments in how the government counts the uninsured). Yet perhaps most striking is not the decrease but, rather, that it took so long to happen and that the overall trend in the past decade remained one of an expanding uninsured population. Since the early 1990s, the United States has enjoyed ideal conditions for an expansion of health insurance. The economy has gone through an unprecedented era of sustained growth, the rates of general inflation and unemployment have remained low, and the rate of health care inflation has moderated. Still, from 1990 to 1998 the number of uninsured people increased by nearly 10 million (Figure 1).

That even these favourable circumstances did not generate any significant expansion of health insurance is disquieting. And future trends are no more encouraging. The US economy slowed in 2000, and the unemployment rate rose. This economic downturn generated new ranks of the uninsured: the recent decline in the uninsured rate has ended. Because most Americans receive health insurance through their employer, a recession would have a strong negative impact on access to insurance.

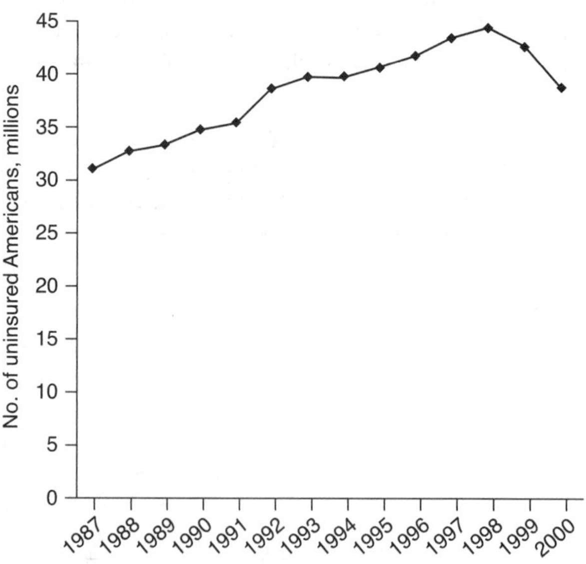

Figure 1 Number of uninsured Americans, 1987–2000.

For the foreseeable future, then, the number of uninsured Americans is likely to continue to grow.

THE POLITICS OF HEALTH REFORM

National health insurance periodically emerged on the US political agenda during the 20th century and was often tantalizingly close to enactment. The most recent failure came in 1994, with the defeat of the Health Security Act, sponsored by President Bill Clinton (and drafted under the guidance of his wife, Hillary). Clinton proposed to achieve universal coverage in the United States by mandating that all employers provide private health insurance to their employees and by giving small businesses and unemployed Americans subsidies with which to purchase insurance. However, the Clinton plan triggered fierce opposition from the insurance industry (which disliked the proposed regulation of behaviours, such as experience rating, which has enabled them to charge higher premiums for sick patients), the business community (which criticized the employer mandate), ideologic conservatives (who saw the plan as an unwarranted nationalization of the health care system) and large segments of the public (who were anxious about the plan's emphasis on moving patients into HMOs). Confronted with this opposition and the lack of a liberal political majority in Congress, the act was defeated. The American Medical Association, which initially endorsed and then waffled on the idea of universal insurance coverage, did not play a prominent role in the 1993/94 debate, a sign of its deteriorating influence on US health politics.

One legacy of the Clinton plan's failure has been caution regarding health policy. Many politicians took the lesson of the plan's demise to be that comprehensive reform — transforming the US system into one of national health insurance, like Canadian medicare — is not politically feasible. Consequently, talk of attaining universal coverage has all but disappeared. Neither of the two major parties' presidential candidates in the 2000 election, Al Gore and George W. Bush, offered plans for universal insurance coverage. None of the plans currently under serious consideration in Congress attempts to cover all of the uninsured. And even one of the few organized advocates for the uninsured, the consumer group Families USA, has toned down its calls for universal coverage in favour of more modest policy goals.

What is remarkable about the absence of proposals for universal coverage in the period 1999–2001 is that the fiscal circumstances of the United States appeared to be conducive to their adoption. After 2 decades of budget deficits, the federal government in 2000 ran a sizeable budget surplus, projected at $5.6 trillion over the next decade.[10] It has long been assumed that the lack of affordability of a public program was a central barrier, particularly in an era of sizeable federal deficits in which large spending initiatives were politically constrained and tax increases taboo. Now, though, the affordability argument has been exposed as a fallacy. Despite the availability of a budget surplus that could be used to pay the costs of covering the uninsured, universal coverage did not emerge as a central political issue in 2000/01. Instead, political attention focused on improving the medical experiences of the already insured through regulation of managed care and expansion of Medicare to cover outpatient prescription drugs.

It is clear that the most relevant fact about US health politics is not that some 15% of the population are uninsured but that about 85% of the population are insured. Those who are insured are generally satisfied with their own medical care, even if they think poorly of the system as a whole; consequently, they are not a strong constituency for change. Indeed, any reform that threatens to alter the medical care arrangements of the insured is likely to provoke public opposition. The formidable constituency against reform is mobilized, wealthy and politically influential. Meanwhile, the uninsured are disproportionately low-income, unorganized and apparently politically expendable. As the Clinton plan exemplified, the political benefits to a president and legislators willing to take on a trillion-dollar health care industry that opposes reform are uncertain, but the costs are certain to be high. The result is that universal coverage remains an elusive reform in the United States, and the uninsured continue to live in an "aura of invisibility."[11]

INCREMENTAL REFORMS

Although there is currently little appetite for comprehensive reforms that would assure universal coverage, there is momentum for incremental measures that would reduce the ranks of the uninsured. Two main pathways to improved coverage have emerged. The first approach is to expand existing public insurance programs, including Medicaid, which provides insurance to about 40% of the poor, and the State Children's Health Insurance Program (SCHIP), which provides insurance to children living in families with incomes up to 200% of the federal poverty line. Proponents of this approach would change eligibility requirements for these programs, opening them up to more of the poor and near-poor (e.g., to parents of children enrolled in SCHIP). One of the more ambitious plans would extend Medicaid and SCHIP coverage, without premiums or cost-sharing, to all persons with incomes below 150% of the federal poverty line and subsidize enrolment for persons with incomes up to 300%.[12] It is estimated that this plan would extend eligibility for public insurance to over 25 million Americans who are currently uninsured. Most plans, however, would not expand coverage so broadly and would thus not reach most of the uninsured.

A second approach — one favoured by the Bush administration — is to adopt tax credits that would help the uninsured purchase private insurance. This approach appears to be especially attractive given the political appeal of tax cuts and the promise of expanded coverage with minimal government involvement. Most tax-credit proposals would target individuals, though some plans have instead focused on credits for employers. Credits could be refundable, so that even low-income persons who do not pay federal income tax would be eligible.

There are several problems, however, with tax-credit proposals in particular and incremental reforms more generally. The main problem with tax credits is the mismatch between the size of the credits that are being proposed and the cost of insurance. The average annual premium of a health insurance policy in the United States is now more than US$6000 (Can$8910) for a family and more than $3000 for an individual. President Bush's proposal would provide a tax credit of only $2000 to a family and $1000 to an individual. It is questionable how much difference these tax credits would make to the uninsured, many of whom have little disposable income. This is especially true because insurance for individuals has much higher administrative costs than group insurance, and consequently higher premiums.

More fundamentally, neither tax credits nor expanded public insurance does anything to control medical care spending. The debate has changed markedly since the early 1990s, when concerns over rapidly rising costs and the economic competitiveness of US firms drove health reform. Politically, the absence of cost containment in the current proposals is hardly surprising. After all, health care costs equal the total incomes of the providers of medical care, a group comprising not merely physicians but also insurers, hospitals, nursing homes, pharmaceutical companies and all those selling medical services and products. Any attempt to restrain national health spending is viewed by providers as an assault on their livelihood, which triggers intense opposition. An understandable reading by US politicians of the Clinton reform debacle is that expanding coverage is difficult; simultaneously mandating spending controls would be political suicide.[13]

Yet there are signs that the moderate medical care inflation that made inattention to cost control comfortable is ending. Absent cost control, then, incremental reforms may become self-defeating, with high rates of medical care inflation leading to higher-than-expected program costs, which could make expansion of insurance coverage less affordable and politically problematic.

THE RISE OF MANAGED CARE

US medical care has long been the most expensive in the world.[14,15] The defeat of comprehensive health reform in 1994 did not obviate the pressures to control health spending; rather, it shifted the engine of control to the private sector. Employers looking to hold down their medical bills embraced managed care and, in a staggeringly short time, managed care became the norm. By 2000, 92% of persons with employer-sponsored insurance were enrolled in a managed care plan.[16] Managed care has also spread to public programs for the elderly, poor and disabled — Medicare and Medicaid — though enrolment in such plans is generally lower than for the employer-sponsored population.[17]

Managed care has come to refer to a wide range of health plans and practices that depart from the traditional US model of insurance. In the traditional model, insured patients chose their physician; physicians treated patients with absolute clinical autonomy; insurers generally paid physicians whatever they billed on a fee-for-service basis; and employers paid premiums for their workers to private insurers, footing the bill regardless of its cost. Managed care has altered all of these arrangements. As a consequence of not having national health insurance, cost control in the United States has focused more on setting limits on the individual medical encounter ("managing care") than on establishing budgetary limits for the entire health care sector.

The rise of managed care has brought about four major changes in US medical care. First is the substantial decline in traditional indemnity-insurance arrangements, which allowed unfettered access to physicians and unregulated delivery of medical care. The proportion of Americans with employer-sponsored indemnity coverage declined from 95% in 1978 to 14% by 1998.[18] This drop was accompanied by an increase in enrolment in a wide variety of managed-care insurance programs, including HMOs, Preferred Provider Organizations (PPOs) and Point of Service plans (POSs). Not only did HMOs grow in enrolment — from 36.5 million in 1990 to 58.2 million in 1995 — but they also changed substantially in form. In particular, there has been rapid growth in for-profit HMOs as well as network and individual-practice association models that contract with providers; in contrast, group or staff-model HMOs (such as Kaiser Permanente) own their facilities, and their physicians work exclusively for them.[19] Yet, while they continue to be regarded as the symbol of managed care, the growth of HMOs has stalled in recent years, and more Americans with job-provided insurance are now enrolled in PPOs (41%) than in HMOs (29%).[16]

Second, patients in managed care receive full coverage for services only if they choose a physician within the plan's network. In the case of HMOs, patients receive no coverage if they see an out-of-network provider. In some plans, patients must go through a gatekeeper, typically a primary care physician, to obtain a specialty referral. The corollary is that most insurers no longer contract with all physicians in a community. Rather, they contract with a limited number of doctors, negotiating price discounts in exchange for guaranteed patient volume and excluding high-cost providers.

Third, physicians' clinical decisions are now regularly subject to external review by insurance plans. Indeed, US physicians probably experience more intrusion into their clinical lives than physicians anywhere in the industrialized world, an ironic development given that the American Medical Association long opposed national health insurance as a threat to clinical autonomy.[20] Under utilization-review arrangements, physicians may have to seek permission from the patient's insurance company for admission to hospital, diagnostic tests or medical procedures. Utilization review and physician profiling may also occur after treatment, with the goal of identifying "inappropriate" or "excessive" care according to the insurer's standards. Proponents of managed care argue that these practices can not only control costs but also enhance quality of care — for instance, by assuring adherence to evidence-based medicine.

Fourth, insurers no longer give physicians a blank cheque; instead, they may dictate not only the price of reimbursement but also the form. This has led to the widespread adoption of predetermined fee schedules for physician payment by managed care plans, which seek discounts from "normal" fees. HMOs have also adopted capitated payment, often focusing on primary care providers. Under capitated payment, physicians receive a set amount for each patient enrolled in their practice, regardless of that patient's actual use of services. The stated aim is to avoid the financial incentive for overtreatment inherent in fee-for-service payment. Another important change in payment arrangements is the introduction of bonuses and other incentives for physicians to meet targets in providing care. Frequently these incentives are aimed at ensuring that physicians hold down costs in a capitated environment; for instance, bonuses may be provided to physicians whose rate of admission to hospital for their patient pool is lower than the insurer's target. Along with capitation, these arrangements put the incomes of many physicians at substantial risk.[21]

THE IMPACT OF MANAGED CARE ON COSTS AND QUALITY

Since the advent of managed care in the early 1990s, health care spending in the United States has slowed. From 1993 to 1998, the share of gross domestic product (GDP) devoted to national health expenditures declined from 13.7% to 13.5%, and premiums for employer-sponsored health insurance actually grew more slowly than the per capita GDP.[22] However, the United States continues to spend far more on medical care than any other nation: in 1998, it spent $4270 per capita, compared with $2400 in Germany, which spent the second-highest amount, and $2250 in Canada.[14,15]

There is substantial disagreement among analysts about the significance of the relative success of the United States in controlling health care spending during the mid-1990s. Some observers believe that this experience demonstrates managed care's effectiveness in controlling costs and the efficiencies inherent in strategies such as selective contracting, utilization review and capitation. Others attribute the slowdown to a one-time switch from indemnity insurance that cannot be duplicated or to temporary circumstances that cannot be sustained, such as marketing strategies that led insurers to underprice their products to expand market share. The long-term cost-containment potential of managed care consequently remains uncertain. However, health care spending in 1999 and 2000 rose at higher rates: insurance premiums increased by 8.3% in 2000,[23] and even larger increases were expected for 2001.[24] This suggests that the era of low medical care inflation is over and that managed care's ability to restrain spending has been exaggerated.

Evidence for the impact of managed care on the quality of care is mixed. Most studies have found little difference in quality of care between traditional insurers and managed care plans, though there is evidence of worse outcomes for chronically ill seniors in HMOs.[25] That quality of care in many cases did not deteriorate despite reduced volume and intensity of services suggests that the previous standard of "unmanaged" care incorporated significant amounts of unnecessary services. However, these findings also cast doubt on the premise that managed care is improving quality through practice guidelines, preventive care, primary care, disease management, integrated delivery systems and other strategies. Too often, these strategies exist more as marketing labels than as workable or proven innovations, though that has not stopped them from being aggressively promoted outside the United States, often to receptive audiences looking for new levers to control costs and improve quality and consumer service. Yet, so far, managed care plans have not consistently implemented these practices, and market competition has not resulted in significant quality improvements. Instead, plans have focused on managing costs, a decision reinforced by employers, who are much more likely to select insurance on the basis of price than on the basis of quality.[26]

THE MANAGED-CARE BACKLASH

Regardless of the evidence, there is strong sentiment among both physicians and patients that managed care is harming quality of care. Consequently, there has been a push to enact patients' bills of rights and other laws that regulate the behaviour of managed care plans.[27] Virtually all of the 50 US states now have such laws on the books, and Congress is debating federal legislation that would permit patients to sue HMOs, guarantee access to specialists and establish procedures for appealing health plan decisions denying coverage or medical care. If adopted, this legislation will no doubt provide political benefits to its sponsors, who can assure the voting public that they are doing something about HMO abuses. Its impact on patients and quality of care is less certain. The legislation is sufficiently vague that it is difficult to know how strictly it will be implemented and how much it will change health plan behaviour. Moreover, the proposed law does not address issues such as financial bonuses for physicians and the incentives of capitation that significantly affect patient care.

CONCLUSION

After a decade of change, the United States appears to be no closer to solving the problems of cost control and access that have characterized its health care system for the past 3 decades. The question is, after the political system takes care of the already insured through managed-care protections and expanded Medicare benefits for the elderly, what will it do for the uninsured?

The September 11, 2001, bombings of the World Trade Center and the Pentagon have triggered a new period in US politics, dominated in the short term by President Bush's war on terrorism. In the aftermath of the terrorist strikes, "United we stand" became a national slogan of solidarity. Some health reformers hope that this communitarian spirit and the renewed faith of Americans in government will give national health insurance a new life. And enactment of incremental expansions of public insurance programs and tax credits for the uninsured is a real possibility. But it is not clear that health reform will move beyond these limited steps, which would leave the bulk of the uninsured population untouched. Absent a sustained economic downturn that makes the middle class anxious about their own coverage, prospects for universal coverage and comprehensive health care reform remain dim. The more things change in US health care policy, the more they seem to stay the same.

REFERENCES

1. Enthoven A, Kronick R. A consumer choice health plan for the 1990s. *N Engl J Med* 1989;320:29.
2. Rublee D. Medical technology in Canada, Germany and the United States. *Health Aff (Millwood)* 1994;13:113–7.
3. Bodenheimer TS, Grumbach K. *Understanding health policy.* Norwalk (CT): Appleton and Lange; 1995.
4. Kemper V. Unlikely coalition declares health-care crisis. *Los Angeles Times* 2002 Feb 13; Sect A:1.
5. US Census Bureau. *Health insurance coverage 2000.* Washington: The Bureau; 2001.
6. Kaiser Commission on Medicaid and the Uninsured. *The uninsured and their access to health care.* Menlo Park (CA): Kaiser Family Foundation; 2001.
7. Ayanian JZ, Weissman JS, Schneider EC, Ginsburg JA, Zaslavsky AM. Unmet health needs of uninsured adults in the United States. *JAMA* 2000;284:2061–9.
8. Crenshaw A. Study cites medical bills for many bankruptcies. *Washington Post* 2000 Apr 25; Sect E:1.
9. Himmelstein D, Woodhandler S. *Bleeding the patient: the consequences of corporate health care.* Monroe (ME): Common Courage Press; 2001. p. 24–5.
10. US Congressional Budget Office. *The budget and economic outlook: fiscal years 2002–2011.* Washington: The Office; 2001.
11. Grumbach K. Insuring the uninsured: time to end the aura of invisibility. *JAMA* 2000;284:2114–6.
12. Feder J, Levitt L, O'Brien E, Rowland D. Covering the low-income uninsured: the case for expanding public programs. *Health Aff (Millwood)* 2001;20:27–39.
13. Oberlander J, Marmor TR. The path to universal health care. In: Borosage RL, Hickey R, editors. *The next agenda.* Boulder (CO): Westview Press; 2001. p. 93–125.
14. Deber R, Swan B. Canadian health expenditures: Where do we *really* stand internationally? *CMAJ* 1999;160(12):1730–4.
15. Anderson GF, Hurst J, Hussey PS, Jee-Hughes M. Health spending and outcomes: trends in OECD countries, 1960–1998. *Health Aff (Millwood)* 2000;19:150–7.
16. Gabel JR, Levitt L, Pickreign J, Whitmore H, Holve E, Hawkins S, et al. Job-based health insurance in 2000: premiums rise sharply while coverage grows. *Health Aff (Millwood)* 2000;19(5):144–51.

17. Health Insurance Association of America. *Source book of health insurance data.* Washington: The Association; 1998.
18. Gabel JR, Ginsburg PB, Whitmore HH, Pickreign JD. Withering on the vine: the decline of indemnity health insurance. *Health Aff (Millwood)* 2000;19(5): 152–7.
19. Gabel JR. Ten ways HMOs have changed during the 1990s. *Health Aff (Millwood)* 1997;16(3):134–45.
20. White J. *Competing solutions: American health care proposals and international experience.* Washington: Brookings Institution Press; 1995.
21. Bodenheimer T. Physicians and the changing medical marketplace. *N Engl J Med* 1999;340:584–8.
22. Levit K, Cowan C, Lazenby H, Sensenig A, McDonnell P, Stiller J, et al. Health spending in 1998: signals of change. The health accounts team. *Health Aff (Millwood)* 2000;19:124–32.
23. Strunk BC, Ginsburg PB, Gabel JR. Tracking health care costs. Washington: Center for Health System Change; 2001. Data Bulletin 21. Available: www.hschange.org/CONTENT/380/ (accessed 2002 June 24).
24. Hogan C, Ginsburg PB, Gabel JR. Tracking health care costs: inflation returns. *Health Aff (Millwood)* 2000;19:217–23.
25. Miller RH, Luft HS. Does managed care lead to better or worse quality of care? *Health Aff (Millwood)* 1997;16:7–25.
26. Dudley RA, Luft HS. Managed care in transition. *N Engl J Med* 2001;344: 1087–92.
27. A patients' bill of rights for Canada? [editorial]. *CMAJ* 2001;165(7):877.

ARTICLE 3

HEALTH INSURANCE COVERAGE: 2000

Robert J. Mills

An estimated 14.0 percent of the population were without health insurance coverage during the entire year in 2000, down from 14.3 percent in 1999. Similarly, the number of people without health insurance coverage declined in 2000, to 38.7 million, down 0.6 million from the previous year.

The estimates in this report are based on the March 2001 Current Population Survey (CPS), conducted by the U.S. Census Bureau. Respondents provide answers to the best of their ability, but as with all surveys, the estimates may differ from the actual values.

HIGHLIGHTS

- The number and percentage of people covered by employment-based health insurance rose significantly in 2000, driving the overall increase in health insurance coverage.
- Mirroring what happened for the total population, the proportion of uninsured children declined in 2000, from 12.6 percent in 1999 to 11.6 percent. The number of uninsured children declined from 9.1 million to 8.5 million.
- For poor people, the uninsured rate also declined in 2000 — from 31.1 percent to 29.5 percent. Although Medicaid insured 12.4 million poor people, 9.2 million poor people still had no health insurance in 2000.
- Compared with the previous year, health insurance coverage rates increased for those with household incomes below $50,000, decreased for those with household incomes between $50,000 and $75,000, and were unchanged for those with $75,000 and higher household incomes.

- Hispanics (68.0 percent) were less likely than White non-Hispanics (90.3 percent) to be covered by health insurance.[1] The coverage rate for Blacks in 2000 (81.5 percent) did not differ statistically from the coverage rate for Asians and Pacific Islanders (82.0 percent).
- American Indians and Alaska Natives were less likely to have health insurance than other racial groups, based on a 3-year average (1998–2000) — 73.2 percent, compared with 80.5 percent of Blacks, 81.2 percent of Asians and Pacific Islanders, and 89.9 percent of White non-Hispanics. However, they were more likely to have insurance than were Hispanics (67.2 percent).[2]
- Among the entire population 18 to 64 years old, workers (both full- and part-time) were more likely to have health insurance (83.8 percent) than nonworkers (76.4 percent), but among the poor, workers were less likely to be covered (54.5 percent) than nonworkers (63.4 percent).
- The foreign-born population was less likely than the native population to be insured — 68.4 percent compared with 88.1 percent in 2000.
- Young adults (18 to 24 years old) were less likely than other age groups to have health insurance coverage — 72.7 percent in 2000 compared with 84.3 percent of those 25 to 64 and, reflecting widespread Medicare coverage, 99.3 percent of those 65 years and over.
- The male population was less likely than the female population to have health insurance coverage — 85.1 percent compared with 86.9 percent in 2000.

Employment-Based Insurance, the Leading Source of Health Coverage, Drove the Increase in Insurance Coverage Rates

Most people (64.1 percent) were covered by a health insurance plan related to employment for some or all of 2000, an increase of 0.6 percentage points over the previous year. The increase in private health insurance coverage largely reflects the increase in employment-based insurance, which increased 0.3 percentage points to 72.4 percent in 2000 (see Figure 1).[3]

The government also provides health insurance coverage, but that coverage rate did not change between 1999 and 2000. Among the entire population, 24.2 percent had government insurance, including Medicare (13.4 percent), Medicaid (10.4 percent), and military health care (3.0 percent). Many people carried coverage from more than one plan during the year; for example, 7.6 percent of people were covered by both private health insurance and Medicare.

1. Hispanics may be of any race.
2. The difference in health insurance coverage rates between Blacks and Asians and Pacific Islanders was not statistically significant.
3. Employment-based health insurance is coverage offered through one's own employment or a relative's.

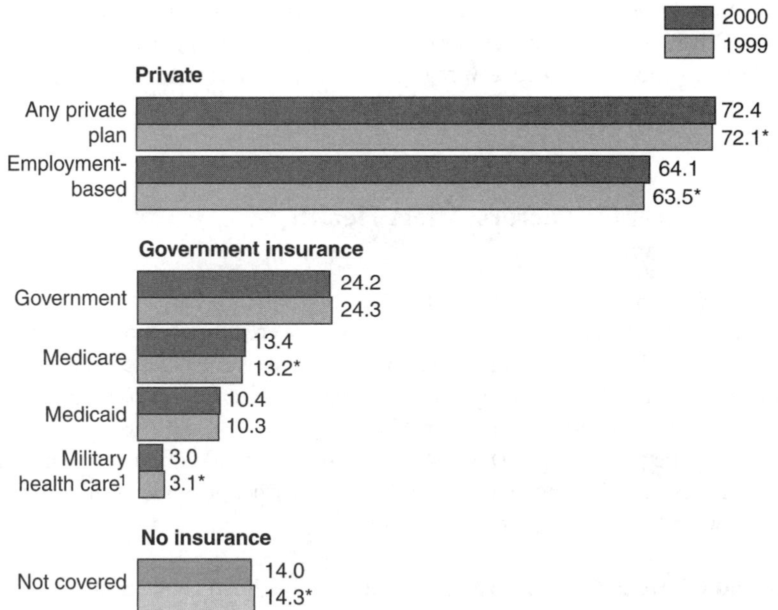

*Statistically significant at the 90-percent confidence level.
[1]Military health care includes CHAMPUS (Comprehensive Health and Medical Plan for Uniformed Services)/ Tricare, CHAMPVA (Civilian Health and Medical Program of the Department of Veterans Affairs), Veterans', and military health care.

Note: The estimates by type of coverage are not mutually exclusive; people can be covered by more than one type of health insurance during the year.

Figure 1 Type of health insurance and coverage status: 1999 and 2000 (in percent). (Source: U.S. Census Bureau, Current Population Survey, March 2000 and 2001.)

While the Uninsured Rate for the Poor Decreased between 1999 and 2000, the Uninsured Rate for the Near Poor Increased

Despite the Medicaid program, 9.2 million, or 29.5 percent, of the poor had no health insurance of any kind during 2000. This percentage — more than double the rate for the total population — did, however, drop from 31.1 percent for the previous year. The uninsured poor comprised 23.8 percent of all uninsured people.

Medicaid was the most widespread type of health insurance among the poor, with 39.8 percent (12.4 million) of those in poverty covered by Medicaid for some or all of 2000. This percentage did not change statistically from the previous year.[4]

Among the near poor (those with a family income greater than, but less than 125 percent of, the poverty level), 26.9 percent (3.3 million people) lacked health

4. Changes in year-to-year Medicaid estimates should be viewed with caution. For more information, see the Technical Note.

insurance in 2000. This percentage increased significantly from 1999, from 24.7 percent. Private health insurance coverage among the near poor (40.3 percent) and government health insurance coverage (44.6 percent) did not change significantly from 1999.

Key Demographic Factors Affect Health Insurance Coverage

Age. People 18 to 24 years old were less likely than other age groups to have health insurance coverage, with 72.7 percent covered for some or all of 2000. Because of Medicare, almost all people 65 years and over (99.3 percent) had health insurance in 2000. For other age groups, health insurance coverage ranged from 78.8 percent to 88.4 percent (see Figure 2).

Among the poor, people 18 to 64 years old had a markedly lower health insurance coverage rate (59.0 percent) in 2000 than either people under 18 (78.5 percent) or 65 years and over (97.6 percent).

Race and Hispanic Origin. The uninsured rate declined significantly in 2000 for Blacks and White non-Hispanics — for Blacks, from 19.6 percent to 18.5 percent and for White non-Hispanics, from 9.9 percent to 9.7 percent. Among Asian and Pacific Islanders, the apparent decline in the uninsured rate from 19.0 percent in 1999 to 18.0 percent in 2000 was not statistically significant.[5] The uninsured rate among Hispanics (32.0 percent in 2000) also did not change significantly from 1999.[6]

The Current Population Survey, the source of these data, samples 50,000 households nationwide and is not large enough to produce reliable annual estimates for American Indians and Alaska Natives. However, 3-year averages (1998–2000) of the number of American Indians and Alaska Natives, their 3-year average uninsured rate, and 3-year average uninsured rates for other race groups show that 26.8 percent of American Indians and Alaska Natives were without coverage, compared with 19.5 percent for Blacks, 18.8 percent for Asians and Pacific Islanders, and

5. The Asian and Pacific Islander population consists of many distinct groups that differ in socioeconomic characteristics, culture, and recency of immigration. Because of differences among them, data users should exercise caution when interpreting aggregate data for this population.

6. Because Hispanics may be of any race, use caution in comparing data for Hispanics and data for racial groups such as Blacks (3.1 percent of whom were Hispanic in 2000) and Asians and Pacific Islanders (1.9 percent of whom were Hispanic in 2000). Furthermore, the Hispanic population consists of many distinct groups that differ in socioeconomic characteristics, culture, and recency of immigration. Because of differences among the individual groups, data users should exercise caution when interpreting aggregate data for this population.

The difference in health insurance coverage rates between Blacks and Asians and Pacific Islanders was not statistically significant.

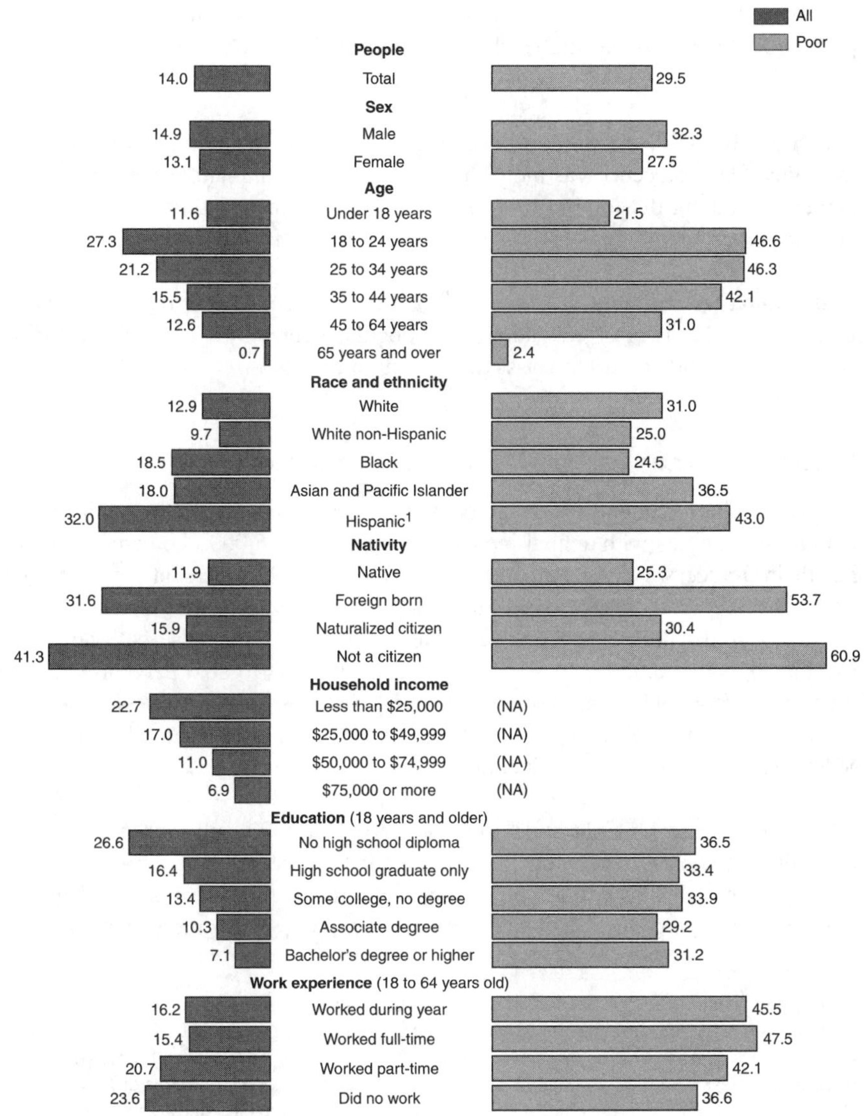

Figure 2 People without health insurance for the entire year by selected characteristics: 2000 (in percent). (Source: U.S. Census Bureau, Current Population Survey, March 2001.)

10.1 percent for White non-Hispanics.[7] The 3-year average uninsured rate for Hispanics (32.8 percent) was higher than the uninsured rate for American Indians and Alaska Natives.[8]

Nativity. In 2000, the proportion of the foreign-born population without health insurance (31.6 percent) was more than double that of the native population (11.9 percent).[9] Among the foreign born, noncitizens were more likely than naturalized citizens to lack coverage — 41.3 percent compared with 15.9 percent.

Educational Attainment. Among all adults, the likelihood of being insured increased as the level of education rose. For the poor, however, health insurance coverage rates did not differ across the education groups.

Economic Status Affects Health Insurance Coverage

Income. The likelihood of being covered by health insurance rises with income. Among households with annual incomes of less than $25,000, the percentage with health insurance was 77.3 percent; the level rises to 93.1 percent for those with incomes of $75,000 or more (see Figure 2).

Compared with the previous year, the coverage rate for those with household incomes below $50,000 increased 0.3 percentage points to 80.5 percent, while for those with household incomes of $50,000 to $75,000, the coverage rate decreased 0.7 percentage points to 89.0 percent. Coverage rates remained the same for those with $75,000 and higher household income.

Work Experience. Of those 18 to 64 years old in 2000, full-time workers were more likely to be covered by health insurance (84.6 percent) than part-time workers (79.3 percent), and part-time workers were more likely to be insured than nonworkers (76.4 percent).[10] However, among the poor, nonworkers (63.4 percent)

---

7. Data users should exercise caution when interpreting aggregate data for American Indians and Alaska Natives (AIAN) because the AIAN population consists of groups that differ in economic characteristics. Data from the 1990 census show that economic characteristics of those American Indians and Alaska Natives who live in American Indian and Alaska Native areas differ from the characteristics of those who live outside these areas. In addition, the CPS does not use separate population controls for weighting the AIAN samples to national totals. See Accuracy of Estimates for a further discussion of CPS estimation procedures. Finally, proportional adjustment was used for the 1998 estimates to account for the verification questions added this year.

8. The difference in health insurance coverage rates between Blacks and Asians and Pacific Islanders was not statistically significant.

9. Natives are people born in the United States, Puerto Rico, or an outlying area of the United States, such as Guam or the U.S. Virgin Islands, and people who were born in a foreign country but who had at least one parent who was a U.S. citizen. All other people born outside the United States are foreign born.

10. Workers were classified as part time if they worked fewer than 35 hours per week in the majority of the weeks they worked in 1999.

were more likely to be insured than workers (54.5 percent). While poor full-time workers appear to be less likely than poor part-time workers to have coverage, the difference was not statistically significant.

Firm Size. Of the 140.4 million workers in the United States who were 18–64 years old, 57.1 percent had employment-based health insurance policies in their own name. The proportion generally increased with the size of the employing firm — 31.6 percent of workers employed by firms with fewer than 25 employees and 69.8 percent for workers employed by firms with 500 or more employees were insured, for example. (These estimates do not reflect the fact that some workers were covered by another family member's employment-based policy.)

The Uninsured Rate for Children Decreased between 1999 and 2000

The percentage of children (people under 18 years old) without health insurance in the United States dropped from 12.6 percent in 1999 to 11.6 percent in 2000. The increase in employment-based insurance accounted for most of the change; no change occurred in government health insurance coverage.

Among poor children, 21.5 percent (2.5 million children) had no health insurance during 2000. This percentage did not change statistically from the previous year. The percentage of poor children with government health insurance or employment-based coverage also did not change. Poor children made up 29.6 percent of all uninsured children in 2000.

Among near-poor children, the proportion without health insurance was 21.9 percent (0.9 million children) in 2000, statistically unchanged from 1999.[11] For this group, private health insurance coverage decreased from 45.2 percent to 38.6 percent, but government health insurance coverage did not change.

The Likelihood of Health Insurance Coverage Varies among Children

- Children 12 to 17 years old were more likely to be uninsured than those under 12 — 12.3 percent compared with 11.3 percent.
- The uninsured rate declined significantly in 2000 for Hispanic, White non-Hispanic, and Black children — from 26.3 percent to 24.9 percent for Hispanic children, from 7.8 percent to 7.3 percent for White non-Hispanic children, and from 16.4 percent to 13.6 percent for Black children. The uninsured rate for Asian and Pacific Islander children in 2000 was 14.2 percent, statistically unchanged from 1999 (see Figure 3).[12]

11. The difference in health insurance coverage rates between poor children and near-poor children was not statistically significant.

12. The difference in health insurance coverage rates between Black children and Asian and Pacific Islander children was not statistically significant.

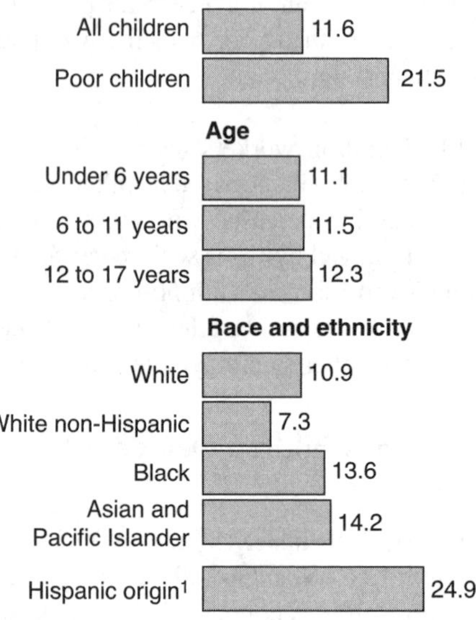

Figure 3 Uninsured children by race, ethnicity, and age: 2000 (in percent). (Source: U.S. Census Bureau, Current Population Survey, March 2001.)

- While most children (70.5 percent) were covered by an employment-based or privately purchased health insurance plan in 2000, one in five (20.4 percent) was covered by Medicaid.
- Black children had a higher rate of Medicaid coverage in 2000 than children of any other racial or ethnic group — 35.8 percent, compared with 32.8 percent of Hispanic children, 18.6 percent of Asian and Pacific Islander children, and 13.2 percent of White non-Hispanic children (see Figure 4).
- Children living in single-parent families in 2000 were less likely to be insured than children living in married-couple families — 84.6 percent compared with 90.3 percent.

Some States had Higher Uninsured Rates Than Others

The proportion of people without health insurance ranged from 6.9 percent in Rhode Island to 22.6 percent in New Mexico, based on 3-year averages for 1998, 1999, and 2000. Although the data presented suggest that New Mexico had the highest uninsured rate, its rate was not statistically different from the rate for Texas. Conversely, the uninsured rate for Minnesota, though seemingly the second lowest, was not statistically different from Iowa, Pennsylvania, New Hampshire, or Missouri.

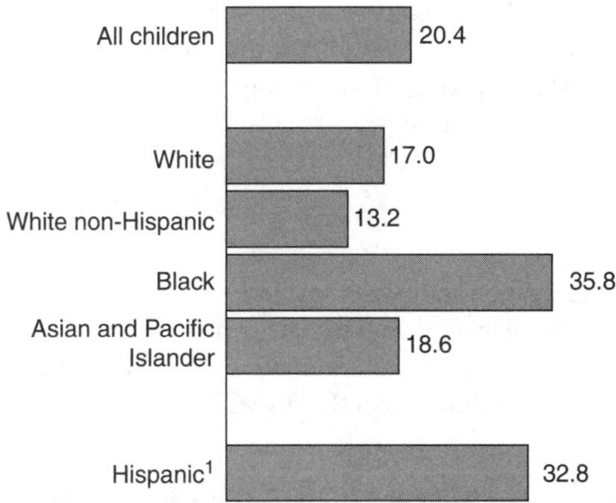

Figure 4 Children covered by Medicaid by race and ethnicity: 2000 (in percent). (Source: U.S. Census Bureau, Current Population Survey, March 2001.)

Comparisons of 2-year moving averages (1998–1999 and 1999–2000) show that the proportion of people without coverage fell in 18 states: Alabama, Arizona, Arkansas, California, Connecticut, Delaware, Georgia, Maryland, Michigan, Mississippi, Nevada, New Hampshire, New Jersey, North Dakota, Pennsylvania, Rhode Island, Texas, and Wisconsin. Meanwhile, the proportion of people without coverage rose in eight states: Alaska, Kansas, Nebraska, New Mexico, Ohio, Oklahoma, Vermont, and Washington.

ACCURACY OF THE ESTIMATES

Statistics from surveys are subject to sampling and nonsampling error. All comparisons presented in this report take sampling error into account and meet the Census Bureau's standards for statistical significance. Nonsampling errors in surveys may be attributed to a variety of sources, such as how the survey was designed, how respondents interpret questions, how able and willing respondents are to provide correct answers, and how accurately answers are coded and classified. The Census Bureau employs quality control procedures throughout the production process — including the overall design of surveys, the wording of questions, review of the work of interviewers and coders, and statistical review of reports.

The Current Population Survey employs ratio estimation, whereby sample estimates are adjusted to independent estimates of the national population by age, race, sex, and Hispanic origin. This weighting partially corrects for bias due to undercoverage, but how it affects different variables in the survey is not precisely known.

Moreover, biases may also be present when people who are missed in the survey differ from those interviewed in ways other than the categories used in weighting (age, race, sex, and Hispanic origin). All of these considerations affect comparisons across different surveys or data sources.

TECHNICAL NOTE

This report presents data on the health insurance coverage of people in the United States during the 2000 calendar year. The data, which are shown by state and selected demographic and socioeconomic characteristics, were collected in the March 2001 Supplement to the Current Population Survey (CPS).

Treatment of Major Federal Health Insurance Programs

The Current Population Survey (CPS) underreports Medicare and Medicaid coverage compared with enrollment and participation data from the Center for Medicare and Medicaid Services (CMS), formerly the Health Care Financing Administration (HCFA).[13] A major reason for the lower CPS estimates is that the CPS is not designed primarily to collect health insurance data; instead, it is largely a labor force survey. Consequently, interviewers receive less training on health insurance concepts. Additionally, many people may not be aware that they or their children are covered by a health insurance program if they have not used covered services recently and therefore fail to report coverage. CMS data, on the other hand, represent the actual number of people who enrolled or participated in these programs and are a more accurate source of coverage levels.

Changes in Medicaid coverage estimates from one year to the next should be viewed with caution. Because many people who are covered by Medicaid do not report that coverage, the Census Bureau assigns coverage to those who are generally regarded as "categorically eligible" (those who received some other benefits, usually public assistance payments, that make them eligible for Medicaid). Since the number of people receiving public assistance has been dropping, the relationship between Medicaid and public assistance has changed, so that the imputation process has introduced a downward bias in the most recent Medicaid estimates.

As a result of consultation with health insurance experts, the Census Bureau modified the definition of the population without health insurance in the March 1998 Current Population Survey. Previously, people with no coverage other than access to Indian Health Service were counted as part of the insured population. Beginning with the 1997 Health Insurance Coverage report, however, the Census Bureau counts these people as uninsured. The effect of this change on the overall estimates of health insurance coverage is negligible.

---

13. CMS is the federal agency primarily responsible for administering the Medicare and Medicaid programs at the national level.

ARTICLE 4

MANAGED CARE IN TRANSITION

R. Adams Dudley and Harold S. Luft

Managed care now dominates health care in the United States. By 1999, only 8 percent of persons with employer-sponsored health insurance coverage had traditional indemnity insurance.[1] This reflects a sea change in the past two decades — not just in the financing of health insurance but also in the way medicine is practiced.

The rapid growth of managed care is not primarily due to enthusiasm for this approach on the part of patients or providers. Patients have had mixed reactions to managed care; they like the low copayments and reduced paperwork but view some managed-care practices as emphasizing cost control over quality. In fact, there is widespread concern among the public, physicians, and legislators about the effect of managed care on the quality of care. In this article, we examine how managed care has made such gains, despite the concern about its effects on quality, and how it may change in the years ahead.

EVOLUTION OF MANAGED CARE

The earliest forms of managed-care organizations were group- or staff-model health maintenance organizations (HMOs), such as Kaiser–Permanente and Group Health Cooperative of Puget Sound. As costs rose in the 1960s and 1970s, policymakers and employers alike began to consider prepayment as an alternative to the fee-for-service system of payment. Under the HMO rubric, prepayment was extended to include not only group- and staff-model organizations but also more loosely organized individual-practice associations.

Initially, insurance companies could not control costs as well as HMOs could. With indemnity insurance, the patient chose a physician from among all those in the community, received care and a bill, and then submitted the bill to the insurer. Insurers had to pay fees that were "usual and customary" in each community, which meant that the local physicians set the fees.

TABLE 1

ENROLLMENT IN HEALTH PLANS AMONG PERSONS WITH EMPLOYER-SPONSORED HEALTH INSURANCE, 1996 AND 1999*

	Enrollment % of persons	
Type of Plan	*1996*	*1999*
Traditional indemnity plan	27	8
Health maintenance organization	31	29
Preferred-provider organization	28	41
Point-of-service plan	14	22

*Data are from Gabel et al.[1]

In 1982, California passed legislation permitting insurers to establish contracts with selected providers. With this new option,[2] insurers could exclude physicians who did not accept their rules and fee schedules. With their extensive experience in negotiating contracts, insurers began to build networks of individual physicians, called preferred-provider organizations. These managed-care organizations were gradually expanded into statewide or even national networks of contracted physicians.

As managed care grew and as more employers provided only managed-care coverage for their employees, some patients complained about the restricted choice of providers. This led to broader networks of preferred providers and to the development of point-of-service plans, which include some coverage for the services of providers who are not part of the network. Table 1 shows the increase from 1996 to 1999 in enrollment in point-of-service plans and preferred-provider organizations, at the expense of indemnity plans, among persons with employer-sponsored insurance.[1]

Insurers have recently begun to offer "multitiered" plans. Enrollment in a multitiered plan gives the patient three options: full coverage in an HMO with a limited number of providers; access to a preferred-provider organization, with slightly higher copayments than those for the HMO; and use of out-of-network providers, with the highest copayments. By combining features of HMOs, preferred-provider organizations, and point-of-service plans, this approach offers a choice between lower copayments for restricted access to providers and higher payments for greater access but allows the patient to make that trade-off at the time of illness rather than during the annual enrollment period. However, to the extent that financial barriers prevent low-income persons from choosing out-of-network providers, multitiered plans may in effect create different classes of coverage for persons with the same employer but different salaries.

Enrollment in managed-care plans grew because managed care costs less than fee-for-service care. Managed-care business practices such as preauthorization of hospital and other services and restricted formularies for medications reduced utilization and cost. As a result of these strategies, managed-care organizations also had healthier enrollees than did fee-for-service plans, because patients switching from fee-for-service care to managed care tended to be healthier than average, and some patients in managed-care plans returned to fee-for-service care when they got sick.[3] This "risk selection" increased the cost advantage of managed care.

Some policymakers supported managed care because they believed that prepayment would improve the quality of care. Fee-for-service payment leads to uncoordinated care, they argued, whereas prepayment for all inpatient and outpatient services allows physicians to allocate resources optimally for each patient. Supporters of managed care also argued that the use of preventive services would increase and that the quality of care for acute and chronic conditions would improve as plans sought to avoid costly complications. Despite this rationale for the superior performance of managed-care organizations, most studies have found little difference in quality between managed care and fee-for-service care. Deficiencies in quality occur in both types of health plans.[4] In addition, purchasers have rarely chosen health plans on the basis of the quality of care. Assuming that accreditation of plans and licensure of providers are sufficient to ensure high quality, they have chosen plans primarily on the basis of price.[5]

EFFECTS OF MANAGED CARE

Effect on Providers

The growth of managed care has profoundly influenced physicians' practices. In 1996, the American Medical Association began tracking the proportion of revenues physicians received from managed care. That year, managed care accounted for 38.4 percent of revenues received by all physicians;[6] by 1999, the proportion was 48.9 percent, and almost all physicians had managed-care contracts (Table 2).[7] About one

TABLE 2

PHYSICIANS' PARTICIPATION IN MANAGED CARE AND CAPITATION, 1996 AND 1999*

Variable	*1996*	*1999*
Physicians with managed-care contracts (% of all physicians)	88.1	90.8
Mean practice revenue from managed care (% of revenue)		
Among all physicians	38.4	48.9
Among physicians with managed-care contracts	43.6	53.9
Physicians with capitation contracts (% of all physicians)	36.7	35.2
Mean practice revenue from capitation (% of revenue)		
Among all physicians	8.4	7.4
Among physicians with capitation contracts	22.9	21.0

*Data are from Gonzalez[6] and Wassenaar and Thran.[7]

third of physicians had capitation contracts. Although capitation accounted for only 7.4 percent of practice revenues among all physicians in the United States in 1999, it accounted for 21.0 percent of revenues among physicians with capitation contracts. Capitation represented a higher proportion of practice revenues in primary care specialties (ranging from 12.2 percent of revenues received by all physicians in general internal medicine to 16.4 percent in pediatrics) and in certain regions of the country (16.8 percent of revenues received by all physicians in Pennsylvania and 14.4 percent in California).[7]

Capitation contracts specify that providers will be prepaid on a per capita basis for an agreed-on list of services (e.g., primary care only, all physicians' services, or hospitalization only) or for all services and drug costs (global capitation). This approach shifts the financial risk from the insurer to the provider. Theoretically, capitation could improve the quality of care if providers focused on prevention and on early diagnosis and treatment and if prepayment resulted in better coordination of care rather than episodic provision of services. However, such improvement is based on four assumptions: that the capitation rate covers all necessary medical care and capital expenses plus enough to cover the occasional case of catastrophic illness, that providers have control over all aspects of care, that they expect to keep patients for a long time, and that they have the managerial skills and infrastructure to respond effectively to the incentives provided through capitation. Although the news media's coverage of problems with capitation has focused on situations in which the capitation rate has been too low to cover all services included in the contract (a violation of the first assumption), there have been cases in which the other assumptions have not held. Thus, most of the reported problems with capitation reflect problems with contracts and with implementation and are probably not sufficient to reject capitation as an approach to the financing of health care.

The relatively low percentage of revenues that physicians receive from capitation and the slight decline in the percentage from 1996 to 1999 suggest that medical groups have not been comfortable with the available capitation arrangements. Some plans have also encountered difficulties in their capitation arrangements with hospitals. In one of the most publicized retreats from hospital capitation, PacifiCare Health Systems decided to restructure some of its contracts in California. In 1998, 91 percent of PacifiCare's California enrollees were covered by plans that included capitation arrangements with hospitals. Under these arrangements, enrollees chose the hospital where they would receive care, if necessary, and the hospital received a fixed payment for each enrollee who chose it. In 1999 and 2000, one third of the hospitals withdrew from the capitation arrangements, citing unbudgeted capital expenditures (e.g., retrofitting of buildings to provide protection against earthquakes), rising operating expenses (e.g., nurses' salaries), or an inability to manage utilization (since physicians, not hospitals, admit and discharge patients). In addition, mergers gave some hospitals enough market power to refuse PacifiCare's capitation rates. PacifiCare continues to have capitation contracts with most of the hospitals and has responded to the rest by negotiating shared-risk contracts and by improving its information and clinical-management systems.

Effect on Patients

Managed care has resulted in major changes for patients and their experience of care. Measures adopted by managed-care organizations to control costs or improve the quality of care, or both, include primary care gatekeeping, preauthorization of referrals, utilization review, profiling of physicians (monitoring of their patterns of utilization or the quality of their care), pharmaceutical restrictions, practice guidelines, case management, and most recently, disease management. (There is no consensus on the definition of disease management, but in general, it involves a multidisciplinary effort to minimize the burden of disease by educating patients, encouraging them to take an active role in their care, and establishing a long-term therapeutic plan.) Patients' reactions to these measures depend primarily on whether they are perceived as attempts to limit expenditures or to ensure proper care. Thus, gatekeeping is often not well received, because people rarely believe its purpose is to maintain or improve the quality of care,[8] whereas disease-management programs may be more acceptable.

The extent to which these measures influence actual care (as opposed to the perception of care) remains uncertain. Attempts to evaluate managed-care practices are complicated by variations in other organizational characteristics, the impossibility of conducting blinded, randomized trials at the organizational level, and inconsistent definitions of each strategy. Studies of the effect of these measures on cost have similar limitations, but there is some evidence that certain measures have little effect. For example, a meta-analysis of studies of physician profiling showed minimal, though statistically significant, reductions in cost.[9]

Experience in the private sector also suggests that some managed-care practices are ineffective, and some insurers are dropping them, especially those perceived as cost-control rather than quality-control measures. In response to patients' complaints about gatekeeping and lack of evidence that it had changed referral patterns, Harvard Pilgrim Health Care, in New England, discontinued its use of gatekeepers in 1997. UnitedHealthcare, a national company, recently stopped requiring preauthorization of referrals, after discovering that requested referrals were denied in less than 1 percent of cases.[10] However, with health care costs rising again, insurers may reconsider cost-control measures.

RESPONSES TO MANAGED CARE

Physicians and Medical Groups

With their purchasing power and negotiating experience, and aided by business and government support for managed care, insurers obtained substantial concessions from providers as managed care grew. These included discounts on fee-for-service rates in some cases, acceptance of capitation arrangements in others, and tolerance of measures to control utilization in almost every case.

One of the primary strategies physicians used to match the purchasing power of managed-care organizations was to affiliate with each other. Table 3 shows the declining

TABLE 3

DISTRIBUTION OF PHYSICIANS ACCORDING TO TYPE OF EMPLOYMENT*

Type of Employment	*% of physicians* 1983	1994	1999
Self-employed			
Solo practice	40.5	29.3	28.4
Group practice	35.3	28.4	33.4
Employed by group practice, managed-care organization, or other organization	24.2	42.3	38.2

*Data are from Wassenaar and Thran[7] and Kletke et al.[11]

percentage of physicians in solo practice from 1983 to 1999 and the rise in the percentage of employed physicians. The change in practice type has been even more pronounced among physicians in their first five years of practice: in 1983, approximately one third of such physicians were employed, as compared with 66 percent in 1994.[11]

Some medical groups also formed larger systems of care. Physician–hospital organizations were created either to accept global capitation or to ensure hospitals a steady stream of admissions. However, differences in the cultures and goals of medical groups and hospitals have limited the growth of these combined organizations. For example, primary care physicians may join a physician–hospital organization to increase their ability to coordinate care and prevent complications. This emphasis on primary care may conflict with the hospital's goals if its reason for forming the organization is to keep the number of admissions high. The most successful physician–hospital organizations tend to be nonprofit organizations involving physicians and hospitals that are prominent in the community and that had established working relationships before the organization was formed.[12]

In the 1990s, some medical groups sold their practices to or signed agreements with practice-management companies.[12] This trend was initially greeted with enthusiasm by Wall Street. At one point, two practice-management companies, MedPartners and PhyCor, proposed a merger that involved 6 percent of all physicians in the United States.[13] However, the growth of practice-management companies slowed substantially as they discovered that buying physicians' practices was easier than changing the way they delivered care. Investors eventually realized that the apparent growth in earnings for MedPartners was due to acquisitions rather than to substantive practice management.[14]

Recently, whether as a result of desperation or confidence, an increasing number of medical groups have rejected or terminated capitation contracts. In California, where many medical groups are on the verge of bankruptcy, Sutter Health, a large network of medical groups and hospitals based in Sacramento, canceled its contract with Blue Cross.[15] Aetna recently had to drop its requirement that physicians who join its preferred-provider organization also accept its HMO contracts.[16]

Employers

Employers have also turned to collective action. Regional coalitions of employers often attempt to negotiate discounts on health care. In addition, many of these coalitions recognize the need to address the problems of risk selection and the lack of incentives for health plans to improve the quality of care.

Some managed-care organizations have used risk selection to reduce their costs, but purchasers now recognize this strategy. The solution is to adjust the premium paid to organizations that enroll patients who are sicker (or healthier) than average. Such an adjustment ensures that managed-care organizations that do not practice risk selection (and hence enroll sicker patients than plans that do practice risk selection) have the resources they need to care for their enrollees and that the plans with healthy enrollees do not receive unwarranted profits. However, risk adjustment requires both data and analytic tools in order to set appropriate rates; the tools have been under development for two decades. Some purchasers believe that adjustment of payments on the basis of diagnoses reported on claims could be an effective approach. Under capitation, however, providers do not submit claims, and it has taken time for some managed-care organizations to develop systems for collecting diagnostic data. Since Medicare adopted a diagnosis-based system of adjustment in 2000, however, the ability of organizations to provide these data has increased.[17] Buyers Health Care Action Groups in Minneapolis, for example, is adjusting payments to delivery systems on the basis of diagnoses recorded at every inpatient or outpatient encounter.

Risk adjustment provides an indirect incentive to improve the quality of care. Some employers are also creating direct incentives. The Pacific Business Group on Health measures the quality of care on several dimensions[18] and uses public recognition (through annual awards), patient volume, and financial bonuses to give plans and providers incentives to improve quality. The Central Florida Health Care Coalition plans to rate the quality of inpatient and outpatient care provided by physicians. The coalition will allow its members to select any physician, but copayments will be lower if they select providers with a high rating for quality of care. In addition, the coalition will make graded fee-for-service payments, with the top-rated physicians receiving a higher payment for any given service than lower-rated physicians. The Leapfrog Group is a national coalition of employers that includes more than 65 Fortune 500 companies and other large employers, with a total of more than 25 million covered employees. The group is trying to use its leverage to foster regional improvement in the quality of care. An example is Leapfrog's involvement with the Michigan Health and Safety Coalition, which includes hospitals, health plans, medical groups, employers, unions, and government agencies. Leapfrog is collaborating with the Michigan coalition to improve the safety of hospitalized patients and to inform patients and providers about issues involving safety.

A parallel initiative by employers is the adoption of a defined-contribution approach, which specifies the amount the employer will pay for an employee's coverage and requires that the employee pay the difference for more expensive coverage. This approach is being used in two different ways. Some employers use it to limit their costs and their involvement in issues concerning the quality of care. Others view it as part of a strategy (along with providing data on the quality of care) to make their employees aware of how plans differ with respect to cost and quality. General Motors makes the largest contributions for the plans it believes offer the highest-quality care. Currently, however, the growth of this approach is limited by a tight labor market and the concern that employees will view defined contributions as a reduction in benefits.

Government

State and federal legislators are responding to public concern about managed care. The major areas of legislative activity are the benefits package (what should be covered), use of emergency room services, the physician–patient relationship, resolution of disputes, and liability (Table 4).[19,20]

Congress has also considered legislation.[20] Passage of the proposed Patient Protection Act has been held up primarily by disagreements over issues involving the liability of health plans — that is, how easy it should be for patients to sue health plans when disputes arise, and whether such suits should be brought in state or federal courts. There is strong public support for a patients' bill of rights, but the prospects for meaningful legislation are unclear.

Managed-care organizations claim they should not be sued for malpractice, even when they deny care. The basis of this claim is that they decide what services are covered but do not make decisions about individual care and that their actions are, in many cases, exempt from state regulation under the federal Employee Retirement Income Security Act. Recent judicial decisions suggest that managed-care organizations, although still protected by the act from claims that they must provide specific services (i.e., they cannot be challenged with respect to the scope of the services they provide), can be held responsible under state laws for the quality of the services that are delivered with their authorization.[21] In addition, managed-care organizations in several states are being sued on the grounds of false advertising. The contention is that although their advertisements state that decisions are made by physicians, in some cases, plans deny coverage for treatments recommended by physicians or require physicians to adhere to guidelines developed by the plans, not by local providers.

THE FUTURE

Health care is not being transformed in isolation. The Internet allows patients to obtain information easily, though many sources of data on the Internet are unreliable. Health care organizations can, however, use the Internet to disseminate data to patients. For example, the Medicare Web site has data on the quality of care provided by each managed-care organization participating in the Medicare program (http://www.medicare.gov/mphcompare/home.asp).

Advances in computer technology have also made the creation of electronic medical records more feasible. The cost of an Internet-based system of medical

TABLE 4

STATE AND FEDERAL CONSUMER-PROTECTION LEGISLATION*

Provision	*No. of States with Provision Enacted as of 9/99*	*Federal Legislation Proposed in 2000*†	
		House	*Senate*
Required benefits			
Referral out of the network if an appropriate provider is not available within the network	18	Yes	No
Option of seeing specialist as primary care provider	12	Yes	No
Standing referral to a specialist for a patient with a chronic disease	20	Yes	No
Direct access to obstetrical–gynecologic services	33	Yes	Yes‡
Continuity of coverage when provider leaves plan	22	Yes	No
Access to nonformulary prescriptions when formulary equivalent is ineffective	14	Yes	Yes
Coverage of routine care during participation in a clinical trial	7	Yes	No
"Prudent layperson" standard for emergency room use§	37	Yes	Yes
Physician–patient relationship			
Full disclosure of all treatment options	48	Yes	Yes
Prohibition of financial incentives for physicians to limit services	23	Yes	No
Dispute resolution			
Independent external review of denial of care at patient's request	28	Yes	No
Independent ombudsperson for patients	10	No	No
Right of patient to sue plan for damages	3¶	Yes	No

*Data are from Families USA.[19,20]

†The House bill covered all health plans, whereas the Senate bill applied only to self-insured plans.

‡The law applies only to physicians, not to midwives.

§The "prudent layperson" standard states that if a patient has symptoms that would lead a prudent layperson to seek emergency care (e.g., chest pain), the health plan must cover the cost of emergency services even if the patient did not call the plan before going to the emergency room.

¶The three states are California, Georgia, and Texas.

records is falling, making it possible to collect and audit data on quality and risk adjustment less expensively, although the issue of privacy must be addressed. Thus, the cost of providing incentives for managed-care plans to improve the quality of care is falling as well.

CONCLUSIONS

The health care market and managed care continue to evolve. There has been legitimate concern about some managed-care practices, and until recently, few attempts had been made to ensure that patients and the quality of care were protected. However, medical groups seem to be assuming a stronger stance in their negotiations with managed-care organizations, and employers, as well as federal and state governments, are becoming more sophisticated in the use of measures to promote and reward high-quality care. Efforts are also being made to prevent managed-care organizations from profiting by selecting healthy patients. Some managed-care organizations are already responding to these changes by eliminating administrative practices that restrict patients' choices and by establishing disease-management programs and other measures that increase the coordination of care.

The future of managed care remains uncertain, however. If employers and federal and state governments continue to emphasize the quality of care, and especially if medical groups and medical societies support these efforts, physicians may be able to spend more time caring for their patients and less time arguing with insurers. This might also help patients regain confidence in a system they have lost trust in. An appropriately designed system of prepayment — with rates that are high enough to cover all appropriate care and the cost of treating catastrophic illness, as well as incentives for providers to plan for the future — could facilitate the coordination of care, which has traditionally been fragmented. On the other hand, medical costs are on the rise again,[1,22] and if the primary focus of the policy debate returns to financial considerations, efforts to improve the quality of care may be postponed.

ACKNOWLEDGMENTS

We are indebted to Eunice Chee, Marchant Wentworth, and Richard Bae for their assistance in the preparation of the manuscript.

REFERENCES

1. Gabel J, Levitt L, Pickreign, J, et al. Job-based health insurance in 2000: premiums rise sharply while coverage grows. *Health Aff* (Millwood) 2000;19(5):144–51.
2. Bergthold L. Crabs in a bucket: the politics of health care reform in California. *J Health Polit Policy Law* 1984;9:203–22.

3. Morgan RO, Virnig BA, DeVito CA, Persily NA. The Medicare-HMO revolving door — the healthy go in and the sick go out. *N Engl J Med* 1997;337:169–75.
4. Dudley RA, Miller RH, Korenbrot TY, Luft HS. The impact of financial incentives on quality of health care. *Milbank Q* 1998;76:511, 649–86.
5. Legnini MW, Rosenberg LE, Perry MJ, Robertson NJ. Where does performance measurement go from here? *Health Aff (Millwood)* 2000;19(3):173–7.
6. Gonzalez ML, ed. Physician marketplace statistics 1996. Chicago: American Medical Association, 1997.
7. Wassenaar JD, Thran SL, eds. Physician socioeconomic statistics: 2000–2002 edition. Chicago: American Medical Association, 2001.
8. Bodenheimer T, Lo B, Casalino L. Primary care physicians should be coordinators, not gatekeepers. *JAMA* 1999;281:2045–9.
9. Balas EA, Boren SA, Brown GD, Ewigman BG, Mitchell JA, Perkoff GT. Effect of physician profiling on utilization: meta-analysis of randomized clinical trials. *J Gen Intern Med* 1996;11:584–90.
10. Shinkman R. UnitedHealth move wins praise: but AAHP study says health plans have chipped away to pre-authorization reviews for years. *Mod Healthc* 1999;29(46):24.
11. Kletke PR, Emmons DW, Gillis KD. Current trends in physicians' practice arrangements: from owners to employees. *JAMA* 1996;276:555–60.
12. Robinson JC. Consolidation of medical groups into physician practice management organizations. *JAMA* 1998;279:144–9.
13. Jaklevic MC. PPMs play big card: MedPartners, PhyCor merger to pool 6% of doctors. *Mod Healthc* 1997;27(44):4, 9.
14. Reinhardt UE. The rise and fall of the physician practice management industry. *Health Aff (Millwood)* 2000;19(1):42–55.
15. Bernstein S. Sutter Health leaves Blue Cross network. *Los Angeles Times*. January 4, 2001:C2.
16. Jackson C. Aetna cuts all-or-nothing arrangements. *AM News* 2001;44(2):1–2.
17. Hash M. Medicare+Choice plans. *JAMA* 2000;284:2988.
18. California Consumer HealthScope. San Francisco: Pacific Business Group on Health, 2000. (See http://www.healthscope.org.)
19. State managed care patient protections. Washington, D.C.: Families USA, October 1999. (See http://www.familiesusa.org/hitmisup.htm.)
20. The 106th Congress: how federal managed care legislation affects you: a comparison of key provisions in the Senate and House bills on managed care. Washington, D.C.: Families USA, July 2000. (See http://www.familiesusa.org/managedcare+u/compare2.htm.)
21. Mariner WK. What recourse? Liability for managed-care decisions and the Employee Retirement Income Security Act. *N Engl J Med* 2000;343:592–6.
22. Blumenthal D. Controlling health care expenditures. *N Engl J Med* 2001;344:766–9.

CHAPTER 8

HEALTH CARE FINANCING: MEDICARE, MEDICAID, AND THE STATE CHILDREN'S HEALTH INSURANCE PROGRAM

This chapter deals with health care financing, particularly with three of the nation's largest health programs — Medicare, Medicaid, and the State Children's Health Insurance Program (SCHIP). Four articles have been included to provide an overview of these programs, challenges faced by policymakers at the federal and state levels, and options for reform.

MEDICARE

Medicare is one of the largest and most popular social programs administered by the U.S. federal government. It now provides medical benefits to 40 million Americans. Created in 1965, Medicare was intended to reduce the economic burden of illness on the elderly and their families and to ensure access to acute medical care for the elderly who were Social Security beneficiaries. While Medicare aimed to alleviate the special situation of the elderly who incurred higher medical expenses, earned less income than workers under age 65 years, and yet were less well insured (only about half had any health insurance), the economic protection of the program and its institutional design were also meant to appeal to younger people who would not only be spared the cost of their parents' medical care, but would also be contributing to the program during their working years in order to be eligible for Medicare when they reached the age of 65.

The principal architects of the program were not only focused on acute medical care for the elderly, but also considered Medicare as a means to commence the journey toward universal health insurance for all Americans. Medicare's benefits were quite limited and not tailored to the chronic medical care needs of the elderly. This reflected the view of its founders that Medicare was merely to serve as the foundation for a more comprehensive and universal system of national health insurance in this country.

Notable changes in the basic characteristics of the Medicare program have occurred during the years since its implementation in 1966, and some overarching trends in the political development of the program have arisen. In Article 1, Marilyn Moon of the Urban Institute provides an excellent overview of the history of the program, its major characteristics, and the current issues.

Changes in Basic Characteristics of the Medicare Program

The size of the population eligible for Medicare has doubled from 19 million in 1966 to 40 million today. The original program extended eligibility only to individuals over age 65 who were eligible for Social Security retirement benefits. Legislation in 1972 extended Medicare coverage to the permanently disabled who had received Social Security benefits for two years and to individuals with end-stage renal disease.

The program originally guaranteed limited coverage of inpatient hospital care, nursing home care, and home health visits to cover acute episodes of illness through the Hospital Insurance program (Part A), all financed by a Social Security payroll tax. It provided voluntary coverage for physician services through the Supplementary Medicare Insurance program (Part B), financed by general revenues and premiums paid by beneficiaries. Over time, Medicare has provided limited additional coverage of home health care, preventive services, rural health clinics, and hospice care. Catastrophic insurance coverage and limited benefits for prescription drugs and other services were adopted in 1988, but most were repealed in 1989.

Federal spending for Medicare more than doubled every five years in the first two decades of the program, rising from $3.7 billion in 1967 to $14.9 billion in 1975 and to $69.1 billion in 1985. This growth has moderated somewhat in the past decade. In 1999, payments for all Medicare services were projected to be $212 billion. Medicare accounted for 3% of the federal budget in 1970 and now accounts for 12%.

Moon (2001) notes the impact of rising costs on the elderly: "In 1965, elderly persons spent an average of about 19% of their income on health care. That share fell to about 11 percent in 1968; today, it is more than 20 percent" (p. 928).

The vast majority of Medicare beneficiaries are enrolled in the fee-for-service portions of the program. In fiscal year 1999, 17% were enrolled in managed care plans paid through capitation contracts or in cost-reimbursed HMOs. Enrollment in managed care grew rapidly in the 1990s, but has slowed dramatically as benefits (especially prescription drugs) have declined and costs have risen.

Today, Medicare is seen by many Americans and policymakers in a very different light from that of 35 years ago. After the elections of 1994, when the Republicans gained control of both the House of Representatives and the Senate, the usual concerns about slowing Medicare spending were joined with an unprecedented battle over the size and role of government and the transformation of Medicare from a defined benefit, which it had been from the beginning, to a defined contribution. The government would provide each beneficiary a fixed amount of money and they could choose among plans. As the largest available source of budget savings (Social Security was technically and politically put off limits by both parties), Medicare became a main focus in a partisan showdown between President Clinton and the new Republican majorities in Congress. Spending, per se, was not the only issue — the fundamental nature of the entitlement to senior citizens was being challenged, as was the division of responsibilities between public and private sectors (see Estes and Linkins [1991] in the Recommended Reading). Two experienced Washington reporters wrote: "It was not consensus politics being practiced in Washington, or even conservative politics as previously defined. This was ideological warfare, a battle to destroy the remnants of the liberal, progressive brand of politics that had governed America throughout most of the twentieth century" (Johnson and Broder, 1996, p. 569). Medicare had entered into the realm of electoral and ideological politics for the first time since 1964, and the simplistic and polarizing policy debate and political deadlock that ensued was regarded as a symptom of a broader breakdown in "the system" of American politics (Johnson and Broder, 1996).

The Medicare debate since 1995 has reflected the bitter debate that was ignited by President Clinton's health care financing and reform proposal in 1993–1994. That debate, as Glied (1997) has pointed out, was fundamentally between those who believe that medical care is a public good (primarily advocates of single-payer plans, including traditional Medicare) and those who believe that medical care should be treated like any other market good (including those who favor competition among health plans and a voucher or guaranteed contribution rather than a guaranteed benefit in Medicare). In the end, the debate surrounding the Clinton health plan became a polarized struggle that the Republicans pursued for partisan political gain, which contributed to their capture of the House of Representatives and the Senate in the 1994 election. The stage was thus set for a showdown in 1995 on the budget and also on reductions in future Medicare increases (often called "cuts") that would be acceptable to the public. Historical shifts such as these are a reminder that the state of the Medicare program cannot be understood apart from developments in American politics.

Beyond the politics of entitlements and privatization are many issues concerning the substantive design of the Medicare program. As Moon noted, "The Medicare benefit package is inadequate because it leaves beneficiaries liable for nearly half of the cost of their acute care" (2001, p. 930). One of the most critical problems for the elderly is the growing cost of prescription drugs and the increasing limits on supplementary coverage for these costs. This issue is dealt with in more detail by Briesacher, Stuart, and Shea in Article 2.

A number of questions are being raised about the Medicare program. Is Medicare serving the economic and health needs of beneficiaries, and is it doing so in an efficient manner? In much of the country, the health care system has been undergoing turbulent changes and, in some cases, has been completely transformed in recent years, with implications for senior citizens as well as the general population (Robinson,

1996; Enthoven and Singer, 1996). In some areas fragmented systems of care are giving way to integrated, coordinated systems. Yet, as fast as these are emerging in some areas, they are collapsing in others (e.g., Southern California). Some argue that Medicare has not kept pace with developments in health care organization and financing. While the private sector has emphasized competition and managed care to control the rising costs of health care, Medicare has emphasized regulation, with prospective payments for hospitals based on diagnosis related groups (DRGs) and a fee schedule for physicians. Does Medicare cover an appropriate range of services and institutional settings for care of the elderly and chronically ill? Should Medicare attempt to move more rapidly into various forms of prepayment and managed care? As noted previously, a variety of analysts have suggested that it may be necessary or appropriate to shift the government's responsibility from covering defined benefits (whatever the cost) to contributing a fixed monetary amount toward each senior citizen's health insurance coverage (see, for example, Aaron and Reischauer, 1995; Fox, Etheredge, and Jones, 1996).

The Balanced Budget Act of 1997 established the Medicare+Choice program (Part C) to expand options for enrollment in managed care, altered the financing of home health services and graduate medical education, and made available medical savings accounts. These were the most significant reforms in the Medicare program since its enactment. The Bipartisan Commission on the Future of Medicare developed proposals to change the nature of the Medicare entitlement and debated adding prescription drug coverage. Reflecting the ideological split within its members, the Commission failed to achieve the support necessary to send formal recommendations to Congress.

Prior to the Balanced Budget Act of 1997, the biggest changes in Medicare were related to payment for hospitals (1983) and payment for physician services (1984–1996). In 1983, Congress mandated the establishment of a system of prospective payment for hospitals based on a standard known as the diagnosis related groups (DRGs). This system dramatically restructured the financial incentives for hospitals by defining specific groupings of conditions for which Medicare patients were hospitalized and setting specific payment amounts for each of these DRGs. This policy overturned the previous method of paying hospitals on the basis of costs incurred in treating patients (cost-based reimbursement), similar in many ways to fee-for-service reimbursement of physicians.

Beginning in 1984, Congress began to regulate direct Medicare payments to physicians as well as the ability of physicians to "balance bill" Medicare beneficiaries. *Balance billing* refers to the practice of charging the beneficiary for any difference between the physician's charge and Medicare's reimbursement payment. This practice became much more limited in the wake of the 1984 reforms. The following year Congress directed the Secretary of Health and Human Services to develop a resource-based relative value scale for physician payment and established the Physician Payment Review Commission to advise Congress and the Department of Health and Human Services (DHHS) on physician payment policies. In 1988, the Commission endorsed the concept of replacing the customary, prevailing, and reasonable (CPR) system of payment with a resource-based fee schedule. In the CPR system, payment was based on the physician's customary charge, modified by the prevailing charge for the same service in the community. In 1989, a resource-based fee schedule with limits on balance billing and an annual expenditure target to restrain rising costs were recommended by the Commission. These recommendations were basically adopted by Congress in 1989, although Congress changed the expenditure target to a volume performance standard. The fee schedule was implemented from 1992 to 1996 (Culbertson and Lee, 1996).

While Medicare was adopting a regulatory approach to both hospital and physician payments, the private sector, driven by employers' desires to slow the rising costs of health care, turned to managed care. The most significant changes have been the shifts from indemnity insurance, with fee-for-service payments to physicians and cost-based payments to hospitals, to capitated payment and managed care, with integration of the financing and delivery of medical care.

Prior to the Balanced Budget Act of 1997, Medicare was gradually expanding its managed care options. At the beginning of the program, Medicare allowed certain prepaid organizations to receive a cost reimbursement, instead of a fee-for-service payment, for Medicare enrollees. After a risk-sharing demonstration project was initiated in the 1980s, Congress authorized managed care payments based on a prospective payment methodology in 1982.

Medicare HMO enrollment increased gradually after risk contracting began in 1985. One million new beneficiaries enrolled in HMOs from 1987 to 1991, and by 1993, three million beneficiaries had enrolled. While the enrollment of Medicare beneficiaries in risk-contracting plans continues to grow, the number of beneficiaries in cost-reimbursement plans has been relatively steady for the past decade. In 1996, nearly 9% of Medicare beneficiaries were enrolled in risk-contracting HMOs. Medicare risk contracting grew rapidly, particularly in California, Oregon, Arizona, and Hawaii. Cutbacks by HMOs eliminated coverage for 934,000 Medicare beneficiaries in January 2001, forcing them to seek alternative HMO coverage or return to traditional Medicare. The HMO option was attractive to many elderly because it often included a prescription drug benefit and limited out-of-pocket expenses.

Medicare reform remains a priority, primarily because of the continual increase in program expenditures and because the baby boom generation will begin to reach age 65 in 2010. A Henry J. Kaiser Family Foundation article, "Medicare: Options for Reform (2002)," provides an analysis of the major issues: (1) cutting federal spending (e.g., trimming payments to doctors and hospitals); (2) asking beneficiaries to pay a greater share of the costs, raising payroll taxes, or raising revenue for other services; (3) improving benefits, particularly those related to prescription drugs; and (4) fundamentally restructuring Medicare. These issues are also dealt with briefly by Moon in Article 1.

This chapter seeks to identify the predominant forces underlying the major episodes of Medicare reform, and to determine the impact those forces have on the structure and operation of the program. It also seeks to identify how Medicare has affected many aspects of the American health care system. Even before it was fully implemented on July 1, 1966, Medicare was used to enforce the 1964 Civil Rights Act in 1965 and

1966 and almost instantly ended racial segregation in the great majority of hospitals in the country. It has substantially underwritten the costs of graduate medical education (e.g., physicians trained in hospitals), affecting the number and degree of specialization of U.S. physicians. Its prospective hospital payment system accelerated the movement toward greater use of ambulatory care settings (e.g., surgicenters, outpatient clinics, and physician offices), resulting in shorter hospital stays, and dramatically changed the economic incentives for hospital care. Physician payment reforms enacted in 1989 and implemented in 1992 had a less dramatic effect, although they did narrow the gap in payments to physicians for procedural and evaluative and management services. The payment methods for hospitals and physicians have been used to bolster health services in rural areas. The failure of Medicare to promote managed care has in many ways left it far behind the private insurance sector in organizational innovation.

MEDICAID

Medicaid is included in this chapter because of its origins with Medicare in 1965 and its growing importance as a source of health care financing for the poor. Medicaid is a federal-state program to finance the care of the poor (originally defined as those who were eligible for federal categorical financial aid such as AFDC or SSI). Because of welfare reform in 1996, Medicaid eligibility is no longer linked to AFDC. Medicaid has been the principal source of payment for medical care for the millions of poor. Its impact on the health of Americans is extensive:

> In 1998, 1 of every 10 people under the age of 65 years was insured through Medicaid, and the program covered a total of 40.4 million persons, including nearly 30 million pregnant women, parents under the age of 65 years, and children, as well as more than 11 million persons with disabilities and elderly persons who had low incomes or who were impoverished because of medical expenses (Rosenbaum, 2002, p. 635).

Although the great majority of Medicaid beneficiaries are single women and their children, the bulk of Medicaid expenditures are for nursing home care for the poor elderly and disabled.

Because of expanded enrollments in recent years, which were mandated by Congress in the late 1980s, costs have continued to rise and have increased the strain on states' discretionary budgets. As a result, the pressures to curtail costs in the Medicaid program led states to turn increasingly to managed care for women and children, described by Roland and Hanson (1996; see Recommended Reading). Several states, including Oregon and Tennessee, used Section 1115 waivers, allowing innovative approaches to bypass federal restrictions to both broaden access for low-income populations and slow the increase in costs. In Tennessee, the emphasis was on managed care. In Oregon, enrollment was expanded and limits were placed on benefits, particularly those that were not considered cost-effective. Bruce Vladeck reviewed the developments in the 1115 waiver program in 1995. The pace of state applications continued after that date, but became unnecessary because of the Balanced Budget Act of 1997.

The rapid shift to managed care creates a number of potential problems. Many of the traditional safety net providers, particularly urban public hospitals, may lose a disproportionate share of funding to cover the costs of serving uninsured populations. There have been concerns expressed about access to care for the chronically ill, the disabled, those with a history of substance abuse and alcoholism, the homeless, and children with chronic illness. If public hospital systems lose Medicaid patients to competing private health plans, their capacity to meet community-wide needs for trauma care and neonatal intensive care services may be compromised.

STATE CHILDREN'S HEALTH INSURANCE PROGRAM

The Balanced Budget Act of 1997 established the State Children's Health Insurance Program (SCHIP) as Title XXI of the Social Security Act. The SCHIP legislation was a milestone that set a priority and provided resources to insure millions of uninsured children in the United States. Over $40 billion was allocated to SCHIP over the next 10 years (U.S. Department of Health and Human Services, 2001). To highlight development and challenges faced at the fifth anniversary of SCHIP implementation, we have included the article "SCHIP Turns 5: Taking Stock, Moving Ahead" by Jennifer M. Ryan (2002).

Design of SCHIP

Under Title XXI, Congress provided states much freedom in designing their SCHIP plans. States were allowed to use SCHIP funds in three ways: (1) to expand Medicaid to cover older children or children from families with incomes too high for them to qualify for regular Medicaid (a "Medicaid expansion" plan), (2) to create an entirely new plan (called a "state-designed" plan) with a benefit package consistent with provisions of Title XXI, or (3) to both expand Medicaid and create a separate plan for different populations (a "combination" plan). "By July 1, 2000, every state implemented a SCHIP plan and, today, 21 states are operating Medicaid expansion programs, 16 states have separate SCHIP programs, and 19 states are operating combination programs" (Ryan, 2002, p. 2).

States that choose to expand Medicaid must follow all Medicaid eligibility rules regarding valuation of family income, geography, residency, and comparability of coverage. States that use SCHIP funds to expand Medicaid must adhere to Medicaid benefit and cost-sharing rules. In the case of states that elect to establish a separate SCHIP plan, the statute authorizes states to offer "child health assistance" that is virtually as broad as that provided to children under Medicaid and also establishes minimum coverage and cost-sharing rules. In addition, states that choose a separate SCHIP plan in part or in whole face numerous choices, including eligibility standards, benefit packages, the form in which child health assistance will be furnished, the conditions of participation for SCHIP providers and entities, and consumer protections.

Program Success

Since the implementation of SCHIP, there has been a steady trend of enrollment growth. From calendar year 1998 through fiscal year 2001, a total of 4.6 million children have been enrolled in SCHIP. In 1998, there were 1.0 million children; in 1999, there were 2.0 million; in 2000, there were 3.3 million; and in 2001, there were 4.6 million. In fact, "as early as 2000, the Census Bureau's report on the *Current Population Survey* noted that the decrease in uninsured children was largely due to the outreach efforts resulting from SCHIP implementation" (Ryan, 2002, p. 3). Such efforts have not only increased enrollment into SCHIP but have also produced increases in regular Medicaid enrollment, particularly through the use of joint application forms and combined SCHIP/Medicaid media campaigns.

Despite these advances, the economic downturn facing our nation threatens the continued success of the program. Many states have implemented strategies to curb or reverse Medicaid and SCHIP spending. Although caps cannot be placed on Medicaid enrollment (because it is an entitlement program), SCHIP is not protected, and some states have considered or even implemented such measures.

Another issue facing the program has been termed the "SCHIP dip." When SCHIP was authorized as part of the Balanced Budget Act of 1997, the program was funded at $40 billion over a 10-year span, and funding was channeled to the states as block grants. Congress "allocated almost $4.3 billion for each of the first four years of the program — 1998 through 2001 — but then decreased the funding by more than $1 billion to $3.15 billion for each of the following years" (Ryan, 2002, p. 4). This funding structure was created as part of the budget-balancing effort; however, it has serious consequences for SCHIP viability and for its beneficiaries. The SCHIP dip translates into a decline in federal funding and a loss of SCHIP coverage for over a million children. As a measure to restore SCHIP funding for fiscal years 2003 and 2004, Senators Jay Rockefeller, Lincoln Chafee, Edward Kennedy, and Orrin Hatch introduced the Children's Health Improvement and Protection Act of 2002. This piece of legislation also proposes to allow states to keep unspent SCHIP monies (instead of returning them to the U.S. Treasury for redistribution among the states) and would create a "caseload stabilization pool that would target the states most likely to have funding shortfalls in the coming years" (Ryan, 2002, p. 5).

Program Innovations

While enrollment was the initial focus of SCHIP planning and implementation in its early years, retention is now seen as the key to its future — for multiple reasons.

> Key eligible children enrolled in health care coverage is important, both administratively for states and in terms of health outcomes for children. Disruptions in coverage can reduce continuity of care, result in missed preventive visits and place families in the tenuous position of trying to pay out-of-pocket for health care costs incurred during periods of uninsurance. In addition, since a significant number of children who are disenrolled return

to public coverage within two months, the costs of re-establishing eligibility and re-enrolling children in health plans can be burdensome for all involved (Ryan, 2002, p. 8).

Because states are free to design their renewal processes, various retention strategies or policies have been adopted. For instance, 42 states reassess eligibility (a process known as *redetermination*) every 12 months for both their Medicaid and SCHIP programs. Seventeen states allow families to maintain their eligibility regardless of income changes or other reasons, which is known as *continuous eligibility.* Some states have adopted *passive renewal* policies, which allow "families to stay enrolled in the program without being required to actively submit new income or other eligibility information to the state" (Ryan, 2002, p. 8).

Another strategy is to expand health care coverage to parents of children in SCHIP through a Section 1115 demonstration waiver. The Urban Institute conducted a study to determine the impact of such expansions among the first four states that received the SCHIP approval (New Jersey, Minnesota, Rhode Island, and Wisconsin) and found that "enrolling parents has led to substantial gains in child enrollment in both Medicaid and SCHIP" (Ryan, 2002, p. 6). Retention is also improved. Additional states (California, Utah, and Arizona) have recently received approval to use SCHIP funding to expand coverage to adults; however, state budget deficits (particularly in California) and other financial barriers may impede such developments.

SUMMARY

This has been a brief introduction to and overview of Medicare, Medicaid, and the State Children's Health Insurance Program. The principal driver of policy in these three programs has been the federal budget, with deficits in the federal and state budgets severely affecting Medicaid and SCHIP. Therefore, major changes in the short term seem very unlikely because of these budget deficits.

REFERENCES

Aaron, H. J., and Reischauer, R. D. (1995). The Medicare reform debate: What is the next step? *Health Affairs, 14* (4), 8–30.

Briesacher, B., Stuart, B., and Shea, D. (2002). *Drug coverage for medicare beneficiaries: Why protection may be in jeopardy* (Issue Brief 505). New York: The Commonwealth Fund.

Culbertson, R., and Lee, P. R. (1996). Medicare and physician autonomy. *Health Care Financing Review, 18* (2), 115–130.

Enthoven, A. C., and Singer, S. J. (1996). Managed competition and California's health care economy. *Health Affairs, 15* (1), 39–57.

Fox, P. D., Etheredge, L., and Jones, S. B. (1996). Addressing the needs of chronically ill persons under Medicare. *Health Affairs, 17* (2), 144–150.

Glied, S. (1997). *Chronic condition: Why health reform fails*. Cambridge, MA: Harvard University Press.

Johnson, H., and Broder, D. S. (1996). *The system: The American way of politics at the breaking point*. Boston: Little, Brown.

Moon, M. (2001). Medicare. *New England Journal of Medicine, 344* (12), 928–931.

Robinson, J. C. (1996). The dynamics and limits of corporate growth in health care. *Health Affairs, 15* (2), 155–169.

Rosenbaum, S. (2002). Medicaid. *New England Journal of Medicine, 346* (8), 635–640.

Ryan, J. M. (2002, August 15). *SCHIP turns 5: Taking stock, moving ahead* (Issue Brief 781, pp. 1–12). Washington, DC: National Health Policy Forum.

U.S. Department of Health and Human Services. (2001, February). *State children's health insurance program: Ensuring Medicaid eligibles are not enrolled in SCHIP*. Washington, D.C.

Vladeck, B. C. (1995). Medicaid 1115 demonstrations: Progress through partnership. *Health Affairs, 14*, 217–220.

ARTICLE 1

MEDICARE

Marilyn Moon

The Medicare program, which serves persons over the age of 65 years and many persons with disabilities, plays a large part in health care in the United States. Since the program was implemented, in 1966, the number of persons served has increased from 19 million to 40 million, and expenditures for Medicare have risen faster than those for any other major federal program. Medicare now insures one of every seven Americans.

Medicare remains at the forefront of political debate because of the aging of the baby-boom generation and the likelihood that health care expenditures will continue to increase. By 2030, the program is expected to serve 77 million people — more than one of every five Americans — and to account for about 4.4 percent of the gross domestic product.[1]

There are three major issues involving Medicare. First, since the late 1970s, legislators have sought to revise the program in order to improve its management and efficiency and thereby slow the growth in federal expenditures. Second, Medicare's benefit package is inadequate. Many beneficiaries rely on supplemental policies, which results in inefficient delivery of care.[2] Medicare does not cover outpatient prescription drugs, and the deductibles and copayments can be very expensive. Thus, about 85 percent of Medicare beneficiaries have some type of supplemental coverage. Even so, Medicare beneficiaries tend to pay more for their health care than do most other Americans — both in absolute dollars and as a share of their total health care expenditures. At present, the average beneficiary pays more than $3,000 out of pocket each year for health care (excluding long-term care).[3] Third, Medicare has not been as well financed as Social Security, leading to numerous fiscal crises.

These three issues overlap. For example, many of those who want to restructure Medicare also propose that the program provide additional benefits, such as coverage of prescription drugs. There are conflicting views about whether restructuring Medicare will fully resolve the financial problems,[4] however, and if the basic benefit package is expanded, the costs will increase even more.

HISTORICAL PERSPECTIVE

In 1965, before the establishment of Medicare, only about half of those in the United States who were 65 years of age or older had health insurance.[5] By 1970, 97 percent of older Americans were enrolled in the program, and that proportion has remained about the same ever since. Part A of Medicare covers inpatient services, skilled nursing care, and home health care. Part B covers outpatient and physicians' services.

The implementation of the Medicare program had two immediate effects. The use of health care services grew, and financial burdens on older Americans and their families declined.[6] Thus, access to health care increased, particularly for those with low incomes who had previously been uninsured. Although the Medicare benefit package has changed little since 1966, the program has generally kept up with changes in medical practice. In some cases, the use of new procedures and devices has grown at a faster pace in the care of older persons than in the care of younger persons.[7]

The increase in life expectancy in the United States since 1965 is undoubtedly attributable in part to Medicare. For a 65-year-old woman, life expectancy increased from 15.8 years in 1960 to 19.2 years in 1998; for a 65-year-old man, it increased from 12.8 years to 15.9 years.[8] In addition, life expectancy has increased at a faster pace for older persons than for the population as a whole. Whereas life expectancy for a 65-year-old man increased by 24.2 percent between 1960 and 1998, life expectancy at birth increased by only 7.6 percent. As life expectancy has increased, disability rates have declined, suggesting that these longer lives are also healthier lives.[9]

In 1965, elderly persons spent an average of about 19 percent of their income on health care. That share fell to about 11 percent in 1968; today, it is more than 20 percent.[3] Medicare copayments and premiums have risen by about 9 percent per year on average, a much faster rate of growth than that of income among beneficiaries.[10] Without Medicare, however, most people would pay even more for health care or go without it.

In the 1980s, Medicare shifted from a cost-based system of paying hospitals and doctors to one in which payments are predetermined, with hospitals receiving a flat rate that is based on the diagnosis. These and other cost-containment efforts, such as restrictions on the use of home health care and skilled nursing care, helped slow the growth in expenditures. As a result, per capita expenditures for Medicare beneficiaries increased more slowly than per capita expenditures for persons with private insurance, particularly in the late 1980s.[11] Moreover, per capita Medicare expenditures grew at a slower rate than per capita expenditures by the private health insurance industry from 1970 to 1997.[6]

In another effort to reduce expenditures, Medicare beneficiaries have been allowed to enroll in private health maintenance organizations (HMOs) instead of remaining in the traditional, fee-for-service program. On average, however, the costs have been higher for HMO enrollees than they would have been if the same enrollees had remained in the traditional program.[12] In 1997, this option was modified to expand the types of plans that could participate in Medicare and to reform the payment system.

In December 2000, 6.3 million Medicare beneficiaries were enrolled in HMOs.[13] This program, called Medicare+Choice, has continued to be problematic. It has not reduced federal spending, nor has it provided stable coverage for those who have chosen it.[14] Even with payments high enough to cover Medicare's basic benefits, private plans have pulled out of some service areas and have restricted benefits. They have also resisted efforts to obtain data on the quality of care and to adjust payments in order to discourage adverse risk selection — that is, the selective enrollment of healthier beneficiaries.

Despite increased payments to Medicare+Choice plans, the problems are likely to continue. On January 1, 2001, about 934,000 people — approximately one of every six Medicare+Choice enrollees — lost coverage from their HMOs, forcing them either to seek coverage from other HMOs or to return to traditional Medicare coverage.[15]

SLOWING THE GROWTH OF PER CAPITA SPENDING

Since the 1980s, slowing the growth of Medicare spending has been a high priority for federal legislators, although the urgency has diminished in recent years as the growth in spending has slowed. In 2000, it was predicted that funds for Part A of Medicare would be exhausted by 2025[1]; in 1996, the estimated date was 2001.[16] Historically, premiums for Medicare and those for private insurance plans have shown similar trends in growth despite the slower rate at which Medicare expenditures have grown. This suggests that Medicare cannot be treated differently from the rest of the health care system over a long period.

Nonetheless, several alternative approaches to reducing per capita Medicare expenditures remain under discussion. These range from incremental changes to major structural reforms that would place Medicare under the control of private health plans. Most of the incremental approaches seek to modernize the fee-for-service portion of Medicare and to reform the way in which Medicare+Choice premiums are set. Critics charge that incremental approaches focus too much on cutting payments for health care services and ignore the need to control their use. But management techniques used by private insurers could be adopted for use in the traditional Medicare program. For example, in 1999, President Bill Clinton proposed that this program contract with a limited number of providers of high-technology procedures, that suppliers of health care products be required to bid for Medicare contracts, and that case-management and disease-management programs become part of traditional Medicare.[17]

The principal proposal for restructuring Medicare is a variant of the 1999 plan considered by the National Bipartisan Commission on the Future of Medicare.[18] Termed "premium support," this approach would require that beneficiaries choose among an array of private plans (with traditional Medicare being just one choice). If the cost of the chosen plan exceeded the national average cost (or some other designated benchmark), the beneficiary would have to pay a higher premium. The goals of this approach are to make beneficiaries more sensitive to the costs of health care and to create stronger incentives for private plans to limit costs. But this approach might lead to adverse risk selection — that is, the traditional Medicare program might become more expensive than private plans because it would serve the patients with the most serious medical disorders. If so, traditional Medicare — now effectively the default plan for many persons — might become unaffordable, forcing beneficiaries to enroll in managed-care plans. Premium-support proposals are based more on theory than on practice, so it is not known whether adjustments to prevent adverse risk selection would be effective.

No proposed reform of Medicare will magically lead to lower costs. What ultimately matters is changing the main determinants of cost: the prices charged for services, administrative costs, and the number of services delivered.

Medicare has always been competitive with the private sector in limiting what it pays for services, particularly in the key areas of payments to hospitals and payments to physicians. Moreover, Medicare has done a better job of controlling administrative costs than private plans have. On the other hand, private plans can be more flexible than Medicare. If a troubling pattern in service delivery is identified, a private plan can decide not to renew contracts with doctors or hospitals.[19] Similarly, private plans can adopt new computer systems or other innovations more rapidly than Medicare can. To operate well, the traditional Medicare program needs more flexibility, but it will probably always have to meet higher standards of due process for providers and patients. Because of this constraint, the Medicare program may remain more costly, but it can also offer legal protection for both providers and beneficiaries.

The most important determinant of cost is the number of services used, particularly if they include expensive new forms of medical technology. Both Medicare and private plans have difficulty distinguishing between appropriate and inappropriate care and then finding ways to reduce the use of services considered to be inappropriate. Under traditional fee-for-service coverage, providers have incentives to offer more rather than fewer services.

In contrast, managed-care organizations should have an advantage in coordinating care, since they have a financial responsibility to keep health care costs within a specific budget. However, many HMOs, particularly those with loose organizational structures, have not made the effort necessary to manage and coordinate care effectively.[20] Over time, some plans may improve their management techniques, thus establishing a case for further privatization of Medicare, but most have not done so. Furthermore, recent problems with Medicare+Choice suggest that private insurance plans are not serving Medicare beneficiaries well. When these plans change the benefits they offer or withdraw from a city or region of the country, they disrupt the health care of the people they serve.

The dissatisfaction of patients and physicians with managed care suggests that Medicare reforms that rely on greater market competition should be undertaken cautiously. Other changes, such as adopting better payment methods for private plans (including adjustments for adverse risk selection) and developing reasonable requirements for reporting on the quality of care, need to be made to ensure the effectiveness of competition.

In addition, improvement in guidelines for care is important, regardless of Medicare's structure. A substantial commitment of public resources may be needed for outcomes research, disease-management programs, information for beneficiaries on the effectiveness of care, and other approaches to improving the quality of care and reestablishing patients' trust in Medicare. Patients also need credible sources of information if they are to choose their health plans wisely. So far, however, there has been little interest in investing in any of these measures.

REDUCING THE NUMBER OF BENEFICIARIES

Another way to reduce Medicare expenditures is to reduce the number of people covered by the program. Increased life expectancy makes each generation of beneficiaries eligible for more years of Medicare coverage. One approach to increased longevity would be to raise the age at which persons become eligible for Medicare. Another approach would be to establish an annual maximal income for eligibility (i.e., means testing). However, both these options are controversial. President George W. Bush promised during the 2000 election not to raise the age of eligibility. Whenever means testing is suggested as a way to exclude persons with high incomes from Medicare coverage, there is strong opposition from advocates of universal coverage, who fear that means testing would undermine support for the entire program.

There are also practical problems with those approaches. Persons who are 65 or 66 years old account for only 5 percent of Medicare beneficiaries. If they were no longer eligible for coverage, the savings would represent only 2 or 3 percent of total Medicare expenditures. Persons in this age group use fewer services and thus are less expensive to insure than those who are older.[21] With means testing, eligibility must be determined. If the criterion for eligibility were an income no higher than $30,000 the most feasible mechanisms for establishing eligibility would be the income tax, an unpopular idea that in the past has killed such proposals. If a lower income level were used, many beneficiaries would lose their Medicare coverage and be unable to afford private coverage. Thus, reforms of the insurance market would be required to guarantee that newly disenfranchised beneficiaries could obtain insurance, and at a reasonable price.

ADDRESSING THE INADEQUACY OF THE BENEFIT PACKAGE

The Medicare benefit package is inadequate because it leaves beneficiaries liable for nearly half the cost of their acute care. The current deductible for hospitalization is $792. In addition, beneficiaries must pay 20 percent of their physicians' fees; there is no annual cap on the amount. Because of these high out-of-pocket expenses, 85 percent of beneficiaries have supplemental insurance.[2] Medicaid (which 15 percent of Medicare beneficiaries have) and employer-sponsored retirement benefits do a good job of filling in the gaps. Employer-sponsored plans are now used by about a third of Medicare beneficiaries but are becoming less available. Private supplemental (Medigap) plans — which serve about one fourth of beneficiaries — are becoming unaffordable for those with an average income. For example, in Dallas, Medigap plans that offered minimal drug coverage for a 65-year-old person ranged in price from $1,500 to $3,900 in 1998. The ranges are similar in other cities, and for older persons the costs are even higher. Premiums for Medigap plans increased by 35 percent between 1994 and 1998.[22]

Medications are a critical part of a comprehensive health care system. Medicare beneficiaries are finding it increasingly difficult to pay for prescription drugs, particularly because they also have other health care expenses. Adding only drug coverage to the benefit package, however, is unlikely to be enough to encourage beneficiaries with traditional Medicare coverage to forgo supplemental insurance. To achieve this goal, further revisions, such as establishing an upper limit on cost sharing and reducing the deductible for hospital services, would be needed. In addition, without a comprehensive benefit package that will attract patients with serious medical conditions as well as those who are relatively healthy, adverse risk selection is likely to undermine competition.[2] Plans with generous prescription-drug benefits, for example, will tend to attract the sick. But if all plans had to offer a basic drug benefit and if payments from Medicare to these plans were increased to reflect the new benefit, competition might improve. Thus, although there is general agreement on the desirability of improving coverage, the higher costs of such changes are still a major impediment.

THE FUTURE OF MEDICARE

Given the conflicting views on how to change Medicare, what direction will Congress and the Bush administration take? Medicare's improved financial outlook and Bush's campaign promise to provide prescription-drug coverage probably mean that cost containment will get little attention. In fact, the fallout from earlier efforts to reduce costs will probably continue, with hospitals and HMOs seeking yet another round of increased payments. The biggest unknown is whether those who seek a structural reform of Medicare will make such changes a condition for enacting prescription-drug coverage. This tactic could stall legislation, since there is little agreement on the best approach to an overall reform of the program. A key issue is how traditional Medicare would be treated under such a reform. If there were no special protection for this part of the Medicare program, political stalemate would be likely. An approach to reform that kept the current system largely intact but established a better way of paying private plans could generate savings and protect the traditional program. The option of increasing competition would remain open. The program is on solid financial footing for the next 10 years, so there is time for incremental changes.

Ultimately, none of the reforms now under consideration are likely to solve the problem of how to finance Medicare after the next decade. The question, then, is who will pay for the health care of older Americans and those who are disabled —

beneficiaries or taxpayers? Even with higher contributions from beneficiaries and successful cost containment, in the long run, Medicare will require additional public funds.[4] Reducing the number of beneficiaries or the scope of coverage would shrink the federal liability but do little to reduce the societal costs of financing health care. The basic issue will be how to share that burden.

REFERENCES

1. Board of Trustees of the Federal Hospital Insurance Trust Fund. Annual report of the Federal Hospital Insurance Trust Fund, Washington, D. C.: USGPO, 2000.
2. Aaron HJ, Reischauer R. D. The Medicare reform debate. What is the next step? *Health Aff (Millwood)*, 1995;14(4):S-30.
3. Maxwell S, Moon M, Segal M. Growth in Medicare and out-of-pocket spending: impact on vulnerable beneficiaries. New York: Commonwealth Fund, January 2001.
4. Gluck M, Moon M. Financing Medicare's future. Washington, D.C.: National Academy of Social Insurance, 2000.
5. Andersen R, Lion J, Anderson OW. Two decades of health services: social survey trends in use and expenditure. Cambridge, Mass.: Ballinger Publishing, 1976.
6. Moon M. Medicare matters: building on a record of accomplishment. *Health Care Financ Rev* 2000;21:9–22.
7. *Idem*. Beneath the averages: an analysis of Medicare and private expenditures. Menlo Park, Calif.: Henry J. Kaiser Family Foundation, September 1999. (See www.kff.org/content/1999/1505/moonbeneath.pdf).
8. National Center for Health Statistics. *Health, United States, 2000*, Hyattsville, Md.: Public Health Service, May 2000.
9. Manton KG, Corder LS, Stallard E. Estimates of change in chronic disability and institutional incidence and prevalence rates in the U.S. elderly population from the 1982, 1984, and 1989 National Long Term Care Survey. *J Gerontol* 1993;48: S153–S166.
10. Medicare and Medicaid statistical supplement, 1999. *Health Care Financ Rev* 1999.
11. Levit K, Cowan C, Lazenby H, et al. Health spending in 1998; signals of change. *Health Aff (Millwood)* 2000;19(1):124–32.
12. Riley GF, Ingber MJ, Tudor CG. Disenrollment of Medicare beneficiaries from HMOs. *Health Aff (Millwood)* 1997;16(5):117–24.
13. Cassidy A, Gold M. Medicare+Choice and Medicare beneficiaries, monthly tracking report for December, 2000. Washington, D.C.: Mathematica Policy Research, January 2001.
14. The Barents Group. How Medicare HMO withdrawals affect beneficiary benefits, costs, and continuity of care. Menlo Park, Calif.: Henry J. Kaiser Family Foundation, November 1999. (See www.kff.org/content/1999/1547/disenrollee11-5-99.pdf.)

15. Thomas J. H.M.O.'s to drop many elderly and disabled people: health experts predict most severe consequences will be loss of prescription drug benefits. *New York Times*. December 21, 2000:A14.
16. Annual report of the Board of Trustees of the Federal Hospital Insurance Trust Fund. Washington, D.C.: USGPO, June 1996.
17. National Economic Council. The President's plan to strengthen and modernize Medicare for the 21st century. Office of the President, July 2, 1999.
18. National Bipartisan Commission on the Future of Medicare. Building a better Medicare for today and tomorrow, U.S. Congress, March 16, 1999.
19. Center for Studying Health System Change. Wall Street comes to Washington: market watchers evaluate the health care system. Issue Brief no. 31, Washington, D.C., September 2000.
20. Lesser CS, Ginsburg PB. Update on the nation's health care system: 1997–1999. *Health Aff (Millwood)* 2000;19(6):206–16.
21. Waidmann TA. Potential effects of raising Medicare's eligibility age. *Health Aff (Millwood)* 1998;17(2):156–64.
22. Medicare: new choices, new worries. *Consumer Reports*, September 1998: 27–38.

ARTICLE 2

Drug Coverage for Medicare Beneficiaries

Why Protection May Be in Jeopardy

Becky Briesacher, Bruce Stuart, and Dennis Shea

Following a period of growth over the last decade, trends suggest that Medicare beneficiaries' access to affordable prescription drug benefits has begun to decline. Since the late 1990s, the engines that had been driving that growth — employer health plans and Medicare HMOs — have been offering increasingly less generous benefits to fewer people. There is no evidence that the private market or current public programs can reverse this decline in the coming years.

This analysis evaluates trends in prescription drug coverage for Medicare beneficiaries during the 1990s as a way to project their future coverage, costs, and needs. Projections are based on data from 1993 to 1998, the most recent year for which published data are available. The results indicate that beneficiary drug coverage peaked in that year, or shortly thereafter, and has been in decline ever since. Even while coverage was expanding, beneficiaries' spending on prescriptions was on the rise: the elderly with drug benefits spent 35 percent more out-of-pocket in 1998 than they did in 1993.

The prescription coverage outlook for Medicare beneficiaries will most likely further deteriorate without concerted and timely government action. If access to affordable drug benefits is not greatly expanded, elderly Americans — most of whom already make do on modest or low incomes — will find it even more difficult to obtain the medications they need.

BENEFICIARY DRUG COVERAGE AND SPENDING 1993–98[1]

Trends in Prescription Coverage

From 1993 to 1998, the number of beneficiaries with some prescription coverage increased from 64.6 percent to 76.0 percent of the Medicare population (Table 1).[2] The most rapid expansion occurred from 1994 to 1997, when coverage grew from 4 to 6 percent per year. The growth rate slowed to less than 2 percent from 1997 to 1998.

This pattern of growth was far from uniform across the various sources of prescription coverage available in the 1990s. Beneficiaries with a single source of prescription benefits in a given year accounted for most of the increase (Table 1). Medicare HMO enrollments accounted for nearly all the growth in coverage for these individuals, rising from just 4 percent of beneficiaries in 1993 to almost 13 percent in 1998. Prescription coverage from employer-sponsored plans represented the single most important source of drug benefits during the period, reaching nearly 29 percent of the beneficiary population by 1998. However, employer plans offered little growth in coverage after 1995. Prescription coverage under self-purchased Medigap plans peaked a year earlier, in 1994, at nearly 10 percent of the Medicare population, but declined to 8 percent by 1998. Even larger declines were recorded for publicly funded plans — Medicaid and other programs such as state pharmacy assistance programs and Veterans Administration programs. Taken together, drug coverage under public plans dropped from 16 percent of the Medicare population in 1993 to less than 13 percent in 1998.

These shifting patterns reflect only one aspect of how prescription coverage for Medicare beneficiaries changed during the 1990s. Table 1 shows that the proportion of beneficiaries with evidence of drug coverage from multiple sources grew from 11 percent to about 14 percent during the period. We estimate that about a third of these

---

1. Our estimates come from the Medicare Current Beneficiary Survey (MCBS) Cost and Use files for 1993–1998. Each annual sample consists of all beneficiaries with full-year Medicare entitlement who live outside of a facility for at least part of the year. (We exclude a small group of people who were newly entitled or died during the year in order to distinguish those with full-year and part-year drug coverage. People who live in facilities are omitted because prescription use is not captured in the MCBS.) We then classified individuals according to whether or not they have any prescription coverage and, if so, the source of coverage. The sources of coverage included employer-sponsored plans, Medicare HMOs, Medigap plans, Medicaid, and "other" coverage sources, including state pharmacy assistance plans, Veterans Administration coverage, and unknown sources of private coverage. In cases where people had more than one source of coverage or had third party payments for prescription fills but did not report the source, we assigned them to a mixed plan category.

2. The estimated coverage rate of 76 percent is 3 percentage points higher than the figure in Poisal and Murray (2001). They base coverage on the full-year and part-year Medicare population while we use only the full-year enrolled population. The difference means that beneficiaries who are not enrolled in Medicare for the entire year have lower drug coverage rates than those who are. This difference was only 1 percentage point in 1996 (see Stuart, Shea, and Briesacher 2000). The implication is that fewer new Medicare enrollees have prescription coverage and that this trend is accelerating.

TABLE 1

PRESCRIPTION DRUG COVERAGE OF MEDICARE BENEFICIARIES BY SOURCE, 1993–1998[a]

Sources of Prescription Coverage	*1993*	*1994*	*1995*	*1996*	*1997*	*1998*	*Percent Change 1993–98*
All sources	64.6%	65.3%	68.9%	71.6%	74.7%	76.0%	17.7%
Beneficiaries with a single source of coverage	53.4	54.0	57.8	58.5	60.0	62.1	16.3
Employer-sponsored	25.6	25.9	27.9	28.2	28.0	28.7	12.2
Medigap	7.8	9.6	8.5	8.9	8.6	8.1	4.1
Medicare HMO	4.1	5.0	7.4	8.2	10.7	12.9	211.6
Medicaid	11.3	11.5	9.9	9.3	9.1	8.9	–21.1
Other public	4.6	4.7	4.2	3.9	3.6	3.6	–22.1
Beneficiaries with multiple sources of coverage[b]	11.2	11.3	11.1	13.1	14.7	13.9	24.1

[a] Noninstitutionalized beneficiaries with full-year Medicare enrollment.
[b] Includes small numbers of beneficiaries with evidence of third-party payments for prescription drugs but no identified benefit plan.
Source: Medicare Current Beneficiary Surveys, 1993–1998.

individuals were able to maintain continuous coverage by switching from one plan to another during the year (Stuart, Shea, and Briesacher 2001), while the rest had sporadic coverage from various sources. However, even larger numbers of beneficiaries were unable (or perhaps unwilling) to maintain continuous prescription coverage from their primary source of drug benefits. In all, 17 to 19 percent of beneficiaries had coverage for only part of the year from 1995 to 1998 (Figure 1).[3] Further, among people with some coverage, those with continuous coverage decreased from 74 percent in 1995 to 72 percent in 1998.

Trends in Prescription Spending

Table 2 presents data from 1993 and 1998 showing changes in total and out-of-pocket prescription spending for Medicare beneficiaries.[4] Total drug expenditures per person increased dramatically regardless of prescription coverage status, although growth in

3. Limitations in MCBS reporting preclude estimating duration of coverage for beneficiaries in 1993 and 1994.
4. In 1998, the MCBS applied a new methodology to estimate prescription payment amounts, which increased per capita total drug spending by about 8 percent more than it would have been under the original methodology. See Poisal and Murray 2001 for a discussion of the new method.

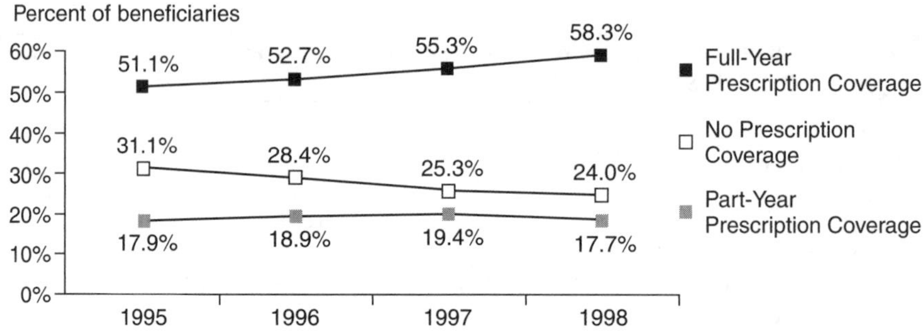

Figure 1 Stability of prescription drug coverage among noninstitutionalized Medicare beneficiaries, 1995–1998. (Source: Medicare Current Beneficiary Surveys, 1995–1998.)

spending was slower for those without coverage. In 1993, beneficiaries with no drug benefits incurred prescription drug expenditures just 60 percent of those of people with some form of coverage. By 1998 that fraction had declined to 55 percent. For beneficiaries with coverage, growth in per-person drug expenditures was greatest for "dual eligible" Medicare/Medicaid recipients and least for those enrolled in other public programs.

For beneficiaries without drug coverage, the increase in their out-of-pocket spending on prescription drugs equaled the change in their total spending on prescriptions — 51 percent. However, those who had benefits paid 35 percent more out-of-pocket in 1998 than they did six years earlier. Clearly, the additional coverage did not protect these beneficiaries from rising prescription costs.

The most dramatic percentage increase in out-of-pocket drug spending occurred among Medicare HMO enrollees. From 1993 to 1998, Medicare HMO enrollees saw their out-of-pocket costs more than double, to 40 percent of their total drug expenditures. Although high, this pales before the 67 percent paid out-of-pocket by beneficiaries with only Medigap coverage in 1998. Medigap policies with prescription benefits covered only one-third of Medicare beneficiaries' prescription drug expenses. The only two sources of drug coverage that provided significant protection to beneficiaries in 1998, compared with 1993, were Medicaid and employer-sponsored plans.

Another way to measure the level of protection that prescription coverage provides is to examine out-of-pocket spending as a percent of beneficiary income. Despite expanding drug coverage in the 1990s, more Medicare beneficiaries spent 5 percent or more of their incomes on prescriptions in 1998 than in 1993. The trend holds regardless of whether they had prescription drug coverage or not. By 1998, almost one-third of all beneficiaries without coverage spent more than 5 percent of their income on prescriptions. A much smaller fraction of people with full-year drug benefits fell into this category, but the trend is upward just the same. Those with part-year drug coverage were about twice as likely to spend 5 percent or more of income on drugs compared with those with full-year coverage.

TABLE 2

Total Prescription Spending and Out-of-Pocket Prescription Spending for Medicare Beneficiaries by Presence and Source of Drug Coverage, 1993–1998[a]

	Total Prescription Spending			*Out-of-Pocket Prescription Spending*			*Out-of-Pocket Spending as a Percent of Total Prescription Spending*		
Presence and Source of Prescription Coverage	*1993*	*1998*	*Percent Change 1993–98*	*1993*	*1998*	*Percent Change 1993–98*	*1993*	*1998*	*Percent Change 1993–98*
No coverage[b]	$368.90	$555.42	50.5%	$368.91	$555.32	50.5%	100.0%	100.0%	0.0%
Any coverage	615.13	1007.08	63.7	241.09	326.49	35.4	39.2	32.4	–30.4
Percent difference	60.0%	55.1%		153.0%	170.1%				
Beneficiaries with a single source of coverage									
Employer-sponsored	$637.36	$1101.97	72.9%	$247.33	$288.04	16.5%	38.8%	26.1%	–32.6%
Medigap	519.08	852.44	64.2	370.47	569.58	53.7	71.4	66.8	–6.4
Medicare HMO	395.90	679.28	71.6	122.02	273.03	123.8	30.8	40.2	30.4
Medicaid	636.38	1223.00	92.2	128.70	174.51	35.6	20.2	14.3	–29.4
Other public	729.24	1116.30	53.1	281.24	484.84	72.4	38.6	43.4	12.6
Beneficiaries with multiple sources of coverage[c]	643.60	1038.19	61.3	277.64	370.96	33.6	43.1	35.7	–17.2

[a] Noninstitutionalized beneficiaries with full-year Medicare enrollment.
[b] Total spending and out-of-pocket spending differ because of the small group of medications covered by Medicare.
[c] Includes small numbers of beneficiaries with evidence of third-party payments for prescription drugs but no identified benefit plan.
Source: Medicare Current Beneficiary Surveys, 1993–1998.

BENEFICIARY DRUG COVERAGE AND SPENDING SINCE 1998

Our empirical analysis ends at what may have been the high point in drug coverage for Medicare beneficiaries. There are good reasons to believe that, if coverage did not peak in 1998, then it did shortly thereafter. Recent developments in premiums and offer rates for private sources of drug benefits from employers, private insurers, and Medicare+Choice managed care plans all point in that direction.

New retirees may not be as fortunate as those in the 1990s. Although employer-sponsored health insurance plans were a stable and generous source of drug benefits at least until 1998, recent data cast doubt on the sustainability of such coverage. Periodic surveys conducted by Hewitt Associates show continued erosion in the number of large employers offering retiree health benefits, dropping from 80 percent in 1991 down to 66 percent by 1999 (Hewitt Associates 1997; 1999). When asked if they are seriously considering further retrenchment, 30 percent of the employers interviewed in 1999 indicated they would consider dropping all retiree coverage in the next three to five years, and 40 percent said they would consider cutting back on prescription benefits (Hewitt Associates 1999). These are particularly ominous findings because large employers have traditionally been much more likely to offer retiree health benefits than small employers. Because employers typically grandfather current retirees when making benefit policy changes (McArdle 2000), the impact of these changes should accelerate with the influx of new retirees into the Medicare system.

Medicare beneficiaries without access to employer-sponsored health benefits can buy individual Medigap policies that offer limited prescription coverage (up to $1,250 after deductible and coinsurance payments for the standard H and I plans, and up to $3,000 for plan J). Some beneficiaries have access to non-standardized policies with more generous drug coverage, either because they live in a state exempt from the 1989 federal law authorizing the standardized plans or because they continued to renew policies purchased prior to July 1992, when the federal law took effect.[5] A recent study by Chollet (2001) found that most Medigap policyholders with drug benefits bought their coverage before 1992. This would help explain the decline in Medigap coverage rates after 1994, noted in Table 1, as older policyholders die and fewer new retirees take up coverage. Indeed, this movement may accelerate in the future if Medigap premium rates continue to climb. From 1998 to 2000, the premiums for Medigap policies with drug coverage rose 37 percent, more than twice the increase for Medigap policies without drug coverage (Weiss Ratings 2001).

Medicare HMOs Drop Out

Medicare HMOs typically included prescription drug benefits in the 1990s, making them an attractive option. As late as 1997, virtually all Medicare+Choice HMO plans offered prescription benefits (Poisal and Murray 2001). But by 2001, only 70 percent

5. Massachusetts, Minnesota, and Wisconsin have such exemptions.

did so (Gold 2001). The cost to beneficiaries enrolling in Medicare+Choice plans has also risen sharply. In 1999, 80 percent of plans offered zero-premium policies (i.e., premiums equal to the Part B monthly amount). By March 2001, only 46 percent of plans had zero premium options (Gold 2001). Compounding the financial burden, the extra premiums buy less coverage today. In 1999, 36 percent of Medicare+Choice plans offered drug coverage with an annual benefit cap greater than $1,000. By 2001, that had dropped to 22 percent (Gold 2001).

These numbers have received less public attention than HMOs dropping out of the Medicare+Choice program in the last two years. More than 300 plans have left the program since 1999, leaving beneficiaries with fewer choices. In 2001, 67 percent of beneficiaries lived in regions served by one or more Medicare+Choice plans, down from 72 percent in 1999. Total Medicare+Choice enrollments dropped by nearly 1 million people during this two-year period (Gold 2001). In an attempt to turn these trends around, Congress passed the Benefits Improvement and Protections Act (BIPA) in 2000. The early evidence suggests that BIPA has had minimal effect (Gold and Achman 2001). The Medicare program anticipates that plan withdrawals will affect several hundred thousand beneficiaries in 2002, as the five largest Medicare HMOs all announced dropping business in next year's Medicare+Choice filings (Appleby 2001). Even if the number of plans stabilizes, the combination of rising premiums and reduced drug benefits will make Medicare+Choice plans a less desirable choice for beneficiaries in search of prescription coverage.

Rising Drug Costs a Major Factor in Declining Coverage

The rising cost of prescription drugs places beneficiaries' coverage in jeopardy. Expenditures on prescription drugs increased an estimated 19 percent from 1999 to 2000, capping four years of double digit increases (NIHCM 2001). Moreover, it is projected that the rate of growth will be about 15 percent annually through 2004 (Mullins et al. 2001). The increases are fueled by price, volume, and, most importantly, a steady shift to newer, more expensive therapies. Our trend analysis showed that Medicare beneficiaries who have no prescription coverage feel the impact of increasing prescription costs most keenly. But even those with coverage feel the effects through higher premiums, reduced benefits, and fewer choices of coverage. If the forecasts prove correct, there is little relief in sight.

Taken together, these findings suggest that the increased availability of prescription coverage in the mid-1990s will not continue and has already begun to decline. There is no evidence that either the private market or public programs as currently designed can solve the problem of prescription coverage for Medicare beneficiaries in the coming decade. In fact, our analysis of the six-year period from 1993 through 1998 showed that out-of-pocket prescription costs rose continually even as prescription coverage was rising.

These data, together with projections for the future, presage a looming crisis in the elderly's access to prescription drugs if nothing is done soon to address the situation. Adding prescription coverage to the Medicare benefit package is the only sure solution.

REFERENCES

J. Appleby, "More HMOs to Drop Medicare Patients," *USA Today* (Sept, 20, 2001): 6B.

D. Chollet, Senate Committee on Finance, Medigap Coverage of Prescription Drugs: Testimony on "Finding the Right Fit: Prescription Drugs and Current Coverage Options," Apr. 24, 2001, 107th Congress, first session.

M. Gold, "Medicare+Choice: An Interim Report Card," *Health Affairs* 20 (Jul./Aug. 2001): 120–138.

M. Gold and L. Achman, "Rising Payment Rates: Initial Effects of BIPA 2000," *Monitoring Medicare+Choice — Fast Facts Number 6* (Washington D.C.: Mathematica Policy Research, Inc., June 2001).

Hewitt Associates LLC, *Retiree Health Coverage: Recent Trends and Employer Perspectives on Future Benefits Reforms* (Menlo Park, Calif.: Henry J. Kaiser Family Foundation, October 1999).

Hewitt Associates LLC, *Retiree Health Trends and Implications of Possible Medicare Reforms* (Menlo Park, Calif.: Henry J. Kaiser Family Foundation, Sept. 1997).

M. A. Laschober et al., "Medicare HMO Withdrawals: What Happens to Beneficiaries?" *Health Affairs* 18 (Nov./Dec. 1999): 150–157.

F. McArdle, "Role of Retiree Benefits in Health Insurance's Future," [Letter] *Health Affairs* 19 (Mar./Apr. 2000): 274–275.

D. Mullins et al., "The Impact of Pipeline Drugs on Drug Expenditure Growth Trends," *Health Affairs* 20 (Sept./Oct. 2001): 210–215.

NIHCM Foundation, *Prescription Drug Expenditures in 2000: The Upward Trend Continues* (Washington, D.C.: National Institute for Health Care Management, May 2001).

J. A. Poisal and L. Murray, "Growing Differences Between Medicare Beneficiaries with and Without Drug Coverage," *Health Affairs* 20 (Mar./Apr. 2001): 74–85.

B. Stuart, D. Shea, and B. Briesacher, *Prescription Drug Costs for Medicare Beneficiaries: Coverage and Health Status Matter* (New York: The Commonwealth Fund, Jan. 2000).

———. "Dynamics in Drug Coverage of Medicare Beneficiaries: Finders, Losers, Switchers," *Health Affairs* 20 (Mar./Apr. 2001): 86–99.

Weiss Ratings, "Prescription Drug Costs Boost Medigap Premiums Dramatically," [Press Release] Mar. 26, 2001, available at www.weissratings.com/NewsReleases/Latest/index.htm.

ARTICLE 3

MEDICAID

Sara Rosenbaum

When Medicaid was enacted in 1965 as a legislative afterthought to Medicare, few would have predicted its evolution into a basic component of the American health care system. In this report, I examine Medicaid, which has become one of the most complex social-welfare programs, and consider prospects for its reform.

OVERVIEW OF THE PROGRAM

Medicaid, codified under Title XIX of the Social Security Act, provides federal financial assistance to states operating approved medical-assistance plans. Unlike eligibility for Medicare, eligibility for Medicaid is means-tested (i.e., there are financial criteria for enrollment); like Medicare, however, Medicaid is an individual legal entitlement.[1,2] In 1999, Medicaid payments accounted for more than 15 percent of national health care expenditures.[3]

In 1998, 1 of every 10 people under the age of 65 years was insured through Medicaid,[4] and the program covered a total of 40.4 million persons, including nearly 30 million pregnant women, parents under the age of 65 years, and children, as well as more than 11 million persons with disabilities and elderly persons who had low incomes or who were impoverished because of medical expenses.[5] The program's impact in certain sectors of the health care system has been enormous: in 1998, Medicaid paid the costs of one third of all births in the United States, nearly half of all nursing home care, and health care for 25 percent of children under the age of five years.[5] Medicaid is the single largest source of financial support for essential community health services. It covers over 45 percent of inpatients in public hospitals and more than a third of patients who obtain care at federally funded community health centers.[6]

TABLE 1

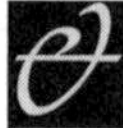

Selected Reforms Introduced through the Medicaid Program
Insurance coverage for low-income, uninsured pregnant women and low-income children[7]
Support for the deinstitutionalization of persons with physical and mental disabilities through community-based, long-term care[8,9]
Insurance coverage for persons moving from welfare to work and their families, for low-income workers without access to coverage provided by an employer, and for the families of such workers[7]
Insurance coverage for persons with disabilities who are able to work if they have adequate medical support[10]
Supplemental insurance coverage for low-income Medicare beneficiaries[11]
A national vaccine-purchasing system to ensure adequate vaccine coverage for low-income, publicly insured or uninsured children[12]
Treatment of tuberculosis[13]
Establishment of managed-care systems for beneficiaries with both basic and complex physical and mental health care needs[14]
Support of institutions participating in the "health care safety net" through special compensation arrangements[15]
Insurance coverage for uninsured women with diagnosed cervical or breast cancer[16]

Although it operates as a single program, Medicaid is actually an agglomeration of programs spanning the full spectrum of health care. Over the years, Medicaid has served as the legislative vehicle for an extraordinary range of reforms (Table 1). Because of the persons it covers and the services it pays for, Medicaid has also become the central source of health care financing for persons with human immunodeficiency virus (HIV) infection or full-blown AIDS.[17]

Federal financing of state Medicaid plans is open-ended. Each participating state is entitled to payments up to a federally approved percentage of state expenditures, and there is no limit on total payments to any state. Payments are calculated according to a federal formula linked to state revenue and range from 50 percent to over 80 percent of approved state medical expenditures.[18] With federal contributions limited only by the size of state programs, Medicaid encourages its own growth and expansion.

In fiscal year 2000, state and federal Medicaid outlays totaled $207 billion — $10 billion more than total Medicare expenditures.[19] As with other health care programs, Medicaid's annual rates of growth have historically exceeded those for nonmedical goods and services. In February 2001, before the recession and the catastrophic events of September 11, it was estimated that the average annual rate of growth over the next decade would be between 8 percent and 9 percent.[19]

STATE FLEXIBILITY AND FEDERAL REQUIREMENTS

Because Medicaid is designed to help the states finance their health care initiatives, the states have considerable discretion with respect to the criteria for eligibility, the services covered, and program administration. In 2000, Medicaid accounted for 50 percent of total state health care expenditures.[20] However, approximately one third of total Medicaid expenditures and 79 percent of all expenditures for long-term care are attributable to state choices rather than federal requirements.[21]

Medicaid is both an entitlement program and a conduit for transferring an enormous amount of federal revenue to state budgets. Consequently, federal law prescribes certain standards for state Medicaid plans. Because Medicaid is an entitlement program, persons wishing to apply for assistance must be allowed to do so without delay and must receive prompt medical assistance once their eligibility has been confirmed.[9] States may not set an upper limit for enrollment, arbitrarily restrict program expenditures under their approved plans, or unreasonably delay the provision of assistance.[22] Since financing is open-ended, during economic downturns enrollment can grow in proportion to need, as persons lose their jobs and thus lose health insurance provided by their employers. The surge in Medicaid enrollment in New York City after the events of September 11 illustrates the program's ability to respond to sudden, unanticipated needs on a large scale.[23] States may reduce their Medicaid expenditures only by formally revising their programs to scale back eligibility, benefits, payments to providers, or other features of their plans.

The eligibility standards for Medicaid, which are legendary in their complexity, are an outgrowth of federal cash welfare programs. There are two basic criteria for eligibility: financial need (as evidenced by low income or impoverishment due to high medical bills) and a federally recognized eligibility category (e.g., a household with dependent children, an age of 65 years or older, and disability). Both criteria must be met for enrollment.

According to federal law, participating states must provide Medicaid coverage for certain groups of persons, with the option to extend coverage to dozens of other groups.[24] The mandatory groups are families that qualify for cash welfare programs for families with dependent children; families in which a parent is making the transition from welfare to work; low-income pregnant women and low-income children (defined as persons under 19 years of age); persons who are elderly or disabled, as defined under the Social Security Act, and who qualify for cash benefits under the Supplemental Security Income program; and certain other low-income Medicare beneficiaries. In the case of pregnant women, children, and Medicare beneficiaries, the definition of low income is tied to the federal poverty level, which in 2001 was an annual income of $8,590 for a single person and $14,630 for a family of three.[25] For families with children whose eligibility is based on their qualification for welfare programs, the states may establish the financial criteria for Medicaid eligibility, and in many states the criteria are extremely restrictive. In 1999, for example, parents who had dependent children and who worked full time at the minimum wage were eligible for Medicaid in only 19 states and the District of Columbia.[4]

The most controversial aspects of Medicaid are evident in the area of coverage. Medicaid resembles insurance in its coverage of defined classes of medical benefits. Because of the groups it covers and the services it pays for, however, the Medicaid program requires that state plans provide much more extensive coverage than that provided by private insurance plans, prohibits nearly all cost sharing by patients, and applies these requirements to virtually all beneficiaries, regardless of their age or status with respect to disability.

Just as federal law mandates coverage of certain groups of people, it establishes the level of coverage that must be provided for all beneficiaries, as well as the exclusions and limitations that can be imposed — two areas in which private insurance plans have nearly total discretion.[26,27] Common restrictions in the coverage provided by private insurance plans, such as the exclusion of coverage for preexisting conditions and a required waiting period for coverage, are prohibited, and the limits on coverage must meet specific criteria for reasonableness. In addition, all federally recognized classes of benefits, whether or not they are provided to adults, must be furnished to children (defined as persons under 21 years of age). The adequacy of coverage for children is determined by tests of reasonableness that emphasize growth, development, and the prevention of disability rather than simply the treatment of illness or injury.[28]

Federal law prohibits arbitrary exclusions and limitations that are based on a diagnosis, such as limits on outpatient and inpatient services for the treatment of mental illness or AIDS, whereas private insurers often single out certain conditions for limitations and exclusions.[26,27] Because Medicaid assists so many persons with serious illnesses and disabilities, discrimination in coverage based on the ability to recover from an illness or injury is prohibited; unlike private insurers, state Medicaid plans cannot stop providing coverage simply because "significant improvement" is not possible.[26,27] In short, whereas private insurers structure their coverage to limit or prevent financial risk, the states are not allowed to do so. Thus, Medicaid is technically not insurance at all but instead a mechanism for financing many forms of health care that would be considered uninsurable and beyond the reach of the commercial market.

MEDICAID ENROLLMENT AND EXPENDITURES

Analyses of beneficiary groups and program expenditures provide very different pictures of the Medicaid program. In 1998, nearly 75 percent of all enrollees were nondisabled, working-age adults and children (Figure 1).[29] However, roughly two thirds of program expenditures were for services provided to elderly or disabled beneficiaries; expenditures for nondisabled working-age adults and children amounted to less than 25 percent of total expenditures (Figure 1).

There are large differences in per capita Medicaid expenditures for acute and long-term care, depending on the basis of eligibility (Figure 2). Per capita payments

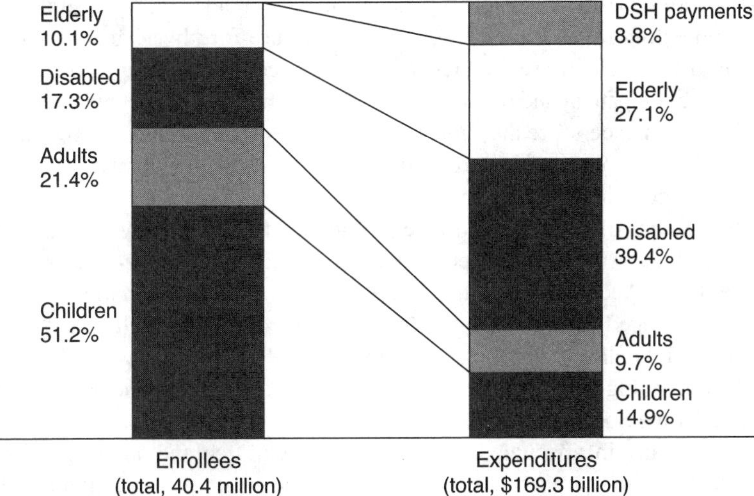

Figure 1 Medicaid enrollment and expenditures according to the beneficiary group, 1998. Total expenditures exclude administrative expenses. DSH denotes disproportionate-share hospitals (i.e., those serving a disproportionate number of low-income and publicly insured persons). Data are estimates prepared by the Urban Institute for the Kaiser Commission on Medicaid and the Uninsured.[29]

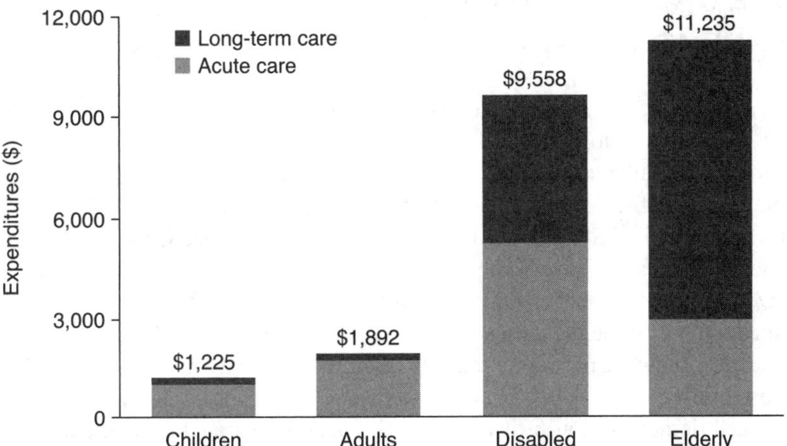

Figure 2 Medicaid expenditures for acute and long-term care per enrollee, 1998. Long-term care includes services provided by nursing facilities, intermediate care facilities for the mentally retarded, mental health services, and home health services. Acute care includes inpatient, physician, laboratory, radiographic, outpatient, clinic, prescription-drug, family-planning, dental, vision, and hospice services; care provided by other practitioners; and early and periodic screening, diagnosis, and treatment. This category of expenditures also includes payments to managed-care organizations and payments to Medicare. Expenditures do not include payments to disproportionate-share hospitals, adjustments of federal payments, or administrative costs. Data are estimates prepared by the Urban Institute for the Kaiser Commission on Medicaid and the Uninsured.[29]

for acute care services for disabled persons far exceed those for nondisabled beneficiaries, reflecting much higher levels of expenditure for physicians' services, prescription drugs (which are subject to especially comprehensive federal rules for coverage), and inpatient and outpatient care. The high per capita payments for persons with disabilities underscore the enormous differences in health status between persons with employer-sponsored coverage through private health plans and those who depend on Medicaid coverage.

The number of persons who receive Medicaid because they are disabled is a substantial underestimate of the prevalence of disability among beneficiaries, particularly children. According to a study that compared Medicaid beneficiaries enrolled in private managed-care plans with other persons enrolled in such plans, the health care costs for Medicaid beneficiaries who were not officially classified as disabled were 25 percent higher than those for non-Medicaid enrollees.[30] The definition of disability under the Social Security Act is so restrictive that it limits coverage to persons who are virtually incapacitated.[31] Consequently, children and adults with mild-to-moderate disabilities are not enrolled unless they meet another criterion for eligibility, such as poverty or qualification for cash welfare for families. Among children covered by Medicaid who have chronic physical or mental conditions or disabilities, about 14 percent qualified for enrollment on the basis of these conditions or disabilities; most qualified for other reasons.[32]

REFORMING THROUGH LEGISLATION AND DEMONSTRATION PROJECTS

Medicaid has had far-reaching achievements, including improved access to health care.[33] Persons who lose Medicaid coverage are three times as likely as insured persons to lack a regular source of health care and twice as likely to have made no visits to a physician's office in a year.[4] In the absence of Medicaid, the number of uninsured people in the United States would increase dramatically, since most Medicaid beneficiaries have no alternative source of coverage.

Despite these achievements, Medicaid has serious problems, although reaching agreement on what the most important problems are turns out to be as politically difficult as resolving them. Some analysts point to the program's limits on eligibility. Because of Medicaid's roots as a cash welfare program, in the absence of a federally sanctioned demonstration project, no public health insurance is available for low-income, nondisabled, working-age adults without children.[34,35] In addition, the restrictive definition of disability under the Social Security Act excludes persons with serious conditions that could be disabling in the absence of medical care (such as children with debilitating mental illness or persons with HIV infection, which is not considered disabling until it becomes AIDS).[35] Medicaid's eligibility and enrollment systems can be daunting because of the length of the application and the difficulty of having to apply at a welfare office. As the recent situation in New York illustrates,[23] when a state eases the process of enrollment, tens of thousands of persons may seek assistance.

Furthermore, coverage can end abruptly because of arbitrary restrictions on eligibility. Finally, since its inception, the program has been plagued by low participation rates among physicians and other providers.[8]

State officials recognize these problems but tend to focus on the program's extensive coverage requirements.[36] Some officials have noted that because Medicaid is an entitlement program, the states must maintain open enrollment even when it is not financially feasible to do so. The states are required to cut back on eligibility rather than impose waiting periods, which is perceived as a less severe means of controlling the number of beneficiaries. State officials also view federal benefit requirements as barriers to the provision of less expensive coverage. With regard to overall spending, the current federal formula is problematic. Despite its relative generosity, state Medicaid expenditures can be burdensome, particularly during an economic downturn, when there is a need for expanded coverage and revenues are diminished. On the other hand, conservative analysts point to Medicaid's status as an entitlement program and its open-ended financing as the basic policy problems. An open-ended entitlement structure limits the ability to control federal expenditures.[37]

The failure to agree on what the most important problems are — the size of Medicaid, its limitations, or the need for greater flexibility — has prevented all but incremental legislative reforms. However, a substantial restructuring of the program, even in the absence of a legislative consensus, is possible through demonstration projects.

Since 1962, the Social Security Act has given the Secretary of Health and Human Services unilateral authority to implement demonstration projects in order to restructure federal grant-in-aid programs, such as Medicaid. This authority is codified in section 1115 of the Social Security Act. This section vests nearly unlimited discretion in the Secretary to decide which types of demonstration projects to pursue and which program requirements to override.[37] On only a few occasions have courts prohibited such projects on the grounds that they exceed the department's authority,[38,39] and Congress has almost never intervened.

Although the executive branch has used section-1115 authority sparingly, the Clinton administration made extensive use of it to permit states to mandate the enrollment of Medicaid beneficiaries in managed-care plans in many states and, in a few cases, to expand eligibility.[39] As of 2000, approximately half of all beneficiaries, including those with disabilities, were enrolled in managed-care plans.

In August 2001, apparently in response to recommendations by the National Governors Association, the Bush administration announced a section-1115 demonstration initiative known as Health Insurance Flexibility and Accountability (HIFA).[40] This program would permit states to provide very limited coverage for low-income persons who are currently ineligible for Medicaid (e.g., coverage restricted to primary care for adults without dependent children), while explicitly permitting reductions in coverage for many groups of current beneficiaries.

The initial purpose of HIFA may have been to permit reductions in coverage as a trade-off for a limited expansion of eligibility. Recent remarks by federal and state officials suggest that the Bush administration may now be willing to consider proposals such as the one from Washington State, which would reduce benefits to low-income beneficiaries, increase cost sharing, and limit enrollment without expanding eligibility to include currently uninsured persons.[41] Because applications for demonstration projects are not routinely made public, it is impossible to know how many states have submitted proposals, what they have proposed, what benefit reductions are under consideration, or what conditions the federal government may impose.

OUTLOOK FOR THE FUTURE

HIFA appears to be an attempt to restructure Medicaid as a program that provides "premium support," with the states subsidizing the enrollment of low-income persons in private insurance plans that offer more limited coverage than the traditional Medicaid program. Were most or all states to apply for participation in the HIFA program (section 1115 does not impose an upper limit on the number of participating states), then eventually the principles of Medicaid coverage would parallel those of private insurance coverage. In 1997, Congress took a step in this direction when it enacted the State Children's Health Insurance Program. This program gives states the option of buying private insurance for uninsured children in families near the federal poverty level, rather than expanding Medicaid to cover them.[42]

The long-term consequences of such changes for the millions of beneficiaries with chronic illness or disability are unclear. As of the end of 2001, Congress had held no oversight hearings on HIFA. Nor has there been congressional scrutiny of the program's emphasis on demonstration projects that help low-income workers buy coverage through their employers when it is available — despite concern about "health insurance crowd-out." This phenomenon occurs when public funds are substituted for employers' contributions to health insurance coverage.[43]

In view of the fundamental disagreement over which features of Medicaid are problematic, much less how to change them, broad congressional action is unlikely in the near future. It remains to be seen whether Congress will permit the Bush administration to transform Medicaid into a premium-support program and to do so with a minimum of oversight.

REFERENCES

1. Rosado v. Wyman, 397 U.S. 397, 1970.
2. Virginia Hosp. Asso. v. Wilder, 496 U.S. 498, 1990.
3. Heffler S, Levit K, Smith S, et al. Health spending growth up in 1999: faster growth expected in the future. *Health Aff (Millwood)* 209;20(2):193–203.
4. Hoffman C, Schlobohm A. Uninsured in America: a chart book. 2nd ed. Washington, D.C.: Kaiser Commission on Medicaid and the Uninsured, March 2000. (Accessed February 4, 2002, at http://www.kff.org/content/archive/1407/.)
5. The Medicaid program at a glance. Washington, D.C.: Kaiser Commission on Medicaid and the Uninsured, 2001.

6. Lewin ME, Altman S, eds. America's health care safety net: intact but endangered. Washington, D.C.: National Academy Press, 2000. Tables 2.1 and 3.4.
7. Schneider A, Fennel K, Long P. Medicaid eligibility for families with children. Washington, D.C.: Kaiser Commission on Medicaid and the Uninsured, 1998.
8. Congressional Research Service. Medicaid source book: background data and analysis. Washington, D.C.: Government Printing Office, 1993.
9. Perkins J, Boyle RT. Addressing long waits for home and community-based care through Medicaid and the ADA. *St. Louis Univ Law J* 2000;45:117–45.
10. Schneider A, Ellberger R. Medicaid-related provisions in the Ticket to Work and Work Incentives Improvement Act of 1999. Washington, D.C.: Kaiser Commission on Medicaid and the Uninsured, April 2000.
11. Schneider A, Fennel K, Keenan P. Medicaid eligibility for the elderly. Washington, D.C.: Kaiser Commission on Medicaid and the Uninsured, May 1999.
12. 42 U.S.C. §1396s.
13. 42 U.S.C. §1396a(a)(10)(a)(ii)(XII) and 1396a(z).
14. 42 U.S.C. §1396u-2.
15. 42 U.S.C. §1396a(a)(13).
16. Westmoreland T. State Medicaid director letter. Baltimore: Health Care Financing Administration, January 4, 2001.
17. *Idem*. Medicaid and HIV/AIDS policy: a basic primer. Menlo Park, Calif.: The Henry J. Kaiser Family Foundation, July 1999.
18. 42 U.S.C. §1396b(a).
19. Congressional Budget Office. The budget and economic outlook: 2002–2011. Washington, D.C.: Government Printing Office, 2001.
20. Milbank Memorial Fund, National Association of State Budget Officers, Reforming States Group. 1998–1999 State health care expenditure report. New York: Milbank Memorial Fund, March 2001.
21. Holahan J. Restructuring Medicaid financing: implications of the NGA proposal. Washington, D.C.: Kaiser Commission on Medicaid and the Uninsured, June 2001. (Accessed February 4, 2002, at http://www.kff.org/content/2001/2257.)
22. Alabama Nursing Home Association v. Harris, 617 F. 2d 388 (5th Cir., 1980).
23. Russakoff D. Out of tragedy, N.Y. finds way to treat Medicaid need: streamlined post-crisis process draws record enrollment through a multilingual grapevine. *Washington Post*. November 26, 2001:A2.
24. Medicaid "mandatory" and "optional" eligibility and benefits. Washington, D.C.: Kaiser Commission on Medicaid and the Uninsured, July 2001. (Accessed February 4, 2002, at http://www.kff.org/content/2001/2256/).
25. Census Bureau. 2001 Poverty estimates. Washington, D.C.: Department of Commerce, 2001.
26. Rosenblatt RE, Law SA, Rosenbaum S. Law and the American health care system. Westbury, N.Y.: Foundation Press, 1997.
27. Rosenblatt RE, Rosenbaum S, Rankford D. Law and the American health care system: 2001–2002 supplement. Westbury, N.Y.: Foundation Press, 2001.

28. Rosenbaum S, Markus A, Sonosky C, Repasch L. Policy brief #2: state benefit design choices under SCHIP: implications for pediatric health care. Washington, D.C.: The George Washington University Medical Center, Center for Health Services Research and Policy, May 2001.
29. Medicaid: a primer. Washington, D.C.: Kaiser Commission on Medicaid and the Uninsured, 2001.
30. Welch WP, Wade M. The relative cost of Medicaid enrollees and the commercially insured in HMOs. *Health Aff (Millwood)* 1995;14(2):212–23.
31. United States House of Representatives, Committee on Ways and Means. Green book. Washington, D.C.: Government Printing Office, 1998.
32. The faces of Medicaid: the complexities of caring for people with chronic illnesses and disabilities. Princeton, N.J.: Center for Health Care Strategies, 2001. (Accessed February 4, 2002, at http://www.chcs.org/publications/cfm-view.html.)
33. Davis K, Schoen C. Health and the war on poverty: a ten-year appraisal. Washington, D.C.: Brookings Institution, 1978.
34. Rowland D. Health insurance for unemployed workers. Washington, D.C.: Kaiser Commission on Medicaid and the Uninsured, 2001. (Accessed February 4, 2002, at http://www.kff.org/content/2001/4018/).
35. Feder J, Levitt L, O'Brien E, Rowland D. Covering the low-income uninsured: the case for expanding public programs. *Health Aff (Millwood)* 2001;20(1):27–39.
36. Policy position statement HR-16: Medicaid policy. Washington, D.C.: National Governors Association, 2001. (Accessed February 4, 2002, at http://www.nga.org/nga/legislativeUpdate/1,1169,C_POLICY_POSITION^D_533,00.html.)
37. Beach WW. The cost to the states of not fundamentally reforming Medicaid. Washington, D.C.: Heritage Foundation, 1996. (Accessed February 4, 2002, at http://www.heritage.org/library/categories/healthwel/cb22.html.)
38. Resenbaum S, Darnell J, Seliger P, Simon L. Section 1115 Medicaid waivers: charting a path for Medicaid managed care reform. In: Lillie-Blanton M, Martinez RM, Lyons B, Rowland D, eds. Access to health care: promises and prospects for low-income Americans. Washington, D.C.: Kaiser Commission on Medicaid and the Uninsured, 1999:179–97.
39. Lambrew J. Section 1115 waivers in Medicaid and the State Children's Health Insurance Program: an overview. Washington, D.C.: Kaiser Commission on Medicaid and the Uninsured, July 2001. (Accessed February 4, 2002, at http://www.kff.org/content/2001/4001/.)
40. Health Insurance Flexibility and Accountability (HIFA) demonstration initiative. Baltimore: Health Care Financing Administration, 2001. (Accessed February 4, 2002, at http://www.hcfa.gov/medicaid/hifa/default.htm.)
41. Kaisernetwork.org. Daily health policy report: Washington State seeks federal approval for 'groundbreaking' Medicaid proposal to add copayments, cap enrollment in some programs. Washington, D.C.: Henry J. Kaiser Family Foundation, December 3, 2001. (Accessed February 4, 2002, at http://kaisernetwork.org/daily_reports/rep_index.cfm?dr_id=8334.)

42. Rosenbaum S, Johnson K, Sonosky C, Markus A, DeGraw C. The children's hour: the State Children's Health Insurance Program. *Health Aff (Millwood)* 1998;17(1):75–89.

43. Dubay L. Expansions in public health insurance and crowd-out: what the evidence says. Washington, D.C.: Henry J. Kaiser Family Foundation, October 1999. (Accessed February 4, 2002, at http://www.kff.org/content/1999/19991112m/).

ARTICLE 4

SCHIP TURNS 5

TAKING STOCK, MOVING AHEAD

Jennifer M. Ryan

October 1, 2002, will mark the five-year anniversary of the effective date of the State Children's Health Insurance Program (SCHIP). The program was the result of bipartisan agreement in the Congress to provide new funding for health insurance coverage for low-income uninsured children. SCHIP was generally targeted at children in families with incomes below 200 percent of the federal poverty level, which equals $36,200 for a family of four in 2002. Therefore, children eligible for the program are often in working families who cannot afford coverage or whose employers do not offer health benefits. States had the opportunity to set up a new, free-standing SCHIP program, to expand their existing Medicaid programs, or to develop a combination of the two approaches. By July 2000, every state and territory had implemented a SCHIP plan and, today, 21 states are operating Medicaid expansion programs, 16 states have separate SCHIP programs, and 19 states are operating combination programs.[1]

States took great pride in the new opportunity to develop their SCHIP programs and reach out to low-income families. They set up marketing campaigns, held outreach events featuring their governors, and came up with catchy names — such as Healthy Kids, Peach Care, and Hoosier Healthwise — for their new programs. Behind the scenes, states also simplified their programs to make them more user friendly. They shortened applications, encouraged families to apply by mail rather than making them come in to the welfare office, and removed some of the burdensome eligibility verification requirements. The federal government did its share as well. President Clinton and other members of the administration hosted many SCHIP events, including the launch of a nationwide outreach campaign, Insure Kids Now, that includes a tollfree number and Web site where families can call and be linked directly with enrollment information for SCHIP in their state.

In addition, in 1997, the Robert Wood Johnson Foundation (RWJF) signaled its strong support for the new SCHIP program by creating a $47 million initiative called

"Covering Kids." The initiative was designed to help states reach out to families and provide them with information about the availability of health coverage through SCHIP and Medicaid. Administered by the Southern Institute on Children and Families, Covering Kids has provided grants to all 50 states and the District of Columbia and has conducted nationwide outreach events as well as large-scale advertising campaigns and an annual back-to-school enrollment drive.

SUCCESSES AND CHALLENGES

Enrollment Growth

Despite initial delays and quandaries in some states about how to structure their new programs, states and their legislatures took a thoughtful approach toward the design and rollout of SCHIP. The result has been a steady trend of significant enrollment growth — over a million children each year — and a wide recognition of success by academics, advocates, and governments alike. The Centers for Medicare and Medicaid Services (CMS) reports that 4.6 million children were enrolled at some point during fiscal year (FY) 2001 (the year ending September 30, 2001) — an increase of 38 percent over the 3.3 million enrolled during the previous fiscal year (Figure 1).[2] These numbers are extremely encouraging, given the stated program goal of reducing the number of uninsured, and several studies have substantiated SCHIP's positive impact on the overall rate of uninsurance in the nation. As early as 2000, the Census Bureau's report on the Current Population Survey noted that the decrease in uninsured children was largely due to the outreach efforts resulting from SCHIP implementation.[3]

In addition, research is beginning to substantiate the anecdotal evidence from states that SCHIP outreach efforts have also resulted in significant increases in regular

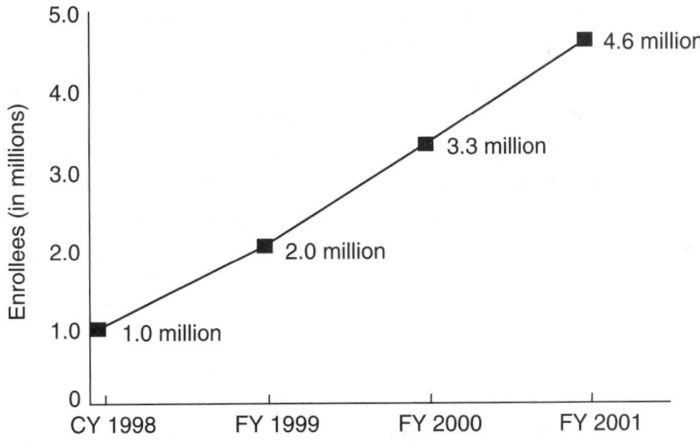

Figure 1 Number of children ever enrolled in SCHIP, calendar year 1998 through fiscal year 2001. (Source: Centers for Medicare and Medicaid Services, "State Children's Health Insurance Program: Fiscal Year 2001 Annual Enrollment Report," U.S. Department of Health and Human Services, Washington, D.C., February 6, 2002.)

Medicaid enrollment. Outreach strategies and simplification efforts have not only made the SCHIP program user friendly, they have encouraged states to streamline their Medicaid programs in ways that begin to step away from the "welfare stigma" from which many states' programs still suffer. Covering Kids has played a significant role in encouraging state innovations with outreach and eligibility simplification activities for both SCHIP and Medicaid. In fact, on May 1, 2002, RWJF announced a new initiative, Covering Kids and Families, and provided an additional $55 million in grants to support and enhance states' outreach and retention efforts over the next four years.

Economic Downturn

The current economic situation has caused states to slow or even reverse some of those efforts in an attempt to control Medicaid spending and enrollment. A few states have considered or implemented similar changes to their SCHIP programs, including capping enrollment for extended periods of time. On the whole, however, states are committed to maintaining their programs and the streamlined processes that have helped them find and enroll uninsured children over the past four years.

These successes must be considered in the context of the number of uninsured children that have not yet been reached, the size of SCHIP compared to that of states' Medicaid programs, and the current fiscal environment. For more than a year, the economy has been a major cause for concern across the board, and nearly all states have reported shortfalls in their budgets. While the direct effect on program enrollment is just beginning to be documented, declines in the economy logically result in more families becoming unemployed, uninsured, and therefore eligible for Medicaid or SCHIP. This influx of eligibles could prove to be problematic for states in a time of even tighter budgets than usual. The Medicaid program already serves 21 million children, and federal funding accounted for an average of 15 percent of states' general revenues in 2001.[4] In addition, even though the SCHIP allotments are a separate and additional funding stream for states, they must contribute a portion of their own funds in order to draw down the federal enhanced match. When there is no state money to be had, the availability of federal matching funds is a small consolation. Finally, while several studies have indicated that SCHIP has had a positive impact on Medicaid enrollment, as well as the overall rate of uninsurance in the nation, the Census Bureau reports that there were still 8.4 million uninsured children in 2000, many of whom are eligible for Medicaid or SCHIP.[5] There is clearly much more work to be done.

The "SCHIP Dip"

When it was authorized as part of the Balanced Budget Act of 1997, the SCHIP program was funded as a block grant to states, providing them $40 billion over ten years to expand health coverage to low-income uninsured children. However, as part of the budget balancing effort, the SCHIP funding was not distributed equally over the ten years. Instead, Congress allocated almost $4.3 billion for each of the first four years of the program — 1998 through 2001 — but then decreased the funding by more

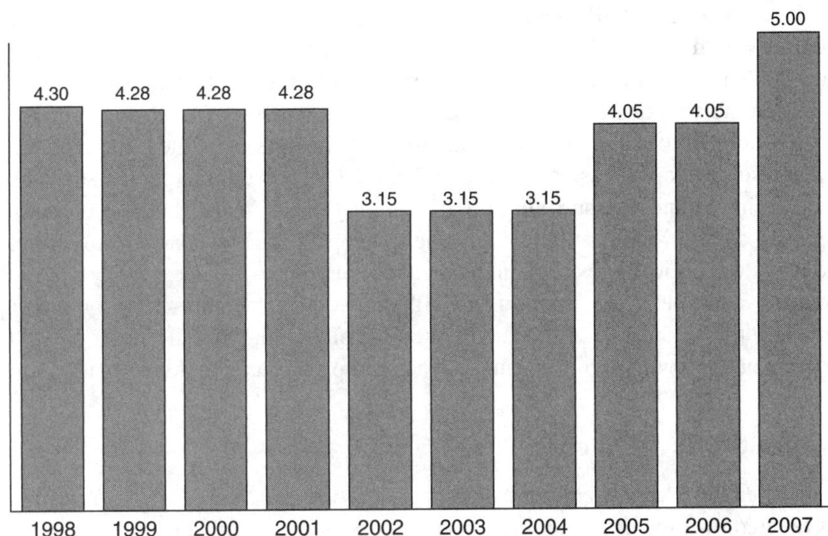

Figure 2 The SCHIP dip: State Children's Health Insurance Program allotments to states, FY 1998–FY 2007 (in billions of dollars). (Source: Centers for Medicare and Medicaid Services, U.S. Department of Health and Human Services, "State Children's Health Insurance Program; Final Allotments to States, the District of Columbia, and U.S. Territories and Commonwealths for Fiscal Year 2002." Notice (CMS-2133-N), Federal Register, 66, no. 208 (October 26, 2001); accessed August 13, 2002, at http://cms.hhs.gov/schip/2133n.pdf)

than $1 billion to $3.15 billion for each of the following three years (Figure 2). So, between 2002 and 2004, states will experience a 26 percent decline in the amount of federal funding that is available to them for the maintenance (or unlikely expansion) of their SCHIP programs. Done with the sole purpose of helping to balance the overall federal budget, this "SCHIP dip" could mean a loss of SCHIP coverage for nearly 1 million children over the next three years.[6]

SCHIP funding is made available to the states through an allocation formula specified in the statute. The statute also includes a provision that requires any unspent SCHIP funds to be redistributed to states that fully expend their allotments at the end of a three-year period. These states would then have one additional year to spend the redistributed funds. In 2001, Congress amended this provision to allow for the redistribution and retention of unused funds for FY 1998 and FY 1999. Any remaining unused funds from these years are scheduled to return to the U.S. treasury at the end of this fiscal year (September 30, 2002). Currently a total of $2.8 billion of unspent federal funding is scheduled to revert to the treasury at the end of FY 2002 and FY 2003.[7]

On August 5, 2002, Sens. Jay Rockefeller (D-W.Va.), Lincoln D. Chafee (R-R.I.), Edward M. Kennedy (D-Mass.), and Orrin G. Hatch (R-Utah) introduced the Children's Health Improvement and Protection Act of 2002 (S.2860), legislation designed to correct the SCHIP dip and help avoid the reduction in SCHIP caseloads that has been anticipated under the current law. The bill would provide additional funding to restore SCHIP allotments for FY 2003 and FY 2004 to the FY 2001 level. The bill would also enable the expiring unspent SCHIP funds to remain with the states, rather than return to the U.S. treasury and continue to allocate unspent SCHIP funds equitably among the states.[8]

In addition to extending the availability of the existing funds, the legislation would also develop a "caseload stabilization pool" that would target the states most likely to have funding shortfalls in the coming years.[9] Analysis suggests that this approach could provide sufficient funding to keep SCHIP caseloads from dropping and may even allow more children to receive coverage over the next five years of the program.[10] Although the future of this bill is uncertain, the administration has supported, in the President's 2003 budget, the goal of keeping SCHIP funding with the program and allowing it to continue to reach more uninsured children and families.

Medicaid Budget Woes

As noted earlier, states' Medicaid budgets have become extremely tight as the economy has faltered over the past year. In response, the Senate, on July 25, 2002, approved a fiscal relief amendment that would provide a total of $5.7 billion in additional Medicaid funding to temporarily increase the Medicaid matching rate for states that stand to have their federal medical assistance percentages (FMAPs)[11] decreased as a result of the strong economy of the late 1990s.[12] The FMAP recalculations are based on a Department of Health and Human Services (DHHS) analysis of three years of Census Bureau data on per capita income growth. Because they are based on the three-year average of these data, the adjustments are not immediately responsive to economic conditions. Consequently, the updated FMAPs, which will take effect on October 1, 2002, will reflect the tremendous economic growth between 1998 and 2000 (rather than states' current budgetary restrictions) and will only further compound their problems. Although the bill passed the Senate with very strong bipartisan support, there is no comparable bill in the House, so the future of this measure is not yet clear.

If these two bills eventually become law, states will gain some additional funds to help them sustain their Medicaid and SCHIP programs. However, the economy will continue to be the deciding factor in determining whether states will be able to further expand their programs to reach more uninsured children and families.

Health Insurance Family Style

The theory that reaching out to and enrolling parents in health coverage will result in more children enrolled has become widely accepted over the past two years. Several states have made this assertion as a basis for an SCHIP Section 1115 demonstration and a means to access unspent SCHIP allotment funds. The Urban Institute looked at the first four states — New Jersey, Minnesota, Rhode Island, and Wisconsin — that received approval to use SCHIP funds to cover parents of children enrolled in the program and found that parents, and indeed their children, are enrolling readily in Medicaid and SCHIP. In fact, enrollment has even exceeded projected targets in some states.

And state officials concluded that enrolling parents has led to substantial gains in child enrollment in both Medicaid and SCHIP, with child enrollment growing more rapidly than it did during the Medicaid child-only coverage expansions of the 1990s.[13]

More recently, states have been afforded even more flexibility to cover new populations and modify benefit packages and cost-sharing structures through a new approach to Section 1115 demonstrations and the new Health Insurance Flexibility and Accountability Initiative (HIFA) announced by DHHS in August 2001. In the past year, three states have received approval to use SCHIP funding to expand coverage to adults using a Section 1115 waiver — California, Utah, and Arizona.[14]

Recently, questions and concerns have been raised regarding the additional flexibility the administration is providing states in using their SCHIP allotments. In particular, Arizona's demonstration, which uses SCHIP funding to provide coverage for childless adults, prompted strong criticism from the General Accounting Office (GAO). The concern is that allowing states to use unspent SCHIP funding to cover childless adults is not consistent with the statutory objective of expanding health coverage to low-income children. In a July 2002 report to the Senate Finance Committee, GAO asserted that DHHS has not, with its recent approvals of waivers under the new flexibility initiatives, consistently ensured that waivers are in line with program goals and are budget neutral. In fact, it concluded that the use of SCHIP funding for adults "is not authorized" under the statute.[15] GAO is further concerned that allowing coverage of childless adults could eventually prevent the redistribution of SCHIP funds to other states that have exhausted their allocations by covering children. The report recommends that the Secretary of Health and Human Services amend the approval of the Arizona waiver to prevent future use of SCHIP funds on childless adults and deny any pending proposals from other states. In addition, GAO recommends that Congress consider amending Title XXI, the SCHIP statute, to specify that SCHIP funds are not available for coverage of childless adults.[16]

In its comments on the GAO report, DHHS disagreed with the assertion that the Arizona waiver is inconsistent with the intent of the SCHIP statute. The agency argued that the Arizona waiver "must be viewed as a comprehensive approach in providing health insurance coverage to those who were previously uninsured, including parents and childless adults, some of whom may indeed be former Medicaid recipients."[17] It is not yet clear whether the administration will accept the GAO's recommendations or how it might respond to further criticisms from Congress. By making the request to GAO for an investigation, Congress does appear to be taking seriously the original intent of the SCHIP statute and the need to protect the funding that accompanies it.

RETENTION: THE KEY TO THE FUTURE

While upward SCHIP enrollment trends have earned the states a reputation for innovation and commitment to the goal of reaching out to the uninsured, very little is known about what happens to families after they reach the end of their initial period of eligibility. Indeed, during the first few years of SCHIP, the main focus was on enrollment strategies: outreach, marketing, eligibility simplification, and cultural competency. Retention has always been a stated goal of SCHIP, but until recently monitoring disenrollment rates and eligibility renewal processes has generally taken a back seat to increasing enrollment.

Keeping eligible children enrolled in health care coverage is important, both administratively for states and in terms of health outcomes for children. Disruptions in health coverage can reduce continuity of care, result in missed preventive visits and place families in the tenuous position of trying to pay out-of-pocket for health care costs incurred during periods of uninsurance. In addition, since a significant number of children who are disenrolled return to public coverage within two months, (suggesting that they did not have access to other coverage), the costs of re-establishing eligibility and re-enrolling children in health plans can be burdensome for all involved.[18]

Retention has been an elusive issue, both semantically and in practice. States are free to design their renewal processes to best suit their own administrative structures and budgets, so comparing policies across states has been difficult. A few common themes have emerged, however, and several terms should be defined in order to clarify the discussion.

Redetermination is the process though which a family's SCHIP or Medicaid eligibility is reassessed. States have flexibility to decide how much information to request and how frequently to conduct redeterminations. Forty-two states have established a 12-month eligibility period in both their Medicaid and SCHIP programs,[19] but only a handful have significantly reduced the information required to redetermine eligibility. Of late, many states have begun to refer to redeterminations as *renewals* to help the program sound more like a commercial insurance product.

Continuous eligibility is a policy that allows families to remain enrolled in SCHIP or Medicaid for the entire eligibility period, regardless of a change in financial or other circumstances. Seventeen states currently provide children with 12 months of continuous eligibility.[20] (Many states have a 12-month eligibility period, but require families to report changes in income to the SCHIP or Medicaid agency, which would lead to an earlier eligibility redetermination and possible discontinuation of coverage.)

Passive renewal is a policy that a few states have implemented that allows families to stay enrolled in the program without being required to actively submit new income or other eligibility information to the state. Instead, the state sends the family a preprinted renewal form and asks them to return the form only if information needs to be updated. Passive renewal is often done in combination with a monthly premium. In this case, at the point of redetermination, states assume the family is still financially eligible and living in the state as long as they continue to make the premium payment.

NASHP and CHIRI — First Looks at Retention

In 2001, with funding from the David and Lucile Packard Foundation, the National Academy for State Health Policy (NASHP) established a SWOT (Strengths, Weaknesses, Opportunities and Threats) Team made up of seven states operating stand-alone

SCHIP programs (Alabama, Arizona, California, Georgia, Iowa, New Jersey, and Utah) that agreed to take an in-depth look at their eligibility renewal processes and corresponding retention rates. NASHP contracted with a national research firm to conduct a study from the families' perspective. Lake Snell Perry and Associates conducted focus groups and a telephone survey with parents of current and past SCHIP enrollees. The study focused on two groups, current enrollees who have been enrolled in SCHIP for at least 6 months and "lapsed families" who had been terminated from the program either for nonpayment of their premiums or for failure to complete the renewal process.

The findings of the survey and focus group discussions include the following:

- Parents appreciate SCHIP and consider it a "high-quality" program. They want to keep their children enrolled (or would like to re-enroll them).
- Both programs and parents play a role in the effectiveness of the retention process — while it is clear that states could do more to make the renewal process more user friendly and less burdensome, many parents reported that they just had not gotten around to sending in the paperwork.
- Most parents consider the premium to be reasonable and say they feel good about contributing toward their children's coverage, but they sometimes have trouble finding the money to pay the premiums.[21]

While the results highlight positive aspects of the programs, they also indicate a few areas for concern and, perhaps most importantly, make it clear that very little is really known about retention at this point. There will undoubtedly be continuing lessons — similar to those states have been able to learn from each other about enrollment and outreach strategies — in finding the most effective and efficient retention strategies.

The Child Health Insurance Research Initiative (CHIRI), led jointly by the federal Agency for Health Care Research and Quality (AHRQ) and the Health Resources and Services Administration (HRSA) and funded by AHRQ, HRSA, and the David and Lucile Packard Foundation, looked at renewal and disenrollment policies in four states — Kansas, Oregon, New York, and Florida. The study examined state policies in more detail and attempted to measure how each state's combination of strategies affected their overall retention rates. The study yielded many interesting findings, some dos and don'ts, and opportunities for further thinking and experimentation by states.

- More than half of the children in New York and Florida were enrolled in SCHIP at the two-year anniversary of their initial enrollment; however, many of these children had been disenrolled at least once during that time.
- Complex and administratively burdensome redetermination requirements can generate large numbers of disenrollments (as many as 50 percent). While some represent transfers to Medicaid or other coverage, 25 percent of those who were disenrolled re-enrolled in SCHIP after two months. This suggests that these children did not obtain other coverage and had likely been disenrolled inappropriately.

- Longer periods of continuous eligibility result in better program retention, but requiring additional paperwork and concrete verification of income still results in spikes in disenrollment at the end of the continuous eligibility period.
- Even in the absence of 12-month continuous eligibility, a passive renewal policy seems to have the most positive effect on program retention.[23]

These two studies and other anecdotal information from states provide interesting opportunities for other states to think about ways to improve their renewal processes and keep children enrolled in SCHIP for as long as they are eligible.

THE FUTURE OF SCHIP: MOVING AHEAD

As SCHIP moves from childhood into adolescence, the successes and challenges, but also the lessons learned, will undoubtedly continue. In the grand scheme of things, federal funding for the program is secured by the statute until 2007, and SCHIP and Medicaid will likely play a role in the continuing debate over universal health coverage. On a more local scale, states will continue to refine their programs and learn from each other about what works best. They will share ideas about enrollment and retention strategies, cost-sharing and benefit structures, and creative financing mechanisms. States will also continue to have opportunities to experiment with their SCHIP and Medicaid programs — expand them to (some) new populations, work with the private sector to blend funding and benefit packages, and continue to reach out to low-income families whose children are in great need of health care coverage.

ENDNOTES

1. Centers for Medicare and Medicaid Services, "State Child Health Insurance Program Plan Activity Map," updated as of August 6, 2002; accessed August 13, 2002, at http://www.cms.hhs.gov/schip/chip-map.asp.
2. Centers for Medicare and Medicaid Services, "State Children's Health Insurance Program Annual Enrollment Report: Fiscal Year 2001: October 1, 2000–September 30, 2001," February 6, 2002; accessed July 30, 2002, at http://www.cms.hhs.gov/schip/schip01.pdf. These data indicate the number of children "ever enrolled" during the course of the year, not to be confused with "point-in-time" enrollment numbers that indicate enrollment during a given month. For example, Vernon Smith, Ph.D., has conducted an ongoing survey of states' enrollment counts for December of each year, finding that 3.5 million children were enrolled in SCHIP in December 2001.
3. U.S. Census Bureau, "Health Insurance Coverage: Consumer Income — 1999," Estimates based on the March 2000 Current Population Survey, September 29, 2000, 9; accessed August 12, 2002, at http://www.census.gov/prod/www/abs/popula.html#income. Mathematica Policy Research, Inc,. and the Urban Institute have also done analysis to further quantify this effect.

4. Kaiser Commission on Medicaid and the Uninsured, "Medicaid 'Mandatory' and 'Optional' Eligibility and Benefits," Washington, D.C., July 2001, 1.
5. U.S. Census Bureau, "Health Insurance Coverage: Consumer Income — 2000," Based on the March 2001 Current Population Survey, Washington, D.C., September 2001, 3; accessed August 13, 2002 at http://www.census.gov/prod/www/abs/popula.html#income. There are a range of estimates regarding the numbers of uninsured children that are actually eligible for Medicaid or SCHIP, but are not enrolled. Urban Institute analysis has estimated that 6.8 million uninsured children are eligible but unenrolled, with 4.6 million eligible for Medicaid and 2.3 million eligible for SCHIP (these estimates account for immigrant children as well). See Lisa Dubay, Jennifer Haley, and Genevieve Kenney, "Children's Eligibility for Medicaid and SCHIP: A View from 2000," Urban Institute, Washington, D.C., March 2002, 3; accessed August 13, 2002, at http://www.urban.org/uploadedPDF/310435.pdf. Another recent analysis, by John Holohan at the Urban Institute, has estimated that nearly 5 million children are eligible for the programs but have not been reached. See also Robert Wood Johnson Foundation, "New Data: Nearly 5 Million Children in America Are Needlessly Uninsured," press release, Washington, D.C., August 1, 2002; accessed August 6, 2002, at http://www.rwjf.org/newsEvents/index.jsp.
6. Office of Management and Budget, *Analytic Perspectives, Budget of the United States Government, Fiscal Year 2003*, 297; accessed August 13, 2002, at http://www.whitehouse.gov/omb/budget/fy2003/pdf/spec.pdf. See also Edwin Park, Leighton Ku, and Matthew Broaddus, "OMB Estimates Indicate that 900,000 Children Will Lose Health Insurance Due to Reductions in Federal SCHIP Funding," Center on Budget and Policy Priorities, Washington, D.C., July 15, 2002; accessed August 8, 2002, at http://www.cbpp.org/7-15-02health.htm.
7. On September 20, 2002, $1.2 billion is scheduled to expire and revert to the treasury; an additional $1.6 billion is expected to expire on September 30, 2003.
8. Office of Sen. Jay Rockefeller, "Fact Sheet on Rockefeller-Chafee-Kennedy-Hatch Children's Health Improvement and Protection Act of 2002, August 1, 2002; accessed August 6, 2002, at http://www.rockefeller.senate.gov/2002/pr080102b.html.

CHAPTER 9

QUALITY OF HEALTH CARE

Previous chapters have addressed several critical financing, organizational, and access issues emerging as the U.S. health care system undergoes unprecedented changes as it enters the 21st century. We now turn our attention to specific concerns about the quality of health care services in the United States, including the underuse of preventive or beneficial services by certain populations, the overuse of technologies and procedures with uncertain health benefits, and physician errors. Initial studies of quality focused on the process of care and the structure of services provided. In recent years, however, policymakers and researchers have turned their attention to whether the care provided is appropriate and effective, and to identifying the specific outcomes of services provided. Without outcome measures for increasingly complex therapies and treatments, it is impossible to determine whether specific approaches are cost-effective and, more important, if they improve the health of patients. Previous emphasis on the process (versus the outcome) of health care services had rendered clinicians, patients, payers, and policymakers uninformed about the efficacy, desirability, and cost-effectiveness of many health care procedures and services that are routinely provided.

The current managed care environment insists on, as a structural mandate, evidence from randomized controlled trials that objectively indicates the efficacy and the cost-effectiveness of care. However, recent studies have revealed that even with this emphasis on evidence-based clinical guidelines, some standard preventive and treatment practices do not confer health benefits. Barbara McNeil discusses the inherent uncertainties of treatment efficacy and clinical outcomes that challenge our ability to assess and to improve quality of care (2001; see Recommended Reading). Articles 4 and 5 in Chapter 10 add to the discussion with recent findings on the inefficacy of estrogen/progestin replacement therapy in reducing coronary disease events (Fletcher and Colditz, 2002) and the uncertain benefit of breast cancer screening due to the high rate of false positives (Ernster, 2002). Even after treatments become standard practice, this does not necessarily indicate that they are beneficial. In combination with knowledge about the efficacy of interventions and the skills needed to deliver care, the movement to contain cost requires prudent application of outcomes data to appropriately provide health care services.

The last edition of *The Nation's Health* included papers that represented recent attempts to better define, describe, and measure the quality, appropriateness, and effectiveness of health care services. This edition includes Article 1 by Bodenheimer (1999) from the previous edition. Article 2 by McGlynn and Brook (2001) focuses on the factors influencing why it is hard to keep quality improvements on the policy agenda and in the public eye, and Article 3 by Davies, Washington, and Bindman (2002) analyzes the limitations of health care quality report cards when applied to vulnerable populations.

Issues related to the quality of health care have been studied intensively in recent years. In April 2002, the Commonwealth Fund produced *Quality of Health Care in the United States: A Chartbook* (Leatherman and Douglas, 2002), which presents a spectrum of data on quality and suggestions for reform:

> It is clear that improvement in six areas of performance could significantly affect the process and outcomes of health care: (1) consistently providing appropriate and effective care, (2) reducing unjustified geographic variation in care, (3) eliminating avoidable mistakes, (4) lowering access barriers, including lack of insurance, (5) improving responsiveness of patients, and (6) eliminating racial/ethnic, gender, socioeconomic, and other disparities and inequalities in access and treatment (p. 12).

The range of problems related to underuse, overuse, or misuse; mistakes in diagnosis; low rates of patient use of effective clinical preventive services (e.g., Pap smears, immunization); errors in medication use; failures of equipment and technologies; and unforeseen complications of treatment have been well documented for decades. However, addressing these shortcomings is not as simple as identifying the problems. Spending more money on health care will not necessarily improve quality in these realms. The United States currently spends more on health care per capita than any other nation in the world despite the nation's 38 to 41 million uninsured. McNeil (2001) illustrates how the increasing adoption and expanding application of new medical technologies in diagnosis and treatment have fueled rising health care costs. Although these technologies have helped to improve the quality of lives and to extend healthy years of life, in some cases we have reached "flat-of-the-curve medicine," where the marginal benefit of using a medical technology is so small that it is not cost-effective (McNeil, 2001, p. 1617). Changes in the U.S. health care system that increase the awareness and involvement of physicians, health care organizations, industry, and patients in improving and sustaining a culture of quality are needed.

In Article 1, Thomas Bodenheimer reviews the magnitude of the problem of quality deficiencies. He documents the organizations concerned with quality assessment, reporting, and maintenance; the difficulties in measuring quality; and the attempts to maintain a standard of quality by pressuring institutions with policy measures from the outside and by creating a culture of quality within institutions.

A multiplicity of professional and consumer-oriented organizations are concerned with accreditation (e.g., National Committee for Quality Assurance), the development of standards (e.g., Foundation for Accountability), and consumer education and advocacy (e.g., American Association of Retired Persons). Despite the efforts of these organizations and others, there is still the view among leaders in the field that "a fundamental change is needed within institutions to bring both a science and a culture of quality to U.S. medicine that are currently lacking in most hospitals and physicians' organizations" (Bodenheimer, 1999, p. 447). To date, there has been little change.

Elizabeth A. McGlynn and Robert H. Brook (Article 2) focus on the problem of how to sustain public and policy attention to improving quality. They stress the important role of both government and the private sector in taking steps to incorporate better quality-monitoring systems and technologies, such as computerized clinical management systems that will reduce preventable medical errors.

One such quality-monitoring system that has become increasingly used to inform purchasers and consumers is standardized public reporting of quality through report cards (Davies, Washington, and Bindman, 2002). However, it remains to be seen if report cards will help to improve access to and use of effective health care services by the populations most in need. A primary focus of quality improvement relates to the Healthy People 2010 objective of eliminating health disparities. Article 3 by Davies, Washington, and Bindman (2002) critically assesses the impact of report cards on vulnerable population subgroups, which are defined as

> those who have difficulty comprehending or making use of report card data (e.g., those with limited education, those for whom English is not their first language, those with literacy problems or learning difficulties as well as those who are seriously sick or mentally unwell) and those who may comprehend but simply have limited maneuverability to act on the information (the uninsured and those who for reasons of plan specification or geography have limited choice) (p. 381).

Although they have not been included in this book because of space limitations, several recent papers add important dimensions to the discussion concerning quality of and access to health care. These papers raise a broad spectrum of continuing issues in the policy arena. These references are listed in the Recommended Reading section because of their importance.

The essay by David L. Sackett and his colleagues from the United Kingdom, Canada, and the United States (1996) discusses the concept of evidence-based medicine and raises important issues relevant across health care disciplines. The overriding theme of this paper is the need to consider important and unique information about individual patients in light of research-based information about populations of possibly dissimilar patients and to make clinical decisions that reflect these considerations. For example, most clinical trials are performed on white males rather than women, children, or ethnic minorities, but often the population being treated for a condition does not reflect the research population. As defined by the authors, "Evidence-based medicine is the conscientious, explicit, and judicious use of current best evidence in making decisions about the care of individual patients" (Sackett et al., 1996, p. 71). Their discussion encourages consideration of how health care professionals can best weigh internal (patient-centered) and external (population-focused) evidence in formulating care decisions that are appropriate and effective for individual patients.

In "A User's Manual for the IOM's *Quality Chasm* report," Donald A. Berwick (2002) sets forth a framework for conceptualizing the health care system as described in the Institute of Medicine's 2001 report *Crossing the Quality Chasm*. Level A is patients' experiences; Level B, the small units of care delivery, or microsystems; Level C, the organizations supporting the microsystems; and Level D, the social and environmental factors that influence activities at Level C. Berwick states that "'True north' in the model lies at Level A, in the experience of patients, their loved ones, and the communities in which they live" (p. 83). The Institute of Medicine (IOM) committee identified six goals: safety, effectiveness, patient centeredness, timeliness, efficiency, and equity. The report suggests important fundamental, organizational, financing, and cultural changes at each of the four levels to shift the system toward health care embodying these six attributes.

Joseph P. Newhouse, in "Why Is There a Quality Chasm?" (2002), uses the IOM *Quality Chasm* report (2001) as a springboard for discussing the economic reasons for why a gap exists between the actual and potential quality of care in the U.S. health care system given its resources and expenditures.

SUMMARY

In recent decades, a number of reports have increased attention to the serious quality deficiencies in our health care system and provided promising suggestions for reform. However, action to address quality concerns has been difficult to pursue at the policy level. Despite the occasional media reports of harm to patients and the known underutilization of critical preventive health services by disadvantaged populations, public interest to date has fallen short of generating enough momentum to take concerted effort to systematically change the health care system in a way that improves quality. Furthermore, although quality improvements are in much need of attention, it is important to remember that medical care services do not equal or necessarily produce the health of the population.

REFERENCES

Berwick, D. A. (2002). A user's manual for the IOM's "Quality Chasm" report. *Health Affairs, 21* (3), 80–90.

Bodenheimer, T. (1999). The American health care system: The movement for improved quality in health care. *New England Journal of Medicine, 340*, 488–492.

Davies, H. T. O., Washington, A. E., and Bindman, A. B. (2002). Health care report cards: Implications for vulnerable patient groups and the organizations providing them care. *Journal of Health Politics, Policy and Law, 27* (3), 379–399.

Ernster, V. (2002, February 14). Mammograms and personal choice. *New York Times,* p. 35.

Fletcher, S. W., and Colditz, G. A. (2002). Failure of estrogen plus progestin therapy for prevention. *Journal of the American Medical Association, 288* (3), 366–368.

Institute of Medicine. (2001). *Crossing the quality chasm: A new health system for the twenty-first century*. Washington: National Academy Press.

Leatherman, S., and McCarthy, D. (2002). *Quality of health care in the United States: A chartbook*. New York: The Commonwealth Fund.

McGlynn, E. A., and Brook, R. H. (2001). Keeping quality on the policy agenda. *Health Affairs, 20* (3), 82–89.

McNeil, Barbara J. (2001). Shattuck lecture—hidden barriers to improvement in the quality of care. *New England Journal of Medicine, 345* (22), 1612–1620.

Newhouse, J. (2002). Why is there a quality chasm? *Health Affairs, 21* (4), 13–25.

Oberlander, J. (2002). The U.S. health care system: On a road to nowhere? *Canadian Medical Association Journal, 167* (2), 163–168.

Sackett, D. L., Rosenberg, W. M. C., Haynes, R. B., and Richardson, W. S. (1996). Evidence-based medicine: What is it and what isn't it? *British Medical Journal, 312* (13), 71–72.

ARTICLE 1

THE AMERICAN HEALTH CARE SYSTEM

THE MOVEMENT FOR IMPROVED QUALITY IN HEALTH CARE

Thomas Bodenheimer

A vibrant movement to improve the quality of health care has sprung up in the United States. Report cards on health plans, hospitals, medical groups, and even individual physicians have appeared on the front pages of newspapers, on television, and on the Internet. Projects to solve problems of quality within health care institutions dot the health care landscape. A small but determined cadre of physician leaders has developed a science of health care quality and is working to transform that science into a national movement.

Two main strategic threads intertwine to create the present and future agenda of the movement to improve quality in health care. First, activists are persuading the purchasers of health care — large employers and the government — to demand high-quality care from managed-care plans and health care providers. Second, leaders are attempting to inspire health professionals to create a "culture of quality" within their health care institutions. A description of these interrelated strategies is the subject of this health policy report. The report is based on interviews with experts on the quality of health care in academic medicine, business, and government and with the leaders of organizations that focus on quality in health care. Before describing the two strategies of the movement, I will briefly review the nation's main problems with the quality of health care, how it is measured, and the most important organizations concerned with the quality of health care.

PROBLEMS WITH QUALITY

Problems with the quality of health care can be categorized as overuse, underuse, and misuse.[1] A number of studies have demonstrated overuse of health care services; for example, from 8 to 86 percent of operations — depending on the type — have been found to be unnecessary and have caused substantial avoidable death and disability.[2]

Underuse is prevalent in the care of patients with chronic disease. For instance, many patients with diabetes do not have regular glycohemoglobin measurements and retinal examinations, and from 1993 through 1995, only 14 percent of patients with cardiovascular disease had achieved the serum lipid levels recommended in national guidelines.[3,4] Underuse also occurs in acute care. The failure to use effective therapies for acute myocardial infarction may lead to as many as 18,000 preventable deaths each year.[1]

Misuse is a pervasive problem. An estimated 180,000 people die each year partly as a result of injuries caused by physicians.[5] Fatal adverse drug reactions in hospitalized patients caused an estimated 106,000 deaths in 1994.[6] Fatal medication errors among outpatients doubled between 1983 and 1993.[7] The quality of care within hospitals has been found to be inferior for blacks and the uninsured.[8,9] To deal with the problem of misuse, the movement for quality has begun to target issues of patient safety.

MEASURING QUALITY

The Institute of Medicine has defined quality as "the degree to which health services for individuals and populations increase the likelihood of desired health outcomes and are consistent with current professional knowledge."[1] How does an individual physician, medical group, or health maintenance organization (HMO) know whether it is providing care of average, below average, or superior quality? The measurement of quality is an elusive but achievable goal.[10,11] Health care is not a single product, like a toaster or a lamp. It includes such diverse components as performing screening mammography in a healthy woman, optimally treating a patient with a myocardial infarction and cardiogenic shock, and counseling a depressed patient. Each intervention requires its own particular measurements of quality; some elucidate the processes of care, and some focus on outcomes. For patients with diabetes, the relevant measures might include the percentage of patients who undergo an annual retinal examination (a measure of process) and the percentage with normal glycohemoglobin levels (a measure of outcome). For patients with coronary heart disease, measures might include the percentage receiving aspirin and beta-blockers (process) and the percentage who have myocardial infarction or sudden death from cardiac causes (outcomes). Even when considering only one health care intervention — for example, coronary-artery bypass surgery — it is treacherous to compare the outcomes of one surgical team with those of another without adjusting for the age of the patients and the severity of their illness.

Different groups in the health care system have different issues of concern regarding the quality of health care and are interested in different measures of performance. Physicians view quality in health care as the application of evidence-based medical knowledge to the particular needs and wishes of individual patients. Patients may place more importance on how clinicians communicate with them, or how long they are kept waiting for appointments, than on the technical accuracy of the advice offered, though a new wave of health-conscious consumers is developing technical sophistication.

HMOs may value patient satisfaction and the use of preventive services above clinical outcomes because satisfied patients are less likely to leave the health plan and because the application of preventive services is a measure on which HMOs are currently judged.

ORGANIZATIONS CONCERNED WITH QUALITY

The National Committee for Quality Assurance (NCQA) was formed in 1979 by managed-care trade associations hoping to fend off federal monitoring of health plans. In 1990, in order to reduce competition from newer, presumably lower-quality HMOs, a group of HMOs in coalition with some large employers engineered a restructuring of the NCQA's board, transforming the organization into something more than a mere advocate for the interests of HMOs.[12]

The NCQA has two main voluntary activities: the accreditation of HMOs and the publication of measures of performance in the Health Plan Employer Data and Information Set (HEDIS). As of October 1998, 48 percent of the nation's approximately 650 HMOs had requested accreditation surveys from the NCQA; 96 percent of those surveyed have received three-year, one-year, or provisional accreditation. Thirty large corporations, including Xerox, General Motors, and IBM, will not contract with health plans that are not accredited by the NCQA, but most employers do not make accreditation a requirement. Employers concerned with the quality of health care tend to be companies that have been forced by international competition to improve the quality of their own products. Forty percent of the NCQA's budget comes from fees paid by HMOs for accreditation surveys; the rest comes from foundation grants, contracts, educational programs, and publications.

The current data set from the NCQA, HEDIS 3.0/1998, includes more than 50 measures of performance, including patient satisfaction, rates of childhood immunization, percentages of enrollees of certain ages receiving screening for cervical and breast cancer, and percentages of patients with diabetes who undergo retinal examinations.[13] Ironically, although employers tend to associate higher quality with lower costs (achieved by reducing overuse and misuse of services), the NCQA's HEDIS measures focus mainly on the underuse of health care, the correction of which raises costs. The NCQA agrees that the HEDIS measures include few items related to chronic illness; the group hopes to add such items for the year 2000 data set.

A health plan can refuse to disclose its HEDIS profile to the public. A total of 329 HMOs (51 percent of all HMOs) allowed the 1996 data to be publicized, but only 292 plans (45 percent) permitted public reporting of the data for 1997. According to the NCQA, the plans that refuse to allow publication of HEDIS data have significantly lower scores than the plans that permit publication.

The Joint Commission on Accreditation of Healthcare Organizations (JCAHO), founded in 1952 under the aegis of the American Hospital Association and the American Medical Association (AMA), has the authority to terminate hospitals' participation in the Medicare program if the quality of care is found to be deficient. Revenues for the commission come chiefly from fees paid by hospitals, home care agencies, and other facilities that it accredits. For years, the JCAHO attempted to launch outcomes-based accreditation standards that would allow the public to compare hospitals. Because of resistance from hospitals, this effort has been scaled down and converted to the ORYX program. ORYX allows a hospital to pick two measures of performance from a long list, including such items as mortality after coronary-artery surgery or the percentage of patients with diabetes who receive dietary counseling, as long as these measures are relevant to 20 percent of the hospital's patient population. Over time, hospitals must report more measures, but there is no requirement for the type of uniform reporting that would help the public compare one hospital with another.

The Health Care Financing Administration (HCFA) is responsible for ensuring that institutions providing services to Medicare and Medicaid beneficiaries meet certain standards of quality. In the past few years, HCFA has accelerated its quality-related activities and may soon be the nation's most influential organization working to monitor and improve the quality of health care. The Quality Improvement System for Managed Care (QISMC), established in 1996, sets quality standards for Medicare and Medicaid managed-care plans. In contrast to the NCQA, which reports HEDIS data only when health plans wish them to be released, HCFA has the authority to make public such data for all Medicare HMOs, but it has not yet done so. HCFA may eventually require hospitals that participate in Medicare to submit data on standardized measures of quality that consumers can use to compare hospitals, bypassing the more cautious approach of the JCAHO. HCFA is considering a similar approach for independent practice associations and group practices.

In 1972, Congress created professional standards review organizations, supplanted in 1982 by peer review organizations (PROs), one in each state, which are authorized to monitor quality in the Medicare program. A 1990 study found that PROs used ineffective punitive methods such as retrospective case review with denials of payment and warnings to physicians.[14] In 1992, HCFA transformed the PROs into organizations with staffs of medical professionals, trained in quality improvement, who analyze patterns of care through the large Medicare database and feed these data back to physicians and hospitals in order to improve care for patients with common illnesses such as myocardial infarction, congestive heart failure, stroke, and pneumonia.[15] PROs review individual cases in the event of complaints from patients and can deny payment for unnecessary services, but these constitute a small proportion of their work. Experts on quality inside and outside HCFA are concerned that Congress, intent on reducing fraud and abuse in the Medicare program, may require the PROs to return to their previous payment-denial practices and thereby compromise their quality-improvement activities.[16]

The Foundation for Accountability (FACCT) in Portland, Oregon, was created in 1995 on the initiative of Paul Ellwood. In contrast to the NCQA, an accrediting organization, FACCT is a think tank and educational vehicle whose purposes are to develop measures of performance that are relevant to consumers and to educate consumers about how to use this information. FACCT persuades the NCQA, JCAHO, HCFA, state governments, and employers to use its measures of performance.

For 10 years, the Institute for Healthcare Improvement (IHI) in Boston, founded by Donald Berwick, has organized an annual National Forum on Quality Improvement in Health Care; it has also developed a Breakthrough Series, bringing together leaders in health care organizations who are committed to solving problems of quality. The Breakthrough Series focuses on several collaborative efforts to improve care within institutions; the goals include reducing waiting times in emergency departments, preventing adverse events due to medications, and improving care for low back pain.

The National Patient Safety Foundation, located at offices of the AMA in Chicago, was established by the AMA in 1997 to change the attitudes of health professionals and the public regarding medical errors.[17] The foundation, with start-up funds from the AMA, sponsors research and educational efforts based on the assumption that errors are not personal failures deserving punishment but, rather, inadequacies of systems, which must be redesigned to help prevent errors. Leaders of the NCQA, JCAHO, FACCT, and IHI sit on the foundation's board of directors.

The National Roundtable on Health Care Quality, involving representatives from academic, business, consumer, provider, governmental, and publishing organizations, was convened by the Institute of Medicine in 1995 to heighten awareness of issues related to quality in health care. Funded by the federal government and private sources, the roundtable's 1998 report concluded that "serious and widespread quality problems exist throughout American medicine."[1] The Institute of Medicine is continuing the roundtable's work, looking at the dual strategies of changing health care institutions internally and fostering an external environment that encourages improvements in quality.

The Consumer Coalition for Quality Health Care in Washington, D.C. — formed in 1993 through the efforts of the American Association of Retired Persons and other consumer groups — represents labor, the elderly, and advocacy organizations and intends to bring the perspective of consumers to legislative and private initiatives to improve the quality of health care.

PRESSURING INSTITUTIONS FROM THE OUTSIDE

Accreditation, whether voluntary or compulsory, makes health care institutions satisfy a minimal standard of quality, thereby placing demands on these institutions to improve. The goal of the publication of performance measures, or report cards, is to put pressure on institutions in two ways. First, low scores on report cards may steer consumers or employers away from health plans, medical groups, or hospitals, and second, physicians within institutions that score poorly on report cards may be embarrassed into doing better.

Leaders in the movement for quality in health care, including those within the NCQA, view the commission's report cards as a first step toward improving quality, but they cite several limitations of the program:

Report cards may not channel most consumers to higher-quality health plans. Forty-seven percent of employees in large companies and 80 percent in small firms have no choice among health plans,[18] data on quality would therefore be of no use to them. Moreover, only 11 percent of 1500 employers recently surveyed relied on data on quality in selecting health plans; cost is the driving factor in most decisions by employers.[19]

Tens of millions of people receive health insurance through preferred-provider organizations, which are not included in the reporting on performance.

Patient satisfaction, an important component of HMO report cards for marketing purposes, is a questionable measure of the quality of care.[20] Patient satisfaction is an unreliable indicator because positive ratings from the great majority of enrollees — who are healthy and rarely use services — can dwarf the legitimate complaints of those who are sick.[21]

Gathering HEDIS data is costly to health plans and provider organizations, and the cost is ultimately shifted to purchasers and consumers. The movement for quality in health care brings profits to consultants as well as to the newest suppliers of health care products: computer and software companies.

If report cards truly channeled patients to higher-quality plans, those plans might attract a sicker, more expensive population of patients. The higher-quality plans would thus be punished rather than rewarded by the market, which does not adjust HMO premiums for severity of illness.

Although the impetus provided by report cards may boost quality within HMOs,[22] **only items measured by HEDIS are affected**. As pressure to reduce costs intensifies and the time patients spend with physicians decreases, overall quality could suffer even as HEDIS scores soar.[20]

What is the community of professionals concerned about the quality of health care doing about these shortcomings?

Some groups of employers, in particular the Pacific Business Group on Health (PBGH) and the Minnesota-based Buyers Health Care Action Group (BHCAG), are publishing report cards on medical groups and integrated care systems rather than focusing solely on health plans. A few purchasers are creating financial incentives aimed at improving the quality of care. PBGH pays health plans more money if they achieve negotiated preventive-services scores on HEDIS.[23] The huge Federal Employee Health Benefits Program is considering a similar move. General Motors reduces premiums for employees who choose high-quality plans.

A far more effective step is for employers to place clauses in contracts with health plans that require specific improvements in quality. This development comes from a leading-edge group called the Leapfrog Group. This is an informal think tank of several large employer organizations, including PBGH, BHCAG, and General Motors, whose goal is to make a direct assault on targeted issues related to patients' safety. The group, whose "epidemiology of opportunities for improving quality" is researched by PBGH medical director Dr. Arnold Milstein, has picked two issues as its initial focus on safety. The first is "evidence-based hospital referral" — that is, the channeling of patients to certain hospitals for conditions and procedures (including coronary angioplasty and bypass surgery, carotid endarterectomy, and repair of abdominal aortic aneurysm) for which clear evidence exists that a higher volume of procedures or teaching status is associated with better outcomes.[24–27] After learning that this program could save 500 to 1000 lives per year in California, PBGH (which is made up of employers that purchase care for a total of approximately 3 million employees and their dependents) is asking its California HMOs to use new performance standards for physician groups, hospital precertification, and enrollee education to advance evidence-based hospital referral for an initial subgroup of these interventions, beginning in urban areas. Although PBGH is beginning this effort with its HMOs, the intention of PBGH and the rest of the Leapfrog Group is to make these changes for all forms of health insurance.

The Leapfrog Group's second focus stems from research suggesting that medication errors at hospitals can be substantially reduced by installing computerized physician-order entry systems that display warnings in cases of drug interactions, known drug allergies, and incorrect dosages.[28] Employers could create contractual requirements, incentives, or consumer expectations for computerized physician-order entry systems.

The Leapfrog Group is intent on pushing the movement for quality forward in two ways: by bringing the safety of patients to the forefront of the consciousness of purchasers, and by going beyond the reporting of performance measures of health plans to make attention to quality improvement part of health plans' and providers' contractual obligations and market rewards.

CREATING A CULTURE OF QUALITY INSIDE INSTITUTIONS

External pressure from private purchasers and government regulators is necessary but not sufficient for improvement in quality.[29] Leaders in the field argue that a fundamental change is needed within institutions to bring both a science and a culture of quality to U.S. medicine that are currently lacking in most hospitals and physicians' organizations.

For years, experts on quality, most prominently Donald Berwick and Lucian Leape, have translated quality-enhancing techniques from other industries to health care.[5,30] Mark Chassin, cochair of the Institute of Medicine's National Roundtable on Health Care Quality, challenges the medical profession to strive toward "six sigma quality."[31] The six-sigma goal means tolerating fewer than 3.4 errors per 1 million events — a rate that lies outside six standard deviations of a normal distribution. Currently, the frequency of deaths during anesthesia has been reduced to 5.4 per million, close to the six-sigma goal. In contrast, 580,000 per million patients with depression (58 percent) are not given the correct diagnosis or treated adequately, and 790,000 eligible survivors of heart attacks per million (79 percent) do not receive beta-blockers; these rates are in the neighborhood of one sigma.[31]

Physicians, nurses, pharmacists, and other care givers cannot individually perform at a six-sigma level of reliability; meeting this goal requires building systems designed to prevent adverse consequences of unavoidable human errors.[5] For example, the use of information-and-reminder systems increases the proportion of patients with diabetes who regularly undergo glycohemoglobin tests and retinal and foot examinations.[32] The implication is that clinical care should be redesigned according to a team approach, so that goals for acute, long-term, and preventive care can all be met.

Some institutions are beginning to strive for six-sigma quality in specific areas. LDS Hospital in Salt Lake City designed computer programs to assist physicians in prescribing antibiotics and thus reduced mortality among patients treated with antibiotics by 27 percent.[33] A northern New England multihospital project used quality-improvement techniques to reduce mortality among patients undergoing cardiovascular surgery by 24 percent in three years.[34] The Community Medical Alliance in Boston has redesigned systems of care for patients with severe chronic disease by providing a wide range of services at home and greatly reducing the need for hospitals, specialists, and ambulances.[29] The IHI's National Forum and Breakthrough Series allow institutions across the country to learn from one another's quality-improvement projects. Given the tens of thousands of hospitals and medical practices in the nation, many of which do not have leaders capable of carrying through major quality-improvement projects, this strategy has had limited effects thus far.[1]

Leaders in the movement for quality in health care emphasize that health plans and providers will work toward six-sigma quality on a large scale only if they are rewarded in the market for doing so; currently, financial rewards favor low cost over high quality. Even with a fundamental change in the market, however, this level of quality is difficult to achieve. Physicians' offices, still the main site of clinical practice, are harder to redesign than larger multispecialty groups, which are more able to invest in information-and-reminder systems and to create team-based clinical care.

CONCLUSIONS

Why is the movement to improve the quality of health care active in the United States at a time when cost containment dominates the health care agenda? To some degree, improved quality can reduce costs, particularly costs due to overuse and misuse of services.[31] But substantial investment is needed to reduce misuse, and more funds are needed to address underuse. One cannot explain the existence of the movement simply as a cost-containment activity. A small number of people, mostly physicians, have brought the movement into being, to some extent against considerable odds. Overall, the movement for quality in health care expresses a human desire to do the right thing.

The movement has major barriers to overcome. Corporate purchasers and governments have reduced rates of reimbursement to providers, leading to reduced staffing in hospitals and less time with physicians for patients. Investor-owned health plans and provider organizations have exacerbated these trends by shifting dollars away from direct health services and toward profits and administration. Nonetheless, the goal of improving the quality of care has gained a prominent place on the nation's health care agenda.

REFERENCES

1. Chassin MR, Galvin RW. The urgent need to improve health care quality. *JAMA* 1998;280:1000–5.
2. Leape LL. Unnecessary surgery. *Annu Rev Public Health* 1992;13:363–83.
3. Weiner JP, Parente ST, Garnick DW, Fowles J, Lawthers AG, Palmer RH. Variation in office-based quality. *JAMA* 1995;273:1503–8.
4. McBride P, Schrott HG, Plane MB, Underbakke G, Brown RL. Primary care practice adherence to National Cholesterol Education Program guidelines for patients with coronary heart disease. *Arch Intern Med* 1998;158:1238–44.
5. Leape LL. Error in medicine. *JAMA* 1994;272:1851–7.
6. Lazarou J, Pomeranz BH, Corey PN. Incidence of adverse drug reactions in hospitalized patients. *JAMA* 1998;279:1200–5.
7. Phillips DP, Christenfeld N, Glynn LM. Increase in US medication-error deaths between 1983 and 1993. *Lancet* 1998;351:643–4.
8. Kahn KL, Pearson ML, Harrison ER, et al. Health care for black and poor hospitalized Medicare patients. *JAMA* 1994;271:1169–74.
9. Burstin HR, Lipsitz SR, Brennan TA. Socioeconomic status and risk for substandard medical care. *JAMA* 1992;268:2383–7.
10. Brook RH, McGlynn EA, Cleary PD. Measuring quality of care. *N Engl J Med* 1996;335:966–70.
11. Eddy DM. Performance measurement: problems and solutions. *Health Aff (Millwood)* 1998;17(4):7–25.
12. Millenson ML. Demanding medical excellence. Chicago: University of Chicago Press, 1997.
13. Epstein AM. Rolling down the runway: the challenges ahead for quality report cards. *JAMA* 1998;279:1691–6.
14. Rubin HR, Rogers WH, Kahn KL, Rubenstein LV, Brook RH. Watching the doctor-watchers: how well do peer review organization methods detect hospital care quality problems? *JAMA* 1992;267:2349–54.
15. Jencks SF, Wilensky GR. The health care quality improvement initiative: a new approach to quality assurance in Medicare. *JAMA* 1992;268:900–3.
16. Prager LO. PROs aim to help curb payment errors. *American Medical News.* December 7, 1998:1, 38.
17. Leape LL, Woods DD, Hatlie MJ, Kizer KW, Schroeder SA, Lundberg GD. Promoting patient safety by preventing medical error. *JAMA* 1998;280:1444–7.
18. Gabel JR, Ginsburg PB, Hunt KA. Small employers and their health benefits, 1988–1996: an awkward adolescence. *Health Aff (Millwood)* 1997;16(5):103–10.
19. Prager LO. Top accreditor ties accountability to higher HMO quality. *American Medical News.* October 19, 1998:10, 13.
20. Brook RH, Kamberg CJ, McGlynn EA. Health system reform and quality. *JAMA* 1996;276:476–80.
21. Angell M, Kassirer JP. Quality and the medical marketplace — following elephants. *N Engl J Med* 1996;335:883–5.

22. Longo DR, Land G, Schramm W, Fraas J, Hoskins B, Howell V. Consumer reports in health care: do they make a difference in patient care? *JAMA* 1997;278:1579–84.
23. Schauffler HH, Rodriguez T. Exercising purchasing power for preventive care. *Health Aff (Millwood)* 1996;15(1):73–85.
24. Jollis JG, Peterson ED, DeLong ER, et al. The relation between the volume of coronary angioplasty procedures at hospitals treating Medicare beneficiaries and short-term mortality. *N Engl J Med* 1994;331:1625–9.
25. Grumbach K, Anderson GM, Luft HS, Roos LL, Brook R. Regionalization of cardiac surgery in the United States and Canada: geographic access, choice, and outcomes. *JAMA* 1995;274:1282–8.
26. Karp HR, Flanders WD, Shipp CC, Taylor B, Martin D. Carotid end-arterectomy among Medicare beneficiaries: a statewide evaluation of appropriateness and outcome. *Stroke* 1998;29:46–52.
27. Hannan EL, Kilburn H Jr, O'Donnell JF, et al. A longitudinal analysis of the relationship between in-hospital mortality in New York State and the volume of abdominal aortic aneurysm surgeries performed. *Health Serv Res* 1992;27:517–42.
28. Bates DW, Leape LL, Cullen DJ, et al. Effect of computerized physician order entry and a team intervention on prevention of serious medication errors. *JAMA* 1998;280:1311–6.
29. Berwick DM. Crossing the boundary: changing mental models in the service of improvement. *Int J Qual Health Care* 1998;10:435–41.
30. Berwick DM. Continuous improvement as an ideal in health care. *N Engl J Med* 1989;320:53–6.
31. Chassin MR. Is health care ready for six sigma quality? *Milbank Q* 1998; 76:565–91.
32. McCulloch DK, Price MJ, Hindmarsh M, Wagner EH. A population-based approach to diabetes management in a primary care setting. *Effective Clin Pract* 1998;1(1):12–22.
33. Pestotnik SL, Classen DC, Evans RS, Burke JP. Implementing antibiotic practice guidelines through computer-assisted decision support: clinical and financial outcomes. *Ann Intern Med* 1996;124:884–90.
34. O'Connor GT, Plume SK, Olmstead EM, et al. A regional intervention to improve the hospital mortality associated with coronary bypass graft surgery. *JAMA* 1996;275:841–6.

ARTICLE 2

KEEPING QUALITY ON THE POLICY AGENDA

Elizabeth A. McGlynn and Robert H. Brook

The United States ranks thirty-seventh in the world in overall health system performance and seventy-second on population health, according to a recent World Health Organization (WHO) report.[1] These rankings are at odds with many Americans' belief that the United States has the best quality of care in the world.[2] Objective information on U.S. health system failures is generally met with a day or two of media flurry and no sustained policy response. By contrast, Congress took immediate steps to identify and correct problems that had led to defective Firestone tires, and the Federal Aviation Administration (FAA) ordered a redesign of faulty rudders on Boeing 737s following a series of reported failures in the 1990s. Policymakers are capable of taking action to protect human life in many other areas, but efforts directed at the health care system remain uncommon. Without sustained public attention to solving the quality deficit problem in health care, little progress will be made.

THE QUALITY OF HEALTH CARE IS SUBSTANDARD

How good is quality of care in the United States? We don't really know, but a review of the best scientific literature reveals the following sobering facts.[3] Only half of the population receives needed preventive care; 70 percent receive recommended care for acute problems, such as colds or stomach pain; and just 60 percent of those with a chronic illness such as diabetes or hypertension get the care they need. On the other hand, about one-third of the care delivered for acute problems is not needed (for example, antibiotics prescribed for the common cold) and may actually be harmful. About one-fifth of the care given to persons with chronic conditions is also unnecessary and possibly harmful. Given the public outcry over a few deaths from bad tires, the lack of public outrage over thousands of preventable deaths in medicine is astounding.

Serious deficits are also manifest in how skillfully care is delivered. Coronary angiography is an invasive test used to diagnose cardiac disease and determine what treatment is appropriate for a patient. Analysis of a random sample of angiographies performed in one state showed that only half of the tests were done competently enough to be accurately interpreted.[4] When the tests were reread by a group of expert cardiologists, one-quarter of patients determined by the original reading to have the most severe disease did not have it. Six percent of persons who were told that their test results were not severely abnormal actually had severely abnormal results. One-third of persons whose bypass surgery was considered necessary or appropriate based on the original interpretation of the angiography results underwent surgery that was of uncertain benefit or inappropriate based on the gold-standard review. Nearly 1.3 million coronary angiographies were performed in 1998 nationally. If the results of this study held nationally, nearly 650,000 tests would be difficult to interpret accurately; at $12,450 per test, that is more than $8 billion in wasted expense.

Countless other examples show that medicine as practiced in the United States today is dangerous. The Institute of Medicine recently estimated that as many as 98,000 people may die in any given year from medical errors.[5] Although stories on errors in medicine continue to appear in the media, serious action to improve the situation has yet to emerge.

Deficits in quality of care are not unique to the United States. A summary of the international literature showed that only about half of what is recommended in medicine gets done.[6] Studies of the appropriateness of various diagnostic and therapeutic surgical procedures in the United Kingdom, Canada, Israel, and Sweden show similar results to those in the United States.[7]

Such statistics point to health care systems that pose real and potential threats to human life far greater than those from defective tires or airplane rudders. Deficits in quality have been noted consistently throughout the past three or four decades, despite changes in how services are paid for (for example, prospective payment under Medicare) or delivered (managed care). Quality deficits are also found in countries with very different organizational and financial structures. Fixing quality requires a fundamentally different policy approach than either increasing or reducing expenditures.

WHY IS IT SO DIFFICULT TO SUSTAIN PUBLIC INTEREST?

The message that there is a problem with the quality of health care around the world is not a new one. Given that poor quality affects whether and how well people live, why is it so difficult to sustain public interest in this problem? We provide several reasons that underscore how the health care system differs from other economic sectors. Strategies to address these barriers should be useful for improving quality in the United States and internationally.

Diffuse Responsibility

When a problem with the processes or outcomes of care is identified, no single or large manufacturer is to blame — no Firestone or Boeing. Research has shown that persons undergoing coronary artery bypass graft surgery have a variable likelihood of survival after the procedure.[8] However, to motivate improved surgical care, problems must be identified and solutions developed in each of thousands of hospitals. There is rarely a credible threat that poor-quality providers will be driven out of business or even suffer a significant loss of revenue.

The Health Care Financing Administration (HCFA) tried in the mid-1980s to create an environment of accountability by developing standardized reports on whether the death rate in each hospital was what one might expect given how sick the patients were at admission. These mortality reports were discontinued in 1993 primarily for political reasons, but they inspired the development of some local organizations (for example, the Northern New England Cardiovascular Disease Study Group) dedicated to improving care. Although some of these efforts have been successful, few such examples exist nationally. Even the Peer Review Organization (PRO) program, which has been overseeing quality in the Medicare program since 1986, has not solved the problem of substandard care.[9]

Cognitive Dissonance

Most people assume that their own doctor is excellent and that any problems identified by researchers, accreditors, the media, or malpractice lawyers affect someone else. Most doctors believe that they deliver care consistent with guidelines and standards. But if the public and the medical profession do not acknowledge that suboptimal care is delivered throughout the medical care system and that significant reengineering is essential, then thousands more lives will be needlessly lost.

Reports on medical errors have come closest in recent times to breaking through this cognitive dissonance. We need to find ways to use the dialogue that has begun around errors to promote a shared understanding of the quality problem without fundamentally undermining trust in the medical care system.

Outmoded System Design

The U.S. health care system is a technological anomaly. We have made amazing advances in the availability of diagnostic machines, chemicals to treat or cure illnesses, and microsurgical techniques to repair the ravages of disease or injury. Yet most physicians and hospitals rely on barely legible, handwritten notes to track what is done to a patient and how the patient responds.

Doctors also are expected to maintain in their individual memories the appropriate approaches to diagnosing and treating a wide variety of diseases as they are manifest in human beings of radically different designs (age, race, height, weight, other health problems). By contrast, airline pilots are only allowed to fly one type of airplane and rely on extensive checklists and computer monitoring to ensure its safe operation. Nonetheless, we are surprised when physicians, using systems from the nineteenth century, and subject to the limitations of being human, fall well short of perfection.

The medical establishment has actively dismissed attempts to introduce systems principles into medical care. Physicians dismiss "cookbook" medical practice as if consistent delivery of known practices is necessarily a bad thing. In many other areas of consumable goods and services, consumers expect to get the same thing (such as a Big Mac or local currency from an automated teller machine anywhere in the world), at the same level of quality, no matter where they are. In medicine, the focus on individually tailored services means that if one has a heart attack, survival is dependent on whether the hospital used — usually the closest one — consistently uses appropriate and timely diagnostic and therapeutic procedures.

Much of the research on quality looks retrospectively at whether care already delivered is consistent with standards. Although these methods are useful for documenting the nature of the problem, they do not offer a solution. We cannot recall defective medical care the way we can recall a defective car. Systems must be in place to guide doctors' actions while the patient is being seen or to bring patients in for routine monitoring.

Information Void

We lack basic, objective information on how well the health system is functioning and what would make it function better. There is no national tracking system for identifying defects and correcting them before someone dies. There are few early warning systems to identify problems before they become widespread. There are no systems in place for ensuring that best practices are consistently implemented. There is almost no systematic information on what reengineering strategies are likely to work on a large scale. Many small projects (including many of the PRO projects) done in one state, one health system, or one hospital have demonstrated that improvement is possible. These individual projects (many of which are never published) have not led to any generalized knowledge of what changes are necessary to improve quality. Randomized trials in this area are rare but can add much to our understanding of generalizable quality improvement techniques.[10]

The Tendency to Shoot the Messenger

Finally, a common response to objective quality-performance results is to insist that the data are inaccurate and do not reflect what is really happening in any particular hospital or doctor's office. This attitude is part of what led to the demise of the HCFA mortality reports. Doctors and system administrators are not only reluctant to use information, they are often reluctant to participate in efforts to obtain good information about performance. This shoot-the-messenger attitude means that more energy is devoted to undermining the findings than to formulating and implementing solutions.

IS CHANGE HOPELESS, OR CAN WE MAKE PROGRESS?

The authors of this essay, perhaps eternal optimists, remain hopeful that change is possible. Because the problem is complex and the solutions require innovative strategies, we must generate sustained public interest to improve quality. Patience and perseverance will be essential, as will cooperation between the private and public sectors. We would like to give an outline of the exact interventions that would work best, but this knowledge does not exist. Leadership is the necessary first step.

Create Quality Champions

Fundamentally, we need a "war on poor quality" that has the same level of public commitment as the war on cancer or the campaign to put a man on the moon. We believe that the subsequent funding of needed research in response to this declaration of war will lead to the development of specific strategies that should be followed. Both the private and public sectors will have to demand a complete overhaul of medical practice, and implementing such change will necessitate leadership from clinicians and a vigilant constituency.

Advocacy organizations have been successful in raising funds for research related to curing specific diseases such as human immunodeficiency virus (HIV) or breast cancer. If such groups added to their mission pressure on health systems and public and private purchasers to pay only for high-quality care that is consistent with best practices, great progress could be made. These advocacy organizations could be champions who would put quality first and insist on design changes that ensure that the health care system gets the fundamentals right.

Medicare could similarly become a quality champion by setting higher standards for public reporting on quality. HCFA does require that managed care plans report data on measures in the Health Plan Employer Data and Information Set (HEDIS). The National Committee for Quality Assurance (NCQA) has demonstrated that managed care plans publicly reporting HEDIS data for three consecutive years have higher quality than plans that do not make data available.[11] But we can no longer tolerate the lack of information on performance in the non–managed care sector.

Develop a Functional Information System

Second, health care professionals and organizations need to embrace computer technologies that can be used to receive and transmit information. The private sector should lead the way by making investment in such systems an allowable expense in calculating health insurance premiums. The government should undertake an evaluation of tax incentives that might further spur the adoption of computer technologies in office-based medical practice. No serious advances in quality of care can be made without a functioning, computer-based information system. Computerized order-entry systems used in hospitals have been shown to reduce adverse events associated with errors in the prescribing and administering of medications.[12]

Right now, nobody is penalized financially for failing to adopt computerized clinical management systems. Regulators and purchasers should use every available tool to provide such a disincentive. Adequate clinical management hardware and software could become a condition of licensure, contracting, malpractice insurance policies, and reimbursement. Although these demands could not be made overnight, compliance within five years would be more than reasonable in the current environment.

Routinely Monitor and Report on Performance

Third, an independent group should routinely compile information into a national report on whether average levels of and variation in quality are increasing or decreasing. There have been scattered attempts to do this, including an effort mandated by Congress, but the amount of funding allocated to these efforts has been grossly inadequate. The New York State Cardiac Reporting System offers an example of the benefits to be had from public reporting. Risk-adjusted mortality rates following bypass surgery have declined significantly in the state since the reporting system was introduced.[13]

To motivate change, public reports on communities, hospitals, health systems, and providers must also be available. Communities could compete to provide the best care to their citizens: If you have a heart attack in Paris, London, or Los Angeles, in which city are you most likely to survive? Families regularly make relocation decisions based on the quality of schools in an area; they might choose to factor quality of medical care into the equation as well.

Ensure Adequate Funding for Quality Measurement

To make all of this work, sustained investments must be made in the tools that are used to set standards, promulgate current and scientifically valid measures for monitoring, provide consistent information to physicians on best practices, make information easily accessible to decisionmakers, and so on. This is not a trivial enterprise.

Developing guidelines for care is difficult and expensive, and it requires the highest level of scientific integrity. If guidelines are promulgated by individuals without much support, they will be done carelessly and will be (properly) ignored. If guidelines are issued by those who stand to benefit financially, they will be suspect and fail to attract necessary consensus. The Agency for Health Care Research and Quality (AHRQ) should have as its primary mission improving quality of care through facilitating use of information systems, developing guidelines and other standards of practice, updating and improving quality measurement tools, producing data for national reports on quality, and developing a strategic plan for quality improvement. This ambitious and essential undertaking will require a few billion dollars of new money each year. This amount pales in comparison with total spending on health care (more than $1 trillion), the size of the proposed tax cut ($1.6 trillion), and the budget of the National Institutes of Health ($19 billion in 2001).[14] AHRQ will have to be insulated from political forces that have previously limited its ability to provide strong leadership.

Where might these steps take us by the year 2010? They could mean that people, especially when they required urgent care, would not have to worry about where they go for care. Patients and their families might not need to be warned, as they are today, that they should carefully monitor what medical services they do and do not receive because their inattention might result in serious problems. The science that the nation spent so much public and private money developing could produce its promised benefits. Waste could be eliminated so that all Americans, not just those who have health insurance, could get the care they need.

These achievements are within our grasp. We spend more money on health care than any country in the world; one of every seven dollars spent in this country goes to medical care.[15] We have sophisticated physicians and social scientists. But we lack the will to reengineer our own health system.

Leadership for this reengineering will have to come from both government and the private sector. The government role is particularly critical, something that has been recognized in all other Western nations except the United States. Reengineering the health care system will be complicated by the fact that we cannot shut down the system and import our health care while we slowly redesign processes and plants. We must develop an incentive structure that promotes reengineering while enabling us to operate a system that is providing care to patients.

We must find a way to keep quality of care at the top of the health policy agenda. After providing insurance to all Americans, there is no issue of equal importance.

ACKNOWLEDGMENTS

An earlier version of this paper was presented at the Ditchley Park Conference on Improving the Quality of Health Care in the United States and the United Kingdom, cosponsored by the Commonwealth Fund and the Nuffield Trust, Oxfordshire, England, 10 June 2000. The authors thank Paul Shekelle for discussions that shaped the arguments presented here and Mary Vaiana for editorial assistance.

REFERENCES

1. World Health Organization, *The World Health Report 2000: Health Systems — Improving Performance* (Geneva: WHO, 2000).

2. R.J. Blendon, M. Kim, and J.M. Benson, "The Public versus the World Health Organization on Health System Performance," *Health Affairs* (May/June 2001): 10–20.

3. M.A. Schuster, E.A. McGlynn, and R.H. Brook, "How Good Is the Quality of Health Care in the United States?" *Milbank Quarterly* 76, no. 4 (1998): 517–563.

4. L.L. Leape et al., "Effect of Variability in the Interpretation of Coronary Angiograms on the Appropriateness of Use of Coronary Revascularization Procedures," *American Heart Journal* 139, no. 1, Part 1 (2000): 106–113.
5. Institute of Medicine, *To Err Is Human: Building a Safer Health System* (Washington: National Academy Press, 1999).
6. J.M. Grimshaw and I.T. Russell, "Effect of Clinical Guidelines on Medical Practice: A Systematic Review of Rigorous Evaluations," *Lancet* 342, no. 8883 (1993): 1317–1322.
7. D. Gray et al., "Audit of Coronary Angiography and Bypass Surgery," *Lancet* 335, no. 8701 (1990): 1317–1320; E.A. McGlynn et al., "A Comparison of the Appropriateness of Coronary Angiography and Coronary Artery Bypass Graft Surgery between Canada and New York State," *Journal of the American Medical Association* 272, no. 12 (1994): 934–940; D. Pilpel et al., "Regional Differences in Appropriateness of Cholecystectomy in a Prepaid Health Insurance System," *Public Health Review* 20, no. 1–2 (1992–1993): 61–74; and S.J. Bernstein et al., "Appropriateness of Referral of Coronary Angiography Patients in Sweden: SECOR/SBU Project Group," *Heart* 81, no. 5 (1999): 470–477.
8. G.T. O'Connor et al., "A Regional Prospective Study of In-Hospital Mortality Associated with Coronary Artery Bypass Grafting: The Northern New England Cardiovascular Disease Study Group," *Journal of the American Medical Association* 266, no. 6 (1991): 803–809; H.S. Luft and P.S. Romano, "Chance, Continuity, and Change in Hospital Mortality Rates: Coronary Artery Bypass Graft Patients in California Hospitals, 1983 to 1989," *Journal of the American Medical Association* 270, no. 3 (1993): 331–337; E.L. Hannan et al., "Improving the Outcomes of Coronary Artery Bypass Surgery in New York State," *Journal of the American Medical Association* 271, no. 10 (1994): 761–766; and W.A. Ghali et al., "Coronary Artery Bypass Grafting in Canada: Hospital Mortality Rates, 1992–1995," *Canadian Medical Association Journal* 159, no. 8 (1998): 926–930.
9. S.F. Jencks et al., "Quality of Medical Care Delivered to Medicare Beneficiaries: A Profile at State and National Levels," *Journal of the American Medical Association* 284, no. 13 (2000): 1670–1676.
10. K.B. Wells et al., "Impact of Disseminating Quality Improvement Programs for Depression in Managed Primary Care: A Randomized Controlled Trial," *Journal of the American Medical Association* 283, no. 2 (2000): 212–220.
11. National Committee for Quality Assurance, *The State of Managed Care Quality* (Washington: NCQA, 1999).
12. D.W. Bates et al., "Effect of Computerized Physician Order Entry and a Team Intervention on Prevention of Serious Medication Errors," *Journal of the American Medical Association* 280, no. 15 (1998): 1311–1316.
13. Hannan et al., "Improving the Outcomes of Coronary Artery Bypass Surgery."
14. C.A. Cowan et al., "National Health Expenditures, 1998," *Health Care Financing Review* 21, no. 2 (1999): 165–210; G. Kessler and E. Pianin, "Bush Tax Cut Faces Spending Pressures," *Washington Post,* 25 January 2001, Al; and

National Institutes of Health Press Briefing on FY 2001 President's Budget, <www4.od.nih.gov/ofm/budget/fy2001pressbriefing.htm> (15 March 2001).
15. Selected national health accounts indicators for all World Health Organization member states, estimates for 1997, Statistical Annex, Table 8, <www.who.int/whr/2000/en/report.htm> (15 March 2001); and Cowan et al., "National Health Expenditures, 1998."

ARTICLE 3

HEALTH CARE REPORT CARDS

IMPLICATIONS FOR VULNERABLE PATIENT GROUPS AND THE ORGANIZATIONS PROVIDING THEM CARE

Huw T. O. Davies, A. Eugene Washington, and Andrew B. Bindman

Health care policy faces perennial tensions and compromises between three key objectives: controlling costs, improving quality, and widening access. Action in any one of these areas may impact detrimentally on progress in one or both of the other two. The past two decades have seen an explosion of work on measuring the quality of care as a precursor to driving through quality improvements. This movement then begs the question of how might attention to the quality part of the triad affect cost control and access?

Some of the debate surrounding the many quality initiatives has been about the potential impact on costs (Blumenthal 2001). Quality improvement may reduce costs by diminishing inappropriate use, ensuring timely preventive interventions, and avoiding iatrogenic harm (and thus unnecessary additional costs). In contrast, quality improvement may *increase* costs by increasing utilization of some expensive technologies and because quality improvement is itself a resource-hungry activity. It is far from clear how these two opposing forces will balance out in different settings, and detailed empirical work is needed to make the "cost-effectiveness case" for quality activities.

An issue that has received much less attention is the potential impact of quality improvement initiatives on patient access in general and equity in particular. Unpacking the implicit logic behind report cards, this study examines in detail the potentially important ways in which such measures of quality could adversely affect access. Specifically, we examine the recent trend toward the public reporting of health care performance data (both process measures and health outcomes) to examine the impact such activities might have on different population subgroups. As we identify many instances where there may be differential and adverse effects, the discussion makes several recommendations as to how these impacts might be clarified or ameliorated.

DEFINING VULNERABLE POPULATION SUBGROUPS

The population subgroups at the center of our analysis are those who, for a variety of reasons, are vulnerable to neglect by the health care system. Included in this category are the poor, the less educated, the uninsured, the chronically sick, and members of minority ethnic and language groups. Of course, the boundaries of these groups are not coterminous, nor are these groups mutually exclusive. Some individuals may possess several of the defining characteristics (bringing multiple problems), whereas others possess just one or none.

Categorizing the vulnerable populations in this way, while having some empirical base, nonetheless reflects a process of social construction, and such social constructions may "*influence the policy agenda and the selection of policy tools, as well as the rationales that legitimate policy choices*" (Schneider and Ingram 1993). In Schneider and Ingram's typology, policy subgroups may be constructed positively (e.g., deserving) or negatively (e.g., undeserving) and are differentiated in terms of power (weak/strong). Importantly, many of the population subgroups we focus on are frequently negatively constructed, often powerless, and are typically already underserved by health care in the United States (and elsewhere). A Rawlsian analysis (Rawls 1972) here would then suggest that because of this vulnerability and a lack of political leverage, researchers and policy makers have a special obligation to pay particular attention to their needs. Thus the possibility that health care report cards may have differential effects on these groups, further exacerbating extant difficulties, poses some important policy questions within this relatively new approach to health care quality.

Our definitions of vulnerable population subgroups thus emerge from a concern to bring to the fore issues germane to the marginalized and the less powerful. However, we do not suggest in our analysis that all vulnerable groups will necessarily be affected by report cards in similar ways, and we describe some of the ways in which the impacts will vary. One way in which we might distinguish relevant subgroups is by differentiating between those who have difficulty comprehending or making use of report card data (e.g., those with limited education, those for whom English is not their first language, those with literacy problems or learning difficulties as well as those who are seriously sick or mentally unwell) and those who may comprehend but simply have limited maneuverability to act on the information (the uninsured and those who for reasons of plan specification or geography have limited choice). Specifying in more detail the constituent subgroups gathered under our overarching label of "vulnerable" might at times refine the arguments (and we do so throughout the text). In general, however, we contend that there is often sufficient commonality to make an analysis of a broad collection of vulnerable groups worthwhile.

One issue to emerge, which is both troubling and frustrating, is the lack of empirical evidence for some of the difficulties that we postulate. Our concern here is that this is simply an absence of evidence of any kind rather than reassurance that the problems suggested are baseless. Indeed, perhaps the biggest single contribution from our analysis is to draw attention to the potential difficulties as a way of focusing future empirical study. We do not, however, underestimate the difficulties of such a task: identifying *any* substantial impacts of report cards has proved troublesome enough (Marshall et al. 2000); searching for subgroup effects will be even more challenging.

THE RISE OF THE REPORT CARD

An important component in the recent strategy for improving the quality of health care is the development and dissemination of health care report cards (U.S. General Administration Organization 1994; Epstein 1995, 1998; Wicks and Meyer 1999). Performance measures, covering the utilization rates of health care interventions as well as subsequent aggregate health outcomes, are used to describe the quality of care provided by medical institutions, health plans, and individual practitioners. Such activities are undertaken by federal agencies (such as the Health Care Financing Administration [HCFA]), state departments of health, as well as private sector, not-for-profit, and for-profit organizations (such as the National Committee for Quality Assurance [NCQA] and various consulting firms). In addition, large business purchasers, acting either individually or in consortia, are demanding much more information about the health care packages that they are purchasing.

A key feature of the report card movement is the public release of judgments on performance (Davies and Marshall 1999). Standardized public reporting on the quality of health care, particularly when it is linked to information on health care costs, offers an opportunity to empower consumers, either directly or through their employers, so that they can make choices that *can* result in better health care for less money. In addition, very public judgments about the quality of services affect the reputation of organizations, and organizations so affected might be expected to respond. There is some evidence that they will do so (Longo et al. 1997; Bentley and Nash 1998; Marshall et al. 2000; Davies 2001), and so report cards can thus feed into organizational learning, redirection, or restructuring.

LIMITATIONS OF REPORT CARDS

Even the most avid proponents of report cards recognize that they have some limitations. Problems arise in three distinct areas. The first concern is about the *relevance* of the measures used (Lansky 1998). Reporting of clinical performance has tended to focus on preventive services that are relatively easy to measure (e.g., mammogram rate) or big-ticket acute episodes (especially cardiovascular disease and elective surgery). Day-to-day primary care and the management of chronic disease have received less attention. A second major issue arises from disputes over the *meaningfulness* of the measures produced: there are many reasons to doubt that the rankings or categorizations used in report cards reflect accurately and robustly underlying true quality performance (U.S. General Administration Organization 1994; Goldstein and Spiegelhalter 1996; Davies and Crombie 1997). Even if the data do have some meaning, managed care plans are "bundled products" and consumers are unable to pick and mix from plans according to the individual indicators (Sullivan 1996). Finally, concerns abound over the *use and misuse* of the data produced: whether the data are accessed and interpreted by stakeholders (Hibbard and Jewett 1997; Hibbard et al. 1997), whether the data produce perverse incentives and dysfunctional effect (Smith 1995; Nutley and Smith 1998), and even whether the data have any impact at all (Davies 1998; Schneider and Epstein 1998).

The purpose of this article is not to reiterate these problems, which are in any case receiving some attention in this fast-moving field. Instead, we wish to assess how some of the potential flaws in clinical performance measurement may have a differential and disproportionate effect on vulnerable population subgroups and to examine how these effects might be ameliorated. The article is structured by examining three key concerns:

- relevance of typical report card measures to vulnerable patient groups;
- meaningfulness of existing aggregate measures to vulnerable patient groups;
- potential for differential effects on vulnerable patient groups and the providers who care for them arising from the dissemination and use of report cards.

Ways of dealing with these concerns and suggestions for future research are identified and elaborated in the concluding section.

RELEVANCE OF REPORT CARD DATA TO VULNERABLE PATIENT GROUPS

Wide acceptance of report cards has been an important indication that one of the major barriers to performance reporting, namely, the lack of consensus about what to measure, appears to have been overcome. Probably the most widely recognized measures are the Health Plan Employer Data and Information Set (HEDIS) indicators developed by the NCQA. However, in reviewing HEDIS and other publicly available report cards, we have to ask whether they accurately and equally capture the problems affecting different population subgroups. Many of the leading causes of death among minority and low-income groups (such as strokes, AIDS, and unintentional injuries) are underrepresented in most report cards. Some diseases that affect minority groups, such as sickle-cell anemia, are not covered at all. Other key health care concerns of vulnerable subgroups, such as nutritional needs and the impact of their living environment on their health, receive scant attention. Not only is it likely that quality problems in all of these areas may go unrecognized, but individuals in groups affected by these problems might not be able to make choices that are relevant to their needs. So while health plans are improving in their ability to report mammography screening rates, readily available data are unlikely to assist in choosing either a primary care provider or selecting providers adept (both clinically and culturally) in managing chronic conditions (such as hypertension) or diseases requiring specialist services (such as AIDS).

It is not just that the clinical spectrum covered by report cards may be largely irrelevant to vulnerable patient groups; the very emphasis on diseases, clinical procedures, and health status may be misplaced. For example, for many individuals with low income, key concerns center around issues of access: physical proximity of services; availability of appointments; extent of financial barriers (co-payments, deductibles, etc.); navigability of the bureaucratic restrictions on pharmacy benefits, referrals, and the like; and the quality of patient-provider communication (Stewart et al. 1999). If patients are to obtain maximal medical benefits, they need low financial and practical barriers, a clear understanding of their medical options, and they must feel comfortable seeking care when it is indicated. In addition, minority populations, particularly those for whom English is not their primary language, are more likely than many other patient groups to have comprehension difficulties and to be discouraged by culturally insensitive care. For these population subgroups, therefore, a key concern is access to "culturally appropriate" care, such as a physician or other health care worker from their own ethnic or language group, and access to culturally specific information and advice. Report card data have little to say on most of these crucial issues.

Whereas *what* is measured may be a problem, there are also concerns about *who* is captured by the report card samples. One disquietude is whether health care report cards sample adequately from vulnerable patient groups. Most obviously, the focus in report cards is almost exclusively on patients in managed care. However, substantial numbers of persons from low-income and minority groups are still not in managed care plans, for example, just over half of Medicaid beneficiaries (see report on-line at www.hcfa.gov/medicaid/mcsten00.pdf) and none of the uninsured. The experiences of these groups will therefore not be captured, further marginalizing an already disenfranchised group. Although the NCQA has attempted to address some of the health care service issues that are unique within the Medicaid population by developing a Medicaid version of the HEDIS, it is unclear what efforts have been made to really address those concerns most central to this group of users, and most of the items have not been validated as measures of quality. Even if these measures are ultimately found to be both relevant and valid, it is not clear that a Medicaid-focused report card would address the concerns of *other* vulnerable population groups that are *not* covered by Medicaid.

Even when persons from low-income and minority groups are in managed care organizations, their contribution to the measurement of quality of care may be underrepresented. A number of the measures of quality of care, such as patient satisfaction, require voluntary responses to surveys from patients. Persons of lower socioeconomic status and certain racial and ethnic minorities tend to be less likely to respond to traditional recruitment efforts (Melton 1993; Holt, Martin, and LoGerfo 1997). Standard approaches to reporting response rates, such as a health plan's overall survey participation rate, are inadequate for determining if there is a reasonable representation of minority populations. For example, a survey conducted with 34,000 Kaiser Permanente members reported an overall response rate of 57 percent but found significantly lower response rates for African Americans and Latinos compared to white and Asian subgroups (Gordon 1995). In addition, if approaches to gathering data for health care report cards deliberately exclude certain subgroups (perhaps for practical reasons), such as Spanish-speaking patients, the potential exists for significantly misrepresenting the quality of care for these populations.

It could be argued that when noncoverage results from selective nonresponse by certain population subgroups, then these groups have abrogated their right to inclusion. However, we need to recognize that declining to participate may be a legitimate response to being on the margins of society — fear of the IRS or the INS, for example, and a sense that one's input is not valued. A Rawlsian understanding of such preexisting inequalities places an obligation on those collating report card data to make additional efforts to ensure that such "hard to reach" groups are adequately represented.

Even when individuals from vulnerable groups *are* included in the samples used to derive report card indicators, the experience and outcomes for these groups could be diluted or even swamped by the inclusion of other larger groups with divergent experience. Aggregation of disparate experiences can lead to summary measures that are typical for no individual or group. In particular, given the extant difficulties faced by many vulnerable patient groups in obtaining adequate care, aggregate measures are likely to overestimate the quality of care received by these groups.

In summary, then, report card data may fail to capture health care issues of key relevance to population groups already typically underserved in health care, especially the poor, ethnic minorities, and those for whom English is not their first language. Minority subgroups may be undersampled (through either noncontact or nonresponse), and any data that are collected may be swamped by inappropriate aggregation. Thus the measures produced may have little relevance to underserved groups and may be unreflective of their experiences (with any analysis suggesting that the actual experience of vulnerable groups will be worse than that depicted by report cards). Such deficiencies may be of limited interest to report card vendors who may not see vulnerable patient groups as key stakeholders. Nonetheless, these concerns do pose some urgent policy questions.

MEANINGFULNESS

Many commentators have described the difficulties associated with making sense of the observational (i.e., nonrandomized) comparative data seen in report cards (*Lancet* 1993; Goldstein and Spiegelhalter 1996; Davies and Crombie 1997). It is not our intention to reiterate all those difficulties here. Nonetheless, there are a number of concerns specific to vulnerable groups that are germane and worthy of further elaboration.

The first point of note is that there may be differential levels to the validity and reliability of the data gathered. For self-reported data, for example, members of minority and low-income groups may be more likely to deliver "socially desirable" answers to questions about the provider-patient interaction, satisfaction, and functional/health status (Aday, Chiu, and Anderson 1980; Ross and Mirowsky 1984).

In addition, observer effects interacting with patient characteristics may further bias data gathered in clinical settings during health care delivery. Lack of blinding in routine data collection remains a concern — for example, studies show that assessors who are aware of previous treatment history may come to different assessments of patient outcomes than those who are not (Noseworthy et al. 1994).

The process used for analyzing health care report card data also holds some potential for introducing into the assessment of quality a bias based on race, ethnicity, or socioeconomic status. Since individuals are not randomly assigned to health plans or providers, there may be quite large differences between plans or providers in their respective pool of patients. For example, one plan might attract mostly white, well-educated, largely healthy people, while another might enroll mostly poor Hispanic individuals with poor initial health status. The statistical process of controlling for various differences between the groups managed by different plans or seen by different providers is called case-mix adjustment. This is necessary to ensure that the findings from report cards are appropriately attributed to quality of care and are not driven instead by variations in underlying patient characteristics (the problem of case mix). There is, however, no gold standard approach to adjusting the risks appropriately. Case-mix adjustment methods vary enormously in complexity and cost, and agreement among them is often poor (Iezzoni et al. 1994). A few states, including New York and California, have developed careful risk adjustment strategies that include patient demographics and clinical conditions (Hannan et al. 1994; Hannan et al. 1995; Romano et al. 1995); however, these are the exception. With few objective data about the validity and reliability of case-mix adjustment approaches, most health care report cards are either using proprietary ad hoc approaches, adjusting merely for age and sex, or (more likely) ignoring case-mix adjustment altogether. This may again lead to an overestimate of the expected outcomes where certain subgroups have, for example, more severe disease, a greater level of co-morbidity, or lower levels of compliance with treatment (some or all of which are likely to apply to various vulnerable patient subgroups). That is, presentations of some "average experience" will overestimate the true situation for patient groups whose individual characteristics make them less likely to achieve good outcomes.

Case-mix adjustment is critical even when quality is assessed using a validated measure of quality. For example, one of the initial HEDIS indicators of quality — asthma hospitalization rates — has been shown at the community level to be inversely associated with reports of access to health care. Patients who live in communities with better access to health care have lower rates of asthma hospitalization (Bindman et al. 1995). However, African American race and poverty are also independently associated with higher rates of asthma admissions. Thus, a health plan with a greater proportion of African Americans or persons of low income might be expected to have a higher rate of admissions for asthma than a plan with lower proportions of these individuals. Reporting health plans' quality on the basis of asthma admission rates without adjusting for underlying membership demographics and socioeconomics will generally make plans with fewer African American patients look like they are doing a better job. This problem is generic. Race, ethnicity, and socioeconomic status have been shown repeatedly to be associated with health service utilization and health outcomes — patients from vulnerable groups having lower levels of utilization and poorer outcomes (Shulman et al. 1995). However, health care report cards are rarely adjusted for these characteristics, in part because many health plans and providers incorrectly believe that they are precluded by civil rights protection from systematically collecting information on their patients' race and ethnicity.

An additional complexity that arises in attempting to adjust measures of quality is that the variables used to make an adjustment can themselves vary according to race and ethnicity. Since many of the indicators of quality included in health care report cards are utilization measures, investigators have recognized the importance of adjusting for health status or need in order to reach a conclusion about quality. For example, with measures such as childhood immunization rates, the determination of need is derived from the age of the child, and it is assumed that if a child of the appropriate age did not receive recommended immunizations that this signifies a quality defect. Other process measures of health care quality are not so easily defined. For example, measures such as the percentage of health plan members who have had a physician visit in a given time period are best analyzed by adjusting for a direct assessment of the patient's need for care. It would be inappropriate to use the same number of physician visits as an indicator of quality in patients who are generally healthy as for those who have chronic conditions such as asthma, AIDS, or cancer. Unfortunately, there has been no consensus reached on what variables should be used in the adjustment for need. In examining six indicators of "need for care," Osmond et al. (1996) found that no single measure provided a valid estimate of the relationship between need for health care and outpatient visits across ethnic groups. There were significant interactions between racial/ethnic group and need measures when used to predict outpatient visits. As a result, applying "need adjustment" to use of health care services without regard for ethnic variability could lead to biased conclusions about quality.

One final difficulty in analyzing report card data arises when these measures focus on processes (utilization) rather than on the outcomes of care. The relationship between the process and outcomes of care can differ by racial and ethnic groups. For example, some data indicate that the response to beta-blockers, diuretics, ACE inhibitors, and beta agonists differs by race (Saunders 1991; Lange et al. 1995), with those from minority groups receiving fewer benefits than whites from application of these therapies. To the degree that value judgments about quality are made about process measures (such as the percentage of patients on particular medications), individuals from minority groups may be misled about the quality of outcomes that they can expect to obtain: anticipated benefits may not, in actuality, accrue.

In short, there are many reasons to suspect that biases in data collection and absent or imperfect case-mix adjustment will lead to measures that provide an inaccurate picture of the true quality of care likely to be received by members of typically underserved groups. These biases, combined with a weaker link between processes and outcomes for these same groups, may conspire to paint an overoptimistic picture of the quality of care — in terms of both process and outcomes — that these groups can expect to receive in reality.

INTERPRETATION AND USE

The belief that report cards can empower consumers is predicated on an assumption that consumers have options between which they have meaningful choice. For the uninsured this is manifestly untrue. Even for those with health insurance the position is little better (Gabel, Ginsburg, and Hunt 1997). The latest survey data from the Kaiser Family Fund (available on-line at www.kff.org) show that, whereas about two-thirds of large firms (greater than 1,000 workers) offer a choice of health plans, less than 10 percent of small firms (fewer than 200 workers) do (data for 2001). Compared to earlier survey findings, these data suggest that employees of larger firms may be getting more choice while those in small firms have seen their chances of choice diminish. Access to choice also varies between socioeconomic groups, with most choice usually available to the affluent and least choice (or no choice at all) being commonplace among the poor (Gawande et al. 1998).

In order for report cards to influence consumer choice, they must be broadly available and contain information that patients value and understand. An AHRQ/ Kaiser Family Foundation national survey in 2000 (on-line at www.kff.org) found that only 27 percent of consumers had seen health care quality data in the past year, and less than half of these said that they had used such information. These figures actually seem to have diminished since earlier surveys (Robinson and Brodie 1997). Of particular concern is whether persons from minority and low-income groups are able to interpret health care report card data and to use this information to achieve high-quality care. Focus groups conducted with thirty-five- to fifty-five-year-old individuals revealed widespread misunderstanding of health care report card data (Jewett and Hibbard 1996). Privately insured individuals were more likely to acknowledge their lack of comprehension of report card data while Medicaid and uninsured patients were more likely not even to know they were misinterpreting the information. For example, Medicaid and uninsured patients believed that providers and health plans that had high rates of hospitalization for asthma were providing high-quality care because it suggested an ability to be hospitalized when needed (in fact, a high asthma hospitalization rate is intended to demonstrate poor-quality delivery of primary care that could have prevented the need for the admission). These findings underscore the potential for report card measures to mislead rather than enlighten consumers, a concern that goes beyond simple literacy issues (Root and Stableford 1999). Cultural, educational, and linguistic barriers cannot but exacerbate these difficulties among vulnerable groups; information brokers or patient advocates may in turn mitigate the identified problems.

Currently there is little evidence that report card data are having any major effects on purchasers or providers (Davies and Marshall 1999; Marshall et al. 2000; Davies 2001). However, such data are in their infancy, and many are hopeful that their impact will increase (Epstein 1998; Wicks and Meyer 1999). In one sense, however, quality data more generally may have a profound impact on services for vulnerable population groups. For example, in the past, decisions to close "safety net" facilities have sometimes been made on the basis that the quality of care has declined to such a point that public interest is best served by closing the institution (e.g., Philadelphia General Hospital [Friedman 1987]). The real reasons for decline (such as financial stringency) get subsumed into more acceptable arguments about quality of care. Thus quality assessment may be a policy tool used to change service configurations, and report cards could be the new vehicle for advancing such arguments.

If report card data do become more significant in the medical marketplace then this may pose additional dangers for vulnerable patient groups already underserved by the health system. Plans and providers that currently provide care to a disproportionate number of minority and low-income populations are in danger of having their quality of care judged as inferior perhaps simply because of the characteristics of their patient population. Recent empirical work emphasizes that these issues are of real concern: adjusting HEDIS measures for sociodemographic variables made little difference to the majority of health plans but had substantial impact on a few (Zaslavsky et al. 2000). Those plans most affected were those that had "*unusually large concentrations of members in areas with characteristics associated with poor performance*" (e.g., high proportion of Hispanic or large proportion receiving public assistance) (ibid.). Without proper risk adjustment, health plans and providers are likely to attempt to avoid minority and low-income patients not only because they could create poor health care report card scores but also because they may be more costly to care for. These exclusions (risk selection) may operate at "corporate" level or at the level of the individual physician.

Discrimination against patients termed "hard to manage" may operate in more subtle ways than simply refusing individuals access to the system. Even when individuals are enrolled with a health plan or are accepted for care by a provider they may be denied the full intensity of care. The temptation to providers worried about report card indicators may be to give greatest effort to those aspects of care and with those individuals where the payback is likely to be commensurate. For example, consider primary care providers wanting to increase their mammography rate. Where should they concentrate their efforts on outreach? Presented with the choice between white middle-class women and the indigent — homeless or rootless — and women with a poor grasp of English, providers can be expected to pursue the options likely to bring the greatest return. The fact that individual physician profiles are very sensitive to changes in the care of just a handful of individuals to shift the profile from "aberrant" to "average" makes such shifts uncomfortably plausible and hard to detect (Hofer et al. 1999).

In summary, for all the hyperbole surrounding the public release of performance data, considerable doubt remains as to whether these data are accessed, are used in decision making, or are otherwise influential (Davies 1998; Marshall et al. 2000). Even if such data do have an effect, there is no guarantee that the effects will be desirable: dysfunctional change, and especially encouragement to select away from disadvantaged groups, is a real possibility. Furthermore the efforts that plans and providers make to improve their monitored processes could be diverting resources from unmonitored clinical areas (Davies 2001). Regardless, whatever the effects that do exist, they are likely to be different for different vulnerable patient groups. In each case such differential effects are likely to run counter to the interests of existing underserved groups.

DISCUSSION: AMELIORATING THE DIFFERENTIAL EFFECTS OF REPORT CARDS

The United States and other developed countries have embarked on a course of making data on health care quality available to the public and other stakeholders. The development and release of health care report cards on specific health plans and providers parallels a movement occurring across other parts of the public sector (especially education) and many parts of private industry. Notwithstanding the concerns about both the technical qualities of the measures used in health care (Goldstein and Spiegelhalter 1996; Davies and Crombie 1997; Iezzoni 1997) and their potential for misuse (Smith 1995; Davies and Lampel 1998), it seems very unlikely that this particular genie can be put back in the bottle. Public interest and freedom-of-information concerns more or less demand that such data be made publicly available. The debate for or against such an approach to health care quality is one that will no doubt continue to rage, but this (often polarized) debate is not the main focus of this analysis.

Instead, our specific concern was to examine the implications of the widespread reporting of clinical performance data for specific population subgroups, especially those vulnerable in the health system and traditionally underserved in health care (the poor, less educated, chronically sick, and ethnic-linguistic minorities). In doing so, we do not seek to apportion blame to the individual players in the system, such as those who create, research, and market report cards. Instead we have sought to develop an overarching analysis of the effects — many unwanted — that have been created by the wide range of activity in this field. Finding empirical support for many of these effects may take considerable time, energy, and ingenuity: even identifying gross effects of report cards has proved difficult (Marshall et al. 2000); assessing subgroup impacts will be more so. Yet framing the correct questions now, and focusing research effort accordingly, could help inform the report card debate before the style and use of such tools becomes too entrenched. We believe that our analysis poses broad policy questions given the current proliferation of report cards.

Four major concerns emerge from this analysis. *First, the public release of clinical performance data may offer little to patients from vulnerable subgroups.* These groups are among those least likely to have health care choices in the first place, they are less likely to access the data for cultural and educational reasons, and they are more likely to have special difficulties making sense of such data. The areas of health care covered by the measures may have only limited relevance to their everyday health care concerns. In addition, patients from vulnerable groups are likely to have been underrepresented in the samples from which the measures are calculated (which may then say little about the sorts of experiences that they can expect). Thus the gap in empowerment and enlightened choice may be further widened between the underserved and the articulate middle classes.

Second, the public release of clinical performance data skewed away from the interests of vulnerable patient groups may further enhance neglect of services for these groups. If it is true that "what gets measured gets attention" and assuming that report cards are able to encourage at least some beneficial performance improvements, then the comparative neglect of measures central to the concerns of vulnerable patient groups may again distract attention from resourcing and improving these services. Thus the health care needs of the underserved may be further marginalized. The growing disinterest on the part of commercial health plans to compete for Medicaid beneficiaries is primarily economic, but it also suggests that even Medicaid beneficiaries (who in many ways are more powerful than other vulnerable groups such as the uninsured) are going to have difficulties getting health plans to take seriously their specific health care quality concerns.

Third, for fear of looking bad in publicly released data sets, health plans and providers can be expected to avoid caring for "hard to manage" individuals. Widespread recognition that caring for individuals from vulnerable patient groups is likely to bias report card results in unfavorable directions provides incentives for risk selection to occur. Thus organizations may seek not only to avoid certain patient groups entirely, but also may discriminate between individuals according to expected levels of compliance and efficacy when allocating service effort. Again, this bias is likely to work against the interests of the underserved.

Fourth, the public release of performance data may be damaging to organizations that service a disproportionate number of vulnerable patients. Organizations providing services to difficult to manage groups may appear as poor performers not because they are intrinsically failing but because the nature of their client population makes success that much harder to achieve. This both damages the prospects of such organizations (for example, reputation may be diminished and contracts may be lost) and consequently provides a perverse incentive for them to de-emphasize the enrollment and care of the most needy groups. Each of these in turn is detrimental to the interests of underserved populations.

RECOMMENDATIONS: LESSENING DIFFERENTIAL EFFECTS

It is an imperative (derived from Rawls's [1972] second principle of justice) that well-meaning attempts at quality improvement do nothing to widen existing health care inequities. That an analysis of report cards from the perspective of vulnerable patient groups should reveal a plethora of worrisome issues may come as little surprise but does deserve attention. The health care system already offers many barriers and obstacles that hamper these groups from obtaining appropriate, effective, and culturally sensitive care. The characteristics that make individuals vulnerable in the health system (poverty, lack of education, inarticulateness, lack of English language) often come together, leading to multiple cumulative problems. This vulnerability, powerlessness, and potential for additional differential disadvantage arising from the proliferation of report cards provide a compelling argument for further policy analysis and action. Indeed, our analysis suggests a number of areas where steps could be taken to ameliorate the potentially deleterious impacts on vulnerable patient groups.

First, a concerted research effort should document any differential effect of report cards on vulnerable patient groups. Existing empirical evidence in this area may be lacking, yet our analysis suggests a number of plausible concerns. Much more focused research is needed to uncover the presence and extent of the problems identified. Perhaps these problems will turn out to be inconsequential in size or effect — but as yet we have little data to provide such reassurance, and we need to look harder. Without such reassurance we should at least be prepared to put in place monitoring systems that can evaluate any deleterious or disproportionate impacts arising from the public release of data.

Second, special efforts are needed to address the information needs of vulnerable patient groups. The range of measures available for comparative performance is growing all the time. As such bodies as NCQA, the Joint Commission on Accreditation of Healthcare Organizations (JCAHO), and HCFA increase the data demands placed on plans and providers, they should ensure that these demands cover at least some of the concerns of vulnerable patient groups. This may involve, for example, the generation of new measures specific to vulnerable groups (for example, sickle-cell disease) and measures that document the extent and impact of other system features (such as access to culturally appropriate care, pharmacy benefit limitations, and the use of co-payments). Some of the latter issues are beginning to be addressed with the Consumer Assessment of Health Plans Project (CAHPS; available on-line at www.ahrq.gov/qual/cahp-six.htm), and AHRQ are also funding further research in this area. In addition, data presentation must be designed to meet the information needs of individuals as well as group purchasers. Special attempts could also be made to connect vulnerable patients to the data, providing, for example, interpretation assistance, information brokers, and advocacy services.

Third, oversampling of minority groups and stratification of the data may help to highlight the care of those with distinctive health care experiences. This would help overcome the danger that these groups get swamped in the aggregation needed for analysis. Further, presentation of data stratified by age, gender, ethnicity, co-morbidity, or socioeconomic status could prove valuable as a means of highlighting the experiences of underserved groups. Current approaches to data presentation based around aggregation and averages offer little to those who are atypical.

Fourth, improvements to risk-adjustment methodologies are needed, but these cannot obviate the need for inherently fair comparisons. The possibility of using risk-adjustment models extended to include, for example, ethnicity and socioeconomic status, needs special mention. Although superficially attractive, this approach nonetheless contains certain dangers. Most crucially, in attempting to get a clearer picture of the performance of those caring for vulnerable patient groups we must be careful not to excuse or institutionalize any poor clinical performance in the care of these patients. That is, using risk adjustment models that include demographic, ethnic, and socioeconomic variables may simply "adjust away" important information on performance that could otherwise be valuable in dragging upward the care of the vulnerable and underserved. This fear suggests that a preferable approach is the presentation of stratified data and the restriction of comparisons to like-with-like, that is, comparisons of the care of similar groups of patients (e.g., African Americans, chronically sick patients) in similar organizations (between, say, public providers).

Finally, reimbursement strategies need to pay further attention to the difficulties and excess costs associated with providing services to hard-to-manage groups. It is ironic that the preceding three recommendations may actually exacerbate the concerns of plans and providers that it is not in their interest to care for patients from vulnerable population subgroups. Thus it becomes essential that concomitant attention is paid to this final recommendation. In particular, payment approaches that involve substantial risk sharing or reimbursement on the basis of health outcomes (Kindig 1997) may need careful scrutiny. Both have the potential to return inadequate recompensation to providers struggling to manage clients with special needs, high levels of concomitant problems, or compliance issues.

Careful balance is needed in all of these suggested approaches to ameliorating the differential effects of report cards on vulnerable patient groups. Hidden dangers include labeling and stigmatizing certain patient groups, oversensitizing plans and providers to the deleterious consequences of caring for these individuals (and so bringing about the very perverse incentives of which we warn), and providing excuses to the health care system for substandard or variable care. However, simply ignoring the special difficulties faced in providing care to certain patient groups is unhelpful. The report card movement needs to embrace this analysis and respond to these concerns.

The process for developing and disseminating health care report cards remains in a relatively embryonic stage (Epstein 1998). Nonetheless, reports have been introduced into the medical market in part with the assumption that this implementation will catalyze the rate of their improvement. While this may be true, patients of today must nonetheless still live with the consequences of existing deficiencies. That the flaws in current health care report cards may not be evenly distributed among plans, providers, and patients is cause for concern and worthy of some attention. Gains in quality for some may be offset by losses in quality for others and may exacerbate access difficulties. At the very least, an opportunity will have been missed to help narrow the health care gap between those already well able to navigate through a complex health system and others, such as vulnerable patient groups, who are not. In summary, clinical performance data may be detrimental to minority and low-income populations and the providers who care for them — providing additional challenges to those interested in equity as well as quality.

ACKNOWLEDGMENTS

The authors gratefully acknowledge support from the Agency for Healthcare Research and Quality (AHRQ) (HS07373) and The Commonwealth Fund. However, the views presented here are those of the authors and not necessarily those of any of the funding bodies. Huw Davies was a Harkness Fellow in Health Care Policy based at the

Institute for Health Policy Studies, University of California, San Francisco, during the preparation of this article and is very grateful to the Institute for its hospitality.

REFERENCES

Aday, L., G. Chiu, and R. Anderson. 1980. Methodological Issues in Health Care Surveys of the Spanish Language Population. *American Journal of Public Health* 70:367–374.

Bentley, J. M., and D. B. Nash. 1998. How Pennsylvania Hospitals Have Responded to Publicly Released Reports on Coronary Artery Bypass Graft Surgery. *Joint Commission Journal on Quality Improvement* 24:40–49.

Bindman, A. B., K. Grumbach, D. Osmond, M. Komaromy, K. Vranizan, N. Lurie, J. Billings, and A. Stewart. 1995. Preventable Hospitalizations and Access to Health Care. *Journal of the American Medical Association* 274:305–311.

Blumenthal, D. 2001. Controlling Health Care Expenditures. *New England Journal of Medicine* 344(10):766–769.

Davies, H. T. O. 1998. Performance Management Using Health Outcomes: In Search of Instrumentality. *Journal of Evaluation in Clinical Practice* 4:150–153.

———. 2001. Public Release of Performance Data and Quality Improvement: Internal Responses to External Data by U.S. Health Care Providers. *Quality in Health Care* 10:104–110.

Davies, H. T. O., and I. K. Crombie. 1997. Interpreting Health Outcomes. *Journal of Evaluation in Clinical Practice* 3(3):187–200.

Davies, H. T. O., and J. Lampel. 1998. Trust in Performance Indicators. *Quality in Health Care* 7:159–162.

Davies, H. T. O., and M. N. Marshall. 1999. Public Disclosure of Performance Data. Does the Public Get What the Public Wants? *Lancet* 353:1639–1640.

Epstein, A. 1995. Performance Reports on Quality — Prototypes, Problems, and Prospects. *New England Journal of Medicine* 333:57–61.

———. 1998. Rolling Down the Runway; the Challenges Ahead for Quality Report Cards. *Journal of the American Medical Association* 279:1691–1696.

Friedman, E. 1987. Demise of Philadelphia General an Instructive Case; Other Cities Treat Public Hospital Ills Differently. *Journal of the American Medical Association* 257:1571–1575.

Gabel, J., P. Ginsburg, and K. Hunt. 1997. Small Employers and Their Health Benefits, 1988–1996: An Awkward Adolescence. *Health Affairs* 16(5):103–110.

Gawande, A., R. Blendon, M. Brodie, J. Benson, L. Levitt, and L. Hugick. 1998. Does Dissatisfaction with Health Plans Stem from Having No Choices? *Health Affairs* 17(5):187–194.

Goldstein, H., and D. J. Spiegelhalter. 1996. League Tables and Their Limitations: Statistical Issues in Comparisons of Institutional Performance. *Journal of the Royal Statistical Society* 159(3):385–443.

Gordon, N. P. 1995. Surveillance of Health, Functional Status, and Satisfaction of Health Plan Members by Mailed Survey: Potential Sources of Bias. *American Public Health Association Abstract* #303.

Hannan, E. L., H. Kilburn, M. Racz, E. Shields, and M. R. Chassin. 1994. Improving the Outcomes of Coronary Artery Bypass Surgery in New York State. *Journal of the American Medical Association* 271:761–766.

Hannan, E. L., A. L. Siu, D. Kumar, H. Kilburn, and M. R. Chassin. 1995. The Decline in Coronary Artery Bypass Graft Surgery Mortality in New York State. *Journal of the American Medical Association* 273:209–213.

Hibbard, J. H., and J. J. Jewett. 1997. Will Quality Report Cards Help Consumers? *Health Affairs* 16:218–228.

Hibbard, J. H., J. J. Jewett, M. W. Legnini, and M. Tusler. 1997. Choosing a Health Plan: Do Large Employers Use the Data? *Health Affairs* 16:172–180.

Hofer, T. P., R. A. Hayward, S. Greenfield, E. H. Wagner, S. H. Kaplan, and W. G. Manning. 1999. The Unreliability of Individual Physician "Report Cards" for Assessing the Costs and Quality of Care of a Chronic Disease. *Journal of the American Medical Association* 281:2098–2105.

Holt, V., D. Martin, and J. LoGerfo. 1997. Correlates and Effect of Non-Response in a Postpartum Survey of Obstetrical Care Quality. *Journal of Clinical Epidemiology* 50(10):1117–1122.

Iezzoni, L. I. 1997. The Risks of Risk Adjustment. *Journal of the American Medical Association* 278(19):1600–1607.

Iezzoni, L., A. Ash, M. Schwartz, J. Daley, J. Hughes, and Y. Mackiernan. 1994. Predicting Who Dies Depends on How Severity Is Measured: Implications for Evaluating Patient Outcomes. *Annals of Internal Medicine* 123: 763–770.

Jewett, J. J., and J. H. Hibbard. 1996. Comprehension and Quality Care Indicators: Differences among Privately Insured, Publicly Insured, and Uninsured. *Health Care Financing Review* 18:75–94.

Kindig, D. A. 1997. *Purchasing Population Health: Paying for Results.* Ann Arbor: University of Michigan Press.

Lancet. 1993. Dicing with Death Rates [editorial]. *Lancet* 341:1183–1184.

Lang, C. C., C. M. Stein, R. M. Brown, R. Deegan, R. Nelson, H. B. He, M. Wood, and A. J. Wood. 1995. Attenuation of Isoproterenol-Mediated Vasodilation in Blacks. *New England Journal of Medicine* 333:155–160.

Lansky, D. 1998. Measuring What Matters to the Public. *Health Affairs* 17:40–41.

Longo, D. R., G. Land, W. Schramm, J. Fraas, B. Hoskins, and V. Howell. 1997. Consumer Reports in Health Care; Do They Make a Difference in Patient Care? *Journal of the American Medical Association* 278:1579–1584.

Marshall, M. N., P. G. Shekelle, S. Leatherman, and R. H. Brook. 2000. The Public Release of Performance Data. What Do We Expect to Gain? A Review of the Evidence. *Journal of the American Medical Association* 283:1866–1874.

Melton, L. J. 1993. Non-Response Bias in Studies of Diabetic Complications: The Rochester Diabetes Neuropathy Study. *Clinical Epidemiology* 46:341–348.

National Committee for Quality Assurance (NCQA). 1999. *HEDIS. The Health Plan Employer Data and Information Set*. Washington, DC: National Committee for Quality Assurance.

Noseworthy, J. H., G. C. Ebers, M. K. Vandervoort, R. E. Farquhar, E. Yetisir, and R. Roberts. 1994. The Impact of Blinding on the Results of a Randomized, Placebo-Controlled Multiple Sclerosis Clinical Trial. *Neurology* 44(1):16–20.

Nutley, S., and P. Smith. 1998. League Tables for Performance Improvement in Health Care. *Journal of Health Services Research and Policy* 3:50–57.

Osmond, D. H., K. Vranzian, D. Schillinger, A. L. Stewart and A. B. Bindman. 1996. Measuring the Need for Medical Care in an Ethnically Diverse Population. *Health Services Research* 31:551–571.

Rawls, J. 1972. *A Theory of Justice*. Oxford: Oxford University Press.

Robinson, S., and M. Brodie. 1997. Understanding the Quality Challenge for Health Consumers: The Kaiser/AHCPR Survey. *Journal on Quality Improvement* 23:239–244.

Romano, P. S., A. Zach, H. S. Luft, J. Rainwater, L. L. Remy, and D. Camoa. 1995. The California Hospital Outcomes Project: Using Administrative Data to Compare Hospital Performance. *Joint Commission Journal on Quality Improvement* 21:668–682.

Root, J., and S. Stableford. 1999. Easy-to-Read Consumer Communications: A Missing Link in Medicaid Managed Care. *Journal of Health Politics, Policy and Law* 24(1):1–26.

Ross, C., and J. Mirowsky. 1984. Socially-Desirable Response and Acquiescence in a Cross-Cultural Survey of Mental Health. *Journal of Health and Social Behavior* 25 (June): 189–197.

Saunders, E. 1991. Hypertension in African-Americans. *Circulation* 83:1465–1467.

Schneider, A., and H. Ingram. 1993. Social Construction of Target Populations: Implications for Politics and Policy. *American Political Science Review* 87(2):334–347.

Schneider, E. C., and A. M. Epstein. 1998. Use of Public Performance Reports: A Survey of Patients Undergoing Cardiac Surgery. *Journal of the American Medical Association* 279:1638–1642.

Shulman, K. A., E. Rubenstein, F. D. Chesley, and J. M. Eisenberg. 1995. The Roles of Race and Socioeconomic Factors in Health Services Research. *Health Services Research* 30 (pt. 2):179–195.

Smith, P. 1995. On the Unintended Consequences of Publishing Performance Data in the Public Sector. *International Journal of Public Administration* 18:277–310.

Stewart, A. L., A. Napoles-Springer, E. J. Perez-Stable, S. F. Posner, A. B. Bindman, H. L. Pinderhughes, and A. E. Washington. 1999. Interpersonal Processes of Care in Diverse Populations. *Milbank Quarterly* 77(3):305–339.

Sullivan, K. 1996. Health Insurance Report Cards Cannot Work. Available on-line at http://www.zmag.org/zmag/articles/dec96sullivan.htm (accessed May 2001).

U.S. General Administration Organization. 1994. *Report Cards Are Useful but Significant Issues Need to Be Addressed*. Washington, DC: Government Printing Office.

Wicks, E. K., and J. A. Meyer. 1999. Making Report Cards Work. *Health Affairs* 18:152–155.

Zaslavsky, A. M., J. N. Hochheimer, E. C. Schneider, P. D. Cleary, J. J. Seidman, E. A. McGlynn, J. W. Thompson, C. Sennett, and A. M. Epstein. 2000. Impact of Sociodemographic Case Mix on the HEDIS Measures of Health Plan Quality. *Medical Care* 38:981–992.

PART VI

WOMEN'S HEALTH AND THE HEALTH CARE SYSTEM

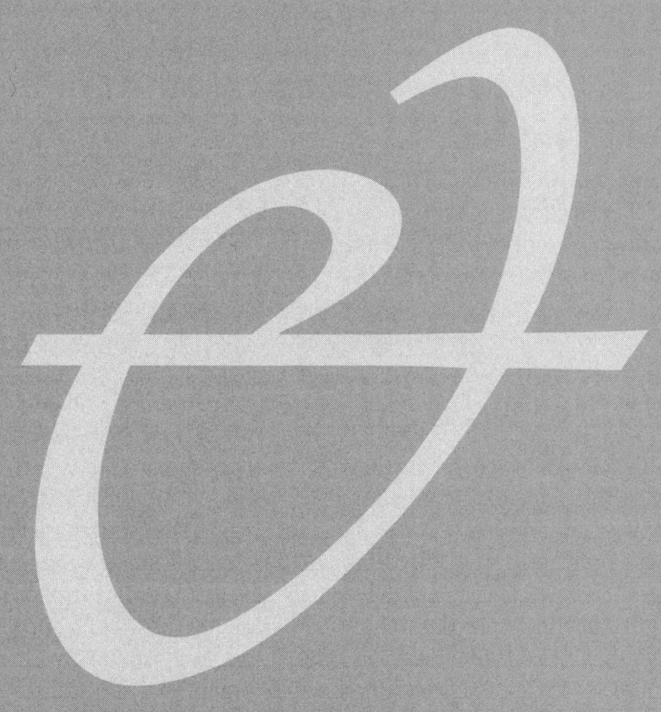

CHAPTER 10

WOMEN'S HEALTH AND THE HEALTH CARE SYSTEM

At the start of the 21st century, health care for women faces a number of critical challenges. New data are challenging old ways of providing care and exposing large disparities in the health status of women. The first results of the Women's Health Initiative have been released, revealing both critical clinical information and the importance of engaging in research on women's health. Reanalysis of old data is calling into question the value of common prevention activities, including screening mammography. Reproductive health services remain highly politicized. In his first act in office, President Bush reinstated the global gag rule prohibiting recipients of U.S. aid from discussing or engaging in activities related to abortion (Hwang, 2002). The domestic push for abstinence-only education is dominating discussions about welfare reform and access to family planning services (Boonstra and Gold, 2002). Access to health care remains limited for millions of women as the numbers of uninsured continue to rise, and the women who most need the care often delay or do not receive it (Salganicoff et al., 2002; Williams, 2002). At this juncture in history we are again reminded of the value of viewing the health care system through a woman's lens as well as the need to pay attention to the biological, social, political, and economic dimensions of health. The articles in this chapter provide only a snapshot of some of the important issues in women's health. Further references are provided in the Recommended Reading list.

HEALTH CONCERNS OF NONELDERLY WOMEN

This chapter begins with the executive summary of an important survey of women's health conducted in 2001 by the Kaiser Family Foundation (KFF) to learn more about the experiences of women with their health plans and their health providers (Salganicoff et al., 2002). The study pays particular attention to those women most likely to fall through the cracks of the health care system: women of color, those without health insurance, and those who are poor. The key findings of this study are that the health care system is not meeting the health needs of a sizable share of women and that those who need health services the most have the hardest time getting care. Costs related to health care continue to present significant problems for women, and the affordability of prescription drugs is a primary concern for many women.

The KFF survey highlights a new area of concern for health care advocates, namely, quality of care. (This new focus of interest is discussed in greater detail in Chapter 9.) As is pointed out in an article by Davies, Washington, and Bindman (2002; see Article 3, Chapter 9), quality concerns are unique for populations traditionally underserved by the health care system. Women are such a population. As the KFF survey results highlight, while one in five women overall (21%) expressed concerns about the quality of the care they received, 40% of women in fair or poor health had significant concerns about the quality of the care they received. For many women, quality of care is compromised because their connection to the health care system is unstable. In the KFF survey, nearly one in three women reported they were uninsured at some point during the past year (Salganicoff et al., 2002).

A special issue of the *Journal of the American Medical Women's Association* (JAMWA, 2002) was devoted to the effects of welfare reform on women's health. In an article included in the Recommended Reading, Boonstra and Gold (2002) reflect on the implications for reproductive health policy, examining the effects of breaking the historic link between eligibility for welfare benefits and eligibility for Medicaid. They raise concerns about ending the long-standing requirement that welfare recipients have access to family planning. They also comment on the use of incentives to reduce out-of-wedlock childbearing and to promote abstinence-only education, questioning efforts to control the reproductive lives of poor women. Five years after the passage of the Personal Responsibility and Work Opportunity Act in 1996, the number of women enrolled in Medicaid is down and the number not covered by insurance is up. Although the intent of the policy change was to protect the Medicaid status of former welfare recipients, the delinking has not worked. Rather, the effort to "end welfare as we know it" has had negative implications for the health of poor women (Chavkin, Wise, and Romero (2002), see Recommended Reading).

HEALTH CONCERNS OF ELDERLY WOMEN

Poor women are also affected by policy efforts targeted at the other end of the age spectrum, as discussed by Rice (1999) in her article "Medicare: A Women's Issue" (see Recommended Reading). Rice highlights women's greater dependency on Medicare, which results from increased longevity, higher rates of poverty, and poorer health status. The greater longevity for women (and men) since 1965 is certainly related to Medicare; since the enactment of Medicare, life expectancy for women aged 65 years has increased from 15.8 years in 1960 to 19.2 years in 1988 (Moon, 2001). Because of their greater longevity, women constitute a larger percentage of Medicare beneficiaries than men and subsequently rely on Medicare for more years.

Despite their increased longevity, women suffer from higher rates of chronic diseases and greater numbers of conditions per individual than men. Consequently, women report lower health status and higher utilization of health services.

Unfortunately, health status is not the only characteristic that declines for women with age. Older women are twice as likely as older men to be poor, and poverty among older women increases with age. Much of this rise in poverty is explained by women's marital status and living arrangements, which change dramatically with age. Current gaps in Medicare, including lack of coverage for prescription drugs and insufficient long-term care, disproportionately affect older women, who consequently have higher out-of pocket costs despite lower incomes. However, as Rice notes, even with the limits of Medicare, women have benefited from its existence. Therefore, efforts to reform Medicare that do not address current gaps or that reduce access to current benefits are potentially detrimental to the health of older women (Rice, 1999).

Weitz and Estes (2001; Article 2) provide greater analysis of the issues specific to older women. These authors note that while the current models for health care delivery, financing, and policy fail to meet the needs of women in general, older women are a vulnerable population that must be examined. To understand the complex interaction of medical, social, and economic factors that affect women's wellness, Weitz and Estes argue for a new paradigm that bridges the gap between those who are concerned about aging issues and those concerned about women's health. This new framework takes account of the institutional structures and relations that greatly influence the economic security of women and their ability to access health resources as they age. To bridge the gap between women's issues and aging concerns, the authors advance three interrelated themes: "(1) there is a gendered relationship between socioeconomic structures and health over time; (2) there are gender-specific implications of health care financing and policy; and (3) there are health consequences to the gendered nature of caregiving" (Weitz and Estes, 2001, p. 4).

THE ROLE OF RACE/ETHNICITY AND SOCIOECONOMIC STATUS

Professor David Williams, a leading scholar on racial/ethnic differences in health, has finally turned his eye to the issue of gender. In Article 3, he emphasizes the importance of attending to diversity in the health profiles and populations of minority women. Williams notes that white women have a life expectancy at birth that exceeds that of their black peers by 5.2 years, and that for the 10 leading causes of death in 1998 for women, there are variations across major racial/ethnic populations. There are also major variations within racial/ethnic classifications that must be attended to. In addition to providing an overview of racial/ethnic disparities in health for U.S. women, Williams discusses the complex interactions between race/ethnicity and socioeconomic status in affecting women's health.

Socioeconomic status is typically assessed by income, education, or occupation (Williams, 2002). Unfortunately, defining and understanding these indices for women are especially difficult (Krieger, Williams, and Moss, 1997; McDonough et al., 1999). For example, research has yet to determine how best to define a married woman's social class in relationship to the social class of her husband or what the relationship is between an unmarried woman's social class and the social class of her parents (Feinleib and Ingster, 1999). However, despite the imprecise nature of these indices, researchers argue that economic structural relationships play a major role in shaping women's health (Moss, 2000). Women with more education and higher income live longer than women with fewer years of schooling and less income, and they are healthier along the way (Moss, 2000). Irrespective of race, women who are poor or near poor are far more likely to describe themselves as in fair or poor health than women with middle or higher incomes (Moss, 2000). A woman's chance of getting medical care depends on her employment and marital status, and she is often disadvantaged compared with a comparably situated man (Benderly and Institute of Medicine, 1997). In his work, however, Williams points out that there is nonequivalence of measures of socioeconomic status across race/ethnicity. Disparities exist in quality of education, the purchasing power of income, the stability of employment, and the health risks associated with working in particular occupations (Williams and Collins, 1995).

THE IMPORTANCE OF RESEARCH

As the social understanding of women's health continues to advance, renewed attention is being paid to the biomedical issues of women's health. In 2002, the Institute of Medicine (IOM) released a provocatively titled report, *Exploring the Biological Contributions to Human Health: Does Sex Matter?*, which argues that many normal physiological functions are influenced directly or indirectly by sex-based differences in biology (IOM Committee on Understanding the Biology of Sex and Gender Differences, Wizemann, and Pardue, 2001). The report concludes that sexually determined characteristics can be found all the way down to the cellular level (Pardue, 2001). Such a sweeping statement is called into question by new scholars in feminist and queer theory who advocate for a more fluid interpretation of the division between the "sexes" (Butler, 1990, 1993; Chase, 1998). The division between "sex" and "gender," once thought to be reflective of the social/biological divide, is seen as increasingly problematic for many of these scholars (Scott, 1999). Regardless of how this theoretical debate progresses, the events of the recent past demonstrate the importance of continued work on biomedical issues of women's health.

The history of biomedical research on women's health is not very old. As Dr. Pardue, the chair of the IOM panel, reminds us, "It's hard to believe that only a little over two decades ago, the US government issued guidelines recommending that pharmaceutical companies exclude women of childbearing age from participating in clinical trials" (IOM Committee, Wizemann, and Pardue, 2001, p. 6). The negative implications of this policy were challenged loudly by women leaders in Congress, who called for change. Responding to this pressure, in 1990 the National Institutes of

Health (NIH) established the Office of Research on Women's Health (ORWH), which established guidelines and policies for the inclusion of women and minorities in clinical studies. In 1991, Dr. Bernadine Healy, then director of the NIH, launched the single largest effort to redress the inadequacy of biomedical research related to women's health. The Women's Health Initiative (WHI) is a large and complex clinical investigation of strategies for the prevention and control of some of the most common causes of morbidity and mortality among postmenopausal women, including cancer, cardiovascular disease, and osteoporotic fractures. The WHI was initiated in 1992, with a planned completion date of 2007. Between 1993 and 1998, the WHI enrolled 161,809 postmenopausal women aged 50 to 79 years in a set of clinical trials. These included trials of low-fat diets, calcium and vitamin D supplementation, and two trials of postmenopausal hormone use, as well as an observational study (Women's Health Initiative Study Group, 1998).

In 2002, the first results of the WHI came in the form of an announcement that the hormone replacement regimen followed by six million American women did more harm than good. As the executive director of the North American Menopause Society said, "This is the biggest bombshell that ever hit in my 30-something years in the menopause area" (D. Wulf Utian, quoted in Kolata and Petersen, 2002). For years, women had taken hormone replacement as a prevention strategy against osteoporosis and heart disease. In 2000, 46 million prescriptions were written for Premarin (conjugated estrogen) and another 22.3 million prescriptions for Prempro (conjugated estrogen plus medroxyprogesterone acetate) (Kreling et al., 2001).

After 5.2 years of follow-up of women in the WHI, the data and safety monitoring board in 2002 recommended stopping the trial of estrogen plus progestin versus placebo because the overall health risks exceeded the benefits from the use of these medications (Writing Group for the Women's Health Initiative Investigators, 2002). Included in this chapter is an editorial (Fletcher and Colditz, 2002; Article 4) from the issue of the *Journal of the American Medical Association* that carried the study results. The clinical implications of the results of this study are profound for millions of women and their health care providers, who must now decide whether to continue or discontinue taking these medications and for what reasons. The implications of these results for clinical medicine as a whole are also acute. Much of medical care is built on a body of knowledge gained over time from observational studies. What the WHI results demonstrate is that long-held assumptions made from this observational data must be questioned and that large clinical studies are needed.

The final article in this chapter addresses another area of women's health that has been thrown into chaos in the last few years. In her thoughtful opinion piece in the *New York Times*, UCSF Professor and leading expert on mammography Virginia Ernster explains the quandary in which women today find themselves as a result of conflicting judgments about the value of routine mammography (Ernster, 2002). Whereas mammography was once thought to be the reason for declining mortality from breast cancer, reanalysis of old data has challenged mammography's contribution to this positive health outcome (Nystrom et al., 2002). Dr. Ernster explains that the evidence is far from perfect and is weaker than previously thought. As a result, women need to make individual choices about risks and benefits. But in order to make these choices, women need accurate information and sensitive health care providers. These have long been the goals of the women's health movement (Weisman, 1998). As the 21st century begins, women's health remains a challenge and a priority.

REFERENCES

Benderly, B. L., and Institute of Medicine. (1997). *In her own right: The Institute of Medicine's guide to women's health issues*. Washington, DC: National Academy Press.

Boonstra, H., and Gold, R. B. (2002). Overhauling welfare: Implications for reproductive health policy in the United States. *Journal of the American Medical Women's Association, 57* (1), 41–46.

Butler, J. P. (1990). *Gender trouble: Feminism and the subversion of identity*. New York: Routledge.

Butler, J. P. (1993). *Bodies that matter: On the discursive limits of "sex."* New York: Routledge.

Chase, C. (1998). Hermaphrodites with attitude — Mapping the emergence of intersex political activism. *Glq — A Journal of Lesbian and Gay Studies, 4* (2), 189–211.

Chavkin, W., Wise, P. H., and Romero, D. (2002). Welfare, women, and children: It's time for doctors to speak out. *Journal of the American Medical Women's Association, 57* (1), 3–4, 10.

Davies, H. T. O., Washington, A. E., and Bindman, A. B. (2002). Health care report cards: Implications for vulnerable patient groups and the organizations providing them care. *Journal of Health Politics, Policy and Law, 27,* 379–399.

Ernster, V. (2002, February 14). Mammograms and personal choice. *New York Times,* p. A35.

Feinleib, M., and Ingster, L. (1999). Socioeconomic gradient in health among men and women. In R. B. Ness and L. H. Keller (Eds.), *Health and disease among women: Biological and environmental influences* (pp. 3–32). New York: Oxford University Press.

Fletcher, S. W., and Colditz, G. A. (2002). Failure of estrogen plus progestin therapy for prevention. *Journal of the American Medical Association, 288* (3), 366–368.

Hwang, A. (2002, January–Februrary). Exportable righteousness, expendable women. *World Watch, 15,* 24.

Institute of Medicine Committee on Understanding the Biology of Sex and Gender Differences, Wizemann, T. M., and Pardue, M. L. (2001). *Exploring the biological contributions to human health: Does sex matter?* Washington, DC: National Academy Press.

JAMWA. (2002). Welfare reform and women's health [Special issue]. *Journal of the American Medical Women's Association, 57* (1).

Kolata, G., and Petersen, M. (2002, July 10). Hormone replacement study a shock to the medical system. *New York Times,* p. A1.

Kreling, D., Mott, D., Wiederholt, J., Lundy, J., and Levitt, L. (2001). *Prescription drug trends: A chartbook update*. Menlo Park, CA: Henry J. Kaiser Family Foundation.

Krieger, N., Williams, D. R., and Moss, N. E. (1997). Measuring social class in US public health research: Concepts, methodologies, and guidelines. *Annual Review of Public Health, 18,* 341–378.

McDonough, P., Williams, D. R., House, J. S, and Duncan, G. J. (1999). Gender and the socioeconomic gradient in mortality. *Journal of Health and Social Behavior, 40* (1), 17–31.

Moon, M. (2001). Medicare. *New England Journal of Medicine, 344* (12), 928–931.

Moss, N. (2000). Socioeconomic inequalities in women's health. In M. B. Goldman and M. Hatch (Eds.), *Women and health* (pp. 541–552). San Diego: Academic Press.

Nystrom, L., Andersson, I., Bjurstam, N., Frisell, J., Nordenskjold, B., and Rutqvist, L. E. (2002). Long-term effects of mammography screening: Updated overview of the Swedish randomised trials. *Lancet, 359* (9310), 909–919.

Pardue, M. L. (2001). Studying differences between the sexes may spur improvements in medicine. *The Scientist, 15* (14), 6.

Rice, D. P. (1999). *Medicare: A women's issue*. Paper presented at the Jacobs Institute and Commonwealth Fund meeting "Women and Medicare: Agenda for Change," Washington, DC.

Salganicoff, A., Beckerman, J. Z., Wyn, R., and Ojeda, V. D. (2002). *Women's health in the United States: Health coverage and access to care* [Executive summary]. Menlo Park, CA: The Henry J. Kaiser Family Foundation.

Scott, J. W. (1999). Some reflections on gender and politics. In M. M. Ferree, J. Lorber, and B. B. Hess (Eds.), *Revisioning gender* (pp. 70–96). Thousand Oaks, CA: Sage.

Weisman, C. S. (1998). *Women's health care: Activist traditions and institutional change*. Baltimore: Johns Hopkins University Press.

Weitz, T., and Estes, C. L. (2001). Adding aging and gender to the women's health agenda. *Journal of Women and Aging, 13* (2), 3–20.

Williams, D. R., (2002). Racial/ethnic variations in women's health: The social embeddedness of health. *American Journal of Public Health, 92* (4), 588–597.

William, D., and Collins, C. (1995). US socioeconomic and racial differences in health: Patterns and explanations. *Annual Review of Sociology, 21,* 349–396.

Women's Health Initiative Study Group. (1998). Design of the Women's Health Initiative clinical trial and observational study. *Controlled Clinical Trials, 19* (1), 61–109.

Writing Group for the Women's Health Initiative Investigators. (2002). Risks and benefits of estrogen plus progestin in healthy postmenopausal women: Principal results from the Women's Health Initiative randomized controlled trial. *Journal of the American Medical Association, 288* (3), 321–333.

ARTICLE 1

WOMEN'S HEALTH IN THE UNITED STATES

HEALTH COVERAGE AND ACCESS TO CARE

Alina Salganicoff, J. Zoë Beckerman, Roberta Wyn, and Victoria D. Ojeda

Women are major consumers of health care services, in many cases negotiating not only their own care, but also that of their family members. Their reproductive health needs, greater rate of health problems, and longer life spans compared to men make their relationships with the health system complex. Their access to care is often complicated by their disproportionately lower incomes and greater responsibilities juggling work and family concerns. Because of their own health needs, limited financial resources, and family responsibilities, women have a vested interest in the scope and type of services offered by health plans, as well as in the mechanisms that fund health care services.

The Kaiser Family Foundation developed the *Kaiser Women's Health Survey* to learn more about the experiences of women with both their health plans and their health providers, with a special focus on the women who are most likely to fall through the cracks in the health care system — women of color, those who are poor, and those who are uninsured. This nationally representative telephone survey was administered to 3,966 women ages 18 to 64 in the Spring and Summer of 2001. Women who were nonelderly Latina, African American, uninsured, low-income, or on Medicaid were over-sampled to improve our understanding of the multifaceted health issues and challenges facing these often underserved groups of women.

KEY FINDINGS

The health care system is not meeting the health needs of a sizable share of women. For women, affordability of care is a major concern. A significant portion of women cannot afford to go to the doctor and fill their doctor's drug prescriptions — even when they have insurance coverage. Women with health problems, who need health care services the most, often have the hardest time getting care because of plan coverage policies, affordability concerns, and logistical barriers, such as transportation. Women also have some important concerns about the quality of care they are receiving. A substantial proportion of women changed doctors because of dissatisfaction with care and concerns about quality. For many women, coverage and access to care is unstable. Health coverage, involvement with health plans, and relationships with doctors are often short lived, resulting in care that can be spotty and fragmented.

Selected crosscutting survey findings include:

- **Costs related to health care present significant problems for nonelderly women.**
  - One-quarter (24%) of nonelderly women delayed or went without care in the past year because they could not afford it, compared to 16% of men.
  - Almost three in 10 (28%) women found out-of-pocket costs to be higher than expected when they went to their doctor, a rate similar to that of men.
  - One-quarter (23%) of women gave their plan a low rating on the out-of-pocket costs they incurred.
- **Affordability of prescription drugs is a primary concern for a sizable share of nonelderly women.**
  - Half of nonelderly women used prescription drugs on a regular basis, compared to 31% of men.
  - Overall, one in five (21%) nonelderly women did not fill a prescription for medication because of the cost, compared to 13% of men. This was a problem for 40% of uninsured women, 27% of women with Medicaid, and 15% of privately insured women.
  - About four in 10 women in fair or poor health (38%) did not fill a prescription in the past year due to cost, as did one-quarter (25%) of women who used prescription drugs on a regular basis.
- **Women in fair or poor health — who have the greatest need for health care services — often experience major problems accessing care.**
  - About one-third of nonelderly women (32%) had a health condition that required ongoing medical treatment, such as asthma, allergies, or arthritis, compared to 26% of men.
  - Of the 16% of women in fair or poor health, half (49%) reported they needed to see a doctor in the past year, but did not.
  - Transportation difficulties resulted in delayed care for about one in five women in fair or poor health (21%), four times the rate of women in better health (5%).
  - Nearly one-quarter of women in fair or poor health (23%) reported that their health plan refused to approve or pay for needed tests or treatment in the past two years; 57% of them either delayed care or never got treatment.
- **Women have significant concerns about the quality of care they receive.**
  - Over one in five women (22%) expressed concerns about the quality of care they got from their physicians or health care providers, compared to 17% of

men. This issue was a particular problem for women in fair or poor health (40%).
    - Almost one in five women (18%) changed providers in the past five years due to dissatisfaction with care, twice the rate of men (9%).
    - Overall, one in seven women (14%) gave their plan a low rating on the number and quality of physicians in the plan, as did the same share of men. This was a major concern for women with Medicaid (28%) and low-income women (21%).
- **Connection to the health system is unstable for many women.**
    - Nearly three in 10 women (28%) reported they were uninsured at some point in the past year. Nearly one in five (19%) were uninsured at the time of the survey and one in 10 (9%) had coverage at the time of the survey, but were uninsured for some period of time in the past year. Rates were similar for men.
    - Half of uninsured women (51%) lacked coverage for over one year.
    - Women experienced churning between plans. Nearly half of nonelderly women had switched plans in the past five years. The leading reasons were employers changing plans (34%) or job changes for women or their spouses (30%). These statistics were similar for men.
    - Among women who switched plans, over one in 10 (13%) left their old provider and changed to a different doctor affiliated with their new plan.
    - Many women had relatively new relationships with their providers; one-third of women with a regular provider had been seeing that provider for two years or less.

These findings highlight the importance of viewing the health system through a woman's lens. Women's health is likely to be a silent victim of the combination of the recent downturn in the economy and rapidly increasing health care costs. In response to these major forces, employers may be more likely to drop dependent coverage, switch to less expensive and/or more limited plans, or raise worker costs for care. Because women are likely to be low-income and also rely on dependent coverage more often than men, they may have much to lose. Stable coverage will thus be likely to continue to elude many women.

With the rapid growth in prescription drug costs and limits on employer-based coverage, affordability barriers for women will undoubtedly rise. Fiscal pressures on employers, insurers, health plans and providers are likely to create even more difficulties for women in affording and obtaining the often basic — and sometimes complex — range of health care services they require.

SURVEY HIGHLIGHTS

The following section summarizes the highlights of the report and presents the findings on women's health status, their health insurance coverage, their satisfaction and experiences with their health plans and providers, and their access and use of health care services.

Women's Health Status

Women's health status is influenced by factors such as age, income, and race/ethnicity. This survey sought to learn more about how these factors affect the health of women. A primary concern was to document the health conditions that women face and the factors associated with poor health among women.

- **Many women had health conditions that necessitated ongoing treatment. The prevalence of most of these chronic conditions increased with age.**
  - Over one in 10 women (13%) had a health problem that limited their ability to participate in everyday activities.
  - Compared to women ages 18 to 44, women ages 45 to 64 were three times as likely to have cancer or heart disease and four times as likely to have arthritis or hypertension.
- **Low-income women were likely to have poor health status and activity limitations.**
  - Low-income women were twice as likely as those with higher incomes to have fair or poor health status (23% and 10%, respectively) and conditions that limit activity (19% and 9%).
  - They were at considerably higher risk for experiencing health problems in their older years, when the combination of increasing age and economic hardship takes its toll. Among low-income women ages 45 to 64, 49% reported arthritis, 41% had hypertension, and 32% had mental health concerns such as anxiety or depression.
- **Health status differentials by race and ethnicity persist.**
  - Latinas were the most likely to report fair or poor health (29%), and African American women were the most likely to report a health condition that limited their activity (16%).
  - Among African American women ages 45 to 64, over half (57%) reported hypertension and 40% had arthritis. One in six Latinas and African American women in this age group were diagnosed with diabetes in the past five years.

Health Insurance Coverage

Health insurance facilitates women's access to care by reducing financial barriers to care. Unfortunately, many women lack insurance or face obstacles in securing health coverage. This survey was designed to learn more about the status of health coverage for nonelderly women, focusing on who has coverage and who is at greatest risk for being uninsured.

- **A significant portion of women lacked health insurance coverage. Certain subgroups of women were at higher risk of going without health coverage than other women.**

    - One in five women ages 18 to 64 was uninsured, with the risk of being uninsured falling disproportionately on women with limited incomes; one-third of low-income women lacked coverage.
    - Latinas were also at very high risk of being uninsured; nearly four in 10 (37%) were without coverage. Younger women (between the ages of 18 and 29), those who were foreign born, and those who lived in the South or West, were the most likely to lack coverage.
    - Half of uninsured women (51%) lacked coverage for more than one year.
    - Six in 10 (57%) uninsured women worked either full- or part-time.
- **Most women with health insurance received it through work situations.**
    - Employer-sponsored insurance was the predominant form of coverage for nonelderly women, with six in 10 covered by their own or their spouse's employer.
    - Women were less likely than men to be covered by their own employers (33% vs. 53%, respectively) and more likely to be insured as a dependent (27% to 13%, respectively).
- **Medicaid, the state-federal health program for the poor, served an important role for low-income women.**
    - Nearly one in 10 nonelderly women (9%) received Medicaid coverage.
    - Medicaid played an especially important role for poor women, covering nearly one-third.

Health Plans

Benefits covered by health plans and how plans operate are particularly important issues for women. Both can affect the types of health providers and health services that women are able to obtain. This survey focused on women's concerns about their health plans and the factors that influenced their decisions and satisfaction with their plans.

- **Women took a leading role making family coverage decisions.**
    - Nearly six in 10 women reported that they were the primary decision-makers in their families about health insurance; 22% made the decisions jointly with their spouses.
    - As they selected health plans, over half of women rated the benefits offered, selection of doctors, cost of plan, and reputation of the plan as "very important" in health plan selection.
    - Most women with insurance were in managed care.
    - The overwhelming majority of nonelderly insured women (82%) were enrolled in a managed care plan, such as a Health Maintenance Organization (HMO) or Preferred Provider Organization (PPO), and 17% were in fee-for-service arrangements.
    - Just over half of privately insured women (53%) were enrolled in a loosely controlled plan where they had some flexibility to self-refer to a specialist

or go out of network at higher cost. One-third of women were in more rigid, tightly controlled plans.

  - Among women enrolled in Medicaid, 82% were members of a managed care plan.

- **The majority of women were generally satisfied with their health plans.**
  - Overall, few women gave their plans low ratings on issues such as the number of benefits (16%), ease of use (15%) and the number and quality of physicians in plan (14%). Out-of-pocket costs were rated poorly by nearly one-quarter (23%) of nonelderly women.
  - On many of these issues, women in poorer health, those on Medicaid, and low-income women had higher rates of dissatisfaction than other women.
- **A sizable share of women faced difficulties in getting needed care because their plans denied payment or approval.**
  - One in seven women reported that their plans denied coverage for care they thought they needed.
  - Lack of plan approval for treatment or tests resulted in nearly one-half of women either delaying or never receiving the services they thought they needed.
  - About half of women (53%) whose insurance denied payment for needed services disputed their plans' decisions.
  - Low-income women were disproportionately affected by plan refusal to pay for services, and were twice as likely as higher-income women not to obtain the treatment they thought they needed (33% vs. 15%).

Health Providers

A woman's relationship and satisfaction with her provider is a critical component of her health care. This survey explored women's relationships with their providers, focusing on both what worked well and women's chief concerns regarding their physicians and other providers.

- **Women's complex mix of reproductive and general health care needs make their relationships with their health care providers very important.**
  - Nearly one in five women (17%) did not have a regular health provider, about half the rate of men (28%). Almost half of uninsured women (46%), one-third of Latinas (31%), and one-quarter of low-income women (24%) lacked a regular provider.
  - About one-half of women had at least two routine providers, typically a primary care provider such as an internist or a general practitioner, along with an obstetrician or gynecologist (Ob/Gyn). The other half of women saw just one provider for regular care, typically a primary care doctor. Only a small fraction of women (7%) relied exclusively on an Ob/Gyn for all of their routine care.
  - Despite the increasing pool of women physicians, only one-third of women saw a female as their regular provider.

- Many women had relatively new relationships with their providers; one-third of women with a regular provider had been seeing that provider for two years or less.
- **A sizable minority of women — particularly those that faced the greatest health challenges — reported that they had difficulty communicating with their providers.**
  - Women in poor health (18%) and Latinas (14%) were the most likely to feel that their doctor did not take the time to answer all their questions.
  - Nearly two in 10 women (17%) left their doctor's office and reported that they did not understand or remember all of the information provided to them at their medical visit. This was particularly a problem for nearly one-third of women in fair or poor health.
- **A significant portion of women have changed doctors because they were dissatisfied.**
  - Nearly one in five (18%) women had changed her doctor at some point in the past five years due to dissatisfaction, double the rate of men (9%).

Access to and Use of Health Care

Women's access and use of the health system is influenced in part by their individual characteristics, health needs, and prior experience with both illness and the health system. It is also strongly influenced by insurance coverage and health system features. This survey examined the characteristics of women who faced the greatest challenges accessing health care and explored the factors that placed them at highest risk for experiencing barriers to care.

- **Most women (87%) had a health care visit in the past year, but where they got their care varied for different subgroups of women.**
  - Latinas and uninsured women, both groups at higher risk for experiencing access problems and barriers to care, were the least likely to have had a doctor visit in the past year (31% and 24%, respectively).
  - Women on Medicaid or who were uninsured (about four in 10 each) as well as African American women and Latinas (27% and 38%, respectively) were more likely to rely on hospital clinics and health centers for medical care than other women.
- **Overall, women fell short of receiving many recommended screening tests. Insurance coverage was a major determinant for whether women received preventive screenings.**
  - Only 35% of women 50 to 64 had a screening test for colon cancer in the past two years, 77% of women in the same age group had a mammogram in the past two years, and 56% of women 18 to 64 had a blood cholesterol test.
  - Uninsured women and, to a somewhat lesser extent, women on Medicaid, were consistently less likely than women with private coverage to obtain many of the recommended preventive screening tests.

- **Women experienced multiple types of barriers to receiving health care.**
  - The cost of care was a significant barrier to obtaining medical attention for vulnerable women. Nearly six in 10 (59%) uninsured women, 42% of women in fair or poor health, and 31% of Latinas delayed or went without care because they could not afford it.
  - Transportation barriers were experienced by 7% of women, but were especially salient for women on Medicaid (23%), Latinas (18%), and uninsured women (12%).
  - Problems in child care contributed to delays and postponement of care for 10% of women with children and ranged from 17% of women on Medicaid to just 8% of privately insured women.

TECHNICAL NOTE

The Kaiser Women's Health Survey reports findings from a national telephone survey of 3,966 women ages 18 to 64 in the United States. A disproportionate stratified random sample was used to over-sample African American women, Latinas, those in low-income households (defined as having incomes below 200% of the federal poverty level), and those who were medically uninsured or Medicaid beneficiaries, so that sample sizes would be adequate to allow for subanalysis of these populations. The sample was then weighted using the Census Bureau Demographic Profile (from the March 2000 Current Population Survey) to adjust for variations in the sample relating to region of residence, sex, age, race, and education to provide nationally representative statistics. Interviews were conducted in either English or Spanish, depending on participants' preference. A shorter companion survey of 700 English-speaking men was conducted for the purposes of gender comparison.

Foundation staff designed the survey in collaboration with Princeton Survey Research Associates (PSRA) and analyzed it with researchers from the University of California, Los Angeles. Fieldwork was conducted by PSRA between March 28 and July 29, 2001. The margin of sampling error is ±2 percentage points for the total women sample, ±4 percentage points for the men, and is larger for subgroups. Note that in addition to sampling error, there are other possible sources of measurement error, though every effort was undertaken to minimize these other sources. A copy of the survey instrument is available upon request.

ARTICLE 2

ADDING AGING AND GENDER TO THE WOMEN'S HEALTH AGENDA

Tracy Weitz and Carroll L. Estes

INTRODUCTION

The current models for health care delivery, financing, and policy fail to meet the needs of women in general, and older women in particular. The complex interaction of medical, social, and economic factors that affect women's wellness requires a new paradigm that bridges the gap between those who are concerned about aging issues and those concerned about women's health. A new paradigm must also take account of the institutional structures and relations that greatly influence the economic security of women and the ability to access health resources as they age.

The current women's health agenda is the result of independent and isolated efforts in the areas of aging, health, and women's issues. To "bridge the gap," old questions need to be examined in new ways, and new questions need to be asked about old assumptions. In this article, we begin this endeavor by advancing three interrelated themes: (1) there is a gendered relationship between socioeconomic structures and health over time; (2) there are gender-specific implications of health care financing and policy; and (3) there are health consequences to the gendered nature of caregiving.

BACKGROUND

Women comprise an increasing segment of the aging population. O'Rand (1996) argues that the older population of the United States is undergoing a feminization. In 1997, 59 percent of persons 65 years of age and over were women. The sex ratio is higher with age; 71 percent of persons 85 years of age and over were women (DHHS, 1999). In 1997, the life expectancy was 79.4 years for women and 73.6 years for men.

Under current mortality conditions, women who survive to age 65 can, on average, expect to live to age 84, and women who survive to age 85 can, on average, anticipate living to age 92 (DHHS, 1999). Despite their increased longevity, older women live under more compromised circumstances than those experienced by men. In general, older women are more likely than men to live in poverty, have less access to a secure retirement, and pay an increased percentage of their income on out-of-pocket health care costs. Likewise, women play substantially different social roles than men and those roles directly impact their health and economic well-being. Women are also more likely than men to suffer from chronic conditions and disabilities that limit their quality of life (Rice & Michel, 1998).

In order to meet the needs of this feminized aging population, the leadership of the aging movement and of the women's health movement must work together to build a paradigm of health that promotes the wellness of older women. The current hesitancy to look at aging issues from a gendered perspective and the historical focus of women's health on reproductive issues have hindered this union.

Despite recent acknowledgements that aging is a women's issue (AAWH, DHHS, & WHO, 1999), discussions surrounding aging continue to lack a gender-lens and confound the difference between the issues that affect both women and men. Fearful of excluding men, advocates have sought to adopt gender-neutral language and agendas. While the role of poverty in health has received attention, the unique aspects of women's poverty as they age remain unexplored. Only minimal attention has been paid to the ways in which policy implications under discussion uniquely affect women (Shaw, Zuckerman, & Hartman, 1998). For example, current efforts to reform social security will affect men and women in distinct and different ways (Estes, 1998; Smeeding, 1999). When, on rare occasion, these differences are explored, policy makers are accused of political pandering, instead of being recognized for highlighting the potential adverse impacts on vulnerable populations (Toner, 1999).

The women's health movement has historically focused on the reproductive health issues unique to women (Ussher, 1992). In fact, the phrase "maternal-child health" is often used synonymously with women's health (Weisman, 1998). Concerns about access to abortion, family planning, prenatal care, and infant mortality dominate the forefront of women's health. While the graying of the baby-boomers has resulted in an expanded interest in midlife women (especially menopause), the current onslaught of welfare reform and abortion restriction legislation has forced advocates to continue to maintain their focus on traditional reproductive health issues with limited inclusion of disease specific interests such as breast cancer.

BRIDGING AGING, GENDER, AND HEALTH: A NEW PARADIGM FOR OLDER WOMEN'S HEALTH

In the Introduction, we suggested three interrelated themes that could provide a foundation for a new paradigm that recognizes the complexities of the medical, social, and economic factors that affect older women's health.

Articulating the Gender-Dependent Relationship between Socioeconomic Structure and Health

A growing body of evidence indicates that socioeconomic status (SES) continues to be a remarkably robust indicator of rates of illness and death (Williams & Collins, 1995). The relationship between SES and health occurs at every socioeconomic level and for a broad range of SES indicators, and cannot be accounted for simply by classic risk factors such as diet and smoking (Adler, Boyce, Chesney, Folkman, & Syme, 1993). The relationship is so strong that each level of SES is associated with better health outcomes. This occurrence, although not completely understood, is referred to as the "SES gradient in health status" (Adler et al., 1994; Adler et al., 1993).

Given the well-established relationship and the existence of the SES gradient, it is critical to view women's economic situation as a component of their health. Currently, the two poorest groups in the United States are women raising children alone and women over sixty-five living alone (Doress-Worters & Siegal, 1994). Understanding the commonalties that influence the economic situations of these two populations of women is the first step to developing public policies that benefit women across the lifespan. For these two groups of women, the economic status is conditioned by gendered work patterns and by social and political policies that link women's economic security to that of men (Estes, 2000; Harrington Meyer, 1996).

The Role of Gendered Work Patterns in Women's Economic Security

Almost three-quarters of the nation's elderly poor are women (Grad, 1998; SSA, 1998) and according to future projections by ICF, Incorporated, by the year 2020 poverty among older people will be almost exclusively poverty among older women (Commonwealth Fund, 1987 as quoted in Friedman, 1994). Lower lifetime earnings produce lower retirement income and higher poverty for older women (Estes & Michel, 1999). The poverty for women of color is a result of the triple threat of race, gender, and age. Reasons for the economic reality of all women include gender-biased economic structures such as the methodology used to calculate Social Security, work patterns that differ between men and women, and women's reduced access to other retirement income.

Women receive substantially less income from all sources, on average, than men. Social Security is the primary source of income for older women, and more women than men are dependent on Social Security as their sole source of income (Estes & Michel, 1999). The current equation used to calculate Social Security benefits is affected by the patterns of women's participation in the labor market. Overall, women are more likely than men to work in the unpaid labor market, thereby receiving no credit toward Social Security, called "zero years" in the workforce in calculating the formula that determines benefits. Additionally, as a result of caregiving responsibilities for both children and adults, women have more "zero years" in the calculation of their Social Security benefits than do men (Ross, 1997). Women average seven "zero years" in the labor force under Social Security compared to just two and a half years for men (Smeeding, 1999). Under the benefit calculation methodology, women are penalized by the Social Security system for their time out of the labor force to provide caregiving (Stone, Cafferata, & Sangl, 1987).

For those women in the paid work force, discrepancies still exist. In 1999, women still made only 74.1 cents to every dollar earned by men (NCPE, 1999); women of color experience the highest wage gap (NCPE, 1999). Since Social Security benefits are calculated as a function of earned income and years in the workforce, women are again disadvantaged under the system. Because of their lower income, even if they have no "zero years" in the workforce, women still receive lower Social Security payments, on average, than men. Access to other retirement income to supplement Social Security is needed to mitigate the impact of this inequity. Unfortunately, due to differences in the types of jobs women and men obtain in the marketplace, and the disparity of benefits associated with those jobs, women are also less likely to be offered private pensions (Housnell, 1998). Men are twice as likely as women to have pension coverage (Hennesey, 1997).

Marital status also is key. Being non-married in old age (widowed, divorced, separated, or never married) renders a woman much more vulnerable to poverty when compared with a married older woman (Estes & Michel, 1999). The mean proportion of income that non-married women receive from Social Security is 72 percent. Fifty percent of non-married women rely on Social Security for 80 percent of their income, and one in four non-married women age 65 and older rely on Social Security for 100 percent. In contrast, married couples receive 55 percent of their income from Social Security (SSA, 1998). Marital status is also predictive of having pension coverage. However, non-married women are more compromised than similar status men: In 1996, 44 percent of non-married men 65 or older had pension coverage, in comparison to 33 percent of non-married women 65 or older (SSA, 1998). The statistics are even worse for women of color; only 23 percent of African-American non-married women and just 13 percent of Hispanic non-married women received private pension income (SSA, 1998).

The women's health movement must understand that the role of SES in health is not solely a function of a woman's present economic situation, but of her past and future SES. The agenda of the women's health movement must include a life-course perspective. Currently, the women's health movement is arguing for greater workplace accommodation and flexibility in supporting women in childbearing and reproduction. While these are worthwhile and positive agendas, the long-term implications for the health of older women (by reducing the contribution to Social Security, increasing the number of "zero years," and limiting access to other retirement pensions and savings) must be addressed within the same policy discussion. Pushing for financial support and job security for women to "take time off" for caregiving is inadequate to promote the long-term economic security and the health of older women because it fails to provide credit toward Social Security or access to private pensions. Likewise, dependence on a spouse's retirement or Social Security is an inadequate solution and dangerously problematic to a woman's economic security.

Linking Women's Economic Security to Men

The threat of poverty associated with being an older woman is not simply a consequence of longer life. When a woman is married over a long period of time, there is greater stability and security in income (Shaw et al., 1998). In 1996, the median annual income for unmarried elderly women alone was $10,859 compared to $14,007 for unmarried elderly men (SSA, 1998). Poverty for women is either created or accelerated by widowhood and divorce. Eighty percent of all widows in poverty become poor only after their husbands die (Burkhauser & Smeeding, 1994) and divorced older women have higher poverty rates than widows of the same age (Harrington Meyer, 1996). Compared with men, elderly women are three times more likely to be widowed (SSA, 1998).

Women also have a higher probability of being divorced. From 1970 to 1997, the proportion of married women declined from 81.4 percent to 67.9 percent. Much of this change is attributable to higher rates of divorce, although an increase has also occurred in the number of never-married women (Urban Institute, 1999, as reported by Steuerle, 1999). The effects of change in marital status were demonstrated by Shaw et al. who examined a group of women over a nine-year time span and found that poverty was relatively rare and did not increase among women who were married at both times in their study. However, the rate of poverty was substantially higher for women whose marital status had changed over the course of the study (Shaw et al., 1998). Married older women have a four to five times lower poverty rate (4.6 percent) than non-married older women (18 to 22.2 percent) (National Economic Council, 1998). Projected increases in the number of divorced, widowed, separated, and never-married women will result in greater economic hardship for older women in general (Estes & Michel, 1999).

The structures that promote women's dependence on men to minimize their threat of poverty are not limited to affecting older women. Recently, there has been increased attention to the need to reduce "unmarried births." Statistics on unmarried births have replaced the policy focus on "teenage pregnancy" (Besharov & Zinsmeister, 1987; Brownstein, 1994; Fulwood, 1993; LAT, 1996; Vobejda, 1995) and because of the national discomfort with abortion, "unmarried" has replaced "unintended" as the marker for federal and state initiatives (Holmes, 1996; NYT, 1998). While this subtle change may not appear to be of importance to those interested in "aging issues," the change is reflective of the same structural issues that link women's economic security to men. The rationale behind the concern about unmarried births is grounded in arguments about the rates of poverty for these families (Besharov & Zinsmeister, 1987). However, rather than addressing the economic structures that perpetuate women's poverty, this rhetorical focus shifts the blame for poverty to the absence of the male. This rationale is similar to the plight of older women whose poverty is attributable to the death of or divorce from a spouse. Again, rather than addressing the fundamental political and economic structures that produce women's poverty, blame can be assigned to the absence of the husband. In framing the problem in this manner, the solution to both scenarios is the necessary presence of the man in the woman's life. Marriage for younger women, and continuing marriage and longevity for the husbands of older women, are therefore made the reigning factors for women's economic security. In understanding the similarities that underlie these two issues for women at opposite ends of the life course, those interested in women's health and older women can begin to address the fundamental structural causes of women's poverty, rather than seeking prevention of that poverty solely through continued or increased dependency on men.

Addressing the Gender-Specific Implications of Health Care Financing and Policy

As with the overall economic structure, the current policy and financing system for both public and private health care is extraordinarily problematic for older women. On the public side, women are more dependent than men on Medicare for coverage (Rice & Michel, 1998), and on the private side, employer-based insurance continues to link access to health care to marital status and formal paid employment (Harrington Meyer, 1996). Additionally, both the public and the private models of health care financing fail to include a long-term care policy, which is critical to the health and well-being of older women (Estes, Swan, & Associates, 1993).

The Gender-Specific Limitations of Medicare and Employer-Based Insurance

The majority of Medicare recipients are women and because of their longer survival, older women depend on Medicare for an average of 15 years compared with seven years for older men (Butler, 1996). In 1996, 59 percent of all Medicaid beneficiaries were women (Rice & Michel, 1998). In 1997, 70 percent of Medicare beneficiaries were women 85 or older (HCFA, 1998).

Although older women have greater need for Medicare coverage, the system is designed to address acute illnesses rather than chronic conditions (Rice, 2000). While the policy is not written with the intent to be gendered, its effect is different for women and men (Hoffman & Rice, 1996). Multiple data sources support the conclusions that there is a true difference in the rate of illnesses between older men and older women; acute illnesses are more common in older men and chronic illnesses are more common in older women. Of the more than 60 chronic conditions monitored by the National Health Interview Survey, almost two-thirds occur with more frequency in women, while only four conditions occur more frequently in men and the remainder are equal (Adams & Marano, 1995). Nine out of ten women aged 65 and over report one or more chronic conditions and almost three out of four have two or more conditions. Among women age 85 and over, 97 percent have one or more conditions and 90 percent report two or more conditions (Estes & Michel, 1999).

There is also a significant relationship between chronic conditions and out-of-pocket health expenses (Blustein, 2000a; Blustein, 2000b; Rice, 2000). Older women who classify their health status as poor or fair spend 28 percent of their income out-of-pocket compared to women with excellent health who spend 17 percent of their income out-of-pocket (AARP & Lewin-VHI Inc., 1994). Moreover, men spend about five percentage points less than women at every level of health from excellent to poor (AARP & Lewin-VHI Inc., 1994). Likewise, older women who have one or more severe limitations in their activities of daily living spend one-third of their income out-of-pocket compared to 20 percent for women with no limitations in their activities of daily living. In contrast, men with one or more functional limitations in activities of daily living spend only 29 percent of their income out-of-pocket. It is important to note that these figures do not include the costs of nursing homes or home health care expenses that are significant and would substantially raise the calculation of out-of-pocket expenses, especially for women (AARP & Lewin-VHI Inc., 1994). As a result of these differences, older women spend an average of 22 percent of their incomes on medical expenses compared to 17 percent for older men (AARP & Lewin-VHI Inc., 1994).

The compromised health status of older women and particularly of low-income older women has further negative effects on economic status, as out-of-pocket health costs are inversely related to the ability to pay for them. Prescription drugs and long-term care are the highest out-of-pocket expenses (Estes & Michel, 1999). Eight of 10 Medicare beneficiaries regularly use prescription medications, which are now an integral component of medical care (Schoen, Neuman, Kitchman, Davis, & Rowland, 1998), and older women suffer disproportionately from chronic conditions that require greater use of prescription medications. Likewise, pharmaceutical prevention strategies (such as hormone replacement therapy) are more frequently recommended for women by health care providers, also resulting in higher out-of-pocket costs for older women. As a result, most women on Medicare, 17 million, use prescription drugs regularly; 29 percent spend over $50 a month for this purpose (Schoen et al., 1998). Traditional Medicare does not cover outpatient prescription drugs and only half of beneficiaries with a private supplement have coverage for their medications (KFF, 1999). As a result, those with high monthly costs put themselves at financial risk or must forego needed medication (Schoen et al., 1998).

Ironically the women's health movement has taken on the issue of prescription drugs within a completely separate sphere. Fueled by the blatant inequity between prompt coverage of sildenafil citrate (Viagra) by most insurance plans and the historical lack of insurance coverage for contraceptives, women's health advocates have campaigned for "contraceptive parity" (Trafford, 1998). "Contraceptive parity" demands that insurers that provide health insurance coverage for prescription drugs or outpatient services provide coverage for prescribed contraceptive drugs and devices or outpatient contraceptive services. By the end of 1999 only ten states had passed contraceptive parity laws (PPWW, 2000) and most efforts have focused on HMOs. Because of the historical reproductive health focus of the women's movement, this fight has remained separate from discussions about the substantial needs of older women for prescription drug coverage through the public insurance plan of Medicare. Joining the activism for contraceptive parity with those pushing for prescription drug coverage under Medicare will lead to a more comprehensive approach regarding access to and coverage of prescription drugs for all women.

When viewed as a population-specific issue, the debate over coverage for prescription drugs obscures the larger issue of lack of insurance coverage for health care in general. Between 1989 and 1997, the number of people without health insurance increased by 10.1 million to 43.4 million (Carrasquillo, Himmelstein, Woolhandler, & Bor, 1999). The percentage of uninsured women also increased while Medicaid enrollment dropped as a result of cutbacks generated by welfare reform (Carrasquillo, Himmelstein, Woolhandler, & Bor, 1999). The greatest increases in uninsured rates were among low-income and Hispanic women (Collins et al., 1999).

While access to health coverage for uninsured women has been an important agenda item for the women's movement, the priority has been narrowly focused on increasing coverage for pregnant women and children. To the credit of those pushing this agenda, the fights for expanded coverage of prenatal care and for increased access to health insurance for uninsured children have been remarkably successful. Unfortunately, recent efforts to limit prenatal care for immigrants have forced advocates to prioritize retaining this limited scope of coverage rather than expanding health care coverage to non-pregnant women.

Those concerned with aging have begun to address deficiencies in Medicare coverage for beneficiaries by focusing on maintaining current benefits and expanding access to supplemental insurance to cover additional benefits such as prescription drugs. There are currently a number of national debates underway about how to "save" Medicare (Day, 1998; Fronstin & Copeland, 1997; Fuchs, 1999; Gundling, 1997; McKusick, 1999; Serafini, 1997; Wilensky, 1996). A central theme of these discussions is cutting costs, increasing managed care, and expanding services through supplemental private insurance (Oberlander, 1997). Many proposed changes may mean even higher out-of-pocket costs which will disproportionately affect women who are less able to pay (KFF, 1999).

In maintaining a bipolar focus on reproductive-aged women and Medicare-eligible women, advocates fail to adequately address the overall deficiency of the piecemeal insurance structure. By coalescing efforts pushing for health coverage of pregnant women and uninsured children, and efforts working to preserve Medicare, an agenda for comprehensive health care coverage can be forged. Without such an approach, efforts to improve health care will continue to narrowly focus on small improvements to the current market-based system rather than more broad-based approaches such as universal health coverage (Blumenthal, 1999).

The Gender-Specific Impact of the Lack of a Long-Term Care Policy

Even the solution of universal coverage by existing health insurance will be inadequate to fully address the health needs of older women. The current reimbursement model for both public and private insurance fails to include sufficient coverage for long-term care, for which elderly women have a disproportionate need (Estes et al., 1993). Women are both the users and the providers of long-term care and thus, failure to address long-term care disproportionately falls on women (KFF, 1999). Because Medicare does not cover long-term care, it can therefore be said that the U.S. policy on long-term care is gendered in multiple ways largely to the detriment of women.

The higher rate and number of chronic conditions among women results in increased disability among women. Regardless of race and age, women spend about twice as many years disabled before death as their male counterparts (La Croix, Newton, Leveille, & Wallace, 1997). Disability greatly influences functional well-being by limiting an individual's ability to perform certain tasks of daily living. Researchers group these tasks into two categories: (1) essential activities of daily living (ADL), such as bathing, eating, and dressing; and (2) the more complex instrumental activities of daily living (IADL), such as making meals, shopping or cleaning. In 1995, among the noninstitutionalized population 70 years of age and over, 10 percent of women and 7 percent of men were unable to do one or more ADL and about 23 percent of women and 13 percent of men could not do IADLs without help (DHHS, 1999). According to 1994 data, the percentage of women needing help or supervision with IADLs more than doubles across each ten-year age category for women: from 6.3 percent to 15.7 percent to 40.8 percent of women aged 65–74, 75–84, and 85 and older, respectively. In each age group, the rates of disability among women exceed those among men (Guralnik, Leveille, Hirsch, Ferrucci, & Fried, 1997). The need to reside in a nursing home, perhaps the most serious form of loss of independence, is also substantially greater among women than men aged 75 and older (Guralnik et al., 1997). In 1996, three-quarters of the residents in long-term care facilities (skilled nursing homes, intermediate care facilities, retirement homes, and institutions for the mentally retarded) were women, and women made up two-thirds of the home health care users and over half of hospice patients (Rice & Michel, 1998).

The government's refusal to provide a publicly financed universal long-term care policy is borne unequally across gender lines. Devolution and increased state-level responsibility for long-term care makes women dependent on 50 state governors and legislatures for remedy. The result is a fragmented and unequal policy across the different states. As discussed in their work, Estes and Linkins view this fragmentation as "the race to the bottom." Because states are in competition with each other for capital and labor, there is economic incentive to eliminate, rather than enhance, coverage of long-term care. Ultimately, it is women who experience the impact of these negative incentives (Estes, 1992, revised and reprinted in Lee, Estes, & Close, 1997).

Unfortunately, Medicare coverage for long-term care does not appear to be on the agenda of advocates, despite the high potential to benefit the health of older women. Likewise, the issue of long-term care has been virtually ignored by the women's health movement. Long-term care must be viewed as an intergenerational issue, and efforts to develop a gender-neutral health care financing policy must include sufficient coverage for long-term care.

Acknowledging the Health Effect of the Gendered Nature of Caregiving

In addition to having a greater need for long-term care, the labor of long-term care, largely informal, is predominately provided by women, without pay and with negative consequences. Women are 75 percent of the caregivers, 80 percent of whom provide unpaid care of four hours per day, seven days per week (O'Rand & National Academy on Aging, 1994). The "typical" caregiver is in her mid-forties (Caregiving & AARP, 1997) but 25 percent are between the ages of 65 and 74 and 10 percent are 75 and over (Estes & Michel, 1999). A 1997 study found that the mid-range estimate for the economic value of informal caregiving was $196 billion (Amo, Levine, & Memmott, 1999). Women care providers, ironically, often outlive anyone to care for them and then are required to "spend down" into poverty in order to qualify for public assistance through Medicaid. Thus, although women often provide care to others at no economic cost, they are required to pay for the care they receive in old age.

Women maintain a particular status in society, in the labor market, and in the family; public policies reinforce and entrench these roles (Estes, 2000). Women play a unique role as society's caregivers. Nearly two-thirds of caregivers of the elderly are themselves older women, many of whom are caring for both children and older family members. Caregiving is a complex and profoundly women's issue. It reflects some of what is best about being a woman: compassion and concern for others. However, the extent to which women engage in caregiving across the lifespan has a direct impact on their own health. Caregiving affects women's long-term economic security, and these negative economic consequences compound the deleterious health consequences of informal caregiving (Alzheimer's Association, 1996; Stone et al., 1987).

Higher rates of stress and depression, use of prescription drugs, lack of attention to personal health conditions, and participating in fewer social and recreational activities are frequently reported for caregivers (Almberg, Jansson, Grafstreom, & Winblad, 1998; Buckwalter et al., 1999; George, 1984; Martire, Stephens, & Atienza, 1997; Schulz et al., 1997; Wilcox & King, 1999). The higher use of prescription drugs among this group again highlights the need for a comprehensive approach for medication coverage for women across the lifespan. Also, since depression has been shown to affect the maintenance of health behaviors needed for prevention (i.e., proper diet and exercise), understanding the role of caregiving in health outcomes is also important.

As with other issues, caregiving is examined in separate spheres of policy making. Childcare is viewed as a "woman's" issue, and eldercare is viewed as an "aging" issue. Lost in these two discussions are the women caring for a spouse or a family member of the same age in addition to the numerous women caring for multiple individuals or generations. Without addressing caregiving in its totality, which includes understanding the gendered nature of the responsibilities, policy solutions will remain elusive.

The desire to maintain caregiving as an individual responsibility is closely linked to the economic structure of our society. There is substantial economic incentive for the government to maintain caregiving as an individual expense, rather than a societal expense. Consequently, policy makers continue to press for more family (i.e., women's) responsibility in the care of older persons. The ideological revolution of the Reagan and Bush presidencies helped to entrench the notion of the family as primacy for caregiving, thereby justifying shifting social responsibilities to the private sector (Estes, 1992, revised and reprinted in Lee et al., 1997). In reinforcing the notion of the role of the family in caring for elders, the public sector is released from obligation to pay for or provide the care. This primacy of family (i.e., unpaid women) as caregiver of choice is being repeated in the discourse about childcare. As reflected in the language of a governmental fact sheet "... the grandmother is the primary caregiver, offering these children the opportunity to grow up in stable homes and communities among their family and friends" (AOA, 1998). Again, the preference for individual-based solutions (even those supported by tax credits such as President Clinton's 1999 proposed legislation) abdicates the public sector from responsibility for developing a universal and adequate solution to the need. Understanding caregiving through gender and across the lifecourse will promote solutions that address the disproportionate burden of caregiving on women.

CONCLUSION

Because of the complexity of the issues and the separation of women's health from concerns about aging, the issue of older women's health and wellness has been missing from the public agenda. This article proposes a new agenda regarding older women's health and advocates for a bridging of the work done on behalf of women's health and older women. Older women's health represents a complex interplay of medical, social, and economic factors that cannot be understood in isolation. Successfully addressing the needs of older women's health requires the participation of both those interested in women's health and those concerned about aging issues to create a new agenda grounded in three tenets: (1) there is a gendered relationship between socioeconomic structures and health over time; (2) there are gender-specific implications of health care financing and policy; and (3) there are health consequences to the gendered nature of caregiving.

REFERENCES

AARP, & Lewin-VHI Inc. (1994). *Aging Baby Boomers: How Secure Is Their Economic Future?* Washington, DC: Forecasting and Environment Scanning Department.

AAWH, DHHS, & WHO. (1999). *Healthy Aging, Healthy Living — START NOW!* (Resource Booklet). Washington, DC: American Association for World Health, US Department of Health & Human Services, Pan American Health Organization, World Health Organization.

Adams, P., & Marano, M. (1995). *Current estimates from the National Health Interview Survey*. National Center for Health Statistics, Vital Health Statistics.

Adler, N. E., Boyce, T., Chesney, M. A., Cohen, S., Folkman, S., Kahn, R. L., & Syme, S. L. (1994). Socioeconomic status and health. The challenge of the gradient. *American Psychologist, 49* (1), 15–24.

Adler, N. E., Boyce, W. T., Chesney, M. A., Folkman, S., & Syme, S. L. (1993). Socioeconomic inequalities in health: No easy solution. *Journal of the American Medical Association, 269* (24), 3140–3145.

Almberg, B., Jansson, W., Grafstreom, M., & Wimblad, B. (1998). Differences between and within genders in caregiving strain: A comparison between caregivers of demented and non-caregivers of non-demented elderly people. *Journal of Advanced Nursing, 28* (4), 849–58.

Alzheimer's Association. (1996). *An Exploration of the Plight of an Alzheimer's Caregiver.*

AOA. (1998). *Older Women: A Diverse and Growing Population* (Fact Sheet). Washington, DC: Administration on Aging.

Arno, P. S., Levine, C., & Memmott, M. M. (1999). The economic value of informal caregiving. *Health Affairs, 18* (2), 182–8.

Besharov, D. J., & Zinsmeister, K. (1987, May 3). Unwed moms are white, too; once again the conventional wisdom has it wrong. *Washington Post,* B5.

Blumenthal, D. (1999). Health care reform at the close of the 20th century. *New England Journal of Medicine, 340* (24), 1916.

Blustein, J. (2000a). Drug coverage and drug purchases by Medicare beneficiaries with hypertension. *Health Affairs, 19* (2), 219–30.

Blustein, J. (2000b). Medicare and drug coverage: A women's health issue. *Women's Health Issues, 10* (2), 47–53.

Brownstein, R. (1994, July 14). Welfare reformers confront out-of-wedlock births: Panel shows bipartisan resolve to reduce pregnancies by unmarried aid recipients. *Los Angeles Times,* A15.

Buckwalter, K. C., Gerdner, L., Kohout, F., Hall, G. R., Kelly, A., Richards, B., & Sime, M. (1999). A nursing intervention to decrease depression in family caregivers of persons with dementia. *Archives of Psychiatric Nursing, 13* (2), 80–8.

Burkhauser, R., & T. S. (1994). *Social Security Reform: A Budget Neutral Approach to Reducing Older Women's Disproportionate Risk of Poverty.* Syracuse: Syracuse University Press.

Caregiving, National Alliance for, & AARP. (1997). *Family Caregiving in the US.* Washington, DC: American Association for Retired Persons.

Carrasquillo, O., Himmelstein, D. U., Woolhandler, S., & Bor, D. H. (1999). Trends in health insurance coverage, 1989–1997. *International Journal of Health Services, 29* (3), 467–83.

Collins, K. S., Schoen, C., Joseph, S., Duchun, L., Simantov, E., & Yellowitz, M. (1999). *Health Concerns Across a Woman's Lifespan: The Commonwealth Fund 1998 Survey of Women's Health.* New York, NY: The Commonwealth Fund.

Commonwealth Fund, The. (1987). *Old, Alone and Poor: A Plan for Reducing Poverty among Elderly People Living Alone* (Report of The Commonwealth Fund Commission on Elderly People Living Alone). New York, NY: The Commonwealth Fund.

Day, B. (1998). How the private sector can save Medicare. *Hospital Quarterly, 1* (3), 64–8.

DHHS. (1999). *Health, United States, 1999: Health and Aging Chartbook* (Chartbook, DHHS PHS 99-1232-1). Hyattsville, MD: Department of Health and Human Services.

Doress-Worters, P. B., & Siegal, D. L. (1994). *The New Ourselves, Growing Older: Women Aging with Knowledge and Power*. New York, NY: Simon & Schuster.

Estes, C. L. (1992, September 19). *Privatization, the Welfare State, and Aging: The Reagan-Bush Legacy*. Paper presented at the 21st Annual Conference of the British Society of Gerontology, University of Kent at Canterbury.

Estes, C. L. (1998). *Social Security and the Older Woman* (Congressional Briefing). Washington, DC: Organized by the Older Women's League for the Economic Security Task Force, National Council of Women's Organizations.

Estes, C. L. (2000). From gender to the political economy of ageing. *The European Journal of Social Quality, 2* (1).

Estes, C. L., & Michel, M. (1999). Social Security and Women. In The America Task Force on Women (Ed.), *Social Security in the 21st Century*. Washington, DC: Gerontological Society of America.

Estes, C. L., Swan, J. H., & Associates. (1993). *The long-term care crisis: Elders trapped in the no-care zone*. Newbury Park, CA: Sage Publications.

Friedman, E. (1994). *An unfinished revolution: Women and health care in America.* New York, NY: United Hospital Fund of New York.

Fronstin, P., & Copeland, C. (1997). Medicare on life support: Will it survive? *Ebri Issue Brief* (189), 1–22.

Fuchs, V. R. (1999). Health care for the elderly: How much? Who will pay for it? *Health Affairs, 18* (1), 11–21.

Fulwood, S., III. (1993, July 14). Out-of-wedlock births rise sharply among most groups. *Los Angeles Times,* A1.

George, L. K. (1984). The burden of caregiving: How much? What kinds? For whom? In Duke University, Center for the Study of Aging and Human Development (Ed.), *Advances in Research* (Vol. 8).

Grad, S. (1998). *Income of the Population 55 and Older, 1996*. Washington, DC: Office of Research, Evaluation, and Statistics; Social Security Administration.

Gundling, R. (1997). Additional spending reductions necessary to save Medicare. *Healthcare Financial Management, 51* (8), 90.

Guralnik, J. M., Leveille, S. G., Hirsch, R., Ferrucci, L., & Fried, L. P. (1997). The impact of disability in older women. *Journal of the American Medical Women's Association, 52* (3), 113–20.

Harrington Meyer, M. (1996). Making claims as workers on wives: The distribution of Social Security benefits. *American Sociological Review, 61* (3), 449–465.

HCFA. (1998). *A Profile of Medicare Chart Book* (Chart Book). Washington, DC: Office of Strategic Planning, Health Care Financing Administration.

Hennesey, M. (1997). *Women and Pensions*. Paper presented at the Gerontological Society of America, Chicago, IL.

Hoffman, C., & Rice, D. (1996). *Chronic Illness*. Princeton, NJ: Robert Wood Johnson Foundation.

Holmes, S. A. (1996, Oct 5). U.S. reports drop in rate of births to unwed women; fewer teen-age mothers; health agency sees decline as part of a general easing of troubling social trends. *New York Times,* 1 (N), 1 (L).

Housnell, C. (1998). *What Every Woman Needs to Know about Money and Retirement* (Booklet): Women's Institute for a Secure Retirement.

KFF. (1999). *Women and Medicare* (Report of The Kaiser Medicare Policy Project: Medical Program). Washington, DC: Kaiser Family Foundation (KFF).

La Croix, A. Z., Newton, K. M., Leveille, S. G., & Wallace, J. (1997). Healthy aging. A women's issue. *Western Journal of Medicine, 167* (4), 220–32.

LAT. (1996, Oct 8). An encouraging downswing: A national drop in unwed births needs to be sustained. *Los Angeles Times,* B6.

Lee, P. R., Estes, C. L., & Close, L. (1997). *The Nation's Health* (5th ed.). Boston, MA: Jones and Bartlett.

Martire, L. M., Stephens, M. A., & Atienza, A. A. (1997). The interplay of work and caregiving: Relationships between role satisfaction, role involvement, and caregiver's well-being. *Journals of Gerontology. Series B, Psychological Sciences and Social Sciences, 52* (5), S279–89.

McKusick, D. (1999). Demographic issues in Medicare reform. *Health Affairs, 18* (1), 194–207.

National Economic Council. (1998, October 27). *Women and Retirement Security.* Paper presented at the Interagency Working Group on Social Security.

NCPE. (1999). *The Wage Gap: 1997* (Fact Sheet). Washington, DC: National Committee on Pay Equity.

NYT. (1998, March 3). Rules set in effort to reduce some births. *New York Times,* A14 (N), A14 (L).

Oberlander, J. B. (1997). Managed care and Medicare reform. *Journal of Health Politics, Policy and Law, 22* (2), 595–631.

O'Rand, A. (1996). The Cumulative Stratification of the Life Course. In R. Binstock & L. George (Eds.). *Handbook of Aging and the Social Sciences* (pp. 188–207). New York: Academic Press.

O'Rand, A., & National Academy on Aging. (1994). *The Vulnerable Majority: Older Women in Transition* (Advisory Panel Report): Syracuse University.

PPWW. (2000). *Fair Access to Contraception (fac) project.* (www.) Planned Parenthood of Western Washington. Available: http://www.covermypills.org/states.html (2000, July 11).

Rice, D., & Michel, M. (1998). *Women and Medicare* (Fact Sheet for the Henry J. Kaiser Family Foundation and OWL: The Voice of Midlife and Older Women). San Francisco, CA: UCSF Institute for Health & Aging.

Rice, D. P. (2000). Older women's health and access to care. *Women's Health Issues, 10* (2), 42–6.

Ross, J. (1997). *Social Security Reform: Implications for Women's Retirement Income* (Report to the Ranking Minority Member, Subcommittee on Social Security, Committee on Ways & Means, House of Representatives). Washington, DC: U.S. General Accounting Office.

Schoen, C., Neuman, P., Kitchman, M., Davis, K., & Rowland, D. (1998). *Medicare Beneficiaries: A Population at Risk* (Findings from the Kaiser/Commonwealth 1997 Survey of Medicare Beneficiaries). Washington, DC: Kaiser Family Foundation.

Schulz, R., Newsom, J., Mittelmark, M., Burton, L., Hirsch, C., & Jackson, S. (1997). Health effects of caregiving: The caregiver health effects study — an ancillary study of the Cardiovascular Health Study. *Annals of Behavioral Medicine, 19* (2), 110–6.

Serafini, M. W. (1997). Brave new world. *National Journal, 29* (33), 1636–9.

Shaw, L., Zuckerman, D., & Hartman, H. (1998). *The Impact of Social Security Reform on Women* (Report). Washington, DC: Institute for Women's Policy Research.

Smeeding, T. (1999). *Social Security Reform and Older Women: Improving the System.* Syracuse, NY: Syracuse University Press.

SSA. (1998). *Fast Facts & Figures about Social Security* (Fact Sheet). Washington, DC: Office of Research, Evaluation and Statistics; Social Security Administration (SSA).

Steuerle, E. (1999). *The Treatment of the Family and Divorce in the Social Security Program* (Report). Washington, DC: U.S. Senate Special Committee on Aging.

Stone, R., Cafferata, G., & Sangl, J. (1987). Caregivers of the frail elderly: A national profile. *The Gerontologist, 27,* 616–627.

Toner, R. (1999, Sept 13). The debate on aid for the elderly focuses on women; face of aging is female; both parties appeal to them, and use them, in lobbying on safety-net programs. *New York Times,* A1 (N), A1 (L).

Trafford, A. (1998, May 19). Viagra and the other sex pill. *Washington Post,* 6.

Ussher, J. M. (1992). Reproductive rhetoric and the blaming of the body. In P. Nicolson, J. M. Ussher, & J. Campling (Eds.), *The Psychology of Women's Health and Health Care* (pp. 31–61). Houndmills, Basingstoke, Hampshire; UK: Macmillan.

Vobejda, B. (1995, Sept 22). Teen births decline; out-of-wedlock rate levels off. *Washington Post,* A1.

Weisman, C. S. (1998). *Women's Health Care: Activist Traditions and Institutional Change*. Baltimore, MD: Johns Hopkins University Press.

Wilcox, S., & King, A. C. (1999). Sleep complaints in older women who are family caregivers. *Journals of Gerontology. Series B, Psychological Sciences and Social Sciences, 54* (3), 189–98.

Wilensky, G. (1996). What it will take to save Medicare (interview by Michael Pretzer). *Medical Economics, 73* (11), 153–4, 157–8, 160.

Williams, D., & Collins, C. (1995). US Socioeconomic and Racial Differences in Health: Patterns and Explanations. *Annual Review of Sociology, 21,* 349–396.

ARTICLE 3

Racial/Ethnic Variations in Women's Health

The Social Embeddedness of Health

David R. Williams

Race/ethnicity, gender, and socioeconomic position are three social status categories that lead to the differential distribution of health risks and thus to variation in the rates of disease in society.[1,2] In this article I provide an overview of racial/ethnic disparities in health for US women. I discuss the role of socioeconomic status (SES) in accounting for these disparities and the complex interactions between race/ethnicity and SES in affecting women's health. Finally, I highlight the ways in which other social structures and processes affect the distribution of disease among American women.

RACIAL/ETHNIC DIFFERENCES IN HEALTH

In the United States, as in other industrialized societies, women have higher levels of multiple indicators of morbidity but lower rates of mortality than men. In 1998, US women had a life expectancy at birth of 79.5 years, which was 5.7 years longer than that of men (73.8 years).[3] Disaggregation of these data by racial and ethnic status was provided only for Blacks (African Americans) and Whites. The gender difference of 7.2 years within the African American population (74.8 vs 67.6) was larger than the 5.5-year gender difference for Whites (80 vs 74.5). Thus, although women of both racial groups outlive their male counterparts, White women have a life expectancy at birth that exceeds that of their Black peers by 5.2 years.

An examination of age-adjusted mortality rates for all causes by race/ethnicity for women reveals that despite declining death rates over time, African Americans have consistently had higher mortality rates than Whites.[3] The Black–White mortality ratio for females declined from 1.7 in 1950 to 1.5 in 1998. These data also highlight the problem of data availability for racial/ethnic groups other than Black and White. Nationally reported data for American Indians and Asians/Pacific Islanders are available only from 1980, and data for Hispanics only from 1985. Coverage of Hispanics has increased from only 17 states and the District of Columbia in 1995 to all 50 states and the District of Columbia in 1997.[3]

American Indian women have mortality rates that are comparable to those of their White counterparts in nationally reported data.[3] However, mortality data from the Indian Health Service (covering American Indians who live on or near reservations) reveal that between 1955 and 1993 the American Indian–White mortality ratios declined but remained large for some causes of death, such as accidents, homicide, tuberculosis, and alcoholism, and increased for others, such as diabetes, liver cirrhosis, and suicide.[4] Asian American and Hispanic women had mortality rates that were lower than those of their White peers in the first year of available data, and both of these groups have maintained this advantage over time. Across all racial/ethnic categories, the mortality rates for women are considerably lower than those for men, but the minority–White mortality ratio for women is very similar to that of men.

The quality of mortality data is much better for Blacks and Whites than for the other racial/ethnic groups, owing to a substantial undercount in the numerator that understates officially reported mortality rates for American Indians, Asians/Pacific Islanders, and Hispanics.[5,6] For example, Sorlie and colleagues[7] compared self-reported race from a personal interview with the race of the decedent as recorded on the death certificate. Race on the death certificate is typically based on observation or proxy reports. High agreement from both sources was evident for Blacks and Whites, but 1 in 4 American Indians and 1 in 5 Asians/Pacific Islanders were classified as belonging to another race (mainly White) on the death certificate. Ten percent of self-identified Hispanics were misclassified as non-Hispanic.

Racial and ethnic disparities in the severity and course of disease also contribute to observed disparities in disease prevalence and mortality. Black–White differences in survival rates from cancer illustrate this.[3] Between 1974 and 1979, 57% of White females, compared with 47% of their Black counterparts, had a 5-year survival rate for cancers from all sites. Data for 1989 to 1995 revealed that the 5-year cancer survival rate increased modestly for White females, to 63%, and only slightly for Black females, to 49%. Thus, the racial difference for cancer survival increased from 10 percentage points in the earliest period for which data are available to 14 percentage points in the most recent one.

There is some variation by specific types of cancer. Racial differences for breast cancer are considerably larger than those for lung cancer and colon cancer. The case of breast cancer is instructive because, compared with Black women, White women have a higher incidence rate but a lower mortality rate. There are racial differences in cancer staging; Black women are likely to have more advanced cancer at the time of diagnosis than their White peers. However, poorer stage-specific survival rates are also evident for Black compared with White women.[8] Not surprisingly, between 1989 and 1995, the 5-year-survival rate for breast cancer was 71% for African American females and 86% for White females.

Comorbid chronic illnesses disproportionately affect minority women, and the sequelae of multiple illnesses are worse for at least some minority populations than for Whites. Among persons with diabetes, both male and female African Americans are more likely than their White counterparts to become blind, to become amputees, to develop end-stage kidney disease, and to die of diabetes.[9] Similarly, hypertension is more strongly associated with the development of renal disease for American Indians and African Americans than for Whites.[10] Other recent data document that in contrast to other US racial/ethnic groups, rates of cardiovascular disease are rising for American Indians and coronary events are more often fatal for this population.[11]

DIVERSITY OF HEALTH PROFILES

The 10 leading causes of death in 1998 for women in each of the major racial/ethnic populations illustrate that there is variation in the major health challenges faced by these groups.[3] These data also hint at some of the morbidity challenges facing US women. Coronary heart disease and cancer, in that order, are the two leading causes of death for all women in the United States except Asian/Pacific Islander women, for whom the order is reversed. Accidents and unintentional injuries are the third leading cause of death for American Indian women, unlike all other women, for whom cerebrovascular disease is third.

Hypertension is a common chronic disease that is a major risk factor for both coronary heart disease and cerebrovascular disease. Rates of hypertension are 1.8 times higher for African American than for White women.[3] Mexican American, Puerto Rican, Native Hawaiian, and American Indian women also have rates of hypertension that are higher than those of their White counterparts.[9] Filipina women aged 50 years and older in California exhibit a rate of hypertension that is slightly higher than that of similarly aged African American women.[9]

Diabetes, a chronic condition that can have an important negative impact on the quality of life, is the fourth leading cause of death for African American, American Indian, and Hispanic women. These three groups have higher diabetes mortality rates than Whites, and these rates have increased in recent years, both absolutely and relative to White rates.[3] One third of Native Hawaiian women are diabetic, and the highest prevalence of diabetes in the United States has been observed for Yaqui Indian women.[9] In this population 50% of women aged 35 to 54 years and 92% of women aged 55 to 64 years have diabetes.

There are also several conditions that are among the 10 leading causes of death for only one population. Suicide is a leading cause of death (ranked 8th) only for Asian/Pacific Islander women. HIV/AIDS is a leading cause of death (ranked 10th) only for African American women, congenital anomalies (ranked 10th) only for Hispanics, and Alzheimer disease (ranked 8th) only for Whites. The leading causes of death for all racial/ethnic groups vary markedly by age, such that a consideration of racial/ethnic differences across major age groupings would reveal an even more complex pattern of heterogeneity.

Table 1 illustrates the complex pattern of racial/ethnic disparities in health for women by presenting age-adjusted mortality rates for Whites and minority–White

TABLE 1

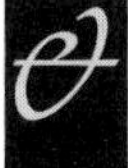

Age-Adjusted Mortality Rate (per 100,000) for Non-Hispanic Whites and Minority–White Ratios for Selected Causes of Death: Women in the United States, 1996–1998

Cause	*White Rate*	*Black–White Ratio*	*AmI-White Ratio*	*API–White Ratio*	*Hispanic–White Ratio*
Heart disease	91.3	1.63	0.80	0.54	0.70
Cancer	108.0	1.21	0.70	0.58	0.60
Homicide	2.2	4.27	2.23	0.95	1.54
HIV/AIDS	0.8	18.75	1.38	0.38	5.00
Suicide	4.7	0.40	1.13	0.70	0.40
Pulmonary disease	19.2	0.68	0.62	0.27	0.35

Note: AmI = American Indian/Alaska Native; API = Asian/Pacific Islander.
Source: National Center for Health Statistics.[3]

ratios for selected causes of death. Several points are noteworthy. First, all of the non-Black minority populations have markedly lower death rates than Whites for heart disease and cancer, the two leading causes of death in the United States. This is a key contributor to the lower death rates for these populations for all-cause mortality. Second, like African Americans, American Indians and Hispanics have higher mortality rates than Whites for some causes of death, such as homicide and HIV/AIDS.

Third, White women have higher death rates than Black and other minority women for some causes of death. Mortality from chronic obstructive pulmonary disease is higher for White women than for all minority women. This probably reflects the earlier onset and increased rates of cigarette smoking among White women.[12] African American and Hispanic women also have markedly lower rates of suicide than White women. Finally, with the exception of homicide, for which their rate is only slightly lower than that of Whites, Asian/Pacific Islander women have death rates that are markedly lower than those of Whites for all causes of death considered.

DIVERSITY OF POPULATIONS

Each racial/ethnic population is characterized by considerable diversity. Data on cancer incidence provides a unique glimpse of the heterogeneity within the Asian/Pacific Islander category.[13] For example, Vietnamese women have a rate of cervical cancer that is considerably higher than that of both Black and White women and about 6 times that of Japanese and Chinese women. Similarly, breast cancer incidence for Native Hawaiian women is higher than that of African American women and more than twice that of Korean and Vietnamese women.

There has been limited attention to diversity within the Black population, but some research suggests there may be important health status variations within this group as well. For example, Fruchter and colleagues[14] found that among Black women, American-born and Haitian-born women had higher rates of cervical cancer than women from the English-speaking Caribbean, but both immigrant groups had lower rates of breast cancer than American-born Black women. Variations within the Black population of the United States have also been reported for birth outcomes[15] and mental health.[16]

Similarly, an overall health statistic for Hispanic women hides the heterogeneity that exists among Latinas. For multiple causes of death, Puerto Rican women have higher mortality rates than other Latinas.[17] Considerable heterogeneity also exists for multiple health behaviors. For example, in 1998, 74% of Hispanic women received prenatal care during the first trimester of pregnancy, compared with 88% of non-Hispanic Whites and 73% of Blacks.[3] However, first-trimester prenatal care use ranged from 92% for Cubans to 73% for Mexican Americans. Smoking during pregnancy is another example. Only 4% of Hispanic mothers smoked during pregnancy in 1998, compared with 16% of non-Hispanic Whites, 10% of African Americans, and 20% of American Indians.[3] However, smoking rates varied from 2% for Central and South Americans and 3% for Mexican Americans to 11% for Puerto Ricans.

UNDERSTANDING RACIAL/ETHNIC DISPARITIES IN HEALTH

Early research on racial differences in health in the United States viewed racial categories as capturing biological homogeneity and racial disparities in health as genetically determined.[18] There is growing recognition that it is scientifically untenable to view race as capturing biological divisions within human populations.[19–22] Our racial categories are more alike than different in terms of biological characteristics and genetics, and they do not capture patterns of genetic variation well. Thus, it is not biologically plausible for genetic differences alone to play a major role in racial/ethnic differences in health.[23] Biological factors (including genetic ones) may, nonetheless, play a small role in accounting for population differences in health. Biology is not static but adapts over time to the conditions of the environment. Thus, for racial/ethnic groups living under different environmental conditions, interaction between biology and socially determined exposures can lead to adaptations that may contribute to population differences in health.

SOCIOECONOMIC STATUS AS A DETERMINANT OF HEALTH DISPARITIES

A growing body of research is focusing on the social context of minority women as reflected in their socioeconomic position. SES is a term conventionally used to refer to an individual's or group's location in the structure of society that determines differential access to power, privilege, and desirable resources. SES is typically assessed

TABLE 2

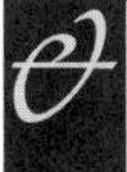

Age-Adjusted Rates for Hypertension and Overweight, by Race/Ethnicity and Average Annual Income: Women in the United States Aged ≥20 Years, 1988–1994

	Hypertension, %			*Overweight, %*		
Income Level	*White*	*Black*	*Mexican American*	*White*	*Black*	*Mexican American*
All (ages 20–74 only)	19.3	34.2	22.0	32.5	53.3	51.8
Poor	30.2	39.9	24.5	42.0	55.0	54.9
Near poor	23.9	35.9	22.4	36.6	51.0	48.7
Middle/high income	20.2	30.0	25.2	30.0	52.4	45.3

Source: National Center for Health Statistics.[85]

by income, education, or occupational status. The major racial/ethnic categories in the United States capture differences in socioeconomic circumstances, and SES plays a large role in accounting for disparities in health.

Table 2 presents age-adjusted rates of hypertension and overweight for White, Black, and Mexican American women in the United States, stratified by income. There are marked racial differences on these two indicators of health status; White women have lower levels of both hypertension and overweight than their Black and Mexican American counterparts. Rates of hypertension are about 1.8 times as high for Black women than for White women, and both African American and Mexican American women are more than 1.5 times as likely to be overweight as White women.

Several patterns are evident in these data. First, income is strongly linked to hypertension for Black and White women and to overweight for White and Mexican American women. Women with lower levels of income have worse health than their economically favored counterparts. However, income was unrelated to hypertension for Mexican American women and was not strongly associated with overweight for African American women.

Second, despite the truncation of the high end of income, differences in hypertension rates by income within the Black and White populations are almost as large as the overall Black–White differences. It is frequently observed, for multiple indicators of health status, that differences between socioeconomic categories within a race are larger than differences between races.[24–26] Third, racial differences persist at every level of SES, emphasizing that race is more than SES. This pattern of findings may reflect complex interactions between racial/ethnic status and migration history or culture, long-term effects of exposure to social and economic adversity during childhood, independent contributions of institutional and individual discrimination, or the noncomparability of SES indicators across racial/ethnic populations.[27,28]

Thus, although SES is, almost universally, a central determinant of variations in health,[29] its effects are conditioned by the presence of other factors. The interplay of migration with SES may underlie the absence of an association between income and hypertension for Mexican Americans. A similar pattern has been observed between SES and blood pressure for Mexican Americans.[30] It is unclear whether this pattern reflects a healthy-immigrant effect, protective effects of an immigrant's culture, or differences in the historical time period between Mexico and the United States in the secular distribution of hypertension and other risk factors for heart disease. The Mexican American population has a large number of immigrants who are low in SES but in relatively good health. At the same time, several health behaviors that adversely affect health status and the prevalence of multiple health conditions increase with acculturation and length of stay.[31]

The absence of an association between overweight and income for Black women highlights the need to better understand the role of culture and interactions between cultural orientations and social conditions. Some evidence suggests that Blacks have more tolerant attitudes toward obesity.[32] It is possible that such a cultural preference could lead to culturally normative elevated rates of overweight among all Black women and thus dampen the expected tendency for income to predict variations in weight.

Alternatively, the absence of a pattern of overweight by income could reflect the impact of the social and economic characteristics of the communities in which African American women reside. Irrespective of household income, Black women are more likely than women of other racial groups to reside in highly segregated neighborhoods with a greater concentration of poor persons.[33,34] These communities tend to have limited exercise facilities and reduced opportunities to engage in physical exercise under conditions of assured safety. Moreover, in addition to having high rates of poverty, Black women are also more likely than women of other groups to be single parents. The combination of these factors can lead to high levels of stress and create constraints on time, financial resources, and access to exercise facilities that can lead to lower levels of leisure-time physical activity.[35]

Table 3 further illustrates the complexity of the associations between race, SES, and health. The percentage of women who smoke cigarettes is only slightly higher for Whites than for Blacks. However, for both groups, the risk of cigarette smoking is strongly patterned by income. Poor White women are 1.7 times as likely as their middle- and high-income peers to smoke, and poor African American women are almost twice as likely as their higher-income counterparts to smoke. Within each racial group, the differences by economic status are large, much larger than the overall difference between races.

At each economic level, African American women report markedly lower levels of smoking than similarly situated Whites. This difference between racial groups suggests the presence of health-enhancing factors within the African American population that reduce the normally expected levels of smoking. The roughly comparable proportions of smokers among Black and White women overall reflects the fact that, compared with their White counterparts, Black women are overrepresented among the poor and underrepresented among middle- and high-income persons.

Infant mortality rates are strongly patterned by educational level for both Black and White women, with increasing years of education predicting lower levels of

TABLE 3

Black–White Differences in Cigarette Smoking and Infant Mortality, by Socioeconomic Status Indicators: Women in the United States, 1995

	White	*Black*	*Black–White Ratio*
Cigarette smokers, %, by income level[a]			
All	23.6	22.8	0.97
Poor	38.6	29.3	0.76
Near poor	31.6	24.9	0.79
Middle/high income	22.2	15.7	0.71
Infant mortality rate, by maternal education[b]			
<12 y	9.9	17.3	1.74
12 y	6.5	14.8	2.28
13–15 y	5.1	12.3	2.41
≥16 y	4.2	11.4	2.71

[a]Age-adjusted, age 18 years and older.
[b]Women aged 20 years and older.
Source: National Center for Health Statistics.[85]

infant mortality. Among Whites, women who did not complete high school have an infant mortality rate that is 2.4 times the rate of women who graduated from college. Similarly, among African Americans, women with less than 12 years of education have an infant mortality rate that is 1.5 times as high as that of college graduates.

However, the racial difference at every level of education is striking. Infants born to Black women in the lowest education category are 1.7 times as likely to die before their first birthday as are infants born to similarly educated White females. At every other level of education, the Black–White ratio is greater than 2. In fact, White women who did not complete high school have a lower infant mortality rate than Black college graduates, and the Black–White ratio for infant mortality increases with level of education: Black college graduates have an infant mortality rate that is 2.7 times the rate of their White counterparts.

NONEQUIVALENCE OF SOCIOECONOMIC STATUS ACROSS RACIAL/ETHNIC GROUPS

This pattern of findings reflects, at least in part, the nonequivalence of measures of SES across race and ethnicity.[27,28] That is, there are group differences in the very nature of SES that make all of the standard SES indicators noncomparable across race. In this article, I provide details on racial/ethnic differences in wealth and income for given levels of education, but similar disparities also exist for the quality of education, the purchasing power of income, the stability of employment, and the health risks associated with working in particular occupations.[27]

Racial/ethnic differences in wealth are considerably larger than those in income, and focusing only on income understates the racial/ethnic disparities in economic status. For example, in 1995, the median wealth (net worth) of White households, $49,030, was almost 7 times that of Black ($7073) and Hispanic ($7255) households.[36] These differences persist at every level of income. White households in the lowest quintile of income had a net worth of $9720, compared with $1500 for Blacks and $1250 for Hispanics. At the highest quintile of income the net worth was $123,781 for White, $40,866 for Black, and $80,416 for Hispanic households. There are also large racial differences in home ownership, a key source of wealth for the average American family. Fewer than half of Black and Hispanic households own their homes, compared with more than 70% of White households.[37]

Among men, the income returns for a given level of education are large, with Black and Hispanic males at every level of income earning considerably less than their similarly educated White counterparts.[38] In contrast, there are only small differences among women in personal earnings at various levels of education. These data mask racial differences in pay.

Analyses of weekly earnings of Black and White women between 1967 and 1997 reveal that the Black–White gap in pay narrowed in the 1960s and early 1970s but has widened since the early 1980s.[37] Women of all races have high rates of employment in technical, sales, and administrative-support occupations. However, while a high percentage of White and Asian women are employed in managerial and professional occupations, a high percentage of Black, Hispanic, and American Indian women are employed in service occupations.

Black families have historically relied more heavily on women's earnings than do other families, and the proportion of female-headed households is highest among Blacks. These racial differences in marital status, and thus in the number of adults contributing to the household income, mean that focusing only on personal income understates racial differences in the flow of economic resources into the household. The racial/ethnic differences in income are now marked. At every level of education, Black and Hispanic women earn considerably less than Whites of similar education. Blacks earn less than Hispanics, and the differences between Blacks and Whites are especially large. For example, Black high school graduates earned 64 cents, and college graduates 74 cents, for every dollar in total household income earned by similarly educated White women.

These data highlight the critical need to comprehensively assess SES in its multiple dimensions and trace its health consequences across the life course. Recent research on economic hardship highlights the fact that there are important racial differences in economic circumstances that are not captured by the traditional measures of SES. Data from the Survey of Income and Program Participation indicated that even after controlling for SES (income, education, transfer payments, home ownership, and employment status) and demographic factors (age, sex, marital status, children, disability, health insurance, and residential mobility), African Americans were more likely than Whites to experience 6 of 9 hardships examined.[39] That is, they were more likely to report being unable to meet essential expenses, being unable to pay full rent or mortgage, being unable to pay full utility bills, having had utilities shut off, having had telephone service shut off, and having been evicted from apartment or home.

Part of this difference in economic hardship is driven by the geographic location of minority women and the resulting cost of housing. African American, Hispanic, Asian, and American Indian households are nearly twice as likely as non-Hispanic White households to spend 50% or more of their income on housing costs.[37] Housing expenditures of less than 30% of income are considered affordable or desirable. High housing costs limit a household's ability to procure other necessities.

TRENDS IN ECONOMIC AND HEALTH DISPARITIES

Analysis of trends in Black–White inequality in economic status and health over the last 50 years reveals that racial disparities in health are sensitive to changes in racial inequality in economic circumstances. During the 1960s and early 70s, the civil rights movement led to improvements in the political and economic situation of Blacks and a narrowing of the Black–White gap in income.[40] Between 1968 and 1978, African American men and women aged 35 to 74 years had a larger decline in overall mortality than Whites in the same age group, on both a percentage and an absolute basis.[41] This pattern was evident across multiple causes of death. For example, the mortality rate for Black women declined by 538 deaths per 100,000 population, compared with a decline of 186 deaths for White women. This was a 29% change in mortality rates for Black women and a 17% change for White women.

However, the narrowing of the Black–White economic gap stalled in the mid-1970s and widened in the early 1980s.[40] The health of poor women and their children worsened in 20 states in the wake of the budget cuts in health and social service spending by the Reagan administration in the early 1980s.[42] Similarly, access to health care declined and levels of blood pressure increased among persons terminated from Medicaid in the state of California.[43]

Not surprisingly, the health of African American men and women declined relative to that of Whites between 1980 and 1991.[44] For example, the Black–White ratio for infant mortality for females increased from 2.0 in 1980 to 2.3 in 1991, and the Black–White gap in life expectancy for females increased from 5.6 years in 1980 to 5.8 years in 1991.

Analyses of the health status of poor Black and White populations during this same time period also document worsening health for Blacks at the local level in multiple locations.[45] For example, between 1980 and 1990, the annual death rate and annual excess deaths for Blacks compared with Whites increased for Black women in Harlem, New York City; the South Side of Chicago, Illinois; the Louisiana Delta; and the "Black belt" of Alabama. At the same time, both the annual death rate and the annual excess number of deaths declined slightly for Black women in central Detroit, Mich, suggesting the need to understand the determinants of variation at the local level.

UNDERSTANDING RACIAL/ETHNIC DISPARITIES IN HEALTH

Understanding the differential distribution of health outcomes across racial/ethnic, gender, and socioeconomic groups requires greater attention to how historical, social, economic, political, and cultural structures and processes shape health-damaging and health-enhancing factors that are typically measured at the level of the individual. Medical care, geographic location, migration and acculturation, stressors and resources, and racism are promising areas for further unraveling the complex ways in which the social position of minority women is linked to health consequences.

Medical Care

Renewed attention to research and policy is needed to understand the role that medical care can play in reducing racial/ethnic disparities in health and to make a new commitment to improving the quality of care for all Americans. Medical care makes a limited contribution to population differences in health.[46,47] A US surgeon general's report concluded that medical care explains only 10% of variation in health status.[48] However, medical care may have a greater impact on the health status of vulnerable populations, such as racial/ethnic minorities and low-SES groups, than on the population in general.[49] Medical care may be an especially important health-protective resource in the context of multiple vulnerabilities.

Minority women face many challenges when it comes to medical care, and they often have a greater need for medical care owing to higher levels of morbidity and comorbidity. Many racial/ethnic minority populations have lower levels of access to medical care in the United States than do Whites. Compared with White women, minority women are less likely to be insured, to have employer-based private insurance coverage, and to have insurance coverage through a spouse's employment, and they are more likely to have public health insurance coverage.[9] They are also more likely than White women to receive care in less than optimal organizational settings (such as the emergency room) and to lack continuity in the health care received.

A recent analysis of racial/ethnic differences in access to and use of health services between 1977 and 1996 concluded that the Black–White gap has not narrowed over time and the gap between Hispanics and Whites has widened.[50] Moreover, this study found that even if income and health insurance coverage were equalized, racial/ethnic differences in ambulatory care would not be eliminated, because one half to three quarters of these disparities are not accounted for by these factors.

The Indian Health Service is a federal agency that provides direct and contract health care services to American Indians who live on or near reservations. The agency has been successful in improving the access of American Indians and Alaska Natives to preventive services such as immunizations and prenatal care,[51] but persisting shortfalls in federal funding and other challenges limit its ability to meet all of the health care needs of its target population.[52]

A large body of evidence documents pervasive racial/ethnic disparities in the diagnosis and treatment of minority persons once they enter the US health care system. These disparities exist across a broad spectrum of therapeutic interventions, ranging from high-technology procedures to the most elementary forms of diagnostic and treatment interventions, and they persist even when adjusted for health insurance coverage, SES, stage and severity of disease, comorbidity, and type of medical facility.[53,54] Moreover, they exist in contexts such as Medicare and the Department of Veterans Affairs health system, where differences in economic status and insurance coverage are minimized. Thus it is likely that greater access to more continuous preventive care and timely and appropriate secondary and tertiary care, from concerned providers, can have an important effect on reducing racial/ethnic disparities in health.[47]

Place and Health

Place is a neglected but critical factor affecting the health of populations. A recent analysis of poor Black and White populations in rural and southern locations and in northern urban areas documented an important interaction among poverty, race, and place.[45] Although African American men and women in rural and southern locations faced economic conditions that were similar to or worse than those of Black populations in northern urban areas, they enjoyed substantially better health. A similar pattern was evident for Whites. In fact, the health profile of poor Whites in some northern urban areas is comparable to that of more economically disadvantaged Blacks in the South.

For example, the 1990 mortality rate of 428 per 100,000 population for White women in Detroit, Mich, was comparable to mortality rates for Black women in east North Carolina (421 per 100,000) and in the "Black belt" of Alabama (425 per 100,000). Similarly, Puerto Rican residents of New York City have higher coronary heart disease mortality than Puerto Ricans living in Puerto Rico and Puerto Rican–born persons elsewhere in the United States.[55] At present it is not clear whether the patterning of health by place reflects the deterioration of social services and the health infrastructure in some urban contexts or the presence of resources, such as a less sedentary and stressful lifestyle and greater social cohesion, in rural areas.[45]

Migration and Acculturation

There is also a critical need to enhance our understanding of the ways in which stressors and resources linked to the process of migration and acculturation relate to each other and combine to affect the health of immigrants. While immigrants of all racial/ethnic groups have lower infant and adult mortality than their US-born counterparts,[56,57] these patterns are complex and not well understood. A good health profile for immigrants may reflect the tendency for immigrants to be selected on the basis of good health or it may reflect a return of at least some ill immigrants to their home countries, but these factors alone do not explain the health profile of immigrants.[58]

Moreover, better health for immigrants does not exist for all outcomes. For example, a study of pregnancy-related mortality between 1991 and 1997 revealed that US-born and foreign-born Black and Hispanic women and foreign-born Asian women had higher pregnancy-related deaths than White women in the United States.[59] In addition, Hispanic and Asian immigrant women had higher pregnancy-related mortality rates than their US-born counterparts. Levels of maternal mortality were especially high for Black women; the pregnancy-related mortality risk of both US-born and foreign-born Black women was 4 times as high as that of White women.

Similarly, although Hispanic women have lower levels of infant mortality than White women, women of all Hispanic immigrant groups have a higher risk of low birthweight and prematurity than do Whites.[60] Analysis of a half century of longitudinal mortality data reveals that for both Mexican immigrants and persons born in the United States of Mexican ancestry, there is a general convergence over time with the health pattern of the White population.[61] Similarly, the advantage in coronary heart disease mortality for Puerto Ricans on the mainland appears to be declining over time.[55]

Clearly, the associations between migration, acculturation, and health are complex. Migration studies of the Chinese and Japanese show that rates of some cancers (e.g., colon cancer) increase when these populations migrate to the United States, while rates of other cancers (e.g., liver and cervical cancer) decline.[62] There is clearly a need to carefully and systematically delineate the harmful and protective factors resident in both immigrant and host cultures and to identify the conditions under which these factors combine over time, across generations, and in particular geographic contexts to affect health.

Stressors and Resources

More generally, we need more comprehensive characterization of the stressors and resources that may have consequences for health.[63] This will require a greater emphasis on a life-course approach that seeks to understand the ways in which resources and adversity accumulate over the lifetime to affect adult health. It will also require greater attention to stressors that are linked to the status of women in society. This includes examination of the physical and mental health consequences of exposure to physical, sexual, and emotional abuse in childhood and adolescence and to the fear of violent victimization and actual experiences of victimization, both within and outside the home, over the life span.[64,65]

At present, we do not clearly understand how the conditions, contexts, burdens, and demands of the multiple-gendered roles that women occupy in society lead to the accumulation of particular configurations of risks and resources that affect their health status.[12] Analyses of state-level data in the United States reveal that higher levels of political and economic status for women are associated with lower morbidity and mortality.[66]

The lower rates of morbidity and mortality that women of all minority groups experience for selected health outcomes highlight the need to understand health-enhancing resources resident within each population that may cushion some of the negative effects of exposure to social and economic adversity. Strong family ties, an extended family system, and religious involvement and participation may reduce some of the negative effects of stress in the lives of minority women. For example, religious involvement and participation can provide supportive social relationships, tangible economic resources, comfort in times of trouble, motivation and support for engaging in healthy behaviors, and belief systems that provide meaning and understanding.[67–71] However, researchers and practitioners should recognize that social relationships and religious involvement can provide both stress and support, and the negative as well as the positive aspects of these potential resources should be assessed.

Racism

Future research on minority women must also give greater attention to the ways in which racism can affect their health. Institutional discrimination plays an important role in restricting economic opportunity for minority women and thus, indirectly, is a key determinant of adult socioeconomic status.[34] Racial residential segregation, a key institutional mechanism of racism, may play a critical role in shaping the adverse health consequences linked to residential location.

In addition, a growing body of research suggests that subjective experiences of discrimination are an important factor in the lives of minority women that may adversely affect physical and mental health.[72–75] Some research suggests that such experiences of discrimination make an incremental contribution to explaining racial differences in health status after SES is considered.[76,77] However, the study of racism and health is still in its infancy, and research is needed that will comprehensively assess racism at its multiple levels of operation and rigorously identify the mechanisms and processes by which it can affect health.[78–83]

CONCLUSION

Like many researchers in this field, in this article I have consistently used White women as the group against which to compare the health experience of minority women in the United States. In race-conscious societies, such comparisons yield useful data, but their limits should be explicitly acknowledged, since the health status of White women is not an optimal benchmark. For example, the infant mortality rate for non-Hispanic Whites was 6.1 per 1000 live births in 1996. Nineteen countries had infant mortality rates for that year that were lower than that of US Whites. Similarly, in 1995, women in 15 countries had longer life expectancies than 79.6 years, which was the life expectancy for White women in the United States.[3]

Thus, despite leading the world in absolute and per capita spending on medical care, the United States does not provide readily achievable levels of health status to even its most advantaged citizens. There is a need for a renewed commitment not only to eliminating racial/ethnic disparities in health care but also to improving the access of all Americans to continuous and comprehensive preventive care.

However, interventions in health care alone will neither eliminate social inequalities in health nor facilitate optimal levels of population health.[47,84] The health of minority women is to an important extent a product of their location in larger historical, geographic, sociocultural, economic, and political contexts. Thus, policies that target and change existing social arrangements can improve the living circumstances and health of minority women.

For example, almost half of all minority children are growing up in poverty.[85] Living in a single-parent household is a strong determinant of exposure to poverty in the United States, but this association is not inevitable. Twenty-one percent of all children in Sweden are in single-parent families, compared with 19% in the United States.[86] However, 55% of American children in single-parent households are growing up poor, compared with 7% of Swedish children in single-parent households.[86] Social policies in Sweden provide a safety net for vulnerable children.

Improving population health and eliminating racial/ethnic and socioeconomic inequalities in health will require a redefinition of health policy to include all societal policies that directly or indirectly affect health and a new commitment to policy changes in a range of areas, including income, education, employment, housing, transportation, and agriculture.[87,88]

Attention to identifying and addressing the fundamental social determinants of health should not obscure the importance of identifying the specific physiological mechanisms and pathways that link social exposures to health and illness. Research is needed to identify how biological factors linked to sex and social factors linked to gender combine with experiences linked to specific racial and ethnic statuses to create particular biological risks and realities. Promising models for understanding and studying these complex processes have been proposed.[83,89]

Finally, some have suggested that the time has come to abandon the assessment of race in public health research and surveillance.[90] However, the data reviewed here indicate that racial/ethnic status remains an important predictor of variations in both the living circumstances and the health of American women. It is necessary not only to continue collecting racial/ethnic data but also to assess these social status categories in their full diversity, with greater attention to assessing the specific factors linked to race/ethnicity that might affect health and appropriately interpreting racial/ethnic data.[76,91–93]

Practitioners should also consider the heterogeneity of each racial and ethnic population and design interventions that are culturally appropriate and that seek to alter not only health beliefs and behaviors but also the living and working conditions in which these beliefs and behaviors are embedded.[94,95] The ultimate goal of such efforts should be to identify the fundamental determinants of disparities in health and the key intervention strategies that are necessary to eliminate racial/ethnic inequalities.

ACKNOWLEDGMENTS

Preparation of this paper was supported by grants MH59575 and MH57425 from the National Institute of Mental Health and the John D. and Catherine T. MacArthur Foundation Research Network on Socioeconomic Status and Health.

I am grateful to Scott Wyatt for research assistance, Kathleen Boyle for preparing the manuscript, and the anonymous reviewers for helpful comments.

REFERENCES

1. Krieger N, Rowley DL, Herman AA, Avery B, Phillips MT. Racism, sexism, and social class: implications for studies of health, disease, and well-being. *Am J Prev Med.* 1993;9(suppl 6):82–122.

2. Lillie-Blanton M, Martinez RM, Taylor AK, Robinson BG. Latina and African American women: continuing disparities in health. *Int J Health Serv.* 1993;23:555–584.

3. *Health, United States, 2000, With Adolescent Health Chartbook.* Hyattsville, Md: National Center for Health Statistics; 2000.

4. *Trends in Indian Health.* Rockville, Md: Indian Health Service; 1997.

5. Hahn RA. The state of federal health statistics on racial and ethnic groups. *JAMA.* 1992;267:268–271.

6. Frost F, Tollestrup K, Ross A, Sabotta E, Kimball E. Correctness of racial coding of American Indians and Alaska Natives on the Washington State death certificate. *Am J Prev Med.* 1994;10:290–294.

7. Sorlie PD, Rogot E, Johnson NJ. Validity of demographic characteristics on the death certificate. *Epidemiology.* 1992;3:181–184.

8. Hunter CP, Redmond CK, Chen VW, et al. Breast cancer: factors associated with stage at diagnosis in Black and White women. *J Natl Cancer Inst.* 1993;85:1129–1137.

9. *Women of Color Health Data Book: Adolescents to Seniors.* Bethesda, Md: Office of Research on Women's Health; 1998. NIH publication 98–4247.

10. Powers DR, Wallin JD. End-stage renal disease in specific ethnic and racial groups: risk factors and benefits of antihypertensive therapy. *Arch Intern Med.* 1998;158:793–800.

11. Howard BV, Lee ET, Cowan LD, et al. Rising tide of cardiovascular disease in American Indians: the strong heart study. *Circulation.* 1999;99:2389–2395.

12. Walsh DC, Sorensen G, Leonard L. Gender, health, and cigarette smoking. In: Amick BC III, Levine S, Tarlov AR, Walsh DC, eds. *Society and Health.* New York, NY: Oxford University Press; 1995:131–171.

13. Miller BA, Kolonel LN, Bernstein L, et al. *Racial/Ethnic Patterns of Cancer in the United States, 1988–1992.* Bethesda, Md: National Cancer Institute; 1996. NIH publication 96–4101.

14. Fruchter RG, Wright C, Habenstreit B, Remy JC, Boyce JG, Imperato PJ. Screening for cervical and breast cancer among Caribbean immigrants. *J Community Health.* 1985;10:121–135.

15. David RJ, Collins JW Jr. Differing birth weight among infants of U.S.-born Blacks, African-born Blacks, and U.S.-born Whites. *N Engl J Med.* 1997;337: 1209–1214.

16. Williams DR. Race, stress and mental health: findings from the Commonwealth Minority Health Survey. In: Hogue C, Hargraves M, Scott-Collins K, eds. *Minority Health in America: Findings and Policy Implications from the Commonwealth Fund Minority Health Survey*. Baltimore, Md: Johns Hopkins University Press; 2000:209–243.
17. Sorlie PD, Backlund E, Johnson NJ, Rogot E. Mortality by Hispanic status in the United States. *JAMA*. 1993;270:2464–2468.
18. Krieger N. Shades of difference: theoretical underpinnings of the medical controversy on black/white differences in the United States, 1830–1870. *Int J Health Serv*. 1987;17:259–278.
19. American Association of Physical Anthropology. AAPA statement on biological aspects of race. *Am J Phys Anthropol*. 1996;101:569–570.
20. Lewontin RC. *Human Diversity*. New York, NY: Scientific American Books; 1982.
21. Cooper RS, David R. The biological concept of race and its application to public health and epidemiology. *J Health Polit Policy Law*. 1986;11:97–116.
22. Williams DR. Race and health: basic questions, emerging directions. *Ann Epidemiol*. 1997;7:322–333.
23. Cooper RS, Freeman VL. Limitations in the use of race in the study of disease causation. *J Natl Med Assoc*. 1999;91:379–383.
24. Sorlie P, Rogor E, Anderson R, Backlund E. Black–white mortality differences by family income. *Lancet*. 1992;340:346–350.
25. Navarro V. Race or class versus race and class: mortality differentials in the United States. *Lancet*. 1990;336:1238–1240.
26. Williams DR. Race, SES, and health: the added effects of racism and discrimination. *Ann N Y Acad Sci*. 1999;896:173–188.
27. Williams DR, Collins C. U.S. socioeconomic and racial differences in health: patterns and explanations. *Annu Rev Sociol*. 1995;21:349–386.
28. Kaufman JS, Cooper RS, McGee DL. Socioeconomic status and health in blacks and whites: the problem of residual confounding and the resiliency of race. *Epidemiology*. 1997;8:621–628.
29. Krieger N, Williams DR, Moss N. Measuring social class in US public health research: concepts, methodologies, and guidelines. *Annu Rev Public Health*. 1997;18:341–378.
30. Sorel JE, Ragland DR, Syme SL, Davis WB. Educational status and blood pressure: the Second National Health and Nutrition Examination Survey, 1976–1980, and the Hispanic Health and Nutrition Examination Survey, 1982–1984. *Am J Epidemiol*. 1992;135:1339–1348.
31. Vega WA, Amaro H. Latino outlook: Good health, uncertain prognosis. *Annu Rev Public Health*. 1994;15:39–67.
32. Kumanyika S. Obesity in black women. *Epidemiol Rev*. 1987;9:31–50.
33. Massey DS, Denton NA. *American Apartheid: Segregation and the Making of the Underclass*. Cambridge, Mass: Harvard University Press; 1993.

34. Williams DR, Collins C. Racial residential segregation: a fundamental cause of racial disparities in health. *Public Health Rep.* In press.
35. Williams DR. Black–white differences in blood pressure: the role of social factors. *Ethn Dis.* 1992;2:126–141.
36. Davern ME, Fisher PJ. *Household Net Worth and Asset Ownership: 1995.* Washington, DC: US Bureau of the Census; 2001. Current Population Reports, Household Economic Studies Series P70–71.
37. *Changing America: Indicators of Social and Economic Well-Being by Race and Hispanic Origin.* Washington, DC: Council of Economic Advisers for the President's Initiative on Race; 1998.
38. *Income by Educational Attainment for Persons 18 Years Old and Over, by Age, Sex, Race, and Hispanic Origin: March 1996.* Washington, DC: US Bureau of the Census; 1997.
39. Bauman K. *Direct Measures of Poverty as Indicators of Economic Need: Evidence from the Survey of Income and Program Participation.* Washington, DC: US Bureau of the Census; November 1998. Population Division Technical Working Paper No. 30.
40. *Economic Report of the President, 1998, With the Annual Report of the Council of Economic Advisers.* Washington, DC: Office of the President; 1998.
41. Cooper R, Steinhauer M, Schatzkin A, Miller W. Improved mortality among U.S. blacks, 1968–1978: the role of antiracist struggle. *Int J Health Serv.* 1981;11:511–522.
42. Mandinger M. Health service funding cuts and the declining health of the poor. *N Engl J Med.* 1985;313:44–47.
43. Lurie N, Ward NB, Shapiro MF, Brook RH. Termination from Medi-Cal — does it affect health? *N Engl J Med.* 1984;311:480–484.
44. *Excess Deaths and Other Mortality Measures for the Black Population: 1979–81 and 1991.* Hyattsville, Md: National Center for Health Statistics; 1994.
45. Geronimus AT, Bound J, Waidmann TA. Poverty, time, and place: variation in excess mortality across selected U.S. populations, 1980–1990. *Epidemiol Community Health.* 1999;53:325–334.
46. Adler NE, Boyce T, Chesney MA, Folkman S, Syme SL. Socioeconomic inequalities in health: no easy solution. *JAMA.* 1993;269:3140–3145.
47. House JS, Williams DR. Understanding and reducing socioeconomic and racial/ethnic disparities in health. In: Smedley BD, Syme SL, eds. *Promoting Health: Intervention Strategies from Social and Behavioral Research.* Washington DC: National Academy Press; 2000:81–124.
48. *Healthy People: The Surgeon General's Report on Health Promotion and Disease Prevention.* Washington, DC: US Dept of Health, Education, and Welfare; 1979.
49. Williams DR. Socioeconomic differentials in health: a review and redirection. *Soc Psychol Q.* 1990;53:81–99.

50. Weinick RM, Zuvekas SH, Cohen JW. Racial and ethnic differences in access to and use of health care services, 1977 to 1996. *Med Care Res Rev.* 2000;57 (suppl 1):36–54.
51. Rhoades ER, D'Angelo AJ, Hurlburt WB. The Indian Health Service record of achievement. *Public Health Rep.* 1987;102:356–360.
52. Noren J, Kindig D, Sprenger A. Challenges to Native American health care. *Public Health Rep.* 1998;113:22–33.
53. Mayberry RM, Mili F, Ofili E. Racial and ethnic differences in access to medical care. *Med Care Res Rev.* 2000;57(suppl 1):108–145.
54. Kressin NR, Petersen LA. Racial differences in the use of invasive cardiovascular procedures: review of the literature and prescription for future research. *Ann Intern Med.* 2001;135:352–366.
55. Rosenwaike I, Hempstead K. Mortality among three Puerto Rican populations: residents of Puerto Rico and migrants in New York City and in the balance of the United States, 1979–81. *Int Migration Rev.* 1990;24:684–702.
56. Singh GK, Yu SM. Adverse pregnancy outcomes: differences between US- and foreign-born women in major US racial and ethnic groups. *Am J Public Health.* 1996:86:837–843.
57. Hummer RA, Rogers RG, Nam CB, LeClere FB. Race/ethnicity, nativity, and U.S. adult mortality. *Soc Sci Q.* 1999;80:136–153.
58. Abraido-Lanza AF, Dohrenwend BP, Ng-Mak DS, Turner JB. The Latino mortality paradox: a test of the "salmon bias" and healthy migrant hypotheses. *Am J Public Health.* 1999;88:1543–1548.
59. Centers for Disease Control. Pregnancy-related deaths among Hispanic, Asian/Pacific Islander, and American Indian/Alaska Native women — United States, 1991–1997. *MMWR Morb Mortal Wkly Rep.* 2001;50:361–364.
60. Frisbie WP, Forbes D, Hummer RA. Hispanic pregnancy outcomes: additional evidence. *Soc Sci Q.* 1998;79:149–169.
61. Bradshaw BS, Frisbie WP. Mortality of Mexican Americans and Mexican immigrants: comparisons with Mexico. In: Weeks JR, Ham-Chande R, eds. *Demographic Dynamics of the U.S.–Mexico Border*. El Paso: Texas Western Press; 1992:125–150.
62. Jenkins CNH, Kagawa-Singer M. Cancer. In: Zane NWS, Takeuchi DT, Young KNJ, eds. *Confronting Critical Health Issues of Asian and Pacific Islander Americans*. Thousand Oaks, Calif: Sage; 1994:105–147.
63. Taylor SE, Repetti RL, Seeman T. Health psychology: what is an unhealthy environment and how does it get under the skin? *Annu Rev Psychol.* 1997;48:411–447.
64. Felitti VJ, Anda RF, Nordenberg D, et al. Relationship of childhood abuse and household dysfunction to many of the leading causes of death in adults. *Am J Prev Med.* 1998;14:245–258.
65. Wyatt GE. The relationship between child sexual abuse and adolescent sexual functioning in Afro-American and white American women. *Ann N Y Acad Sci.* 1988;528:111–122.

66. Kawachi I, Kennedy BP, Gupta V, Prothrow-Stith D. Women's status and the health of women and men: a view from the States. *Soc Sci Med.* 1999;48:21–32.
67. Idler EL. Religious involvement and the health of the elderly: some hypotheses and an initial test. *Soc Forces.* 1987;66:226–238.
68. Griffith EE, Young JL, Smith DL. An analysis of the therapeutic elements in a black church service. *Hosp Community Psychiatry.* 1984;35:464–469.
69. Chatters LM. Religion and health: public health research and practice. *Annu Rev Public Health.* 2000;21:335–367.
70. Wallace JM, Forman TA. Religion's role in promoting health and reducing risk among American youth. *Health Educ Behav.* 1998;25:721–741.
71. Williams DR, Griffith EE, Young J, Collins C, Dodson J. Structure and provision of services in New Haven black churches. *Cultural Diversity Ethn Minority Psychol.* 1999;5:118–133.
72. Amaro H, Russo NF, Johnson J. Family and work predictors of psychological well-being among Hispanic women professionals. *Psychol Women Q.* 1987;11:505–521.
73. Krieger N. Racial and gender discrimination: risk factors for high blood pressure? *Soc Sci Med.* 1990;30:1273–1281.
74. Noh S, Beiser M, Kaspar V, Hou F, Rummens J. Perceived racial discrimination, depression, and coping: a study of Southeast Asian refugees in Canada. *J Health Soc Behav.* 1999;40:193–207.
75. Kessler RC, Mickelson KD, Williams DR. The prevalence, distribution, and mental health correlates of perceived discrimination in the United States. *J Health Soc Behav.* 1999;40;208–230.
76. Williams DR, Yu Y, Jackson J, Anderson N. Racial differences in physical and mental health: socioeconomic status, stress, and discrimination. *J Health Psychol.* 1997;2:335–351.
77. Ren XS, Amick B, Williams DR. Racial/ethnic disparities in health: the interplay between discrimination and socioeconomic status. *Ethn Dis.* 1999;9:151–165.
78. Krieger N. Embodying inequality: a review of concepts, measures, and methods for studying health consequences of discrimination. *Int J Health Serv.* 1999;29:295–352.
79. Williams DR, Williams-Morris R. Racism and mental health: the African American experience. *Ethn Health.* 2000;5:243–268.
80. Williams DR, Neighbors H. Racism, discrimination and hypertension: evidence and needed research. *Ethn Dis.* 2001;11:800–816.
81. Harrell FE, Merritt MM, Kalu J. Racism, stress and disease. In: Jones RL, ed. *African American Mental Health.* Hampton, Va: Cobb & Henry Publishers; 1998:247–280.
82. Jones CP. Levels of racism: a theoretic framework and a gardener's tale. *Am J Public Health.* 2000;90:1212–1215.
83. Clark R, Anderson NB, Clark VR, Williams DR. Racism as a stressor for African Americans: a biopsychosocial model. *Am Psychol.* 1999;54:805–816.

84. Kaplan G, Everson SA, Lynch JW. The contribution of social and behavioral research to an understanding of the distribution of disease: a multilevel approach. In: Smedley BD, Syme SL, eds. *Promoting Health: Intervention Strategies from Social and Behavioral Research*. Washington DC: National Academy Press; 2001:37–79.
85. Pamuk E, Makuk D, Heck K, Reuben C. *Health, United States, 1998 With Socioeconomic Status and Health Chartbook*. Hyattsville, Md: National Center for Health Statistics; 1998.
86. UNICEF. *A League Table of Child Poverty in Rich Nations*. Florence, Italy: Innocenti Research Center; 2000.
87. Acheson SD. *Independent Inquiry into Inequalities in Health Report*. London, England: The Stationery Office; 1998.
88. Newman KS. After Acheson: lessons for American policy on inequality and health. In: Auerbach JS, Krimgold BK, eds. *Income, Socioeconomic Status, and Health: Exploring the Relationships*. Washington, DC: National Policy Association; 2001.
89. McEwen BS. Protective and damaging effects of stress mediators. *N Engl J Med*. 1998;338:171–179.
90. Fullilove MT. Abandoning "race" as a variable in public health research — an idea whose time has come. *Am J Public Health*. 1998;88:1297–1298.
91. Zambrana RE, Carter-Pokras O. Health data issues for Hispanics: implications for public health research. *J Health Care Poor Underserved*. 2001;12:20–34.
92. Burhansstipanov L, Satter DE. Office of Management and Budget racial categories and implications for American Indians and Alaska Natives. *Am J Public Health*. 2000;90:1720–1723.
93. Srinivasan S, Guillermo T. Toward improved health: disaggregating Asian American and Native Hawaiian/Pacific Islander data. *Am J Public Health*. 2000;90:1731–1734.
94. Syme SL. Drug treatment of mild hypertension: social and psychological considerations. *Ann N Y Acad Sci*. 1978;304:99–106.
95. Syme SL. The social environment and health. *Daedalus*. 1994;123:79–86.

ARTICLE 4

FAILURE OF ESTROGEN PLUS PROGESTIN THERAPY FOR PREVENTION

Suzanne W. Fletcher and Graham A. Colditz

Approximately 38% of postmenopausal women in the United States use hormone replacement therapy.[1] In 2000, 46 million prescriptions were written for Premarin (conjugated estrogens), making it the second most frequently prescribed medication in the United States and accounting for more than $1 billion in sales, and 22.3 million prescriptions were written for Prempro (conjugated estrogens plus medroxyprogesterone acetate).[2] While US Food and Drug Administration–approved indications for hormone therapy include relief of menopausal symptoms and prevention of osteoporosis, long-term use has been in vogue to prevent a range of chronic conditions, especially heart disease. Estrogen alone was the dominant hormone until the increased risk of endometrial cancer led to the addition of progestins for women with an intact uterus. Since the mid-1980s, combined estrogen/progestin use has steadily increased.[3]

Evidence on the potential risks and benefits of combined estrogen/progestin has slowly accumulated, suggesting that the combination acts differently than estrogen alone. Several studies found a link between duration of estrogen/progestin use and breast cancer risk.[4-8] Addition of progestins may increase risk above that observed with estrogen alone, as mitotic activity in the breast during normal menstrual cycles is greatest when progesterone levels are highest.[9]

Early evidence from studies of unopposed estrogen suggested it lowered risk of cardiovascular disease, consistent with results from studies of intermediate markers that showed beneficial changes.[10] However, recent evidence from secondary prevention trials and observational studies using combined estrogen/progestin therapy showed increased risk of coronary heart disease in the first year.[11–13] This may reflect prothrombotic and proinflammatory effects of progestins that outweigh any effects of estrogens on atherogenesis and vasodilatation.

Now, the surprising results of the Women's Health Initiative (WHI) are reported in this issue of the journal.[14] The WHI is the first randomized primary prevention trial of postmenopausal hormones, and the part of the study that compared estrogen/progestin with placebo was terminated early. The data and safety monitoring board (DSMB) recommended stopping the trial because women receiving the active drug had an increased risk of invasive breast cancer (hazard ratio [HR], 1.26; 95% confidence interval [CI], 1.00–1.59), and an overall measure suggested that the treatment was causing more harm than good (global index, 1.15; 95% CI, 1.03–1.28). The decision to stop the trial after an average follow-up of 5.2 years (planned duration, 8.5 years) was made when these results met predetermined levels of harm. However, several other outcomes also suggested harm, including increased coronary heart disease (HR, 1.29; 95% CI, 1.02–1.63), stroke (HR, 1.41; 95% CI, 1.07–1.85), and pulmonary embolism (HR, 2.13; 95% CI, 1.39–3.25). Beneficial results included decreases in colorectal cancer (HR, 0.63, 95% CI, 0.43–0.92) and hip fracture (HR, 0.66; 95% CI, 0.45–0.98). Numbers of overall deaths in the estrogen/progestin and placebo groups were statistically and clinically similar in this short-duration study. Most adverse outcomes began appearing within 1 to 2 years, but increased breast cancer risk did not begin until 3 years. Results were remarkably consistent in subgroup analyses, suggesting that there is not a subgroup that the drug benefits.

The DSMB did not recommend stopping the other portion of the hormone replacement trial, which compared estrogen alone with placebo in women with hysterectomies, so it is reasonable to assume that to date, estrogen alone may be safer than combination estrogen/progestin.

The methods of the WHI study appear strong. A total of 16,608 women entered the randomized double-blind trial, and the active treatment group and the placebo group appeared to be comparable at baseline. It is interesting that such a large number of women were willing to participate in a study of a commonly used and accepted drug, and perhaps equally remarkable that only 3.5% were lost to follow-up. Clinicians were unblinded for 40.5% of women in the active treatment group and 6.8% of the placebo group, usually because of persistent vaginal bleeding. The types of outcomes and standardized procedures for measurements make it unlikely that this degree of unblinding affected results. During the study, 42% of women receiving active drug and 38% of those receiving placebo stopped taking their assigned medications, and 6.2% and 10.7%, respectively, initiated hormone therapy. Therefore, as the authors suggest, the reported findings of the intention-to-treat analysis may have underestimated the true effects. Also, if duration of treatment is important, as appears to be the case with breast cancer risk, and if compliance decreases over time, 5-year results may underestimate longer-term treatment effects. The investigators took into account competing risks of therapy and created a global index of major medical events to give an overall assessment of benefits and harms.

The authors present both nominal and rarely used adjusted CIs to take into account multiple testing, thus widening the CIs. Whether such adjustments should be used has been questioned,[15] but nominal CIs are appropriate for breast cancer, coronary heart disease, and the global index outcomes because they were the preselected major outcomes of the trial. Also, the consistency of the results over the 5 years of the study, as shown in Table 4 of the article and in the figures, argues against spurious statistical results.

Overall, the results of the WHI study are consistent with the growing body of literature on the effects of combination estrogen/progestin. The increasing risk of breast cancer with duration of use and the reductions in risk of colon cancer and fractures are in the expected direction and magnitude. Risk for stroke and venous thromboembolism continued throughout the 5 years of therapy, whereas the elevated risk of coronary heart disease was largely limited to the first year of therapy, as occurred in the Coumadin Aspirin Reinfarction Study[12] and the Heart and Estrogen/progestin Replacement Study.[11,16]

How should practicing clinicians and the millions of women taking an estrogen/progestin combination react to the unexpected and disquieting results of this study? First, although the trial results are reported primarily in terms of relative risk, which is appropriate for studies of cause, when applying the results to practice, they must be translated into absolute risk. The absolute risk of harm to an individual woman is very small. As the authors point out, the increased risk of the estrogen/progestin combination means that in 10,000 women taking the drug for a year (10,000 must be used to register risks in whole integers), there will be 7 more coronary heart disease events, 8 more invasive breast cancers, 8 more strokes, and 8 more pulmonary emboli, but 6 fewer colorectal cancers and 5 fewer hip fractures. Nevertheless, when counting all events over the 5.2 years of the trial, the excess number of events in the active drug group was 100 per 10,000 (or 1 in 100 women). This is still a small risk, but it demonstrates that risks from the drug add up over time.

Second, the whole purpose of healthy women taking long-term estrogen/progestin therapy is to preserve health and prevent disease. The results of this study provide strong evidence that the opposite is happening for important aspects of women's health, even if the absolute risk is low. Given these results, we recommend that clinicians stop prescribing this combination for long-term use. Primum non nocere applies especially to preventive health care. The results are for a single dosing regimen (1 daily tablet containing 0.625 mg of conjugated equine estrogen plus 2.5 mg of medroxyprogesterone acetate) and other regimens may have different results, but the three studies reported to date in the United States with other regimens have all found an increased risk of breast cancer.[5,6,17]

How can women be protected against osteoporosis? The results from the WHI and from numerous other studies have shown protection with hormone replacement therapy. Fortunately, there are alternative preventive strategies, at least one of which also lowers the risk of breast cancer (although to date, cardiovascular effects are not clear).[18] What about short-term use for managing menopausal symptoms? The WHI trial does not specifically address this question, but the results suggest short-term use (≤1 year) of the combination has risks for coronary heart disease and thromboembolic disease. The possibility of these small absolute risks must be balanced against the severity of symptoms and benefit of treatment.

Common preventive therapies require rigorous evaluation. For hormone replacement therapy, which is used by millions of patients, even rare adverse effects can harm substantial numbers of women. Although prevention trials are difficult and expensive (the expense often pales compared with drug expenses over time), these studies have produced important results for health care, as demonstrated by the WHI, the Breast Cancer Prevention Trial,[19] and the Multiple Outcomes of Raloxifene Evaluation study.[20] The WHI provides an important health answer for generations of healthy postmenopausal women to come — do not use estrogen/progestin to prevent chronic disease.

REFERENCES

1. Keating N, Cleary P, Aossi A, Zaslavsky A, Ayanlan J. Use of hormone replacement therapy by postmenopausal women in the United States. *Ann Intern Med.* 1999;130:545–553.

2. Kreling D, Mott D, Wiederholt J, Lundy J, Levitt L. Prescription drug trends: a chartbook update. Menlo Park, Calif: Kaiser Family Foundation; November 2001.

3. Wysowski DK, Golden L, Burke L. Use of postmenopausal estrogens and medroxyprogesterone in the United States, 1982–1992. *Obstet Gynecol.* 1995;85:6–10.

4. Bergkvist L, Adami HO, Persson I, Hoover R, Schairer C. The risk of breast cancer after estrogen and estrogen-progestin replacement. *N Engl J Med.* 1989;321:293–297.

5. Schairer C, Lubin J, Troisi R, Sturgeon S, Brinton LA, Hoover R. Menopausal estrogen and estrogen-progestin replacement therapy and breast cancer risk. *JAMA.* 2000;283:485–491.

6. Ross RK, Paganini-Hill A, Wan P, Pike M. Effect of hormone replacement therapy on breast cancer: estrogen versus estrogen plus progestin. *J Natl Cancer Inst.* 2000;92:328–332.

7. Colditz GA, Hankinson SE, Hunter DJ, et al. The use of estrogens and progestins and the risk of breast cancer in postmenopausal women. *N Engl J Med.* 1995;332:1589–1593.

8. Persson I, Weiderpass E, Bergkvist L, Bergstrom A, Schairer C. Risks of breast and endometrial cancer after estrogen and progestin replacement. *Cancer Causes Control.* 1999;10:253–260.

9. Pike MC, Spicer DV, Dahmoush L, Press MF. Estrogens, progestogens, normal breast cell proliferation, and breast cancer risk. *Epidemiol Rev.* 1993;15:17–35.

10. Mendelsohn M, Karas R. The protective effects of estrogen on the cardiovascular system. *N Engl J Med.* 1999;340:1801–1811.

11. Hulley S, Grady D, Bush T, et al. Randomized trial of estrogen plus progestin for secondary prevention of coronary heart disease in postmenopausal women. *JAMA.* 1998;280:605–613.

12. Alexander K, Newby L, Hellkamp A, et al. Initiation of hormone replacement therapy after acute myocardial infarction is associated with more cardiac events during follow-up. *J Am Coll Cardiol.* 2001;38:1–7.

13. Grodstein F, Manson JE, Stampfer MJ. Postmenopausal hormone use and secondary prevention of coronary events in the Nurses' Health Study: a prospective observational study. *Ann Intern Med.* 2001;135:1–8.

14. Writing Group for the Women's Health Initiative Investigators. Risks and benefits of estrogen plus progestin in healthy postmenopausal women: principal results from the Women's Health Initiative randomized controlled trial. *JAMA*. 2002;288:321–333.
15. Rothman KJ. *Modern Epidemiology*. Boston, Mass/Toronto, Ontario: Little Brown & Co; 1986:147–150.
16. Grady D, Herrington D, Bittner V, et al. Cardiovascular disease outcomes during 6.8 years of hormone therapy: Heart and Estrogen/progestin Replacement Study follow-up (HERS II). *JAMA*. 2002;228:49–57.
17. Chen CL, Weiss NS, Newcomb P, Barlow W, White E. Hormone replacement therapy in relation to breast cancer. *JAMA*. 2002;287:734–741.
18. Delmas PD. Treatment of postmenopausal osteoporosis. *Lancet*. 2002;359:2018–2026.
19. Fisher B, Costantino JP, Wickerham DL, et al. Tamoxifen for prevention of breast cancer — report of the National Surgical Adjuvant Breast and Bowel Project P-1. *J Natl Cancer Inst*. 1998;90:1371–1388.
20. Cummings SR, Eckert S, Krueger KA, et al. The effect of raloxifene on risk of breast cancer in postmenopausal women. *JAMA*. 1999;281:2189–2197.

ARTICLE 5

MAMMOGRAMS AND PERSONAL CHOICE

Virginia L. Ernster

Conflicting judgments about the value of routine mammography have left women in a quandary. Some experts say the evidence that mammography reduces breast cancer death rates by detecting cancer early is substantial, while others believe that routine mammograms provide very little, if any, benefit. As a fiftysomething woman and an epidemiologist tracking the data, I believe that for now women 50 to 69 should stay the course and continue to have regular mammograms. But we ought not to dismiss concerns about flaws in the existing data, and women should know why experts are not speaking with a single voice.

The evidence is far from perfect. That is not the same as saying there is good evidence that mammography doesn't work. Rather, the evidence that mammography does work is weaker than we used to think. We also need to recognize that each of us weighs benefits and risks differently.

A patient may reasonably ask what harm screening mammography can do, even if the evidence of benefit is flawed. While the downsides to mammography may seem minor, they are common. With each round of mammography, about 4 percent to 10 percent of women are found to have some sort of abnormal result; depending on the findings, the ensuing recommendations range from simply going for another mammogram to having a biopsy to rule out cancer. Various studies find that 80 percent to 95 percent of mammographic abnormalities turn out not to be cancer. Not having cancer is obviously good news, but with an estimated 28 million women having mammograms each year, that translates into hundreds of thousands going through the anxious experience of an abnormal test until the final result is known. One study estimated that after 10 mammograms the cumulative risk of a false positive result is 49 percent and the cumulative risk of biopsy in women who don't have cancer is 18.6 percent. Thus, false positives and follow-up tests are common. At the same time, we also know that about 15 to 25 percent of breast cancers are missed by mammography.

Another potential consequence is "overdiagnosis" — that is, the detection of some breast cancers that may never have progressed to become symptomatic during a patient's lifetime. Since we don't know which of those cancers will progress and which will not, essentially all women with screening-detected breast cancer are treated surgically, with or without radiation. This may result in unnecessary surgery for some women, but even this serious consequence seems acceptable if the test is saving the lives of other women.

The existing studies, which have recently been challenged, show that women from 50 to 69 who are screened have about a 25 percent lower risk of dying of breast cancer than unscreened women do. This does not mean that all women whose breast cancers are detected by mammography have their lives saved as a result. Some of the mammographically detected cancers might never progress; others would progress but are so nonaggressive that they could still be cured when detected later as breast lumps; and some women whose breast cancers are detected by mammography will still die of breast cancer. Thus advocacy groups and researchers are eager to find better ways of preventing breast cancer, detecting it early and treating it. Breast cancer still kills almost 40,000 women in the United States each year.

In the meantime, women should consider several factors in deciding whether to be screened. Is a patient's risk for the disease — based, for example, on her age — sufficient to warrant her being screened? (We don't screen men or adolescent girls for breast cancer because their risk is so low.) In particular, patients should be informed of the likelihood of false positives and told there is a chance of overdiagnosis.

Most people can tolerate the false positives and the attendant clinical work-ups that go along with screening if a test is effective in reducing mortality, is relatively noninvasive and inexpensive, and has few downsides. However, when many people are tested relative to the number who benefit, and where downsides are common, the policy threshold for recommending testing of all individuals in certain categories should be higher, and an individual's decision about whether to be screened must be an informed one. A woman whose dear friend has just died of breast cancer might ignore the downsides altogether in deciding to be screened. And a woman might decline if she reasons that for her personally, the chance of false positives is high and the absolute possibility of benefit is low. The answer may be different — yet still rational — for women weighing benefits and risks differently.

Despite the recent controversy over mammography, the decline in breast cancer death rates in the United States during the past decade is clear. It seems hard to believe that screening is not at least partially responsible for this decline, although some researchers attribute much if not most of it to improved treatment instead.

If you are a fiftysomething woman, should you get a mammogram? My answer is probably yes, even though my justification would not be that it can't do any harm. Pending further analysis of the existing data, which is essential, recommending mammography for women aged 50 to 69 is still sound public policy for the age group as a whole. But given the uncertainties about benefits and the relatively high frequency of false positives, the decisions of individual women about mammography may understandably differ.

PART VII

AGING AND LONG-TERM CARE

CHAPTER 11

LONG-TERM CARE

This new chapter describes the U.S. long-term care system that provides for the daily living needs of a growing number of older and disabled adults, many of whom have multiple chronic health care needs. Although a broad range of the population is served through a variety of settings and services, this chapter primarily focuses on older adults in long-term care, given their projected growth in numbers, their predominance as users, and the attention given to them in policy discussions and research activities. We have selected a group of articles that provides an overview of the U.S. long-term care system and its challenges, related public policy debates, quality concerns in nursing homes, and growing interest in consumer empowerment initiatives.

In Article 1, Wallace and colleagues (2001) review the long-term care literature, drawing attention to how the dominant policy debates and research agenda have been framed by financial priorities. The authors first describe characteristics, public funding, and recent developments affecting the types of providers and residents served in nursing facilities. Attention is given to the catastrophic private costs and rising public expenditures for nursing home care. Although some attention has been given to the complex issues of quality care, more effort has been devoted to investigating alternative reimbursement methods and policy options for reducing the growth of Medicaid expenditures and nursing home utilization.

Today a large number of older adults with long-term care needs remain at home receiving services from a combination of formal community-based providers, such as adult day care and home health, and informal providers such as family members and friends. Limited public funding for such services exists through Medicare and Medicaid, as described in Chapter 8. An increasing but nevertheless small percentage of Medicaid expenditures is being used by states to provide less expensive services in the community in hopes of reducing Medicaid nursing home spending. Research efforts have focused on identifying programs that can contain costs through institutional diversion efforts while targeting individuals at high risk of nursing home placement.

Policy concerns about the substitution effects of increased public benefits have led to studies that find that "formal services supplement rather than supplant informal care" (Wallace et al., 2001, p. 209). The authors discuss the attention that has been given to "woodwork effect" concerns surrounding the development of new (or expansion of existing) community-based services.

Particular attention is given to the variations in the need and use of formal and informal long-term care services, which are associated with race, ethnicity, gender, and class. Although each of these factors independently affects the need for long-term care services, their cumulative effect creates a disproportionately greater risk of dependency for lower income, nonwhite women. Research and policy activities have rarely addressed the social and economic conditions that contribute to the higher likelihood of women to enter a nursing home. Some research has begun to address the underrepresentation of nonwhites in nursing homes and other variations in long-term care use attributable to access barriers. The authors note how public reimbursement and other social policies have contributed to the creation of a two-class system that is characterized by lower quality of care for Medicaid recipients, discrimination by payment source, inequitable distribution of community-based services, and differential resources to secure informal assistance.

Inequalities may become even more apparent when considering recent initiatives to expand reliance on private-sector financing, such as long-term care insurance, home equity conversions, individual medical accounts, and continuing care retirement communities. Although these programs may be accessible to those who are well off, many are inaccessible to lower- and middle-income elderly, and they may have the unintended effect of undermining limited support for existing public programs. Wallace and colleagues also review the literature regarding informal care, which is disproportionately provided by women without adequate state support and which creates significant physical, emotional, social, and financial burdens. Research has also looked at the inadequate wages and benefits received by long-term care workers, resulting in high rates of turnover among providers and poor living and work conditions for these caregivers.

Given the considerable increase in public financing needed to provide adequate long-term care services in the future, we have included a short commentary by Judith Feder (2001; Article 2) that was written in response to a paper by Robyn Stone (2001). Feder takes up the ongoing debate about public and private responsibility for long-term care, arguing that action is limited by the lack of consensus about the government's role in ensuring that people who need long-term care are adequately insured. First, the need for long-term care is unpredictable and the costs are unmanageable, even when privately insured. Second, the author addresses the shortcomings of both private insurance proposals and the current public safety net funded by Medicaid. Feder discusses skepticism associated with the government's ability to distribute "benefits appropriately, equitably, and efficiently" and addresses the substituting versus supplementing effects of expanded public benefits. Finally, policymakers face the current and future challenge of increasing demands on public resources. How society responds to these needs and distributes the benefits of economic growth will really be a matter of political will.

In Article 3, Charlene Harrington (2001) explores the persistence of quality problems in U.S. nursing facilities despite three decades of efforts to improve them. As many as one third of the 16,500 nursing homes in the United States have serious care problems that threaten the health and safety of older and disabled residents. In more than three fourths of the poorly performing facilities, subsequent state surveys continue to find problems. With two thirds of facilities owned by for-profit organizations and more than half being part of a chain, Harrington explores the impact of investor ownership on quality care. As discussed in this article and reported in greater depth by Harrington and colleagues (2002), for-profit facilities average more deficiencies and have lower nursing-to-resident staffing ratios than nonprofit and government-operated nursing homes.

Harrington describes how persistent quality problems are related to the way federal standards are unevenly carried out by state agencies through monitoring activities, as well as delayed and often lax enforcement mechanisms. Poor care is further associated with the inadequate staffing levels and the poor mix of skills required by federal standards to meet complex health care needs. The author describes legislative efforts to improve required staffing levels in nursing homes at the state and federal levels. Finally, inadequate public reimbursement at the state and federal level through Medicaid is shown to be a major deterrent to increased staffing in nursing homes. With less than 36 cents of every dollar going toward care in nursing homes, Harrington notes the absence of government control over how public funds are used for shareholder return, executive salaries, and capital and administrative costs.

In Article 4, Lynch, Estes, and Hernandez (2002) discuss consumer issues related to chronic and long-term care. Consumers of all ages have increasingly shown an interest in gaining control over the services that they receive, and evidence supports the value and need for care that is more centered on consumer needs and preferences. The authors summarize different models of consumer direction and existing consumer control initiatives that are in various stages of development and evaluation across the United States for both long-term care services and managed care plans. Consumer interests, those of informal caregivers, and functionally oriented long-term care services are juxtaposed with chronic care services that are oriented toward a professionally controlled medical model. Lynch and colleagues review findings related to the impact and costs associated with informal care and its relationship to innovative programs that integrate medical and community-based services. The authors conclude with several recommendations for additional research on chronic disease management, the creation and expansion of self-care and beneficiary education efforts, and broader integration of home and community-based programs with Medicare.

This chapter's Recommended Reading list includes a small sampling of work by some of the leading scholars in the field, who address a wide range of aging and long-term care issues. For example, Robyn Stone (2000) provides an extensive review of current long-term care policies and trends. As noted in Article 2, Stone points out how debates continue about the appropriate roles and responsibilities of the public (state and federal government) and private (for-profit and nonprofit providers) sectors in meeting the financial and service needs of the elderly with chronic care needs:

> Policymakers now face three significant questions: (1) Who should pay for long term care, and how? (2) How should services to elders with disabilities and their families be designed, and who should deliver them? (3) How can the labor force delivering that care be recruited, trained, and maintained? For long term care policymakers in the United States, this is the triple knot. Each of these three strands demands equal attention if sound, appropriate policy is to be developed (Stone, 2000).

Also included in the Recommended Reading list is the recent Institute of Medicine (IOM) report on quality in long-term care (Wunderlich and Kohler, 2001). The IOM committee found that the quality of care in nursing homes had generally improved since the implementation of reforms enacted by the Omnibus Budget Reconciliation Act of 1987, despite the increased frailty of the population served. However, quality of care problems persist in nursing homes, and quality of life has shown less improvement. Additionally, the authors address concerns regarding uneven quality of care in residential care settings such as assisted living and home care. A number of recommendations are provided regarding access to appropriate services; quality assurance and external oversight; workforce strengthening; organizational capacity improvement; and public reimbursement policy.

REFERENCES

Feder, J. (2001). Long-term care: A public responsibility. *Health Affairs, 20* (6), 112–113.

Harrington, C. (2001). Regulating nursing homes: Residential nursing facilities in the United States. *British Medical Journal, 323* (7311), 507–510.

Harrington, C., Woolhandler, S., Mullan, J., Carrillo, H., and Himmelstein, D. U. (2002). Does investor-ownership of nursing homes compromise the quality of care? *International Journal of Health Services, 32* (2), 315–325.

Lynch, M., Estes, C. L., and Hernandez, M. (2002). *Consumer empowerment issues in chronic and long-term care*. San Francisco: Institute for Health and Aging, University of California San Francisco.

Stone, R. (2000). *Long term care for the elderly with disabilities: Current policy, emerging trends, and implications for the 21st century. Milbank Memorial Fund.* Available: http://www.milbank.org/0008stone/.

Stone, R. I. (2001). Providing long-term care benefits in cash: Moving to a disability model. *Health Affairs, 20* (6), 96–108.

Wallace, S. P., Abel, E. K., Stefanowicz, P., and Pourat, N. (2001). Long-term care and the elderly population. In R. M. Andersen, T. H. Rice, and G. F. Kominski (Eds.), *Changing the US health care system: Key issues in health services, policy, and management* (2nd ed.). San Francisco: Jossey-Bass.

Wunderlich, G., and Kohler, P. O. (Eds.). (2001). *Improving the quality of long term care*. Washington, DC: National Academy Press, Institute of Medicine.

ARTICLE 1

LONG-TERM CARE AND THE ELDERLY POPULATION

Steven P. Wallace, Emily K. Abel, Pamela Stefanowicz, and Nadereh Pourat

The health service needs of people in the United States have changed dramatically during the past century as a result of the shift from acute to chronic conditions and an increasing life span. In 1900, the major health problems stemmed from acute infectious diseases such as typhoid fever and smallpox. People usually recovered or died rapidly from those diseases. By midcentury, three chronic conditions alone — heart disease, cancer, and stroke — accounted for more than 50 percent of deaths; today, chronic illnesses are the predominant cause of death. People with chronic illness frequently experience disability and require assistance over an extended period. Disabilities can affect people of any age, but the rate increases with age. Only 2.4 percent of people under sixty-five need any assistance with daily activities, compared to almost half of those eighty-five and over.[1]

Long-term care is the set of health and social services delivered over a sustained period to people who have lost (or never acquired) some capacity for personal care; ideally, it enables recipients to live with as much independence and dignity as possible.[2] Provided in institutional, community, and home settings, long-term care encompasses an array of services ranging from high-tech care to assistance with such daily activities as walking, bathing, cooking, and managing money. The care can be furnished by paid providers (formal care) or unpaid family and friends (informal care), or by a combination of the two. Long-term care differs from most topics discussed in this volume because it includes social as well as medical services.

This chapter reviews the recent literature on long-term care, showing how financial considerations have framed the dominant policy debates and research agenda. Policy makers frequently view nursing homes as a low-cost alternative to a hospital and consider community services and family care as less expensive substitutes for a nursing home — neglecting quality-of-life issues. Both policy makers and researchers also tend to ignore the diversity among older Americans, as well as the problems faced by low-income women who serve as caregivers (whether in a paid or an unpaid capacity).

NURSING HOMES

The term *nursing home* covers a variety of institutions, including skilled nursing facilities (SNFs), which offer twenty-four-hour nursing care; and residential care facilities (RCFs), which provide some personal care but no licensed nursing care. Nursing homes as predominantly medical institutions emphasize the nursing over the home.

At the most acute end, such policy changes as Diagnosis-Related Group (DRG) hospital reimbursement and the growth of HMOs have contributed to the growth of "subacute" care. This type of nursing home care is designed to shift care from hospitals into nursing homes, both reducing hospital costs and capturing extra Medicare reimbursement. The reimbursement formula for nursing home care in general encourages for-profit enterprises; three-quarters of freestanding nursing homes now are profit-making.[3]

Although most older people assume that Medicare covers nursing home stays, it accounts for only 14 percent of total nursing home expenditures. The program pays for one hundred days of post-hospital recovery care in a nursing home; it provides no coverage for custodial care. Medicaid, by contrast, pays for custodial as well as skilled nursing care and has thus become the primary funding source. It finances 42 percent of nursing home expenditures for the elderly and represents three-quarters of the total $48.5 billion government spending on nursing homes.[4] Although about 40 percent of nursing home users enter facilities paying privately, many of them become eligible for Medicaid after "spending down" or depleting their resources. The annual cost of a nursing home stay in 1993 was $37,000, a sum that exceeded the incomes of four-fifths of elderly people.[5] Nursing home spend-down has attracted policy attention because those who spend down account for a significant proportion of Medicaid nursing home expenditures, and because the phenomenon is a demonstration of the catastrophic costs of long-term care.

Nursing homes dominate long-term care spending. The rapid and unexpected rise in government expenditures for nursing homes during the 1960s and 1970s contributed to the policy focus on containing costs. Research has distinguished two types of nursing home user: (1) someone with a short stay, typical of post-hospital use; and (2) someone with a longer stay, typical of more custodial use.[6] The long-stay residents consume most nursing home funds.[7]

Other research has concentrated on designing, implementing, and evaluating alternative reimbursement methods.[8] Studies suggest that although various techniques, especially prospective payment, have slowed the increase in costs, they also have reduced access for Medicaid patients and limited the supply of beds below needed levels in some areas.[9] To discourage nursing homes from taking only the least disabled (and least expensive) Medicaid patients, some states have tried reimbursement formulae that pay more for the care of the most disabled. But this system may have the unintended consequence of reducing access for those needing only custodial care. One group of researchers concluded that reimbursements often reflect state budget balances and overall state resources more than the actual costs of providing nursing home care or improving quality.[10]

Although economic issues dominate research and policy, widespread concern about the treatment of nursing home residents (especially after highly publicized scandals) has kept some attention on quality-of-care issues.[11] The definition of *quality* has changed over the years. Initially, regulations defined it in terms of such "structural" features as conforming to fire and safety codes. Regulations then began to include measures of "process," such as whether a bed-bound patient is repositioned frequently enough to prevent pressure sores. Most recently, federal nursing home regulations have broadened to cover some "outcome" measures, such as change in functional status and psychosocial well-being as indicators of quality.

Some researchers have shown how nursing homes can reduce accidental falls, urinary incontinence, decubitus ulcers, and use of physical restraints and psychotropic drugs.[12] Others have examined quality differences between for-profit and not-for-profit nursing homes, finding that the latter generally provide better care.[13] Studies documenting high use of chemical and physical restraints, inadequate supervision of care by physicians and professional nurses, and the poor quality of life in many institutions helped inform the federal 1987 Omnibus Budget Reconciliation Act's (OBRA) detailed language on nursing home quality. OBRA included national standards for training nursing home aides, presence of social work staff, and delivery of medical care in nursing homes, but poor-quality facilities remain common.

COMMUNITY-BASED SERVICES

For many, long-term care conjures up the image of bedridden elderly residents in nursing homes. But most older people with functional limitations remain at home, often receiving assistance from family and friends as well as community agencies. Community-based services include adult day care, transportation, and congregate meals. Home care includes high-tech equipment, home-delivered meals, visiting nurses, home health aides with some training who can provide basic personal care such as help with bathing, and homemakers or untrained workers who assist with housecleaning and some personal care. We refer to both in-home and out-of-home services as "community-based" services in this chapter.

Public funding for community-based services remains limited. Medicare emphasizes medically oriented, postacute home care, not the ongoing social support services many people need to live independently in the community. Recipients must be homebound, under the care of a physician, and in need of part-time or intermittent skilled nursing or physical or speech therapy. The way these rules were interpreted was loosened in the early 1990s, leading to rapid growth in Medicare expenditures for home health care. In reaction, Congress severely restricted reimbursements in 1997, leading to a 45 percent drop in expenditures the following year.[14]

Unlike Medicare, Medicaid does not limit community-based services to postacute care. The government's concern with reducing Medicaid nursing home spending encouraged expansion of Medicaid coverage of community-based services. Legislation passed in 1981 gave states the option of applying for waivers from existing Medicaid rules in order to provide case management, personal care, respite care, and adult day care. Regulations sought to ensure that such services substituted for, and cost less than, nursing home placement. Largely as a result of these waivers, Medicaid spending on community-based services doubled between 1989 and 1993. Nevertheless, 9 percent of Medicaid's $122 billion budget is spent on community-based services, compared to 24 percent on nursing homes.[15]

Two other major federal programs that fund services for elderly people in the community are Title III of the Older Americans Act (OAA) and the Social Services Block Grant (SSBG). Both have fixed annual budgets that are substantially smaller than the amount spent by Medicaid on community-based services; both programs thus sometimes run out of money before the end of the year and refuse to accept new clients. Moreover, the amount of assistance provided to each recipient tends to be even lower than that furnished by Medicaid programs.[16]

The policy focus on cost containment has shaped the direction of research on community care. Evaluators have concluded that some highly disabled clients would not enter institutions even without access to community services.[17] Thus, although community-based services are usually cheaper than nursing home care for a single individual, total costs tend to be higher because more persons are served by community-based care than would have been served by nursing homes. These findings, coupled with rising Medicaid costs, have stimulated research on identifying clients at imminent risk of institutionalization or those inappropriately placed in nursing homes so that community services can be targeted to them alone. Drawing primarily on the Andersen model of health services utilization,[18] researchers have identified characteristics of elderly people that increase the probability of nursing home placement: advanced age, poorer health status, increased functional impairment, being white, living alone, and not owning a home.[19]

Another body of research addresses the policy concern that publicly funded care not substitute for care provided "free" by family and friends. Such a concern is based on the premise that formal (paid) and informal (unpaid) services are interchangeable and that an hour of paid care results in one less hour of care by family members. Most studies of the intersection of formal and informal services focus exclusively on allocating tasks between family caregivers and formal providers. Family members, however, typically conceptualize caregiving as a complex relationship, not simply as a set of discrete tasks. It is thus unsurprising that researchers consistently find that formal services supplement rather than supplant informal care.[20]

A similar line of research arises from the fear that large numbers of elderly people will come out of the woodwork to use new services because such community-based services as household cleaning, unlike nursing homes, are believed to lack built-in limitation on consumption. This fear, too, appears to be misdirected. Although the potential pool of clients of community-based services is vast, a critical issue for some community agencies is *recruiting* clientele, not controlling intake. Some elderly people postpone assistance until they are extremely disabled in order to maintain a sense of independence. Some elderly people also may cling to housekeeping chores as a way of separating themselves from their more severely impaired counterparts.

As Alan Sager comments, "The notion of a horde of greedy old people and lazy family members anxious to soak up new public benefits appears to be more a projection by a few wealthy legislators accustomed to domestic and hotel and restaurant service than it is a realistic image of our nation's elderly citizens."

Those who fear that the expansion of community services will open the floodgates implicitly acknowledge that the elderly are drastically underserved. Only 36 percent of the 5.6 million functionally impaired elderly people living in the community receive any formal care.[21] More than half of those with the severest disabilities receive no formal help.[22]

Policy on the quality of existing community-based care is at least fifteen years behind similar nursing home policy. Research is just beginning to define quality in community settings and develop a methodology for measuring it.

VARIATIONS IN THE NEED FOR FORMAL SERVICES

As the previous two sections have shown, the research and policy focus on financial considerations has overshadowed other public health concerns such as equity, adequacy, and quality. Understanding variations by race, ethnicity, gender, and class can help identify critical research and policy issues that previously have received inadequate attention.

The elderly population is becoming increasingly African American, Latino, Native American, and Asian American. These groups constituted approximately 16 percent of the elderly population in 2000 and are expected to represent approximately 34 percent by 2050.[23] Thus, programs aimed at the types and levels of functional disability of elderly whites may become less appropriate. Elderly African Americans have the highest rate of death and functional limitation, caused in part by high rates of hypertension, diabetes, circulatory problems, and arthritis. Elderly African Americans also are more likely to rate their health as fair or poor.[24] Research on the functional disabilities of Latinos is inconsistent. Some studies show that Latinos have fewer disabilities than all other groups, some report a similar level, and some find a higher level. Older Latinos have a lower death rate than whites overall, but higher death rates from diabetes, accidents, and chronic liver disease.[25] The health status of Asian American elderly generally is similar to that of white elderly. Aggregate data, however, mask the increasing diversity within Asian American communities. Some Asian Americans groups, especially recent immigrants, have long-term care needs that differ dramatically from those of whites.[26]

Women constitute 59 percent of the elderly population and 71 percent of those eighty-five and over.[27] Women at every age experience more functional limitations than men. Women also have a disproportionate need for formal long-term care because many live by themselves. Seventy-eight percent of elderly people living alone are women.[28]

Class also influences the need for long-term care. Research outside the United States suggests that class position has a direct impact on health status, independent of access to health care. A Swedish study of people eighty-five and over reported that former blue-collar workers are twice as likely as former white-collar workers to experience limitation in activities of daily living.[29] In the United States, functional limitations are highest among elderly people with relatively low income, even after controlling for age and race.[30]

Race and ethnicity, gender, and class interact, intensifying the need for long-term care and aggravating access barriers. The disability rate is highest among older African American women, being about 50 percent higher than that among older white males.[31] Those with the greatest need for long-term care have the least ability to pay for it. In 1997, elderly men's median income was $17,768, while elderly women's was $10,062. The median income for white men sixty-five and over was $15,276, two and a half times that of elderly African American and Latina women ($6,220 and $5,968, respectively).[32] Approximately 84 percent of African American elderly people enter nursing homes on Medicaid, compared to less than 44 percent of whites.[33]

VARIATIONS IN USING LONG-TERM CARE

The elderly population is a heterogeneous group. Characteristics such as gender, race, ethnicity, and class exert a significant influence on the use of LTC services.

Gender

Women are much more likely to enter nursing homes than men; 70 percent of nursing home residents are women, and women are twice as likely as men to use a nursing home at some point in their lives.[34] The imbalance in nursing home utilization occurs not only because women have more disabilities but also because they frequently outlive their husbands and thus lack the social support needed to stay at home. The cruel irony is that, after a lifetime of caring for others, many women are bereft of essential support when they are most in need. Policy makers and researchers rarely address the social and economic policies responsible for the predominance of women in nursing homes.

Race and Ethnicity

In 1990, 25.8 percent of whites age eighty-five and over were in nursing homes, compared to 16.7 percent of African Americans, 11.0 percent of Latinos, and 12.1 percent of Asian Americans.[35] Differences persist even after controlling for other predictors of nursing home use.

The relatively little research on the relation between race and ethnicity and use of community services is contradictory. Some studies report that minority elderly people use community-based care at the same rate as whites (or a higher rate) after controlling for need and resources.[36] Other studies find that African Americans and Latinos are less likely to use community services.[37]

Several reasons could account for the racial and ethnic differences in long-term care utilization. Some studies suggest that minority elderly people are less knowledgeable than whites about the types and functions of many community-based services, others suggest that nursing homes have discriminatory admission policies, and still others suggest that health professionals are less likely to refer minority elderly people to formal services.[38] This racial and ethnic variation is typically overlooked by policy makers who design programs for the "average" elder who is white and middle class.

Class

Some observers argue that social policy for older persons in the United States creates a two-class system. Low-income elderly rely on Medicaid and other poverty programs, while those who are better off benefit from tax preferences and universal programs such as Medicare. Poverty programs are the most vulnerable to cuts because their constituency lacks political and economic clout.

Specific research on class factors in long-term care is sparse and primarily deals with the problems faced by Medicaid recipients. Some evidence suggests that many nursing homes discriminate against Medicaid patients. High occupancy rates (averaging 95 percent nationwide) enable nursing homes to be choosy about admissions. Because the Medicaid reimbursement rate is lower than the amount nursing homes charge private-pay residents, facilities prefer clients who can pay out of pocket.[39] Hospital discharge planners in California estimate that it is four to seven times more difficult to place Medicaid patients in nursing homes than privately funded patients.[40]

The quality of life of Medicaid nursing home residents appears to be especially poor. Medicaid recipients tend to be relegated to institutions that, according to some measures, offer the worst-quality care.[41] Even within a facility, residents relying on Medicaid sometimes receive less care than private-pay residents. Medicaid also does not pay for "incidentals," such as laundering personal clothing or making a phone call. All such expenses must come from the $30–70 per month (varying by state) that Medicaid recipients are allowed to keep.

Class also affects distribution of community-based services. Because most people who receive such care pay privately, utilization varies directly with income. Not surprisingly, people with higher incomes spend far more than others on care. Moreover, self-pay clients receive more hours of home health care than those who rely on public funds.[42] Although Medicaid increases access to community-based services, 71 percent of noninstitutionalized older persons with poverty level incomes do not receive Medicaid.[43] Other elderly people, called "tweeners," have incomes just above the poverty level and therefore do not qualify for Medicaid but are too poor to pay privately for services.

Recent developments have accentuated the class bias of noninstitutional care, especially home health care. First, the deregulation and cost-containment measures of the 1980s eased Medicare restrictions on proprietary home health agencies. By 1998,

56.7 percent of home health agencies were proprietary.[44] For-profit agencies seek out the best-paying (privately insured) patients, leaving other patients for nonprofit and government agencies. Second, large multihospital systems looking for a relatively inexpensive way to expand have been eager to acquire home health agencies. Third, for-profit chains have expanded. Currently, 81.6 percent of the thirty-eight largest home care organizations are members of for-profit chains.[45] These changes have increased the competitiveness of the home health care system, putting agencies under growing pressure to generate revenue by focusing on the most remunerative patients and the best-paid services, thus decreasing access for those whose care is less profitable. Little research has attempted to determine if the quality of care varies by type of payment or ownership or affiliation of the home health agency.

The greatest difference of class may lie in services provided outside the bounds of established organizations. Although most studies ignore the vast network of helpers recruited through ad hoc, informal arrangements, some evidence suggests that disabled elderly people rely disproportionately on this type of assistance. Abel's study of fifty-one predominantly white, middle-class women caring for elderly parents found that just fifteen used services from a community agency, but twenty-eight hired helpers who were unaffiliated with formal agencies. Nine of the unaffiliated home care aides worked forty hours a week, and sixteen provided around-the-clock care.[46] The help from such workers typically is not included in government statistics; however, it constitutes a major source of assistance to the affluent that is not available to others.

PRIVATE SECTOR FINANCING INITIATIVES

The inequities in long-term care may become even more apparent if initiatives to rely more on private sector financing win increased support. Such initiatives take two forms. Some, such as home equity conversions and individual medical accounts, seek to promote private saving, which can then be used to finance long-term care. Other mechanisms include private long-term care insurance and continuing-care retirement communities.

Advocates of such programs argue that the growing segment of the elderly population that is sufficiently well off to be able to pay for long-term care should not rely on limited government funds. Critics charge that expansion of the private sector would sharpen the divide between rich and poor. Most private sector approaches are beyond the reach of low- and middle-income elderly people. Many elderly have neither enough equity in their homes to pay for extended long-term care nor enough income to pay for comprehensive private long-term care insurance. In 1995, a policy paying $100 a day for nursing home and $50 a day for home care cost an average annual premium of $1,881 at sixty-five and $5,889 at seventy-nine.[47] Entry fees for continuing-care retirement communities can be as high as $440,000 for a two-bedroom house for a couple, with monthly fees of $4,267. Increased private financing may also dissolve whatever popular support public programs currently enjoy.

INFORMAL CARE

Research offers overwhelming evidence to refute the enduring myth that families abandon their elderly relatives. Shanas was one of the first scholars to show that elderly people remain in close contact with surviving kin.[48] More recent studies demonstrate that this contact translates into assistance during times of crisis. Families and friends deliver 70–80 percent of the services disabled elderly people receive.[49]

Informal care continues to be allocated on the basis of gender. Women represent 72 percent of all caregivers and 77 percent of children providing care.[50] Daughters are more likely than sons to live with dependent parents and to serve as the primary caregivers.[51] Sons and daughters also assume responsibility for different tasks. Sons are more likely to assist parents with household maintenance and repairs, while daughters are far more likely to help with housework, cooking, shopping, and personal care.[52]

Research on informal care typically focuses on the burden it imposes. Studies have found that caregivers experience a range of physical, emotional, social, and financial problems. In many cases, caregiving responsibilities reignite family conflict, impose financial strain, and encroach on both paid employment and leisure activity.

Despite the many reports of caregiver burden, limited assistance is available. The dominant concern of policy makers is that caregivers will unload responsibilities on the state. As a result, policy makers support social services and financial assistance for caregivers only insofar as they serve to postpone or prevent institutionalization. The major demand of many caregivers is respite services, which provide temporary relief from care.[53] Although most states have established respite programs, they tend to be grossly underfunded, able to serve a small number of families and offering very few hours of care. State programs to reimburse caregivers for their services typically limit payment to those caring for patients deemed most vulnerable to institutionalization. Stringent eligibility criteria often exclude caregivers who are spouses, children over the age of eighteen, relatives who live apart from the care receivers, and relatives with income over a certain amount. The level of reimbursement tends to be low.

The policy response to the conflict between wage work and care also has been limited. The Family and Medical Leave Act (FMLA), passed with widespread acclaim in 1993, covers leave of no more than twelve weeks, provides no remuneration, excludes part-time and contingent workers and those employed in small firms, and defines family narrowly. Workers who are white, middle-class, and married are most likely to be able to take advantage of the act.[54] Employer-based programs to accommodate family caregivers tend to be narrow in scope and concentrated in large businesses.

Unlike respite services, financial compensation, and workplace reforms, programs enhancing the ability of caregivers to adapt to their responsibility enjoy enthusiastic support. The low cost of such programs partly explains their appeal. In addition, many caregivers attest to the benefit of such programs. Support groups alleviate the intense isolation surrounding caregiving. Educational programs that dispense information about the disease process or the new equipment dispatched to the home boost competence and confidence. Counseling services help caregivers disentangle unresolved emotional issues from the process of delivering care. A major disadvantage of these programs is that they reinforce the belief that our primary goal should be to help caregivers adjust to their unavoidable burdens rather than to make care for the dependent population more just and humane.

WORKERS IN THE LONG-TERM CARE SYSTEM

Paid as well as unpaid caregivers suffer from the failure to fund long-term care adequately. Nursing homes, home health agencies, and the elderly themselves seek to save money by keeping wages low. In New York City, 99 percent of home care workers are women, 70 percent are African American, 26 percent are Latina, and almost half (46 percent) are immigrants. A high proportion are single mothers with three or four children. They typically earn less than $5,000 a year. Eighty percent cannot afford adequate housing, and 35 percent often cannot buy enough food for their families.[55] Home care work also is characterized by inadequate supervision and training and few opportunities for advancement. National studies of nursing home assistants show that they receive poor wages and few benefits and in large, metropolitan areas are overwhelmingly women of color and immigrants.[56] One qualitative study found that even though most assistants took extra jobs to make ends meet, staff conversations centered "on not having enough money for rent or transportation or children's necessities."[57]

Most research on home care workers addresses the concerns of home health agencies regarding training, supervision, and especially retention of workers. The high turnover rate of nursing home assistants, estimated to be 40–75 percent annually, has led to a similar focus in the nursing home literature.[58]

Some studies report that nursing home assistants enjoy helping and caring for patients, but that rules and regulations designed to protect patients' rights, ensure quality, and promote efficiency frustrate their efforts. Racial and ethnic differences between workers, administrators, and patients further undermine positive relationships.[59] The racial, ethnic, and class composition of the home care labor force similarly creates serious problems. Many workers complain that they are treated like "maids," asked to perform tasks they consider inappropriate and demeaning. Overall, the challenges facing wage workers in the long-term care system receive scant attention in the research literature.

CONCLUSION

The rapid growth of the older population will put new strains on our long-term care system. We can confidently predict that this cohort will be disproportionately widowed women with high rates of disability and poverty; many will be members of racial and ethnic minorities.

Although the priority in both policy and research is typically on cost containment, the most critical issue is how we can provide adequate and high-quality long-term care services equitably to this growing and diverse population. The limited financial resources of many older people create a need for a universal Medicare type of social insurance for long-term care. The considerable new public financing needed to establish such a system has stymied consideration of such policies in the past. Since the underlying long-term care needs will not disappear simply because public policy fails to come to terms with them, it behooves us to reform our current medical care system so that resources can be allocated to address the pressing needs of the twenty-first century.

REFERENCES

1. National Center for Health Statistics. *Health, United States, 1999, with Health and Aging Chartbook.* Hyattsville, MD: National Center for Health Statistics, 1999.
2. Kane, R. A., Kane, R. L., and Ladd, R. C. *The Heart of Long-Term Care.* New York: Oxford University Press, 1998.
3. Aaronson, W. E., Zinn, J. S., and Rosko, M. D. "Do For-Profit and Not-for-Profit Nursing Homes Behave Differently?" *Gerontologist,* Dec. 1994, *34*, 775–786.
4. U.S. Congressional Budget Office. *Projections of Expenditures for Long-Term Care Services for the Elderly.* Washington, D.C.: U.S. Congress, Mar. 1999.
5. Kane, Kane, and Ladd (1998); Reschovsky, J. D. "The Roles of Medicaid and Economic Factors in the Demand for Nursing Home Care." *Health Services Research,* 1998, *33*(4), 787–813.
6. Liu, K., McBride, T., and Coughlin, T. "Risk of Entering Nursing Homes for Long Versus Short Stays." *Medical Care*, 1994, *32*, 315–327.
7. Kemper, P., Spillman, B. C., and Murtaugh, C. M. "A Lifetime Perspective on Proposals for Financing Nursing Home Care." *Inquiry*, 1991, *28*, 333–344.
8. Schelenker, R. e. "Comparison of Medicaid Nursing Home Payment Systems." *Health Care Financing Review*, Fall 1991, *13*, 93–109.
9. Davis, M. A., Freeman, J. W., and Kirby, E. C. "Nursing Home Performance Under Case-Mix Reimbursement: Responding to Heavy-Care Incentives and Market Changes." *Health Services Research*, 1998, *33*(4), 815–834.
10. Davis, Freeman, and Kirby (1998).
11. U.S. General Accounting Office. *California Nursing Homes: Federal and State Oversight Inadequate to Protect Residents in Homes with Serious Care Violations.* GAO/T-HEHS-98-219. Washington, D.C.: U.S. General Accounting Office, 1998.
12. Starer, P., and Libow, L. S. "Medical Care of the Elderly in the Nursing Home." *Journal of General Internal Medicine*, May–June 1992, *7*, 350–362.
13. Aaronson, Zinn, and Rosko (1994).
14. Pear, R. "Medicare Spending for Care at Home Plunges by 45%." *New York Times*, Apr. 21, 2000.
15. U.S. Health Care Financing Administration. "Table 5. Medicaid Vendor Payments by Type of Service." [http://www.hcfa.gov/medicaid/mnatstat.htm.] Dec. 1999.

16. Wallace, S. P. "The No Care Zone: Availability, Accessibility, and Acceptability in Community-Based Long-Term Care." *Gerontologist*, 1990, *30*, 254–261.
17. Weissert, W. G., Cready, C. M., and Pawelak, J. E. "The Past and Future of Home- and Community-Based Long Term Care." *Milbank Quarterly*, 1988, *66*, 309–388.
18. Andersen, R. M. "Revisiting the Behavioral Model and Access to Medical Care: Does It Matter?" *Journal of Health and Social Behavior*, Mar. 1995, *36*, 1–10.
19. Wallace, S. P., Levy-Storms, L., Kington, R. S., and Andersen, R. M. "The Persistence of Race and Ethnicity in the Use of Long-Term Care." *Journals of Gerontology, Series B, Psychological Sciences and Social Sciences*, 1998, *53*(2), S104–S112; Wallace, S. P., Levy-Storms, L., Andersen, R. M., and Kington, R. S. "The Impact by Race of Changing Long-Term Care Policy." *Journal of Aging and Social Policy*, 1997, *9*(3), 1–20.
20. Jette, A. M., Tennstedt, S., and Crawford, S. "How Does Formal and Informal Community Care Affect Nursing Home Use?" *Journals of Gerontology, Social Sciences*, Jan. 1995, *50B*, S4–S12; Spector, W. D., and Kemper, P. "Disability and Cognitive Impairment Criteria: Targeting Those Who Need the Most Home Care." *Gerontologist*, Oct. 1994, *34*, 640–651; McFall, S., and Miller, B. H. "Caregiver Burden and Nursing Home Admission of Frail Elderly Persons." *Journals of Gerontology, Social Sciences*, 1992, *47*, S73–S79.
21. Short, P. F., and Leon, J. *Use of Home and Community Services by Persons Ages 65 and Older with Functional Difficulties*. (National Medical Expenditure Survey Research Findings, 5, Agency for Health Care Policy and Research.) Rockville, MD: Public Health Service, 1990; Prohaska, T., Mermelstein, R., Miller, B., and Jack, S. "Functional Status and Living Arrangements." In J. F. Van Nostrand, S. E. Furner, and R. Suzman (eds.), *Health Data on Older Americans: United States, 1992*. Hyattsville, Md.: National Center for Health Statistics, 1993.
22. Agency for Health Care Policy and Research. "The Elderly with Functional Difficulties: Characteristics of Users of Home and Community Services." AHCPR publication no. 92-0112. Rockville, Md.: Public Health Service, July 1992.
23. Day (1996).
24. Blesch, K. S., and Furner, S. E. "Health of Older Black Americans." In Van Nostrand, Furner, and Suzman (1993).
25. Wallace, S. P., and Lew-Ting, C.-Y. "Getting by at Home: Community-Based Long-Term Care of Latino Elders." *Western Journal of Medicine*, Sept. 1992, *157*, 337–344.
26. Park-Tanjasiri, S., and Wallace, S. P. "Picture Imperfect: Hidden Problems Among Asian Pacific Islander Elderly." *Gerontologist*, Dec. 1995, *35*, 753–760.
27. Day (1996).
28. U.S. Census Bureau. "National Households and Families Projections, May 1996." (Public-use data file and documentation.) [http://www.census.gov/population/www/projections/nathh.html.] Dec. 1999.
29. Parker, M. G., Thorslund, M., and Lundberg, O. "Physical Function and Social Class Among Swedish Oldest Old." *Journals of Gerontology, Social Sciences*, July 1994, *49*, S196–S201.

30. House, J. S., and others. "The Social Stratification of Aging and Health." *Journal of Health and Social Behavior*, Sept. 1994, *35*, 213–234.
31. Taeuber, C. M., and Allen, J. "Women in Our Aging Society: The Demographic Outlook." In J. Allen and A. Pifer (eds.), *Women on the Front Lines: Meeting the Challenges of an Aging America*. Washington, D.C.: Urban Institute Press, 1993.
32. U.S. Census Bureau. *Money Income in the United States: 1998*. (Current Population Reports, P60-206). Washington, D.C.: U.S. Government Printing Office, 1999.
33. Dalaker, J. *Poverty in the United States: 1998*. (U.S. Census Bureau, Current Population Reports, Series P60-207.) Washington, D.C.: U.S. Government Printing Office, 1998; Pourat, N. "Racial/Ethnic Differences in Utilization of Long-Term Care Services Among the Elderly." UMI Dissertation Services, 1995.
34. Laditka, S. B. "Modeling Lifetime Nursing Home Use Under Assumptions of Better Health." *Journals of Gerontology, Series B: Psychological Sciences and Social Sciences*, 1998, *53*(4), S177–S187.
35. Damron-Rodriguez, J., Wallace, S. P., and Kington, R. "Service Utilization and Minority Elderly: Appropriateness, Accessibility and Acceptability." *Gerontology and Geriatrics Education*, 1994, *15*, 45–64.
36. Miller, B., McFall, S., and Campbell, R. T. "Changes in Sources of Community Long-Term Care Among African American and White Frail Older Persons." *Journals of Gerontology, Social Sciences,* Jan. 1994, *49*, S14–S24; Wallace, S. P., Levy-Storms, L., and Ferguson, L. R. "Access to Paid In-Home Assistance Among Disabled Elderly People: Do Latinos Differ from Non-Latino Whites?" *American Journal of Public Health*, July 1995, *85*, 970–975; Mauser, E., and Miller, N. A. "A Profile of Home Health Users in 1992." *Health Care Financing Review,* 1994, *16*(1), 17–33; Wallace, S. P., Snyder, J., Walker, G., and Ingman, S. "Racial Differences Among Users of Long-Term Care: The Case of Adult Day Care." *Research on Aging*, Dec. 1992, *14*, 471–495.
37. Kemper, P. "The Use of Formal and Informal Home Care by the Disabled Elderly." *Health Services Research*, Oct. 1992, *27*, 421–451; Bass, D. M., and Noelker, L. S. "The Influence of Family Caregivers on Elders' Use of In-Home Services: An Expanded Conceptual Framework." *Journal of Health and Social Behavior*, 1987, *28*, 184–196; Wallace, S. P., Levy-Storms, L., Kington, R. S., and Andersen, R. M. "The Persistence of Race and Ethnicity in the Use of Long-Term Care." *Journals of Gerontology, Series B, Psychological Sciences and Social Sciences*, 1998, *53*(2), S104–112.
38. Falcone, D., and Broyles, R. "Access to Long-Term Care: Race as a Barrier." *Journal of Health Politics, Policy, and Law*, 1995, *19*, 583–595; Wallace, S. P. "The Political Economy of Health Care for Elderly Blacks." *International Journal of Health Services*, 1990, *20*, 665–680.
39. Ettner, S. L. "Do Elderly Medicaid Patients Experience Reduced Access to Nursing Home Care?" *Journal of Health Economics*, Oct. 1993, *12*, 259–280.
40. Lewin and Associates, Inc. "An Evaluation of the Medi-Cal Program's System for Establishing Reimbursement Rates for Nursing Homes." (Submitted to the Office of the Auditor General, State of California, 1987).

41. Rivlin, A. M., and Wiener, J. M. *Caring for the Disabled Elderly: Who Will Pay?* Washington, D.C.: Brookings Institution, 1988; Cohen, J. W., and Spector, W. D. "The Effect of Medicaid Reimbursement of Quality of Care in Nursing Homes." *Journal of Health Economics*, 1996, *15*(1), 23–48.
42. Liu, K., Manton, K. G., and Liu, B. M. "Home Care Expenses for the Disabled Elderly." *Health Care Financing Review*, 1985, *7*, 51–58; Kane, N. M. "The Home Care Crisis of the Nineties." *Gerontologist*, 1989, *29*, 24–31.
43. U.S. Select Committee on Aging. *Aging America: Trends and Projections*. Washington, D.C.: U.S. Department of Health and Human Services, 1991.
44. Hoechst Marion Roussel. *Managed Care Digest Series*. Kansas City, Mo.: Hoechst Marion Roussel, 1999.
45. Hoechst Marion roussel (1999)
46. Abel, E. K. *Who Cares for the Elderly? Public Policy and the Experiences of Adult Daughters*. Philadelphia: Temple University Press, 1991.
47. U.S. General Accounting Office. Baby Boom Generation Presents Financing Challenges. GAO/T-HEHS-98-107. Washington, D.C.: U.S. General Accounting Office, 1998.
48. Shanas, E. "The Family as a Social Support System in Old Age." *Gerontologist*, 1979, *19*, 169–174.
49. See Abel (1991), pp. 3–4.
50. Stone, R. I., Cafferata, L., and Sangl, J. "Caregivers of the Frail Elderly: A National Profile." *Gerontologist*, 1987, *27*(5), 616–626.
51. Robinson, K. M. "Family Caregiving: Who Provides the Care, and at What Cost?" *Nursing Economics*, 1997, *15*(5), 243–247.
52. Stephens, S. A., and Christianson, J. B. *Informal Care of the Elderly*. Lexington, Mass.: Lexington, 1986.
53. Montgomery, R. J. V. "Respite Care: Lessons from a Controlled Design Study." *Health Care Financing Review* (Annual Supplement), 1988, 133–138; and Wallace (1990). Respite programs take the form of either homemaker and home health services in the home or adult day care and foster care homes in the community.
54. Gerstel, N., and McGonagle, K. "The Limits of the Family and Medical Leave Act." Paper presented at the American Sociological Association Meeting, San Francisco, Aug. 1998.
55. Donovan, R. "We Care for the Most Important People in Your Life: Home Care Workers in New York City." *Women's Studies Quarterly*, 1989, *17*, 56–63.
56. Quinlan, A. *Chronic Care Workers: Crisis Among Paid Caregivers of the Elderly*. Washington, D.C.: Older Women's League, 1983.
57. Diamond, T. *Making Gray Gold: Narrations of Nursing Home Care*. Chicago: University of Chicago Press, 1992, pp. 44–45.
58. See Foner, N. *The Caregiving Dilemma: Work in an American Nursing Home*. Berkeley: University of California Press, 1994; Heliner, F. T., Olson, S. F., and Heins, R. I. "Strategies for Nurse Aide Job Satisfaction." *Journal of Long-Term Care Administration*, Summer 1993, *21*, 10–14.
59. Foner (1994).

ARTICLE 2

LONG-TERM CARE
A PUBLIC RESPONSIBILITY

Judith Feder

Robyn Stone's paper focuses policymakers' attention on the kind of insurance benefits people who need long-term care ought to get. That is an important policy question, and Stone's consideration of cash payments — a disability approach — rather than payments for a defined set of services — a health insurance approach — is a valuable contribution to the policy debate. But to produce action, that debate must address an even more fundamental challenge: achieving consensus that government should assure that people who need long-term care get insurance in the first place. Misconceptions and skepticism stand in the way of that guarantee.

RISK OF LONG-TERM CARE NEED

First is the misconception that the need for long-term care is both inevitable and manageable. In fact, the need for long-term care is far from a necessary concomitant of aging. Rather, people of all ages face some risk that they will need long-term care. Although this risk increases as people age, about half of those who need long-term care are under age sixty-five.[1] And the extent and the costliness of people's needs vary considerably among older as well as among younger persons with disabilities. When people actually do need long-term care, managing its burdens is far from easy. Family support imposes sacrifices in employment, health status, and quality of life and cannot always meet needs. Also, the purchase of extensive long-term care entails costs that exceed most individuals' and families' ability to pay. Given the reality that long-term care is an unpredictable need for an unmanageable expense, insurance makes sense.

PUBLIC VERSUS INDIVIDUAL RESPONSIBILITY

Second, even when risk is acknowledged, there is widespread skepticism regarding the need for societal rather than individual responsibility to cope with it. Why not just save in case you need it, or rely on private insurance? Reliance on savings alone is inefficient and will not work; given the unpredictability and variability of the need for long-term care, people will either save too much or too little to cover expenses. Private insurance is also limited as a means to spread long-term care risk. It is not available to those who already have long-term care needs; is not even advocated as a means of protecting young persons against risks; and is acknowledged as unaffordable or insufficient to protect the substantial segment of elderly persons, now and in the future, with low and modest incomes. Public intervention and public financing are essential to assure that people are insured against long-term care risk.

Current public policy falls far short of assuring insurance protection. Medicare, which provides health insurance to many who need long-term care, covers very little long-term care. Medicaid is our long-term care safety net. But Medicaid protections differ considerably from what we think of as "insurance." Medicaid provides invaluable coverage of long-term care expenses, but only after people have exhausted virtually all of their own resources. As a result, Medicaid does not protect against financial catastrophe; it finances services only after catastrophe strikes. Meaningful insurance protection for long-term care requires more expansive public protections.

Historically, critics have questioned the legitimacy of such protections as inappropriately providing "estate preservation." That objection has always seemed peculiar, given acceptance of Medicare's "estate preservation" for older (and some disabled) persons who need medical care. Indeed, as Robert Kuttner has argued, recent repeal of the estate tax now makes Medicaid long-term care requirements for the "spending down" of resources perhaps the only estate tax that still exists.[2] In light of this new tax policy, objections to better long-term care insurance protection have become even less defensible.

GOVERNMENT'S ABILITY TO DISTRIBUTE BENEFITS

A third area of skepticism toward a government role questions government's capacity to provide benefits appropriately, equitably, and efficiently. Key issues include government's ability to target benefits to persons who need (rather than just want) service, to provide benefits in a sufficiently flexible form to promote quality of life, and to balance the desire to support family care with the reluctance to replace it.

Stone's paper illustrates that we have some choices here as well as some experience. State governments and private insurers have become more sophisticated in managing benefit distribution. "Crowding out" of private (especially employer-sponsored) insurance by public insurance is not the problem here that it is in efforts to expand public financing for health insurance (since private long-term care insurance barely exists). Indeed, the private expenditures for which public financing might substitute are primarily out of pocket and widely recognized as "catastrophic." Further, evidence suggests that the availability of insurance benefits does not eliminate family care, and deciding how much to alleviate family burdens or, as Stone suggests, even to encourage family care by paying for it is a matter of policy choice and, of course, willingness to make resources available.

SPREADING FINANCIAL RISK

That brings us to the final and perhaps most daunting challenge in pursuing public responsibility for long-term care: reluctance to gather and redistribute resources to spread the risk of long-term care financing. Current policy concentrates burdens on those who need long-term care. Policies to more effectively spread risk can take a variety of forms, but all will require additional public resources. Indeed, an aging society will require additional public resources even to sustain the limited protection that Medicaid now provides.

Fears about an aging society have raised questions about the availability of resources to meet existing commitments to Social Security, Medicare, and Medicaid, let alone an expanded commitment to spread the risk of long-term care. However, the future holds not only the prospect of an aging society but also of a growing economy. Future political choice — not the nature of people's needs or the limits to our policy skills — will determine how we distribute the benefits of economic growth to spread rather than concentrate risks, or, more specifically, whether and how we live up to our public responsibilities in long-term care.

REFERENCES

1. J. Feder, H. L. Komisar, and M. Niefeld, "Long-Term Care in the United States: An Overview," *Health Affairs* (May/June 2000): 42.
2. R. Kuttner, "What We Need Is Pre-Death Tax Relief," *New York Times*, 15 April 2001.

ARTICLE 3

REGULATING NURSING HOMES

RESIDENTIAL NURSING FACILITIES IN THE UNITED STATES

Charlene Harrington

Poor quality care has been an enduring feature of many of the 16,500 residential nursing facilities that provide care to 1.6 million people in the United States.[1] Despite three decades of public concern, government surveys and data collected by the federal government continue to show that residents of nursing homes experience problems in their care. In 1998 and 1999, 25–33% of nursing homes had serious or potentially life threatening problems in delivering care and were harming residents.[3,4] In 1999, state inspectors found that 26% of the nation's nursing facilities had poor food hygiene; 21% provided care that was inadequate; 19% had environments that contributed to injuries in residents; and in 18% pressure sores were treated improperly. The eight most common deficiencies identified in 1999 are shown in [Table 1].[2] About 77% of facilities that were performing poorly had problems in subsequent surveys conducted by state licensing and certification agencies.[2]

Between 1993 and 1999, there was an increase in the number of residents developing contractures, pressure sores, and incontinence; being bedbound; and receiving psychotropic drugs.[2] In a study of nursing home residents who had died, more than half had received unacceptable care that endangered their health or safety; this care included failure to properly treat pressure sores, failure to manage pain, and some had had a dramatic, unplanned loss of weight.[4] Given the scale and chronic nature of quality of care issues and the failures in resolving them, what can the United Kingdom learn from the experiences of the United States?

OWNERSHIP AND QUALITY OF CARE

Of the nursing homes for older people in the United States, 67% are run by profit making organisations, and 52% are part of an organisation that owns more than one facility.[2] The six largest providers of residential care in the United States also own a

TABLE 1

MOST COMMON VIOLATIONS FOUND IN US NURSING HOMES, 1999[2]

Violation	*Percentage of facilities*
Improper use of restraints	11
Inadequate care plans	13
Inadequate attention to activities of daily living	14
Respect for personal autonomy and privacy	16
Improper care of pressure sores	18
Unsafe environment that contributes to injuries	19
Poor quality of care	21
Inadequate food hygiene	26

large number of facilities internationally.[1] The table shows the companies that own the greatest number of facilities. Sun Healthcare Group, one of the largest companies, had revenues of $2.5bn (£1.8bn) in 1999, and operated 145 long term care facilities with 8320 beds in the United Kingdom, had 1640 licensed beds in Spain, 3339 in Australia, and 1217 in Germany.[5] It also owned hospitals, pharmacies, providers of rehabilitation services, and respiratory therapy services.

Non-profit nursing homes are associated with better staffing and higher quality services[6] as well as with residents having a lower probability of death and infection.[7] Facilities owned by investors have fewer nurses and higher rates of violations, or deficiencies, on annual surveys of nursing homes.[8,9] Profit making facilities were found to have 30% more violations of standards assessing quality of care and more deficiencies in measures assessing quality of life than non-profit facilities.[9]

Not surprisingly, litigation is increasing. In 2000, the Supreme Court of Texas upheld an $11m judgment against the Horizon Health Care Corporation for the death of a resident.[10] In Florida, Extendicare, another nursing home operator, was fined $17m in punitive damages and $3m in compensation for negligent care.[11]

FEDERAL REGULATION

Under federal regulations, each state has a licensing and certification agency that inspects facilities that have a contract with the federal government. This is analogous to regulations in the Care Standards Act 2000 in the United Kingdom except that in the United Kingdom a central agency handles inspection and enforcement; this will be discussed in the third paper in the series.[12] In the United States, federal regulations require each nursing facility to conduct standardised, comprehensive assessments of all patients when they are admitted and periodically thereafter and to implement care plans that meet the individual needs of residents.

Prompted by scandals in care in nursing homes, the US Senate Special Committee on Aging held a series of hearings between 1963 and 1974. These led to reform of the federal and state laws regulating nursing facilities.[15,16] When the Reagan administration attempted to deregulate the nursing home industry in 1982, Congress asked the Institute of Medicine to study the regulations. The institute's report showed that there were widespread problems in the quality of care provided[17]; Congress's investigative agency, the General Accounting Office, also issued a report. The office's report found that over one third of the nation's nursing homes did not meet federal standards.[18] In 1987, Congress passed a bill, the Omnibus Budget Reconciliation Act of 1987, that brought important reforms to the regulation of nursing homes. This act established federal regulations for all facilities serving clients whose care was publicly funded, such as those on Medicare (which pays for care for elderly people and disabled people) and Medicaid (which pays for care for poor people). The federal regulations have three parts: the standards, the survey or monitoring procedures, and the enforcement procedures.

Figure 1 Reform of regulations.

The survey, which is carried out by state agencies, requires that residents be interviewed or assessed and that observations be made to evaluate whether some 185 quality requirements (in 17 different categories) and "life safety" requirements have been met. The surveys examine both the process and the outcomes of care to ensure that minimum standards are met.[13] Data on compliance with regulations and the characteristics of individual nursing homes are collected centrally and published on the internet, where they are available to the public.

The 1987 law [see Figure 1] established new enforcement procedures that use intermediate sanctions (penalties that fall short of closing nursing homes) against facilities that fail to meet federal standards[14]; these sanctions include the ability to issue fines, deny payment for newly admitted residents, and bring in managers from outside. If these sanctions are not effective, the federal government can issue a notice of immediate termination and decertification — that is, withdraw federal payments. The intermediate sanctions, however, were not implemented until 1995.

STAFFING

Two of the fundamental causes of problems with the quality of care in US nursing homes are inadequate staffing and a poor mix of skills. Federal regulations require only that one registered nurse is on duty eight hours a day for seven days a week and

TABLE 2

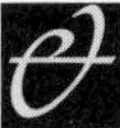

AMOUNT OF TIME NURSES SPEND IN NURSING HOMES PER RESIDENT PER DAY, 1999[2]

Registered nurses — 124 minutes
Licensed vocational nurses — 42 minutes
Nursing assistants — 44 minutes

that a registered nurse or a licensed practical nurse (also known as a licensed vocational nurse) is on duty during other shifts regardless of the size of the facility.[2] (Registered nurses have between two and four years of training and licensed practical nurses have one year of training.) Numerous studies have recommended that standards for staffing should be higher[14,19,20] and have found enormous variation in staffing within and across states.[14,20]

On average, nursing assistants care for 12 residents, and registered nurses and licensed vocational nurses oversee 32 to 34 residents [see Table 2].[2,20] Since nursing facilities report on their own staffing levels, these levels may actually be lower than reported, and facilities commonly increase the number of staff during surveys.[14] Profit making facilities have 20% fewer staff than non-profit and government run facilities. Poor quality care in nursing homes is associated with low wages and few benefits, high rates of employee turnover, and heavy workloads.[21]

Many states have proposed legislative changes to increase the number of staff required in nursing homes (for example, in 1999 California passed legislation requiring a total of 3.2 hours of direct care for each resident each day). In 2000 President Clinton proposed allocating $1bn in new funds for staffing for nursing homes so that states could voluntarily address staffing problems.[22] Additionally, legislation was introduced in the Senate, through the Nursing Home Improvement Act 2000, to require the Health Care Financing Administration (a government agency responsible for administering public funds for Medicare and Medicaid) to set minimum staffing requirements for nurses and to boost staffing in nursing facilities by spending $1bn over two years. There is growing concern, however, that the Health Care Financing Administration will not increase the minimum levels to those that are necessary to ensure quality because of the high cost to government of setting higher standards, in terms of funding for Medicare and Medicaid.

ENFORCEMENT

The weakness of the standards on staffing is made worse by an ineffective system of survey and enforcement in which responsibility is devolved to the states. Those who do the surveys are responsible for visiting nursing facilities every 9 to 15 months to conduct surveys and investigate complaints.[13] The General Accounting Office has found that those conducting surveys are unable to detect serious problems in the quality of care particularly in terms of the number of preventable hospitalisations, deaths, falls that led to fractures, and infections and pressure, as well as the inappropriate use of restraints, the failure to dress and groom residents, and malnutrition.[3,4]

At the 1998 hearings of the US Senate Special Committee on Aging, which examined the General Accounting Office's findings, the committee criticised the Health Care Financing Administration's survey and enforcement efforts, and President Clinton announced a new initiative to improve the enforcement process by introducing stronger oversight of state inspections.[23]

REIMBURSEMENT

The government's payment policies are important to the nursing home industry: they account for 62% of the $87bn earned in revenue by nursing homes in 1998.[24,25] Under the federal Medicare prospective payment system (which covers short term care for elderly people and disabled people), reimbursement to nursing homes is made on the basis of the estimated amount of staff time and the skill mix needed to care for each resident, but facilities are under no obligation to provide the staff time for which they are paid or to provide care that exceeds minimum standards. Medicare payments (which were $264–385 per resident per day in 1999)[1] and payments by private payers, which are the same for profit making, non-profit, and governmental facilities, are significantly higher than payments made by Medicaid (about $95 per day in 1998). Medicaid pays for 54% of the total number of private and public expenditures.

The low level of federal payments and state Medicaid payments are major deterrents to nursing homes increasing staffing.[25] It has been estimated that increasing the total average time spent with a resident from 3.5 hours per resident per day to 4.55 hours per day would cost at least $6bn.[25]

The lack of government control over public funds is a cause for concern. Currently, less than 36 cents in every dollar spent on nursing facilities is spent directly on care.[26] No limits are set on the amount of returns that can be allocated to shareholders, on salaries for chief executive officers, or on spending on capital and administrative costs. Robert Elkins, the former chief executive officer and founder of Integrated Health Systems (which runs a large number of nursing homes whose stock value dropped by 78% between 1997 and 1999) made over $14m in salary and stock bonuses annually[27] and received a package worth $55m when he left the company.[27]

Financial fraud is not uncommon because there are no strong mechanisms of accountability for spending public funds. Beverly Enterprises, which runs the nation's largest chain of nursing homes (561 facilities in 30 states) has agreed to pay $175m to settle US Department of Justice charges of defrauding Medicare of $460m between 1992 and 1998; employees were found to have fabricated records to make it appear that nurses were devoting more time to Medicare patients than they actually were.[28] Vencor, another operator of nursing homes, settled a fraud case brought by the government for $1.3bn and agreed to have an independent monitor for five years to ensure that quality standards are maintained and fraud is avoided.[29]

When Congress passed a new prospective payment system for Medicare in 1997, which used the case mix of residents (known as acuity) to control spending on care in

TABLE 3

CHARACTERISTICS OF THE SIX LARGEST CORPORATIONS RUNNING NURSING HOMES IN THE UNITED STATES, 1999[1]

Company (Headquarters)	*No. of Beds*	*No. of Facilities*	*Revenue** *Percentage of Funds from Federal and State Governments*	*Total Operating Revenue*
Beverly Enterprises (Fort Smith, Arizona)	62,293	562	74	$2.8bn
Mariner Post-Acute Network (Atlanta, Georgia)	49,656	416	67	$1.5bn
HCR Manor Care (Toledo, Ohio)	47,138	297	51	$2.2bn
Sun Healthcare Group (Albuquerque, New Mexico)	44,941	397	83	$2.5bn[5]
Integrated Health Services (Owning Mills, Maryland)	44,302	380	56	$3bn
Vencor (Louisville, Kentucky)	38,362	291	60	$3bn

*$1.40 = £1.00.

nursing homes,[30] some 2000 of the companies running the largest number of nursing homes filed for bankruptcy.[31] Among them were Sun Healthcare Group, which reported losses of $700m in 1998 and $90m in 1999, and Vencor, which reported losses of $563m in 1998 and $612m in 1999.[31] Sun Healthcare Group sold its holdings in the United Kingdom to management for $1 in a buyout and then reduced their workforce from 80,700 in 1999 to 57,100 in 2000.[5]

Although these corporations blamed Medicare's payment policies for their losses, the General Accounting Office found little evidence to support this, instead ascribing the companies' financial difficulties to "high capital-related costs" and substantial non-recurring expenses and write offs [Table 3].[32] Nonetheless, the nursing home industry was successful in its lobbying, and in 2000 Congress and the president implemented the Benefits Improvement and Protection Act which restored many of the cuts made to Medicare reimbursement.

LESSONS FOR THE UNITED KINGDOM

Over the past three decades, the poor qualify of care in nursing homes in the United States has continued to be a problem. The nursing home industry is increasingly controlled by large and politically powerful multinational corporations. These corporations have wide discretion over the spending of large amounts of public funds, but at the same time there is little financial accountability. Fraud and financial mismanagement are widespread throughout the industry as is poor quality care.

Although strong federal quality standards were established by law in 1987, the crucially important standards for staffing continue to be weak; staffing accounts for the largest share of the cost of care. Small numbers of staff, who are paid low wages and have few benefits, and high turnover rates are recognised features of the industry. The delayed implementation of enforcement and the weak sanctions available have yet to improve care because state survey systems are weak and government regulatory bodies are subject to lobbying by the industry. There is also a reluctance to use the enforcement penalties and sanctions available.

The government is reluctant to impose higher standards for staffing because of concerns over cost. Although the government pays 62% of nursing home bills,[24] financial accountability for expenditure does not extend to rules governing the services to be provided, the types of services, how much profit can be made, and how much is spent on administrative costs and other expenditures.

The story of long term care in the United States holds lessons for the United Kingdom. Because the market is increasingly dominated by profit making corporate providers, the government must be prepared to intervene in areas that affect profit margins and must also retain control over the expenditures of providers in the areas of staffing, skill mix, training, and services provided. Failure to do this leaves regulation in the realm of symbolism and vulnerable, frail elderly people at risk of serious harm.

REFERENCES

1. American Health Care Association. *Facts and trends 1999: the nursing facility sourcebook.* Washington, DC: AHCA, 1999.

2. Harrington C, Carrillo H, Thollaug S, Summers P. *Nursing facilities, staffing, residents, and facility deficiencies, 1993–99.* San Francisco: University of California, 2000. (Available at www.hcfa.gov/medicaid/ltchomep.htm.)

3. US General Accounting Office. *California nursing homes: care problems persist despite federal and state oversight.* Washington, DC: GAO, 1998. (Report to the Special Committee on Aging, US Senate. GAO/HEHS-98-202.)

4. US General Accounting Office. *Nursing homes: additional steps needed to strengthen enforcement of federal quality standards.* Washington, DC: GAO, 1999. (Report to the Special Committee on Aging, US Senate. GAO/HEHS-99-46.)

5. US Securities and Exchange Commission. *SUN Healthcare Group Inc. Annual Report for FY ended December 31, 1999.* Washington, DC: SEC, 2001. (No 1-12040.)

6. Aaronson WE, Zinn JS, Rosko MD. Do for-profit and not-for-profit nursing homes behave differently? *Gerontologist* 1994:34:775–86.

7. Spector WD, Seldon TM, Cohen JW. The impact of ownership type on nursing home outcomes. *Health Economics* 1998:7:639–53.

8. Harrington C, Woolhandler S, Mullan J, Carrillo H, Himmelstein D. Does investor-ownership of nursing homes compromise the quality of care? *Am J Public Health* (in press.)
9. Harrington C, Zimmerman D, Karon SL, Robinson J. Beutel P. Nursing home staffing and its relationship to deficiencies. *Journal of Gerontology: Social Sciences* 2000;55B:S278–86.
10. Supreme Court upholds $11 million Horizon judgment. *McKnight's Long-Term Care News* 2000;22:14.
11. Extendicare says it will appeal $20 million lawsuit. *McKnight's Long-Term Care News* 2000;22:14.
12. Kerrison SH, Pollock AM. Regulating the quality of nursing care for older people in the private sector. *BMJ* (in press).
13. US Department of Health and Human Services, Health Care Financing Administration. *2001 state operations manual. Provider certification.* Washington, DC: DHHS, 1995.
14. US Health Care Financing Administration. *Report to Congress: appropriateness of minimum nurse staffing ratios in nursing homes.* Vol 1–3. Baltimore, MD: HCFA, 2000.
15. US Senate Special Committee on Aging. *Nursing home care in the US: failure in public policy.* Washington, DC: US Senate, 1974. (Supporting paper No. 11.)
16. Vladeck B. *Unloving care: the nursing home tragedy.* New York: Basic Books, 1980.
17. Institute of Medicine, Committee on the adequacy of nurse staffing in hospitals and nursing homes. *Nursing staff in hospitals and nursing homes: is it adequate?* Washington, DC: National Academy Press, 1986.
18. US General Accounting Office. *Medicare and Medicaid: stronger enforcement of nursing home requirements needed.* Washington, DC: GAO, 1987. (Report to the chairman, Subcommittee on Health and Long-Term Care, Select Committee on Aging, House of Representatives.)
19. Wunderlich GS, Sloan FA, Davis CK for the Institute of Medicine, Committee on the Adequacy of Nurse Staffing in Hospitals and Nursing Homes. *Nursing staff in hospitals and nursing homes: is it adequate?* Washington, DC: National Academy Press, 1996.
20. Harrington C, Kovner C, Mezey M, Kayser-Jones J, Burger S, Mohler M, et al. Experts recommend minimum nurse staffing standards for nursing facilities in the United States. *Gerontologist* 2000:40:5–16.
21. Cohen JW, Spector WD. The effect of Medicaid reimbursement on quality of care in nursing homes. *J Health Econ* 1996:15:23–8.
22. Pear R. President asks for more aid for elder care. *New York Times* 2000 September 9:A26.
23. US Department of Health and Human Services. *Assuring the quality of nursing home care.* Washington, DC: Health Care Financing Administration, 1998. (HHS fact sheet.)

24. US Health Care Financing Administration. *National health expenditures 1960–1998*. Washington, DC: HCFA, 2000.
25. Wunderlich GS, Kohler P, eds. *Improving the quality of long-term care*. Washington, DC: National Academies of Science, 2001.
26. HCIA, Arthur Andersen. *1998–99: the guide to the nursing home industry*. Baltimore, MD: HCIA, Arthur Andersen, 1998.
27. Nursing home CEO gets departure deal: Elkins led IHS chain to boom, bankruptcy. *Baltimore Sun* 2001 January 13:10C.
28. Hilzenrath DS. Nursing home firm settles fraud case. *Washington Post* 2000 Feb 4:G3.
29. Vencor agrees to improve standards. *McKnight's Long-Term Care News* 2000;21:6.
30. Medicare program; prospective payment system and consolidated billing for skilled nursing facilities. *Federal Register* 1998;63(228):65561–2.
31. Nakhnikian E. Long term care provider.com extends its bankruptcy coverage. www.longtermcareprovider.com. (Accessed 6 April 2001.)
32. US General Accounting Office. *Skilled nursing facilities: Medicare payment changes require provider adjustments but maintain access*. Washington, DC: GAO, 1999. (Report to the Special Committee on Aging, US Senate. GAO/HEHS-00-23.)

ARTICLE 4

CONSUMER EMPOWERMENT ISSUES IN CHRONIC AND LONG-TERM CARE

Marty Lynch, Carroll L. Estes, and Mauro Hernandez

INTRODUCTION

Consumer empowerment has been brought squarely into health and long-term care policy in four ways: (1) disability advocates promoting the Independent Living Movement and the Americans with Disability Act (ADA), for which consumer direction and empowerment are cornerstone principles (Wiener, Estes, Goldenson, & Goldberg, 2001); (2) research evidence on the importance of behavioral and environmental risk factors and work of the Assistant Secretary for Health and the Surgeon General in setting national health promotion and disease prevention goals (U.S. Department of Health & Human Services, 1998); (3) research on inequality and health highlighting the independent effects on health of social factors such as race and racism (Collins & Williams, 1999); and (4) work on the "medicalization" of social problems (Conrad & Schneider, 1992) that points to many potentially modifiable nonmedical factors that are key to these problems. Estes & Binney (1989) discuss the biomedicalization of aging, where normal aging processes are constructed in medical terms, with control of these processes shifting to the medical profession or health care industry and rendering the patient more dependent and powerless. Increasing privatization and rationalization (Estes, Wallace, Linkins, & Binney, 2001) of health care delivery also shifts the domain of caring for the elderly into the business sector, where financial and bureaucratic (e.g., managed care) interests play a more dominant role, with potentially disempowering effects on consumers.

Arguments for the "empowerment imperative" for the disabled, chronically ill, and elderly (Estes, Casper, & Binney, 1993) have been made, not only on political and ideological grounds, but also with the knowledge that the acute care model is woefully inadequate (and too expensive) to deal with the largely social supportive and personal care needs of millions of these individuals. With the sociodemographics of aging and chronic disease, the nation can ill afford to "produce" more (or new) dependencies in patients because of what we do and do not finance and what is excluded from coverage (e.g., reimbursement limits on rehabilitation and prevention). Under the paradigm of patient passivity and compliance, there is a risk that health policy may actually contribute to the unnecessary dependency of the chronically ill by what it does not cover. This could be a form of iatrogenically produced dependency.

The recent Institute of Medicine (IOM) study, *Improving the Quality of Long-Term Care* (Wunderlich & Kohler, 2001), distinguished between "consumer-centered care" and "consumer-directed services." *Consumer-centered care* is patient-centered health care that is "closely congruent with and responsive to patients' wants, needs, and preferences (Gerteis, Edgman-Levitan, Daley, & Delbanco, 1993) ... [and] refer[s] to a shift from a more professional-driven health care system to one ... incorporat[ing] an individual patient's perspectives (Laine & Davidoff, 1996 in Wunderlich & Kohler, 2001, p. 28). *Consumer-directed services* consider the capacity of individuals to "assess their own needs, determine how and by whom these needs should be met and monitor the quality of services they receive" (National Institute on Consumer-Directed Long-Term Services, 1996, p. 1, in Wunderlich & Kohler, 2001, p. 29).

In the end, the quality of long-term care depends on the adoption of consumer-centered approaches, according to Rosalie Kane, Joshua Weiner, and five other IOM committee experts. "[T]he evidence ... supports the value of and the need for consumer centered care," and what is needed is research on "barriers to access and barriers to consumer-centered care." They urge states, providers, and consumers to provide community-based long-term care options in which individual consumers are "afforded the opportunity to specify the degree of control and influence that they are able to or wish to assume over the direction of their care." (Wunderlich & Kohler, 2001, Appendix B, p. 289).

MODELS OF CONSUMER DIRECTION IN CHRONIC AND LONG-TERM CARE

The Institute of Medicine study (Wunderlich & Kohler, 2001) identifies four types of consumer-directed long-term care models:

> (1) consumer selection, training, and supervision of caregivers and providers of service; (2) individualized supports essential to maintaining the consumer's health and quality of life in the community (e.g., personal assistance, assistive devices, environmental modifications, consumer education, service coordination, and family and social supports); (3) consumer involvement in the development and approval of support plans and the authorization of payment; and (4) consumer monitoring of the quality of care (DeJong, Batavia, & McKnew, 1992; Fenton et al., 1997 in Wunderlich & Kohler, 2001, p. 29).

Most existing consumer-directed programs have been developed through state-level Medicaid waivers and personal assistance programs. The Veterans Administration also has a program (Stone, 2000).

Many chronic care initiatives — whether integrating acute and long-term chronic care services or improving disease management for specific conditions — are placed in capitated health plan settings or in academic or hospital settings subject to financial utilization incentives. From a consumer point of view, these incentives raise questions as to whether the interests of the consumer are primary rather than the financial interests of the health plan, hospital, or medical center (Bodenheimer, 2000). Ideally, chronic disease initiatives could combine the best interests of both: the use of flexible financing to support preventive and self-care activities while saving dollars spent on inappropriate utilization. What chronic disease sufferer wouldn't want his or her disease controlled better or appreciate some involvement in managing his or her care or want access to a broader range of chronic care services? Despite earlier beliefs that consumer control was primarily an issue for younger disabled people, recent survey data (Coleman, 2001) suggest that even for elderly consumers, a significant and growing number would prefer some level of control over services they receive. The authors did not find data on the relative involvement of for-profit or nonprofit health plans or health systems in these innovative programs. The initiatives described do, however, indicate the involvement of large nonprofit health plans such as Kaiser and Group Health. Consumers might rightly fear the bottom-line motivation driving for-profit systems unless regulatory controls assured appropriate chronic care management in all Medicare-funded settings.

Existing consumer control initiatives focus on disabled consumers controlling the hiring, supervising, and perhaps training of their own personal care workers (Mahoney, Simone, & Simon-Rusinowitz, 2000) or are initiatives like the RWJ Cash and Counseling program, where disabled consumers have some control over how a community service benefit is expended (35 of 50 states have some type of program). The authors are not familiar with models where consumers have control over medical decisions or a budget for chronic disease interventions. These management and utilization decisions remain in the sphere of the physician, insurance carrier, or health plan, except for the very few who are essentially self-funded for their medical care. The Social Health Maintenance Organization demonstration uses a set dollar benefit for home and community-based care services managed by a care coordinator. This approach hints at the possibility that a care coordinator/case manager and a beneficiary could be jointly responsible for a set budget or benefit level for some range of services, perhaps with a reinsurance mechanism for emergent needs outside of the original care plan.

Research on the outcomes of consumer-directed care is limited. Doty and colleagues (1999) compared worker and client outcomes for those participating in a California independent provider program (In-Home Supportive Services, or IHSS) with those receiving case-managed services from a California county agency. Results from this study for the Department of Health and Human Services show that the consumer-directed model produced more positive client outcomes in three areas than did the model of professionally managed services: satisfaction with services, feelings of empowerment, and perceived quality of life. There were no significant differences in client safety and unmet needs. Agency-based program workers received better hourly wages than independent providers and were more likely to have health insurance and other benefits, although there were no significant differences in job satisfaction between workers in both models. However, independent providers had better client relationships than agency-based workers (Doty, Benjamin, Matthias, & Franke, 1999; Stone, 2000).

In addition, there are multiple other initiatives designed to promote consumer involvement in managed care and other health programs, including those serving persons dually eligible for Medicaid and Medicare (Mollica & Riley, 1997; Office of Disability Aging and Long-Term Care Policy, 2001). Although many of these projects address the chronically ill, Medicare, and Medicaid populations, few are research-based or part of comparative outcome studies of different models of care.

Groups such as AARP, the Older Women's League, and the Center for Medicare Education have all attempted to build beneficiary influence by educating Medicare beneficiaries about their rights and entitlements under the program and how to take advantage of certain rights they may have under appeals procedures. These activities have focused on policy and regulatory protections rather than demands in the arena of beneficiary influence on providers or plans. These organizations variously advocate for the addition of certain chronic care benefits just as they have advocated (unsuccessfully) for the inclusion of pharmacy benefits and long-term care benefits in the Medicare program.

An example of a micro-level beneficiary empowerment effort is available from Kaiser Northern California and is probably replicated in other regions of Kaiser and perhaps other plans. Advocacy efforts of the Gray Panthers, a senior advocacy group, led Kaiser (under threats of picketing and demonstrations) in the 1980s to establish a geriatric advisory committee, which meets with top-level health plan officials to design responses to chronic care and other elderly health problems (Tarail, 2001).

INFORMAL CARE

Informal care issues are critical in examining consumer concerns in the current chronic and long-term care delivery system. In 1994, over 90% of elderly disabled persons in the United States were receiving long-term care services from family and other informal caregivers, with approximately one in four households providing such care in 1997 (Liu, Manton, & Aragon, 2000; Pandya & Coleman, 2000). The great majority of these informal caregivers are women, who suffer significant financial and personal costs of providing care (Coleman, 2000). A study by Arno, Levine, and Memmott (1999) suggests that the labor value of informal caregiving, estimated at $196 billion for 1997, far exceeded the combined national spending for formal home health and nursing home care by about $81 billion. The Medicare and Medicaid programs rely heavily on these informal caregivers to supplement the limited publicly funded system of care and perhaps shift the true cost of chronic and long-term care to women in the informal sector. Although some states have respite care programs to relieve stress or improve the financial burdens of informal caregivers, these programs are limited in funding and size, are not readily available to consumers, and have a great deal of programmatic, funding, and eligibility inconsistency across states (Coleman, 2000).

The Program of All Inclusive Care for the Elderly (PACE) and other innovative programs that provide both medical and home and community-based services could theoretically reduce some of this burden insofar as they coordinate chronic care services and provide some respite and home care. However, we would not expect disease management programs to substantially diminish the need for or use of informal care. An important unanswered question is whether HMOs and other managed care providers actually increase the burden on informal caregivers by reducing hospital stays and their length (Estes & Linkins, 1997). However, participation in PACE does not seem to have a significant, negative effect on informal care utilization provided by family and friends (Chatterji, Burstein, Kidder, & White, 1998). Existing disease management models may assist informal caregivers insofar as they employ case managers or care coordinators. On the other hand, they may shift some additional burden onto caregivers insofar as they rely on improved self-care and a shift of services away from the health system and toward the individual or family. It is also possible that disease management programs that operate in managed care settings may be, in some ways, alleviating the burden faced by caregivers because chronic conditions are better controlled, while at the same time utilization controls inherent in the managed care system may be reducing home care services as compared with fee-for-service Medicare (Shaughnessy, Schlenker, & Hittle, 1994) and thus increasing caregiver burden. In general, we would expect that integrated medical and long-term care models provide some limited assistance to caregivers, but it is harder to predict the effect of medical model disease management programs on informal caregivers.

FUNCTIONAL/SOCIAL VERSUS BIOMEDICAL MODELS

The Independent Living Movement (Hanson, 1999) has also expressed ongoing concern about medical control of services for the disabled, with related fear of being institutionalized by well-meaning medical professionals. This movement promotes consumer control of necessary attendant and other community-based services as an alternative to medically controlled care.

In the arena of elder care, these concerns are reflected by the development of aging services such as social case management targeted toward helping consumers find and organize home and community services that speak not to medical but to functional needs. To a certain extent, the PACE approach also falls at least partially into this arena, since social workers, drivers, and other team members play an important role in care decisions. Aging programs have typically focused on functional status as measured by Activities of Daily Living (ADLs) (Katz, Ford, Moskowitz, Jackson, & Jaffee, 1963). Disease management programs focus more heavily on clinical measures related to diseases, such as "hemoglobin A1c levels" as an indicator of diabetic control. These two very different approaches not only represent varying philosophies of how to approach caring for the disabled or elderly, but also represent a challenge in designing programs for chronic care that can meet both the clinical and functional needs of consumers.

It is possible that for younger, non–functionally disabled beneficiaries suffering from chronic conditions, clinical disease management approaches can take a primary role. For older and/or more functionally disabled beneficiaries, functional and social services oriented interventions may be primary. For midrange levels of age and disability, both approaches are critical. Disease management may be further complicated by the large number of comorbid conditions suffered by those disabled elders who live in nursing homes or assisted living facilities (Gambassi et al., 2000). The authors found few reports on disease management approaches that could be successfully implemented for three, four, or five chronic conditions occurring at the same time.

CONCLUSION

Given the lack of consensus on approaches to chronic disease management, more research is needed. New initiatives representing creative thinking in disease management for multiple comorbid conditions as well as the application of disease management principles within long-term chronic care programs — both in the community and in residential settings — are also clearly needed. Programs that place heavier emphasis on clinical control must be approached with some sensitivity to concerns that social aspects of chronic care will be lost. This is of particular concern for the Medicare program, which has focused on medical care perhaps to the detriment of functionally oriented chronic care, which is often seen as either in the province of Medicaid, family caregivers (usually women), or, for a very few, private insurance. Medicare may be able to improve chronic disease management for beneficiaries, but is unlikely, in the short term, to bridge the gap between disease management and functionally oriented care, thus dooming the very old and functionally disabled to further frustration in meeting their chronic care needs.

Growing numbers of consumers have indicated a preference to have some control of services they receive. Self-care education has also been an important part of disease management approaches. The authors recommend that the Centers for Medicare and Medicaid Services (CMS) initiate a beneficiary education program using major elder and disabled advocacy organizations, insurance counseling programs, and foundation-sponsored programs like the Center for Medicare Education to develop user-friendly materials about chronic disease self-care, necessary clinical testing, and advice for interacting with their physician or health plan. Beneficiaries should also receive more education about their rights as consumers and about Medicare appeals processes.

In the long run, CMS should work toward integrating home and community-based care services, which respond to the functional needs of consumers who have chronic conditions, into the Medicare program. Such an effort would reduce cost shifting between the Medicare and Medicaid programs while improving the quality and accessibility of care for the disabled and elderly with chronic problems. Nevertheless, consumer empowerment remains problematic in an environment where non-medical chronic care services remain uncovered by public insurance for the majority of people who need them and where the services that do exist are fragmented and difficult to access.

REFERENCES

Arno, P. S., Levine, C., & Memmott, M. M. (1999). The economic value of informal caregiving. *Health Affairs (Millwood), 18*(2), 182–188.

Bodenheimer, T. (2000). Disease management in the American market. *British Medical Journal, 320*(7234), 563–566.

Chatterji, P., Burstein, N., Kidder, D., & White, A. (1998). *Evaluation of the Program of All-Inclusive Care for the Elderly (PACE) demonstration: The impact of PACE on participant outcomes*. Washington, DC: HCFA Office of Strategic Planning.

Coleman, B. (2000). *Helping the helpers: State supported services for family caregivers*. Washington, DC: AARP Public Policy Institute.

Coleman, B. (2001). *Consumer-directed services for older people* [Issue Brief]. Washington, DC: AARP Public Policy Institute.

Collins, C., & Williams, D. (1999). Segregation and mortality: The deadly effects of racism. *Sociological Forum, 14*, 495–523.

Conrad, P., & Schneider, J. W. (1992). *Deviance and Medicalization* (Rev. ed.). Philadelphia: Temple University Press.

DeJong, G., Batavia, A. I., & McKnew, L. (1992). The independent living model of personal assistance in national long-term-care policy. *Aging and Disability,* 89–95.

Doty, P., Benjamin, A. E., Matthias, R. E., & Franke, T. M. (1999). *In-home supportive services for the elderly and disabled: A comparison of client-directed and professional management models of service delivery*. (Nontechnical Summary Report). Washington, DC: US Department of Health and Human Services.

Estes, C. L., & Binney, E. A. (1989). The biomedicalization of aging: Dangers and dilemmas. *The Gerontologist, 29*(5), 587–596.

Estes, C. L., Casper, M., & Binney, E. A. (1993). Empowerment imperative. In C. L. Estes, J. H. Swan, & associates (Eds.), *The long term care crisis*. Newbury Park, CA: Sage.

Estes, C. L., & Linkins, K. W. (1997). Devolution and aging policy: Racing to the bottom in long-term care. *International Journal of Health Services, 27*(3), 427–442.

Estes, C. L., Wallace, S. P., Linkins, K. W., & Binney, E. A. (2001). The medicalization and commodification of aging and the privatization and rationalization of old age policy. In *Social Policy & Aging*. Thousand Oaks, CA: Sage Publications.

Fenton, M., Entrikin, T., Morrill, S., Marburg, G., Shumway, D., & Nerney, T. (1997). *Beyond managed care: An owner's manual for self-determination*. Concord, NH: Self-Determination for Persons with Developmental Disabilities.

Gambassi, G., Forman, D. E., Lapane, K. L., Mor, V., Sgadari, A., Lipsitz, L. A., & Bernabei, R. (2000). Management of heart failure among very old persons living in long-term care: Has the voice of trials spread? The SAGE Study Group. *American Heart Journal, 139*(1 Pt 1), 85–93.

Gerteis, M., Edgman-Levitan, S., Daley, J., & Delbanco, T. L. (Eds.). (1993). *Through the patient's eyes: Understanding and promoting patient-centered care*. San Francisco: Jossey Bass.

Hanson, S. (1999). Applying independent living principles to state health care programs for people with disabilities. *Independent Living and Disability Policy Issue Brief, 1*(2).

Katz, S., Ford, A., Moskowitz, R., Jackson, B., & Jaffee, M. (1963). Studies of illness in the aged. The index of ADL: A standardized measure of biological and psychosocial function. *Journal of the American Medical Association, 185*, 94–101.

Laine, C., & Davidoff, F. (1996). Patient-centered medicine: A professional evolution. *Journal of the American Medical Association, 275*(2), 152–156.

Liu, K., Manton, K. G., & Aragon, C. (2000). Changes in home care use by disabled elderly persons: 1982–1994. *Journals of Gerontology, Series B, Psychological Sciences and Social Sciences, 55*(4), S245–253.

Mahoney, K. J., Simone, K., & Simon-Rusinowitz, L. (2000). Early lessons from the cash and counseling demonstration and evaluation. *Generations, 24*(3), 41–46.

Mollica, R., & Riley, T. (1997). *Managed care for low income elders dually eligible for medicaid and medicare: A snapshot of state and federal activity*. Portland, ME: National Academy for State Health Policy.

National Institute on Consumer-Directed Long-Term Services. (1996). *Principles of consumer-directed home and community-based services. National Council on Aging*. Available: http://www.mcare.net/ltprinc.html [2001, Oct. 6].

Office of Disability Aging and Long-Term Care Policy. (2001). *Independent choices: A National Symposium on consumer-direction and self-determination for the elderly and persons with disabilities*. Washington, DC: U.S. Department of Health & Human Services. Available: http://aspe.os.dhhs.gov/daltcp/reports/01cfpack.htm [Oct. 1, 2001].

Pandya, S. M., & Coleman, B. (2000). *Caregiving and long-term care* (FS82). Washington, DC: AARP Public Policy Institute.

Shaughnessy, P. W., Schlenker, R. E., & Hittle, D. F. (1994). Home health care outcomes under capitated and fee-for-service payment. *Health Care Financing Review, 16*(1), 187–222.

Stone, R. (2000). *Long term care for the elderly with disabilities: Current policy, emerging trends, and implications for the 21st century*. Milbank Memorial Fund. Available: http://www.milbank.org/0008stone/ [2000, Dec. 5].

Tarail, T. (2001). Personal communication with Ted Tarail, Chair, Kaiser Oakland Senior Advisory Committee. Oakland, CA.

U.S. Department of Health and Human Services. (1998). *Healthy People 2010.* Washington, DC: Public Health Service.

Wiener, J. M., Estes, C. L., Goldenson, S. M., & Goldberg, S. C. (2001). What happened to long-term care in the health reform debate of 1993–1994? Lessons for the future. *Milbank Quarterly, 79*(2), 207–252.

Wunderlich, G., & Kohler, P. O. (Eds.). (2001). *Improving the quality of long term care*. Washington, DC: National Academy Press, Institute of Medicine.

Recommended Reading

CHAPTER 1

Collins, K. S., Hall, A., and Neuhaus, C. (1999). *U.S. minority health: A chartbook* (pp. 2–5, 24, 25, 32–35, 50–51, 80–83, 86–89). New York: The Commonwealth Fund.

Pamuk, E., Makuc, D., Heck, K., Reuben, C., and Lochnen, K. (1998). Highlights. In *Socioeconomic status and health chartbook: Health, United States, 1998* (pp. 3–20). Hyattsville, MD: National Center for Health Statistics.

U.S. Department of Health and Human Services. (2000). *Healthy People 2010: Understanding and improving health* (2nd ed.). Washington, DC: U.S. Government Printing Office.

CHAPTER 2

Adler, N., and Newman, K. (2002). Socioeconomic disparities in health: Pathways and policies. *Health Affairs, 21* (2), 60–76.

Adler, N. E., Marmot, M., McEwen, B. S., and Stewart, J. (Eds.). (1999). *Socioeconomic status and health in industrial nations: Social, psychological, and biological pathways*. New York: The New York Academy of Sciences.

Case, A., and Paxson, C. (2002). Parental behavior and child health. *Health Affairs, 21* (2), 164–178.

Colgrove, J. (2002). The McKeown thesis: A historical controversy and its enduring influence. *American Journal of Public Health, 92* (5), 725–729.

Deaton, A. (2002). Policy implications of the gradient of health and wealth. *Health Affairs, 21* (2), 13–30.

Evans, R. (2002). *Interpreting and addressing inequalities in health: From Black to Acheson to Blair to…?* London: Office of Health Economics.

Evans, R. G., Barer, M. L., and Marmor, T. R. (Eds.). (1994). *Why are some people healthy and others not? The determinants of health of populations*. Hawthorne, NY: Aldine de Gruyter.

Evans, R. G., and Stoddart, G. (1990). Producing health, consuming health care. *Social Science and Medicine, 31* (2), 1347–1363.

Kaplan, G. A., Pamuk, E. R., Lynch, J. W., Cohen, R. D., and Balfour, J. L. (1996). Inequality in income and mortality in the United States: Analysis of mortality and potential pathways. *British Medical Journal, 312,* 999–1003.

Kuh, D., and Ben-Shlomo, Y. (Eds.). (1997). *A life course approach to chronic disease epidemiology*. Oxford and New York: Oxford University Press.

Lasker, R. D. (2002). Do all roads lead to Jerusalem? The biomedicalization of the determinants of health. In D. P. Chinitz (Ed.), *The changing face of health systems*. Jerusalem: Gefen Publishing.

Mechanic, D. (2002). Disadvantage, inequality, and social policy. *Health Affairs, 21* (2), 48–59.

Power, C., and Hertzman, C. (1997). Social and biological pathways linking early life and adult disease. *British Medical Bulletin, 53* (1), 210–221.

U.S. Department of Health and Human Services. (1980). *Ten leading causes of death in the United States in 1977.* Atlanta, GA: Centers for Disease Control and Prevention.

CHAPTER 3

Barr, D. A. (2002). *Introduction to U.S. health policy: The organization, financing, and delivery of health care in America.* San Francisco: Benjamin Cummings.

Bodenheimer, T., and Grumbach, K. (1995). *Understanding health policy: A clinical approach.* Stamford, CT: Appleton & Lange.

Jacobson, P. D., and Warner, K. E. (1999). Litigation and public health policy making: The case of tobacco control. *Journal of Health Politics, Policy and Law, 24* (4), 769–804.

Kingdon, J. W. (1995). *Agendas, alternatives, and public policies* (2nd ed.). New York: Addison-Wesley.

Longest, B. B. (2002). *Health policymaking in the United States* (3rd ed.). Chicago: Health Administration Press.

McCool, D. (1995). Discussion. In D. McCool (Ed.), *Public policy theories, models, and concepts: An anthology* (pp. 380–385). Englewood Cliffs, New Jersey: Prentice Hall.

Parmet, W. E. (2002). After September 11: Rethinking public health federalism. *Journal of Law, Medicine, and Ethics, 30,* 201–211.

Sabatier, P. A. (1998). An advocacy coalition framework of policy change and the role of policy-oriented learning. *Policy Sciences, 21,* 129–168.

CHAPTER 4

Cater, D., and Lee, P. R. (Eds.). (1972). *Politics of health.* Huntington, NY: Robert E. Krieger.

Glied, S. (1997). Medicalists and marketists. In *Chronic condition: Why health reform fails* (pp. 17–35). Cambridge, MA: Harvard University Press.

Hacker, J. S., and Skocpol, T. (Summer 1997). The new politics of U.S. health policy. *Journal of Health Politics, Policy and Law, 22* (2), 315–338.

Lee, P. R., and Benjamin, A. E. (1993). Health policy and the politics of health care. In S. J. Williams and P. R. Torrens (Eds.), *Introduction to health services* (4th ed.). Albany, NY: Delmar.

Marmor, T. R. (2000). *The politics of Medicare* (2nd ed.). New York: Aldine de Gruyter.

McGinnis, M. J., Williams-Russo, P., and Knickman, J. R. (2002). The case for more active policy attention to health promotion. *Health Affairs, 11* (2), 78–93.

Nestle, M. (2002). *Food politics: How the food industry influences nutrition and health.* Berkeley: University of California Press.

Oliver, T. R. (2001). State health politics and policies: Rhetoric, reality, and the challenges ahead. In R. B. Hacker and D. A. Rochefort (Eds.), *The new politics of state health policy* (pp. 273–289). Topeka: University of Kansas Press.

Skocpol, T. (1996). *Boomerang: Clinton's health security effort and the turn against government in U.S. politics.* New York: W.W. Norton.

CHAPTER 5

Afifi, A. A., and Breslow, L. (1994). The maturing paradigm of public health. *Annual Review of Public Health, 15,* 223–235.

Bruce, T. A., and McKane, S. U. (Eds.). (2000). *Community-based public health: A partnership model.* Washington, DC: American Public Health Association.

Centers for Disease Control and Prevention. (1999). Achievements in public health, 1900–1999: Family planning. *MMWR, 48* (47), 1073–1080.

Centers for Disease Control and Prevention (1999). Achievements in public health, 1900–1999: Improvements in workplace safety — United States, 1900–1999. *MMWR, 48,* 461–469.

Centers for Disease Control and Prevention. (1999). Achievements in public health, 1900–1999: Safer and healthier foods. *MMWR, 48* (40), 905–913.

Centers for Disease Control and Prevention (1999). Impact of vaccines universally recommended for children — United States, 1900–1999. *MMWR, 48,* 243–248.

Centers for Disease Control and Prevention (1999). Motor-vehicle safety: A 20th century public health achievement. *MMWR, 48,* 369–374.

Centers for Disease Control and Prevention. (1999). Achievements in public health, 1900–1999: Tobacco use — United States, 1900–1999. *MMWR, 48* (43), 986–993.

Centers for Disease Control and Prevention. (1999). Achievements in public health, 1900–1999: Fluoridation of drinking water to prevent dental caries. *MMWR, 48* (41), 933–940.

Fielding, J. E. (1999). Public health in the twentieth century: Advances and challenges. *Annual Review of Public Health, 20,* xiii–xxx.

Israel, B. A., Schulz, A. J., Parker, E. A., and Becker, A. B. (1998). Review of community-based research: Assessing partnership approaches to improve public health. *Annual Review of Public Health, 19,* 173–202.

Lasker, R. D., and the Committee on Medicine and Public Health. (1997). *Medicine and public health: The power of collaboration.* Chicago: Health Administration Press.

Lasker, R. D., and Miller, R. (2001). Partnership synergy: A practical framework for studying and strengthening the collaborative advantage. *Milbank Quarterly, 79* (2), 179–205.

Lee, P. R., and Paxman, D. (1997). Reinventing public health. *Annual Review of Public Health, 18,* 1–35.

Szreter, S. (1988). The importance of social intervention in Britain's mortality decline, c. 1850–1914: A reinterpretation of the role of public health. *Social History of Medicine, 1,* 1–37.

CHAPTER 6

Centers for Disease Control and Prevention. (2000). Biological and chemical terrorism: Strategic plan for preparedness and response. Recommendations of the CDC Strategic Planning Workgroup. *MMWR, 49* (RR-4), 1–14.

Chyba, C. F. (2002). Toward biological security. *Foreign Affairs, 81* (3), 122–136.

Committee on Science and Technology for Countering Terrorism, National Research Council. (2002). *Making the nation safer: The role of science and technology in countering terrorism.* Washington, DC: National Academy Press.

Evans, R. G., Crutcher, J. M., Shadel, B., Clements, B. Bronze. M. S. (2002). Terrorism from a public health perspective. *The American Journal of the Medical Sciences, 323* (6), 291–298.

Gostin, L. O., Sapsin, J. W., Teret, S. P., Burris, S., Mair, J. S., Hodge, J. G., and Vernick, J. S. (2002). The model State Emergency Health Powers Act: Planning for and response to bioterrorism and naturally occurring infectious diseases. *Journal of the American Medical Association, 288* (5), 622–628.

Knobler, S. L., Mahmoud, A. A. F., and Pray, L. A. (Eds.). (2002). *Biological threats and terrorism: Assessing the science and response capabilities.* Washington, DC: National Academy Press.

Manning, F. J., and Goldfrank, L. (Eds.). (2002). *Preparing for terrorism: Tools for evaluating the metropolitan medical response system program.* Washington, DC: National Academy Press.

Schuster, M. A., Stein, B. D., Jaycox, L. H., Collins, R. L., Marshall, G. N., Elliott, M. N., Zhou, A. J., Kanouse, D. E., Morrison, J. L., and Berry, S. H. (2001). A national survey of stress reactions after the September 11, 2001, terrorist attacks. *New England Journal of Medicine, 345* (20), 1507–1512.

CHAPTER 7

Davis, K. (2002). *Work in America: New challenges for health care* (pp. 3–15). New York: The Commonwealth Fund.

Glied, S. (2001). Health insurance and market failure since Arrow. *Journal of Health Politics, Policy and Law, 26* (5), 957–965.

Goldberg, B. W. (1998). Managed care and public health departments: Who is responsible for the health of the population? *Annual Review of Public Health, 19,* 527–537.

Goody, B., Mentnech, R., and Riley, G. (2002). Changing nature of public and private insurance. *Health Care Financing Review, 23* (3), 1–7.

Gray, B. (1991). *The profit motive and patient care: The changing accountability of doctors and hospitals.* Cambridge, MA: Harvard University Press.

Kaiser Commission on Medicaid and the Uninsured. (2002, May). *Children's health — Why health insurance matters* (Fact sheet no. 4055). Washington, DC: The Henry J. Kaiser Family Foundation.

Kaiser Commission on Medicaid and the Uninsured. (2002, July). *Underinsured in America — Is health coverage adequate?* (Fact sheet no. 4060). Washington, DC: The Henry J. Kaiser Family Foundation.

Salmon, J. W. (1995). A perspective on the corporate transformation of health care. *International Journal of Health Services, 25* (1), 11–42.

Shroeder, S. A. (2001). Prospects for expanding health insurance coverage. *New England Journal of Medicine, 344* (11), 847–852.

Starr, P. (1982). *The social transformation of American medicine.* New York: Basic Books.

CHAPTER 8

Adams, A. S., Soumerai, S. B., and Ross-Degnan, D. (2001). The case for a Medicare drug coverage benefit: A critical review of the empirical evidence. *Annual Review of Public Health, 22,* 49–61.

Culbertson, R., and Lee, P. R. (1996). Medicare and physician autonomy. *Health Care Financing Review, 18* (2), 115–130.

Enthoven, A. C., and Kronick, R. (1991). Universal health insurance through incentive reform. *Journal of the American Medical Association, 265* (19), 2532–2536.

Estes, C. L., and Linkins, K. W. (1991). Decentralization, devolution, and the deficit: The changing role of the state and the community. In J. G. Goyna (Ed.), *Resecuring Social Security and Medicare: Understanding privatization and risk* (pp. 37–44). Washington, DC: Gerontological Society.

Heffler, S., Smith, S., Won, G., Clemens, M. K., Keehan, S., and Zezza, M. (2002). Health spending projections for 2001–2011: The latest outlook. *Health Affairs, 21* (2): 207–218.

Iglehart, J. K. (2001). The Centers for Medicare and Medicaid Services. *New England Journal of Medicine, 345* (26), 1920–1924.

Iglehart, J. K. (2002). Medicare's declining payment to physicians. *New England Journal of Medicine, 346* (24), 1924–1930.

Laschober, M. A., Kitchman, M., Neuman, P., and Strabic, A. A. (2002, February 27). Trends in Medicare supplemental insurance and prescription drug coverage, 1996–1999 [Online]. *Health Affairs,* W127–W138. Available: http://www.healthaffairs.org/WebExclusives/Laschober_Web_Excl_022702.htm.

Levit, K., Smith, C., Cowan, C., Lazenby, H., and Martin, A. (2002). Inflation spurs health spending in 2000. *Health Affairs, 21* (1), 172–181.

Lyons, B. (2002). *Medicaid's role for seniors: Challenges in a fiscally constrained environment.* Menlo Park, CA: The Henry J. Kaiser Family Foundation.

Kaiser Commission on Medicaid and the Uninsured. (2001, April). *Medicaid facts: Medicaid's role for the disabled population under age 65* (Fact sheet no. 2171). Washington, DC: The Henry J. Kaiser Family Foundation.

Kaiser Family Foundation. (2002). Medicare options for reform. Washington, DC: Kaiser Family Foundation.

Kaiser Family Foundation. (2001, June). *Medicare at a glance.* Washington, DC: The Henry J. Kaiser Family Foundation.

Kaiser Family Foundation. (2001, September). *Medicare+Choice* (Fact sheet no. 2052-03). Washington, DC: The Henry J. Kaiser Family Foundation.

Roland, D., and Hanson, K. (1996). Medicaid: Moving to managed care. *Health Affairs, 15* (3), 150–152.

CHAPTER 9

Becher, E. C., and Chassin, M. R. (2001). Improving quality minimizing error: Making it happen. *Health Affairs, 20* (3), 68–90.

Bergman, D. A., and Homer, C. J. (1998). Managed care and the quality of children's health services. *Children and Managed Care, 8* (2), 60–75.

Berwick, D. M. (2002). A user's manual for the IOM's "Quality Chasm" report. *Health Affairs, 21* (3), 80–90.

Breslow, L. (1990). The future of public health: Prospects in the United States for the 1990s. *Annual Review of Public Health, 11,* 1–28.

Derose, S. F., Schuster, M. A., Fielding, J. E, and Asch, S. M. (2002). Public health quality measurement: Concepts and challenges. *Annual Review of Public Health, 23,* 1–21.

Lansky, D. (2002). Improving quality through public disclosure of performance information. *Health Affairs, 21* (4), 52–62.

Leatherman, S., and McCarthy, D. (2002). *Quality of health care in the United States: A chartbook.* New York: The Commonwealth Fund.

McNeil, B. J. (2001). Shattuck lecture — Hidden barriers to improvement in quality of care. *New England Journal of Medicine, 345* (22), 1612–1620.

Newhouse, J. P. (2002). Why is there a quality chasm? *Health Affairs, 21* (4), 13–25.

Pawlson, L. G., and O'Kane, M. E. (2002). Professionalism, regulation, and the market: Impact on accountability for quality of care. *Health Affairs, 21* (3), 200–207.

Sackett, D. L., Rosenberg, W. M. C., Haynes, R. B., and Richardson, W. S. (1996). Evidence based medicine: What is it and what isn't it? *British Medical Journal, 312* (13), 71–72.

Tropy, J. M. (2002). Raising health care quality: Process, measures, and system failure. *Journal of the American Medical Association, 287* (2), 177–178.

CHAPTER 10

Boonstra, H., and Gold, R. B. (2002). Overhauling welfare: Implications for reproductive health policy in the United States. *Journal of the American Women's Medical Association, 57* (1), 41–46.

Brindis, C. (1999). Building for the future: Adolescent pregnancy prevention. *Journal of the American Women's Medical Association, 54* (3), 129–132.

Chavkin, W., Wise, P. H., and Romero, D. (2002, Winter). Welfare, women, and children: It's time for doctors to speak out. *Journal of the American Women's Association, 57* (1), 3–5.

Cornelius, L. J., Smith, P. L., and Simpson, G. M. (2002). What factors hinder women of color from obtaining preventive health care? *American Journal of Public Health, 92* (4), 535–539.

Estes, C. L. (2002). Sex and gender in the political economy of aging. In C. L. Estes and associates (Eds.), *Social policy and aging* (pp. 119–135). Thousand Oaks, CA: Sage Publications.

Goldman, M. B., and Hatch, M. (Eds.). (2000). *Women and health.* San Diego: Academic Press.

Grimes, D. A., Raymond, E. G., and Scott Jones, B. (2001). Emergency contraception over the counter: The medical and legal imperatives. *Obstetrics and Gynecology, 98* (1), 151–155.

Institute of Medicine Committee on Understanding the Biology of Sex and Gender Differences, Wizemann, T. M., and Pardue, M. L. (2001). *Exploring the biological contributions to human health: Does sex matter?* Washington, DC: National Academy Press.

Johnson, P., and Fulp, R. (2002). Racial and ethnic disparities in coronary heart disease in women: Prevention, treatment, and needed interventions. *Women's Health Issues, 12* (5), 252–271.

Ness, R. B., and Kuller, L. H. (1999). *Health and disease among women: Biological and environmental influences.* New York: Oxford University Press.

Ratcliff, K. S. (2002). *Women and health: Power, technology, inequality, and conflict in a gendered world.* Boston: Allyn and Bacon.

Rice, D. P. (1999, September 16). *Medicare: A women's issue.* Paper presented at the Jacobs Institute and Commonwealth Funding meeting "Women and Medicare: Agenda for Change," Washington, DC.

Ro, M. (2002). Moving forward: Addressing the health of Asian American and Pacific Islander women. *American Journal of Public Health, 92* (4), 516–519.

Tjaden, P. G. (2000). *Extent, nature, and consequences of intimate partner violence*. Washington, DC: U.S. Department of Justice, Office of Justice Programs, National Institute of Justice.

United States Public Health Service. Office of the Surgeon General. (2001). *Women and Smoking: A report of the Surgeon General*. Washington, DC: U.S. Dept. of Health and Human Services, Public Health Service, Office of the Surgeon General.

Weitz, R. (1998). *The politics of women's bodies: Sexuality, appearance, and behavior*. New York: Oxford University Press.

Weitz, T. A., Freund, K. M., and Wright, L. (2001). Identifying and caring for underserved populations: Experience of the National Centers of Excellence in Women's Health. *Journal of Women's Health and Gender-Based Medicine, 10* (10), 937–952.

CHAPTER 11

Charlton, J. I. (1998). *Nothing about us without us: Disability oppression and empowerment*. Berkeley: University of California Press.

Coleman, B., Fox-Grage, W., and Folkemer, D. (2002). *State long-term care: Recent developments and policy directions*. Washington, DC: National Conference of State Legislatures.

Davis, K., and Raetzman, S. (1999). *Meeting future health and long-term care needs of an aging population*. Washington, DC: The Commonwealth Fund.

Estes, C. L., and associates. (2001). *Social policy and aging: A critical perspective*. Thousand Oaks, CA: Sage Publications.

Feder, J., Komisar, H. L., and Niefeld, M. (2000). Long-term care in the United States: An overview. *Health Affairs, 19* (3), 40–56.

Kane, R. A., Kane, R. L., and Ladd, R. C. (1998). *The heart of long term care*. New York: Oxford University Press.

LeBlanc, A. J., Tonner, M. C., and Harrington, C. (2000). Medicaid 1915(c) home and community-based services waivers across the states. *Health Care Financing Review, 22* (2), 159–174.

Newcomer, R., Swan, J., Karon, S., Bigelow, W., Harrington, C., and Zimmerman, D. (2001). Residential care supply and cognitive and physical problem case mix in nursing homes. *Journal of Aging and Health, 13* (2), 217–247.

Stone, R. I. (2000). *Long-term care for the elderly with disabilities: Current policy, emerging trends, and implications for the twenty-first century*. New York: Milbank Memorial Fund. Available: http://www.milbank.org/0008/stone/index.html.

Tilly, J., and Wiener, J. M. (2001). Consumer-directed home and community services program in eight states: Policy issues for older people and government. *Journal of Aging and Social Policy, 12* (4), 1–26.

U. S. Department of Health and Human Services, Administration on Aging. (2001). *A profile of older Americans: 2001*. Washington, DC: U.S. Department of Health and Human Services.

Walker, A. (1999). Public policy and theories of aging. In V. Bengtson and K. W. Schaie (Eds.), *Handbook of theories of aging* (pp. 361–378). New York: Springer.

Wolf, D. A. (2001). Population change: Friend or foe of the chronic care system? *Health Affairs, 20* (6), 28–42.

Wunderlich, G., and Kohler, P. O. (Eds.). (2001). *Improving the quality of long term care*. Washington, DC: National Academy Press.

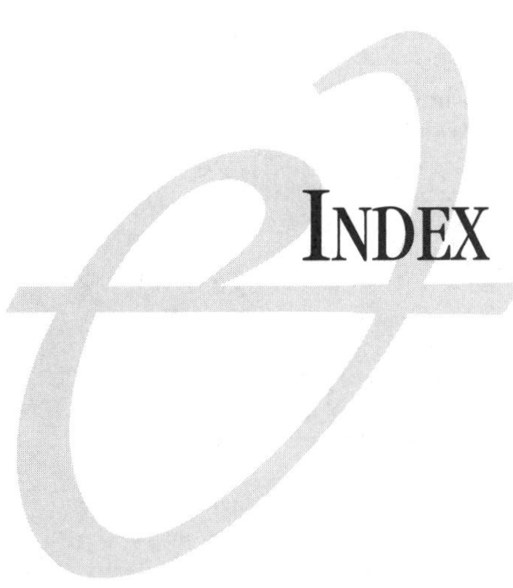

INDEX